The
PAULSON
AND
KRESS
COLLECTIONS
of
Ellen G. White
LETTERS

TAKEN FROM THE PRIVATE COLLECTIONS
OF
DAVID PAULSON M. D.
AND
DANIEL HARTMAN KRESS M. D.

Published by

DIGITAL INSPIRATION

1481 Reagan Valley Road

Tellico Plains, TN 37385

deluxeelectronicbooks@vsdigitalinspiration.com

www.vsdigitalinspiration.com

PREFACE

DAVID PAULSON (1868-1916) and Daniel Kress (1862-1956) were both early Seventh-day Adventist physicians whose lives overlapped that of Ellen G. White by 48 and 53 years respectively. Both married Adventist women physicians—Mary Wild and Lauretta Eby respectively.

Drs. Mary and David Paulson founded and built up the work of the Hinsdale Sanitarium in the Hinsdale suburb of Chicago, Illinois. Earlier Dr. David had been an instructor in the American Medical Missionary College at Battle Creek, Michigan and in 1899 he had taken charge of Battle Creek Sanitarium's medical missionary work in Chicago.

Drs. Lauretta and Daniel Kress labored first at the Battle Creek Sanitarium and then were instrumental in establishing the Church's health work in England, New Zealand, and Australia. In 1907 they returned to the United States where Dr. Daniel became the first medical superintendent of the newly established Washington Sanitarium and Hospital.

Because of the important leadership roles played by these two physician couples, they both received direct communications from the Lord's servant Ellen White. Their collection of such personal letters, as well as copies sent to them of letters directed to other individuals, make up this present publication. There are 183 entries from Dr. Paulson's collection and 43 from that of Dr. Kress.

For reference purposes, material between sets of numbers in curly brackets—e.g. {123} and {124}— are considered to be from the page of the first number.

The Publisher

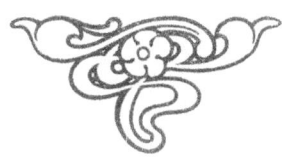

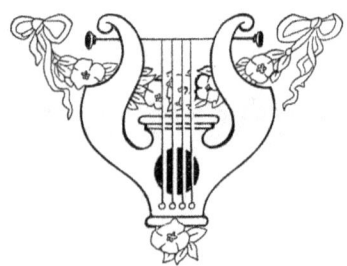

Table of Contents

THE KRESS COLLECTION

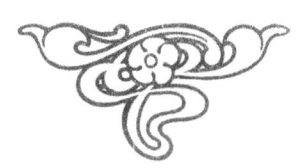

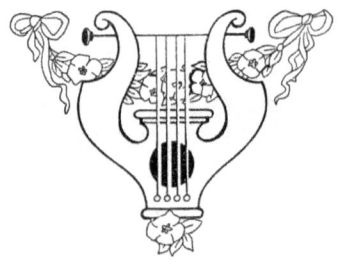

THE PAULSON COLLECTION OF ELLEN G. WHITE LETTERS

DEAR BRETHREN AND SISTERS

July 16, 1901
(B-83-'01)
St. Helena, California, July 15, 1901

YOU ASK IN REGARD to meat-eating. I will say that it is quite true that nearly all animal flesh is diseased. Many people are eating meat filled with consumption and cancerous germs. At the present day animals are suffering from all kinds of deadly diseases.

The Lord has been teaching His people that it is for their spiritual and physical good to abstain from flesh-eating. There is no need to eat the flesh of dead animals.

After the curse was pronounced upon the human family, God permitted man to eat flesh-meat. This He did that life might be shortened. The punishment of death has been pronounced upon the race, and the permission to eat flesh-meat was one of the means used by God to inflict this punishment.

When the Lord took His people from Egypt, He did not give them flesh-meat to eat till they mourned and wept in His ears, saying, "Who shall give us flesh to eat? We remember the flesh, which we did eat in Egypt freely; the cucumbers, and the melons, and the leeks, and the onions, and the garlic; but now our soul is dried away; there is nothing at all beside this manna, before our eyes." Then the Lord gave them flesh to eat. He sent them quails from heaven, but we read, "While the flesh was yet between their teeth, ere it was chewed, the wrath of the Lord was kindled against the people, and the Lord smote the people with a very great plague."

The light God has given His people is that by eating the flesh and blood of dead animals, man becomes animalized. His lower passions are greatly strengthened by such a diet.

Worldly physicians cannot account for the rapid increase of disease among the human family. But we know that much of this suffering is caused by the eating of dead flesh.

Over thirty years ago I was often in great weakness. Many prayers were offered in my behalf. It was thought that flesh-meat would give me vitality, and this was therefore my principal article of diet. But instead of gaining strength I grew weaker and weaker. I often fainted from exhaustion. Light came to me, showing me the injury men and women were doing to the mental, moral, and physical faculties by the use of flesh-meat. I was shown that the whole human structure is affected by this diet, that by it man strengthens the animal propensities and the appetite for liquor.

I at once cut meat out of my bill of fare. After that I was at times at or in places where I was compelled to eat a little meat. But for many years not a morsel of the flesh of dead animals has passed my lips. Neither has meat been placed upon my table. My visitors have been given wholesome, nourishing food, but no meat.

Wise counsel and righteous practices are needed now, if the people of God succeed in preserving clear minds and healthy bodies. We must give {2} close attention to eating, drinking, and dressing. The entire body of believers needs to make a decided reform. A high profession, followed by a disregard of the laws of life, shows a faithless life. Lack of fidelity, want of stability, slavery to wrong habits,—this is the sure result of such a course. Those who follow this course are not consistent Christians. Salvation means deliverance from every habit which tends to drag humanity down. Transgression of the laws of our being is transgression of the laws of God.

COUNSELS REPEATED

June 19, 1908
(MS. 73, '08)

AGAIN REPRESENTATIONS HAVE been made to me that all who have the care of the sick, in our sanitariums, should bear in mind that these institutions are established for a special work, and are to be conducted in a way that will bring honor to God.

Our sanitariums should be established in retired places, that are free from all noise and confusion, such as the rumbling of carriages and street cars.

The Lord has taught us that great efficacy for healing lies in a proper use of water. These treatments should be given skillfully. We have been instructed that in our treatment of the sick we should discard the use of drugs. There are simple herbs that can be used for the recovery of the sick, whose effect upon the system is very different from that of those drugs that poison the blood and endanger life.

The number of our lady physicians should be increased. Care should be taken that lady nurses have the care of lady patients, and gentleman nurses of gentleman patients.

I would say to our physicians, Never allow your patients to think that in the human being is power to heal the sick. You are to depend much more than you have done on the co-operation of the Great Physician in the work of healing disease. Your faith is to lay hold upon the efficacy of Christ to make effectual the effort put forth for the recovery of the sick.

There are some in our institutions who claim to believe the principles of health reform, and yet who indulge in the use of flesh-meats and other foods which they know to be injurious to health. I say to such in the name of the Lord, Do not accept positions in our institutions while you refuse to live the principles for which our institutions stand; for by doing this you make doubly hard the work of teachers and leaders who are striving to carry the work on right lines. Clear the King's highway. Cease to block the way of the message He sends.

I have been shown that the principles that were given us in the early days of the message are to be regarded as just as important by our people today as they were then. There are some who have never followed the light given us on the question of diet. It is time now to take the light from under the bushel, and let it shine forth in clear, bright rays. {3}

Some who are not willing to receive the light, but who prefer to walk in ways of their own choosing, will search the Testimonies to find something in them to encourage the spirit of unbelief and disobedience. Thus a spirit of disunion will be brought in; for the spirit which leads them to criticize the Testimonies will also lead them to watch their brethren to find in them something to condemn.

Satan's rebellion shut him out from the courts of heaven, and all who engaged with him in warfare against Christ were cast out with him. The exercise of Satan's seductive arts against the government of heaven did not cease with his expulsion from the presence of God. Year by year they have grown more deceptive, more subtle, more determined. Every additional evidence rejected increases his power to resist the government of God and of Christ. And every ray of hope resisted, helps to create for him and his followers a hopeless future.

Satan has turned men from the worship of the true Sabbath, which at the creation of the world God sanctified and blessed, and which on Mt. Sinai He repeated amid terrible majesty to His people. All who reject the sacred message regarding the requirements of the law of God, reject truth. God's obedient people are to hold fast to truth in every line. This is the only hope of the soul when Satan seeks to take control of heart and mind.

The resistance of truth leaves men captive to the will of Satan. Those who today hold fast to erroneous ideas, and feel satisfied with popular errors, rejecting a plain "Thus saith the Lord," reveal that had they lived in the days of Christ, they would have helped to swell the cry of the murderous mob, "Crucify Him! Crucify Him!"

God requires continual advancement from His people. They need to learn that indulged appetite is the greatest hindrance to mental improvement and soul sanctification. As a people, with all our profession of health reform, we eat too much. Indulgence of appetite is the greatest cause of physical and mental debility, and lies largely at the foundation of feebleness and premature death. Intemperance begins at our tables, when we use an unwise combination of foods. Let the individual who is seeking to possess purity of spirit, bear in mind that in Christ there is power to control the appetite.

DEAR BROTHER AND SISTER SIMPSON

December 28, 1904
S-343-'04
"Elmshaven," Sanitarium, California
December 27, 1904

I CAN NOW FEEL AT REST in regard to the positions that you have been chosen to fill in the Glendale Sanitarium. Those bearing the chief responsibilities in that in-

stitution can be a great help to one another if they will seek to understand the Lord's instruction. I have great hope that as you and Brother and Sister Burden fill your important places, you will realize the presence of a spiritual helper, One who is ever ready to be the head of your councils. I pray that you will feel His divine presence. Under His guidance none of you need become discouraged.

I am sure that you will find Brother Ballenger a great help to your Board. {4} He visits many places, and his influence will work for the upbuilding of the two Southern California sanitariums.

The strength of the combination of workers in the Glendale Sanitarium depends on their souls being imbued with heavenly love. Christ clothed His divinity with humanity that human beings might lay hold upon His merits, and that they might recognize obedience to God's law as the virtue of the covenant of grace.

Worldly policy plans are not to be woven into the pattern that the Lord's people have been given. To those who receive Him, Christ gives power to become the sons of God, even to as many as believe on His name. God declares, "I will put My laws in their minds." David's prayer expresses this same precious assurance: "Blessed are the undefiled in the way, who walk in the law of the Lord. Blessed are they that keep His testimonies, and that seek Him with the whole heart. They also do no iniquity, they walk in His way. Thou hast commanded me to keep Thy precepts diligently. Then shall I not be ashamed, when I have respect unto all Thy commandments. I will praise Thee with uprightness of heart, when I shall have learned Thy righteous judgments. Wherewithal shall a young man cleanse his way? By taking heed thereto according to Thy word. With my whole heart have I sought Thee; O, let me not wander from Thy commandments."

Here is our strength. The Lord will just as surely lead the workers in the Glendale Sanitarium, as He led David, if they will unite to do His will.

There is a great work to be done in bringing the principles of health reform to the notice of the people. Public meetings should be held to introduce the subject, and schools should be held in which those who are interested can be told more particularly about our health foods and how a wholesome, nourishing, appetizing diet can be provided without the use of meat,

tea, or coffee.

Thus we did in the early history of our work. We taught the people by demonstration that we can safely depend for the sustenance of life upon the productions which God gave our first parents in Eden.

Let men engage in this work who can speak on the principles of health reform. You need not feel that you must depend upon Dr. Kellogg or upon any other man from afar. No, no. At the dedication of the Glendale Sanitarium, let your most intelligent speakers on the subject of health reform come to the front. And remember that God would have the workers in the two Southern California Sanitariums lean wholly upon His wisdom.

Make as much as possible of the dedicatory services to arouse an interest in health reform. Press home the temperance question with all the force of the Holy Spirit's unction. Show the need of total abstinence from all intoxicating liquor. Show the terrible harm that is wrought in the human system by the use of tobacco and alcohol. Explain your methods of giving treatment. Let the talks given be such as will enlighten your hearers. God has mercy on the unrighteous. This service will be an opportunity to tell what health reform really is.

Such services will give the Sanitarium a publicity that will be a great {5} help to it in its work. We must study Christ's methods. He accepted invitations to feasts given by wealthy men. He went to these feasts because He knew that there He would have opportunity to present the truth. We must study how to reach the masses with the truth for this time. As we strive to do this, God will bring to the minds of those not of our faith convictions that cannot be turned aside with a joke. They will be convinced that we have the truth.

Tell them of the principles that we hold, and of why we have established the Sanitarium,—that, under the guidance of God, it may be a help in relieving suffering humanity. Tell them that medical missionary work is to prepare people for the mansions that Christ has gone to prepare for those who are true and loyal to His commandments. Let it be understood that the love of God alone can keep His people true in the self-denial and self-sacrifice that they are called to endure for Christ's sake. Repeat often the first three verses of the fourteenth chapter of John. This scripture is a panacea for trouble, disappointment, and affliction. A conviction that the hope of eternal life is sure causes the heart to overflow with gratitude and thanksgiving.

DEAR BROTHER AND SISTER BELDEN

January 3, 1906
B.-16-'06
"Elmshaven," Sanitarium, Cal.
Nov. 26, 1905

THE PAST NIGHT I HAVE slept better than I have for years. I have no pain. My mind is clear, and I can do much work if I have a chance. I am now seventy-eight years old. I am grateful to my heavenly Father that I am able to do my writing. My appetite is excellent. We have been favored with Brother and Sister King to be our helpers. Both are very useful workers. Sister King is my cook, and the food comes on to the table in an appetizing shape for my workers. This is what we need: simple food prepared in a simple, wholesome and relishable manner. We have no butter and no meat on our table. We do not think fried potatoes are healthful, for there is more or less grease or butter used in preparing them. Good baked or boiled potatoes served up with cream and a sprinkling of salt are more healthful. The remnants of Irish and sweet potatoes are prepared with a little cream and salt and rebaked, and not fried; they are excellent. I have had a good appetite and relish my food, and am perfectly satisfied with the portion which I select, which I know does not injure my digestive organs. Others can eat food which I cannot, such as lentils and beans. We are favored with the services of Brother and Sister King; they are a blessing to us, and we are thankful for their help. Sister Nelson was highly prized as our housekeeper and cook, and we would have kept her if she would have remained. She wished to perfect her education as a nurse, which position she will fill and do good service. This was understood when she came to us. We were troubled at the thought of her leaving us, as she had done good service and was an excellent caretaker both indoors and out of doors. We thought it would be difficult to supply her place, but it would not be doing Sister Nelson justice to keep her here when she desired a change and we considered that she ought to have it. So I let her go. I am glad and thankful that we have secured Sister King, as the matron of our home, and her husband to be a care-taker outside of the home and inside when needed. They

served one year at {6} Healdsburg College and gave good satisfaction. So we are doing well notwithstanding our fears.

I am grateful to my heavenly Father for the preservation of my health for the close application to prepare a repetition of the experiences we have had in the past, as we have prepared testimonies in regard to our first labors and the matter is in print. We have a large amount of matter which the Lord has given me, which light and instruction should not be hid under a bushel or under a bed. The warnings and the messages that the Lord has graciously given me to correct the errors that would come in, and to set things in order, the people should have, for the enemy will continue to work to bring in false theories and to mingle with the truth strange suppositions. These appear as light to those who receive them, but they are deceptive theories that will be brought in as tares sown among the wheat. The Lord has for the last fifty years been instructing me when the seducing theories would arise that they were not to be received, and I must do as did Moses and Joshua: Repeat the errors of the past and the gracious working out of the Lord's will. I praise His holy name.

The sadness of my heart is beyond expression because I must show directly to all the medical missionaries that they are not fulfilling their calling. The Lord has been speaking to Dr. Kellogg through His word, but he would not understand that word. He would not change his course of action, and for the last thirty years especially, my message has been given to him, which message he has in strongest assertions professed to believe. But when the plain reproofs came to him through the messenger God has chosen, just prior to the time of the conference at South Lancaster, he decidedly stated that I was no longer his friend because I stated the facts as they had been presented to me by the Lord. But he had set his mind upon a course of action that the Lord would not sustain him in pursuing. His mistakes were presented before him; likewise the dangers growing out of these mistakes. Our ministers were tempted. They must be on guard, and not in any way be seduced from the straight line of the work God had given them to do, but stand firm like men. Be strong, yea, be strong. Then the Doctor became set and determined, and for a time he had been losing the balance of his mind. He went to Europe and we urged him to come to Australia; to throw off care for a

time and have nothing to do to weary and depress his mind. But although he received the message sent him, he did not accept the invitation. At that time his financial outlook was anything but favorable.

Warnings had been given me for twenty years that Doctor Kellogg was embracing too much. He could not have a well-balanced mind, and he lost patience and brotherly kindness if interrupted in carrying out his purpose and intentions. The Lord sent him warnings that he was endangering himself. Warnings had come to him that unless he guarded his mind he would become overwrought and make mistakes in speech and mistakes in selecting his men to be his helpers and he would not take kindly to any one that questioned his course.

Dr. Kellogg had been represented to me as chosen for a physician. My husband and myself united in taking three promising young men from their humble labors, and placing in the hands of each one thousand dollars to obtain an education in medical lines. This had been the selection that the Lord put into the mind of my husband. The Lord had given light and preference to these three youth, and they were to give themselves to the work of physicians. {7}

Urgent invitations are sent me to visit Washington, to attend an important meeting. Several are urging my presence. I would gladly attend these meetings, but a great work is before me, and I must keep at this work; for it is of great importance. This work is the bringing out of the warnings that have been given me for Dr. Kellogg. As he will present anything and everything possible to make of no effect the testimonies that the Lord has given me, I must do my part to meet the situation just now.

I thought I would take this matter up before, but light came that Dr. Kellogg, united with his associates, was doing a special work. Their plans were being laid, and I was to allow them to make the first move; for then there would be a necessity to "meet it," and I would be saved from much blame.

After this light came, I said to my son, "I will heed this warning. I can see the force of it."

In the visions of the night, I was in an assembly of physicians, and I saw the work that was being planned. Then I said to my son, "I must get everything in readiness; for soon we shall see the necessity of having the armor on, ready for action. In that meeting many things were said which

I can and must meet. I must work now." And we did work.

Letters copied from my diary were sent to Elders Daniells and Irwin, and they were prepared for the issue. You will see by the copies enclosed what took place in Battle Creek. I need not go over the same ground.

(signed) Ellen G. White

FRAGMENTS

August 13, 1912
MS 59-1912

Dear Brother Kress:

IN THE PAST YOU HAVE practiced health reform too rigorously for your own good. Once, when you were very sick, the Lord gave me a message to save your life. You have been too strenuous in restricting your diet to certain articles of food. While I was praying for you, words were given me for you to set you in the right path. The message was sent that you were to allow yourself a more generous diet. The use of flesh meat was not advised. Directions were given as to the food to be taken. You followed directions given, rallied, and are still with us.

I often think of the instruction then given you. I have been given so many precious messages to bear to the sick and the afflicted. For this I am grateful, and I praise the Lord. . . . {8}

Work in the Cities

I have been pleading with the Lord to roll the burden on the watchmen. Presidents of Conferences and church elders must work. Two and two laborers are to be sent forth into the unworked cities. No man is to be authorized to carry the work alone.

I am charged to repeat the warnings given in the past,—that it is not by making a great display that the work in New York and other places is to be carried forward. In the past mistakes have been made in the work in New York, mistakes which placed an erroneous stamp on the work, and left a wrong impression on the minds of those who witnessed the wonderful performance. Much time has thus been lost, and many false impressions made, regarding our work and the truth we believe.

(signed) Ellen G. White

PER ARDUA, WILLIAMS ST., GRANVILLE, N.S.W.

April 23, 1894
MS. -24-a.

THE LORD WOULD HAVE everyone acknowledge that He is the rightful owner of all the goods which He has lent us to trade upon. He says to us, Render back to Me the tithes and gifts and offerings, as a token of your loyalty to Me, and of your dependence upon Me, and I will bless you, and you shall be channels of blessing. Your gratitude offerings will be a token of your sense of obligation to Me. The gratitude that ends simply in words, has no particular value; for faith is made perfect by works, and without works your profession of faith is of no worth. God is continually giving, and the human agent is continually receiving. When we become weary of returning to the Lord His own, His blessing will be withheld from us. As long as we are dependent upon God's bounty, our obligations to render gratitude offerings to Him are upon us.

(signed) Ellen G. White

LABOR TO BE GIVEN TO LAKEPORT AND THE SURROUNDING SETTLEMENTS

June 9, '08
(MS.-65-'08)

THE LORD IS CALLING HIS people to go forth into the highways and byways, and call men and women to come to the gospel feast. If His servants will put their hearts into the work of proclaiming the truth to those who know it not, they may be assured that angels who minister unto those who shall be heirs of salvation, will give them grace and power and efficiency for their labors, and that the Spirit of God will go before them to impress hearts to respond to their efforts. The Lord will work through those who will open the Scriptures to the people who have made their homes in these retired places of the country. I appeal to my brethren and sisters to unite in doing this good work, and carry it to completion...

The people who live in the country places are often more easily reached {9} than are those who dwell in the thickly populated cities. Here among the scenes of nature, Christian character is more easily formed than amid the wickedness of city life. When the truth takes hold of the hearts of the simple-hearted, and the Spirit of God works upon their minds, leading them to respond to the proclamation of the Word, there will be some raised up to help support the cause of God both by their means and their labors...

From the camp-meeting we may take with us a better understanding of our home duties. There are lessons to be learned here regarding the work the Lord would have our sisters do in their homes. They are to learn to cultivate politeness of speech when speaking to husband and children. They are to study how they may help to bring every member of the family under discipline to God. Let fathers and mothers realize that they are under obligation to make home pleasant and attractive, and that obedience is not to be obtained by scolding and threats. Many parents have yet to learn that no good is accomplished by outbursts of scolding. Many do not consider the need of speaking kindly to the children. They do not remember that these little ones are bought with a price, and are the purchased possession of the Lord Jesus...

In our labors at the camp-meetings more attention should be given to the work of teaching the principles of health and temperance reform; these questions are to take an important place in our efforts at this time. My message is, Educate, educate on the question of temperance. In our schools let only those teachers be employed who will exert a reformatory influence in matters of eating and drinking and dressing. Encourage the spirit of self-denial and self-sacrifice. In all our sanitarium and school work, let matters pertaining to health reform take a leading part. The Lord desires to make our sanitariums an educating force in every place. Whether they are large or small institutions, their responsibility remains the same. The Saviour's commission to us is, "Let your light so shine before men, that they may see your good works, and glorify your Father which is in heaven."...

There are many of our people who, if they would go out of the cities, and begin to labor in these byways, and also highways, would recover physical health. I urge our brethren to go out as missionaries, two and two, to these country places. Go in humility. Christ has given an example, and the Lord will certainly bless the efforts of those who will move out in the fear of God, bearing the message the Saviour gave to the first disciples, "The Kingdom of God is come nigh unto you."

(signed) Ellen G. White.

REGARDING THE TESTIMONIES

October 10, 1911
(Ms. 23—1911)

REGARDING THE TESTIMONIES, nothing is ignored; nothing is cast aside; but time and place must be considered. Nothing must be done untimely. Some matters must be withheld because some persons would make an improper use of the light given. Every jot and tittle is essential and must appear at an opportune time. In the past, the testimonies were carefully prepared {10} before they were sent out for publication. And all matter is still carefully studied after the first writing.

Accusations

Tell them to eat the flesh and drink the blood of the Son of God. Place His Word before them. There will be those who will misinterpret and misrepresent. Their eyes have been blinded, and they will set forth the figures and interpretations that Satan has worked out for them, and entirely wrong meaning will be placed upon the words that Sister White has spoken. Satan is just as verily claiming to be Christ's child as did Judas, who was on the accusing side. They have educated themselves in Satan's school of misstating. A description of them is given in the third chapter of Zechariah. Nothing in the world is so dear to God as His church. Satan has worked upon human minds, and will continue to betray sacred trust in a spurious way.

... I can see plainly that should everyone who thinks he is qualified to write books, follow his imagination and have his productions published, insisting that they be recommended by our publishing houses, there would be plenty of tares sown broadcast in our world. Many from among our own people are writing to me, asking with earnest determination the privilege of using my writings to give force to certain subjects which they wish to present to the people in such a way as to leave a deep impression upon them.

It is true that there is a reason why some of these matters should be presented; but I would not venture to give my approval in using the testimonies in this way, or to sanction the placing of matter which is good in itself in the way which they propose.

The persons who make these propositions, for aught I know, may be able to conduct the enterprise of which they write in a wise manner; but nevertheless I dare not give the least license for using my writings in the manner which they propose. In taking account of such an enterprise, there are many things that must come into consideration; for in using the testimonies to bolster up some subject which may impress the mind of the author, the extracts may give a different impression than that which they would were they read in their original connections....

I am not prepared to advise that we make the matter of meat eating a test question with our people. There are some things on this subject that I can write out to be read before the churches, which it is essential for believers to understand; but when it comes to making this a test question, I dare not place it before the people in that positive way. There are those who would stumble over such a presentation, and there are others who would make of it a stone of stumbling.

Let us give this matter due consideration. I am prepared to stand for some things; but not yet are we as a people fully ready for this issue. There should be first a fair representation of the subject, and it should be considered in all its bearings. Read carefully the record of Genesis 18:6-8.

The Lord has given us much instruction on the subject of meat-eating; and from the light He has given we should not prepare meat and place it on our tables for our families. If meat is not placed before them the temptation to eat it is removed.

(signed) Ellen G. White

FROM A LETTER TO ELDER J. A. BURDEN

November 25, 1908
(File No. B-332—1908) {11}

CHRIST WILL INSTRUCT THOSE who manifest a teachable spirit. Among those who heed His instruction He will raise up men and women to act as His agents. But those who follow their own wisdom, fearing to walk in harmony with the revealed plans of the Lord, can be but a hindrance to the work He desires to be performed. You, Brother Burden, have seen how the Lord has wrought when men have not placed themselves directly in the way of the working of His plans.

We are engaged in an important and an essential work. We must carry on an aggressive warfare. We are to stand for the true Protestant principles; for the policies of the papacy will edge their way into every place possible, to proscribe liberty of conscience. Every eye must now be single to the glory of God. Those who have been seeking to undermine the confidence of our people in the testimonies that God has given for their benefit, and in the leadings of Providence in our work, will someday be revealed as having acted a part similar to that acted by Judas.

Judas was tempted and tried, but not rising above his temptations and trials, he lost ground, and finally went so far as to betray his Lord. Christ permitted him to go with the other disciples on their evangelistic tours, but he often manifested a spirit of superiority. He sought to exercise authority over his brethren. This spirit, unchecked and unrestrained, opened the way for the enemy to work upon his mind and heart, until at length he went so far as to betray his Lord and Saviour with a treacherous kiss.

There are today, among the professed people of God, some who are walking in the same path as did Judas. Unless they are converted, they will someday be numbered among the open enemies of God's work for this time.

DEAR BRETHREN IN THE MINISTRY AND THE MEDICAL MISSIONARY WORK

April 10, 1905
File B. 317—1905

THE CLOUD OF DIVINE WRATH was gathering over Jerusalem. Christ saw the city beleaguered. He saw it lost. In a voice full of tears He exclaimed, "If thou hadst known, even thou, at least in this thy day, the things which belong unto thy peace! but now they are hid from thine eyes."

I present this feeble representation of a terrible picture, to those who today are going over the same ground, refusing the messages of the grace of God, rejecting the warnings against a course of wickedness. The ground trodden by the Jewish leaders is being trodden today by those who have made light of the warnings from heaven, with looks, with words, with gesticulations. I have heard the ridicule of the warnings sent them and refused by them, I know that the same spirit that existed in the days of Christ exists today. The blessings that the Saviour longs to bestow He is forced to withhold, because of the contempt manifested by the men who give proof in their lives that they reject all warnings, all entreaties, all efforts for their salvation. They know not the day of their visitation. They despise the evidence of God's working, and history is being repeated. {12}

FROM A LETTER TO DR. GEORGE A. HARE

December 2, 1903
File H. 260—1903

WE WANT THE WASHINGTON sanitarium to be established upon different principles, and conducted upon different plans from those that have been followed in the Battle Creek Sanitarium. We shall not, therefore, go to Battle Creek to receive counsel regarding the establishment of this institution. The time has come when we must move under the direction of our great Leader, the divine Commander.

Please do not delay. Consecrate yourself to God, and He will be to you a present help in time of need. By doing the work that awaits your presence and assistance, depending entirely upon God for guidance and direction, you will obtain an invaluable experience.

God always has men of His appointment to step into the places where work needs to be done, men with whom and by whom He can work. A special work is committed to each one of God's workers. To every man the Lord has entrusted talents, gifts that correspond to the needs of some place.

The Lord will give understanding to everyone who will fully connect with His work. We are not left to trust in human wisdom. In the Lord is wisdom, and it is our privilege to look to Him for counsel.

To no one man is given all the qualifications for every branch of the Lord's work. We are all members of God's family, in all in a greater or less degree entrusted with God-given talents, for the use of which we are held responsible. Whether our talent be great or small, we are to use it in God's service, and we are to recognize the right of every one else to use the gifts entrusted to them.

Never should we disparage the smallest physical, intellectual, or spiritual capital. Some may trade in pennies and farthings, and by God's blessing, and unwearied diligence, these humble ones may make successful investments, and make a gain proportionate to the capital entrusted to them. No one should make light of any humble worker, who is filling his place, and is doing a work that some must do, however small that work may seem.

O how my heart is grieved, as I see men who have had great opportunities, seeking to place in a circumscribed sphere, someone who, with encouragement, might develop to fill a position of great usefulness. The Lord makes use of vessels both large and small. Many whose lives are filled with activity and earnestness need from others counsel and encouragement, and words of approval. God looks with pleasure upon the improvement made by His children as they help and encourage one another.

All, whether entrusted with a few or with many talents, are to blend together in unity. We need more of the spirit of the Saviour that we may help those who have been restricted and hindered. How much we may help them in their efforts to rise will never be known till it is made manifest in the judgment. We should have a word of encouragement to speak to all, remembering that there are a diversity of gifts. Some who desire to fill a large place and do some great service, overlook the little things that must be done by somebody, and forget that those who do these things need encouragement. {13}

If we pray much as we work, we shall gain more than if we give ourselves entirely to seeking for the wisdom that comes by experience. The Master-workman is supervising His workers. When, as I write, a new thought comes into my mind, I reverentially thank God for the appropriate word or sentence brought to my mind.

ON THE TRAIN FROM NORWICH TO BOSTON

Aug. 28, 1898
(File MS. 106, pg.3, 1898)
En route for Lynn, Massachusetts

THOSE WHO HAVE A HOLD of the truth theoretically, with their fingertips, as it were, who have not brought its principles into the inner sanctuary of the soul, but have kept the vital truth in the outer court, will see nothing sacred in the past history of this people which has made them what they are and has established them as earnest, determined missionary workers in the world. The truth for this time is precious, but those whose hearts have not been broken by falling on the Rock, Christ Jesus, will not see and understand what is truth. They will accept that which pleases their ideas and will begin to manufacture another foundation than that which is laid. They will flatter their own vanity and esteem, thinking that they are capable of removing the pillars of our faith.

This will continue to be as long as time shall last. Anyone who has been a close student of the Bible will see and understand the solemn position of those who are living in the closing scenes of this earth's history. They will feel their own inefficiency and weakness, and will make it their first business to have not merely a form of godliness, but a vital connection with God. They will not dare to rest until Christ is formed within, the hope of glory. Self will die; pride will be expelled from the soul, and they will have the meekness and gentleness of Christ.

FROM A LETTER WRITTEN, TO ELDER GEORGE I. BUTLER

December 14, 1903
(File B -43, 1903)

WE ARE ON THE EARTH as combatants. This is no time or place for us to be negligent, indifferent, or careless. We have a heaven to win and a hell to shun. There is frequently presented to me a scene of conflict and of determined opposition. How can it be otherwise when we are in an enemy's country?

"THE WORK IN MELBOURNE"

June 29, 1905
(File No. MS -76, pg. 2, 3, 1905)

LET CENTERS BE NO LONGER made in the cities. Let children no longer be exposed to the temptations of the cities that are ripe for destruction. The Lord has sent us warning and counsel to get out of the cities. Then let us make no more investments in the cities. Fathers and mothers, how do you regard the souls of your children? Are you preparing the members of your families for translation into the heavenly courts? Are you preparing them to become members of the royal family? children of the heavenly King? What shall it profit a man if he gain the whole world, and lose his own soul? {14} How will ease, comfort, convenience, compare with the value of the souls of your children?

There is not one family in a hundred who will be improved physically, mentally, or spiritually, by residence in the city. Faith, hope, love, happiness, can far better be gained in retired places, where there are fields, and hills and trees. Take your children away from the sights and sounds of the city, away from the rattle and din of street cars and teams, and their minds will become more healthy. It will be found easier to bring home to their hearts the truth of the word of God.

The Lord would have the believers

in Melbourne consider the example set by Battle Creek, and not pattern after it. God has sent warning after warning that our schools and publishing houses and sanitariums are to be established out of the city, in places where the youth may be taught most effectively what is truth. Let no one attempt to use the Testimonies to vindicate the establishment of large business interests in the cities. Do not make of no effect the light that has been given upon this subject.

Men will arise speaking perverse things, to counter-work the very movements that the Lord is leading his servants to make. But it is time that men and women reasoned from cause to effect. It is too late, too late, to establish large business firms in the cities,—too late to call young men and women from the country to the city. Conditions are arising in the cities that will make it very hard for those of our faith to remain in them. It would therefore be a great mistake to invest money in the establishment of business interests in the cities.

WRITTEN AT "SUNNYSIDE," COORANBONG

Aug. 25, 1897
(Manuscript, No. 86)

YOUR LETTER TO ME, under date of February 12, is received. Your question is, "Is it advisable to employ a good, Christian physician, who treats his patients on hygiene principles? In urgent cases, should we call in a worldly physician, because the Sanitarium doctors are all so busy that they have no time to devote to outside practice? Some say that when the Sanitarium doctors do use drugs, they give larger doses than ordinary doctors."

If the physicians are so busy that they cannot treat the sick outside of the institution, would it not be wiser for all to educate themselves in the use of simple remedies, than to venture to use drugs, that are given a long name to hide their real qualities? Why need any one be ignorant of God's remedies,—hot water fomentations and cold and hot compresses? It is important to become familiar with the benefit of dieting in case of sickness. All should understand what to do themselves. They may call upon someone who understands nursing, but everyone should have an intelligent knowledge of the house he lives in. All should understand what to do in case of sickness. Were I sick, I would just as soon call in

a lawyer as a physician from among general practitioners. I would not touch their nostrums, to which they give Latin names. I am determined to know, in straight English, the name of everything that I introduce into my system. {15}.

Those who make a practice of taking drugs sin against their intelligence and endanger their whole after life. There are herbs that are harmless, the use of which will tide over many apparently serious difficulties. But if all would seek to become intelligent in regard to their bodily necessities, sickness would be rare instead of common. An ounce of prevention is worth a pound of cure.

You say, "The reason why I advise with you is because there are some who have never heard of the principles of health reform. Converts of the S.D.A. faith, whom one would naturally suppose would be easily led to see the beauty of hygienic remedies for the sick, are being taught to take the Lord for their Healer, without even using simple means and heaven-blessed agencies for the recovery and preservation of health. These agencies are excluded by close rooms and a neglect to procure pure water."

TAKEN FROM DIARY

April 25, 1999
(1999-6- File 68)

THE BUILDING WORK ON OUR hospital has not yet commenced, but the land is being cleared preparatory to building. We need a hospital so much. On Thursday Sister Sara McEnterfer was called to see if she could do anything for Brother Palmer's little son, who is eighteen months old. For several days he has had a painful swelling on the knee, supposed to be from the bite of some poisonous insect. Pulverized charcoal, mixed with flaxseed, was placed upon the swelling, and this poultice gave relief at once. The child had screamed with pain all night, but when this was applied, he slept. Today she has been to see the little one twice. She opened the swelling in two places, and a large amount of yellow matter and blood was discharged freely. The child was relieved of its great suffering. We thank the Lord that we may become intelligent in using the simple things within our reach to alleviate pain, and successfully remove its cause.

Some matters have been deeply impressed upon my mind, and one is the necessity for much better facilities in the

bathrooms. This is where impressions will be made upon minds. We must have conveniences in these rooms—massage tables, and a cot on which to give packs. All these things make their impression. Conversation will sometimes arise, and words will be spoken that will open a flood of light to the patient as to the best methods of caring for the human body, the temple of God. Therefore, the greatest care should be taken to observe decency and strict purity in conversation and in every action. A small, crowded bathroom leaves on the mind an impression of cheapness and commonness, and this should not be.

FROM A LETTER TO ELDER W.C. WHITE

August 18, 1903
File W. 186, 1903

THE MINISTERIAL EVANGELIST who engages in the canvassing work is performing a service fully as important as that of preaching the gospel before a congregation Sabbath after Sabbath. God looks upon the faithful evangelistic canvasser with as much approval as He looks upon any faithful minister. Both workers have a light, and both are to shine in their respective spheres of influence. God calls upon every man to cooperate with the great Medical {16} Missionary Worker, and to go forth into the highways and byways. Each man in his particular line of service, has a work to do for God. Such laborers, if converted, are true missionaries.

Missionaries are needed in workshops. As they toil, they may realize that they are representing Christ and His mission on this earth. In every phase of physical labor God requires His agencies in missionary lines of effort to speak a word at the right time, to caution, to warn, to learn how to adapt themselves to the situation in which they find themselves, and in every respect to be representatives of Christ's great medical missionary work.

When Christ was living on this earth, how surprised would have been His associates, if, after becoming acquainted with Him, they had heard Him utter one word of impatience, one word of accusation or of faultfinding! He expects those who love Him and believe in Him, to represent Him in character.

Although a man may be able to educate others to act as they should, yet if he does not glorify God himself with his lips, he had better first reveal in word and deed that he has received power to become a child of God, an heir of the kingdom, before attempting to teach others. After receiving his life-insurance papers as a member of the elect of God, his great desire henceforth will be to reveal Christ's presence to his fellow men in missionary fields.

Only those whose hearts are filled with the love of God and who reveal that Christ has given them His grace to adorn their office-work as missionaries for Him, should make application to engage in medical missionary work. Those who take up this line of missionary effort should look upon their work as a high and holy calling. This work is committed to them as a sacred trust; and wherever they may be, the Lord expects them to reveal the excellency of their mission.

To Brother and Sister Kress

June 24, 1903
(File K. -116, 1903)

ICERTAINLY THINK THAT AT present it would not be wise to invest two or three thousand dollars in electric light baths and in machinery to operate them. The prosperity of the Sanitarium is not dependent on electric light baths. It is dependent on the prayers and faith and labors of the workers...

Strike the true keynote in the Sanitarium. When Jesus sent out the twelve disciples, He said, "As ye go, preach, saying, The kingdom of heaven is at hand. Heal the sick, cleanse the lepers, raise the dead, cast out devils; freely ye have received, freely give."

Let there be in the Sanitarium much prayer for the healing of the sick. We must depend more decidedly upon the great Healer. It is the miracle-working power of God that will give efficiency to the gospel message. As believers, are we not sons and daughters of God? Is not Christ our Elder Brother? Then shall we not believe that He will reveal His power in restoring the sick to health? Tell Him your wishes and desires, and plead the promise, "Let him take hold of My strength, that he may make peace with Me, and he shall make peace with Me." Christ cannot too often be reminded of His pledged word. {17}

Let us not take ourselves out of the hand of God. Our medical missionary work should bear the similitude of the greatest Missionary this world has ever seen. Present the Lord Jesus, the great Healer, as the One upon whom you depend. The instruction that you give the patients in your parlor lectures will be received much more readily if you send to heaven a petition for the power that is above all human power.

Encourage the patients to breathe the fresh air. Teach them how to breathe deep and how to exercise their muscles. Teach them to use the abdominal muscles in breathing. Encourage them to spend much time in the open air. Make the grounds so attractive that they will want to be out of doors. Provide some pleasant, easy work for those who are able to work. Show them how agreeable and health-giving this out-of-door work is. This is an education that will be invaluable to them after they return to their homes.

Use nature's remedies,—water, sunshine, and fresh air. Do not use drugs. Drugs never heal; they only change the features of the disease.

Do not allow the helpers to overwork. Let the patients see nurses that are cheerful and bright, not nurses who, because they are overworked, are discouraged and downhearted. It is most inconsistent with the principles on which our sanitariums are founded for the nurses to be allowed to break down in their work.

The workers are to practice the principles of health reform in all that they do,—standing, walking, breathing, eating, and dressing. They are to surround themselves with an atmosphere of praise. They are to cultivate the voice, keeping it pleasant and sympathetic. No word of discouragement is to be heard. Let the nurses and physicians face the light. Let them open the windows of the heart heavenward, that it may be flooded with the beams of the Sun of Righteousness.

To Brethren Kilgore and Jacobs

June 26, 1902
(File No. K -95, 1902)

IN A CERTAIN PLACE, preparations were being made to clear the land for the erection of a sanitarium. Light was given that there is health in the fragrance of the pine, the cedar, and the fir. And there are several other kinds of trees that have medicinal properties that are health-promoting. Let not such trees be ruthlessly cut down. Better change the site of the building than cut down these evergreen trees.

...Our sanitariums should be surrounded with choice flowers, that by their growth and beauty they may reveal the advantages of culture. They teach us that it is our privilege to improve. God desires us to bring fragrance into our life-work. We are to be the plants of the Lord, serving Him in whatsoever way He wills. Let us do all in our power to beautify our characters.

The Lord has entrusted His garden to skillful tenders whose work it is to care for His beautiful plants. Tender care must be given {18} to the delicate plants. The useless off-shoots must be taken away. The bruised parts must be carefully bound up. So those who are weak in the faith must have fostering care. We are to bind to our stronger purposes the weaklings in the Lord's garden, giving them support.

From the endless variety of plants and flowers, we may learn an important lesson. All blossoms are not the same in form or color. Some possess healing virtues. Some are always fragrant. There are professing Christians who think it their duty to make every other Christian like themselves. This is man's plan, not the plan of God. In the church of God there is room for characters as varied as are the flowers in the garden. In His spiritual garden there are many variety of flowers...

Do that which presents itself in its time, demanding the first attention. Do not pass by the first duty to do the second. One duty accomplished prepares the way for the next. Readiness to engage in the second known duty brings the Lord's blessing. And the second duty is more easily done if the first has been faithfully performed. The burden is off the soul. The heart is filled with the peace and gladness of Christ.

"The Time of the End"

Oct. 9, 1903
(File No. MS -122, 1903)

GOD MAY SPARE MY LIFE, that I may still work in His cause. Physically, I have always been as a broken vessel; and yet in my old age the Lord continues to move upon me by His Holy Spirit to write the most important books that have ever come before the churches in the world. The Lord is evidencing what He can do through weak vessels. The life that He spares I will use to His glory. And, when He may see fit to let me rest, His messages shall be of even more vital force than when the frail instrumentality through whom they were delivered, was living.

FROM A LETTER TO MRS. S.M.I. HENRY

December 1, 1898
(File, H., 118)

IN THE NIGHT I AM AROUSED from my sleep, and I write in my diary many things that appear as new to me when read as to any who hear them. If I did not see the matter in my own handwriting, I should not think my pen had traced it...

In the providence of God you have been led to the light, to obtain a knowledge of the truth, and the education you have received in the grand temperance work, in connection with your sister workers, is the education you need to bring into the work with men whose hearts are softened by the Spirit of God, and who are searching for the truth as for hidden treasure. For twenty years I have seen that the light would come to the women workers in the temperance lines. But with sadness I have discerned that many of them are becoming politicians, and that against God. They enter into questions and debates and theories of many things that they have no need to touch. {19}

FROM A LETTER TO J. E. WHITE

January 5, 1903
(File W -11, 1903)

I CANNOT, AT MY OWN IMPULSE, take up a work and launch out into it. I have to be impressed by the Spirit of God. I cannot write unless the Holy Spirit helps me. Sometimes I cannot write at all. Then again I am aroused at eleven, twelve, and one o'clock; and I can write as fast as my hand can move over the paper...

Our missions and commissions are all different. No two persons are given precisely the same work. Each has his own manner of performing his work, and that manner must be Christ-like.

God must show us every step of the way. Every hour we must have the new impulses of His Spirit. Love for Him should be the mainspring of our actions. Every hour has its duties, and every moment its cares. Let a controlling power from above check the hasty speech. Let your heart be filled with the kindest, most tender compassion. Never allow yourself to be ruled by impulse. Never get out of patience. New scenes are opening before us, and we need to hear a voice from heaven, directing us to the right or to the left, saying, "This is the way; walk ye in it." God's will, not ours, is to control. "A man's heart deviseth his way; but the Lord directeth his steps."

"MY DEAR GRANDDAUGHTER MABEL"

November 16, 1905
(W -329 A, 1905)
From a letter
written November 16, 1905

I HAVE THE MOST PRECIOUS matter to reproduce and place before the people in testimony form. While I am able to do this work, the people must have these things, to revive past truth, without one heretical sentence, in that which I have written. This, I am instructed, is to be a living letter to all in regard to my faith....

We have every encouragement that if we daily surrender our wills to God, the promise will be fulfilled, "And of His fullness have we all received, and grace for grace." Every revealing of the grace of Christ in our behalf is for us. We are to reveal His grace in our lives, in thought, word, and deed. Let us not lose our opportunity to speak and act Christ Jesus. We are to represent the mercy, the love, and the power of Christ,—the power that He has given us. "God is our refuge and strength, a very present help in trouble. Therefore will not we fear, though the earth be removed, and though the mountains be carried into the midst of the sea."

Were it not for the power received through Christ, we would have no strength. But Christ has all power. "Jesus came and spake unto them, saying, All power is given unto me in heaven and in earth. Go ye therefore, and teach all nations, baptizing them in the name of the Father, and of the Son, and of the Holy Ghost; teaching them to observe all things whatsoever I have commanded; and lo, I am with you alway, even unto the end of the world." Here is our power, our comfort. Of ourselves we have no strength. But He says, "I am with you alway," helping you to perform your duty, guiding, comforting, sanctifying, and sustaining you, giving you success in speaking words that will draw the attention of others to Christ, and awaken in their minds the desire to understand the hope and meaning of {20} the truth, turning them from darkness to light and from the power of sin to God.

It is a wonderful thought that human beings can speak the word of God, in simple words of comfort and encouragement. The humblest instruments will be used of God to sow the seeds of truth, which may spring up and bear fruit, because the one in whose heart they were sown needed help,—a kind thought, a kind word, made effective by the One who has said, "Lo, I am with you alway, even unto the end of the world."

SANITARIUM

September 1887
(File No. MS.-22)
Battle Creek, Michigan

I HAVE RECEIVED LETTERS from different states asking me to answer their inquiries in regard to the wisdom of investing means in building sanitariums, where the sick may be treated, and where there could be a right influence exerted, to point sick souls to Jesus, who is the great Physician of the soul as well as of the body. This is a question that cannot be answered in quick, Italian fashion with "Yes" or "No." There are many sides to the question.

Letters have come to me from Ohio. They have erected a health institution there. Some of our ministers and leading men in Ohio have acted a prominent part in the building of this institution, and now they find that they have no one that is able to run such an institution. There was moneyed men, I have been told, who would put thousands into this institution, but could not be induced to invest means in our home or foreign missions. I came fresh from Europe, where I had seen fields open before us on every side. Hearts were being softened, and were longing for the truth. Calls were constantly coming from all countries for books and for preachers. All was done that could be done, but there was an empty treasury, and a want of qualified men who had experience to do a good work in wisdom, presenting the truth as it is in Jesus. I attended camp-meetings. I tried to set the condition of things before the people, and besides that, wrote to several for means, either to loan or to donate. One of these returned answer that his means were invested in the Sanitarium in Ohio, and he could do nothing. Of some ten letters that we sent, only one was responded to. Brother Smouse, of Mount Pleasant, Iowa, sent one hundred dollars.

The building of health institutions is in itself well enough, if the matter has been duly considered, if there has been prayerful, thoughtful investigation of the subject, and if those who enter upon the enterprise are discerning, careful, prayerful managers, and they begin to build, fully counting the cost, so they know whether they are able to finish that which they enter upon, or not.

Have these brethren in Ohio unselfishly looked to God for light and wisdom how to invest as wise stewards the Lord's money for the upbuilding of His cause and the advancement of His kingdom? Have they decided that the Lord's means was in their hands? Or have they followed their own inclination, and in the place of selling and giving alms, or, in short, investing in the very work that is most essential to open the Word of God to all nations, tongues, and peoples, have they invested their means where they will be sure to get either honor or returns? The judgment will reveal the matter as it is. Every man's work will be tested and proved by the Lord. {21}

If small institutions can be built in some localities, and there are discreet men and women to conduct these institutions, then we will say, Let them be built, if in so doing the cause is not in any way crippled for means to send missionaries to foreign countries, according to the commission Christ gave His disciples. They were to go to all nations, tongues, and peoples, beginning at Jerusalem, and He gave them promise: "Lo, I am with you alway, even to the end of the world."

I have found it no easy matter to secure means to invest in health institutions. But it has proved a still more difficult matter to secure persons who were qualified to conduct such institutions. It requires thoroughly balanced characters to do this work, not men who have some strong traits of character, but who are weak as children in other points. Plenty of physicians can be obtained who ceased to be students when they received their diplomas, who are self-inflated, who feel that they know all that is worth knowing, and what they do not know is not worth knowing. But this class are not the ones we want. When a physician enters upon his work as a practitioner, the more genuine, practical experience he has, the more fully will he feel his want of knowledge. If self-sufficient, he will read articles written in regard to disease and how to treat them without nature's aid; he will grasp statements and weave them into his practice, and without deep research, without earnest study, without sifting every statement, he will merely become a mechanical worker. Because he

knows so little, he will be ready to experiment upon human lives, and sacrifice not a few. This is murder, actual murder. He did not do this work with evil design, he had no malicious purposes; but life was sacrificed on account of his ignorance, because he was a superficial student, because he had not had that practice that would make him a safe man to be entrusted with human lives. It requires care-taking, deep, earnest taxation of the mind to carry the burden a physician should carry in learning his trade thoroughly. Every physician who has received a thorough education will be modest in his claims. It will not do for him to run any risk upon experimenting on human life, lest he be guilty of murder, and this be written against him in the books of heaven. There should be a careful, competent physician who will deal scarcely ever in drugs, and who will not boast that powerful poisons are far more effective than a smaller quantity carefully taken, It is true, it kills, if it does not cure; but drugs never cure. They change the order of difficulties, but never heal them, never remove the cause.

We have deeply regretted that there were not a large number of institutions working from the hygienic principles that are now in existence. All these cannot be prepared upon a large scale, involving large expense; but the question is, will they preserve the principles of hygiene, or will they use the easier method of using drugs, to take the place of treating diseases without resorting to drug medications? There could be many hygienic institutions in all parts of our world, if there were plenty of means and plenty of persons who had the qualifications to manage such institutions. The physicians who shall be employed should not only have a book knowledge, but a practical experience to understand disease and its causes, and will feel the necessity, as soon as they are brought into positions of trust, to commence the work of carrying the burden necessary for them to bear, in order to do the most careful, thorough work. They will, if they are not closely connected with God, become careless and venturesome. The first labors of a physician should be to educate the sick and suffering the very course they should {22} pursue to prevent disease. The greatest good can be done by our trying to enlighten the minds of all we can obtain access to, as to the best course for them to pursue to prevent sickness and suffering, and broken constitutions, and premature death; but those who do not care to undertake work

that taxes their physical and mental powers will be ready to prescribe drug medication, which lays a foundation in the human organism for a two-fold greater evil than that which they claim to have relieved.

A physician who has the moral courage to peril (imperil) his reputation in enlightening the understanding by plain facts, in showing the nature of disease and how to prevent it, and the dangerous practice of resorting to drugs, will have an up-hill business, but he will live and let live. He will not use his powerful drug medication, because of the knowledge he has acquired by studying books. He will, if a reformer, talk plainly in regard to the false appetites and ruinous self-indulgence, in dressing, in eating and drinking, in overtaxing to do a large amount of work in a given time, which has a ruinous influence upon the temper, the physical and mental powers. Knowledge is what is needed. Drugs are too often promised to restore health, and the poor sick are so thoroughly drugged with quinine, morphine, or some strong health-and-life-destroying (word illegible), that nature may never make sufficient protest, but give up the struggle; and they may continue their wrong habits with hopeful impunity. Right and correct habits, intelligently and perseveringly practiced will be removing the cause of disease, and the strong drugs need not be resorted to. Many go on from step to step with their natural indulgences, which is bringing in just as unnatural condition of things as possible.

Diseases of every stripe and type have been brought upon human beings by the use of tea and coffee and the narcotics, opium and tobacco. These hurtful indulgences must be given up, not only one, but all; for all are hurtful, and ruinous to the physical, mental, and moral powers, and should be discontinued from a health standpoint. The common use of the flesh of dead animals has had a deteriorating influence upon the morals, as well as the physical constitution. Ill-health in a variety of forms, if effect could be traced to the cause, would reveal the sure result of flesh eating. The disuse of meats, with healthful dishes nicely prepared to take the place of flesh meats, would place a large number of the sick and suffering ones in a fair way of recovering their health, without the use of drugs. But if the physicians encourage a meat-eating diet to his invalid patients, then he will make a necessity for the use of drugs. Nature will want some assistance to bring things to their proper condition, which may be found in the simplest remedies, especially in the use of nature's own furnished remedies,—pure air, and with a precious knowledge of how to breathe; pure water, with a knowledge of how to apply it; plenty of sunlight in every room, if possible, in the house, and with an intelligent knowledge of what advantages are to be gained by its use. All these are powerful in their efficiency, and the patient who has obtained a knowledge of how to eat and dress healthfully, may live for comfort, for peace, for health; and will not be prevailed upon to put to his lips drugs, which, in the place of helping nature, paralyzes her powers. If the sick and suffering will do only as well as they know in regard to living out the principles of health reform perseveringly, they will, in nine cases out of ten, recover from their ailments.

The feeble and suffering ones must be educated line upon line, precept {23} upon precept, here a little, and there a little, until they will have respect for, and live in obedience to, the law that God has made to control the human organism. Those who sin against knowledge and light, and resort to the skill of a physician in administering drugs, will be constantly losing their hold on life. The less there is of drug-dosing, the more favorable will be their recovery to health. Drugs, in the place of helping nature, are constantly paralyzing her efforts. The health institutions for the sick will be the best places to educate the suffering ones to live in accordance with nature's laws and cease their health-destroying practices in wrong habits in diet, in dress, that are in accordance with the world's habits and customs, which are not at all after God's order, they are doing a good work to enlighten our world.

Drugs always have a tendency to break down and destroy vital forces, and nature becomes so crippled in her efforts, that the invalid dies, not because he needed to die, but because nature was outraged. If she had been left alone, she would have put forth her highest efforts to save life and health. Nature wants none of such help as so many claim that they have given her. Lift off the burdens placed upon her, after the customs of the fashion of this age, and you will see in many cases nature will right herself. The use of drugs is not favorable or natural to the laws of life and health. The drug medication gives nature two burdens to bear, in the place of one. She has two serious difficulties to overcome, in the place of one. There is now positive need even with phy-

sicians, reformers in the line of treatment of disease, that greater painstaking effort be made to carry forward and upward the work for themselves, and to interestedly instruct those who look to them for medical skill to ascertain the cause of their infirmities. They should call their attention in a special manner to the laws which God has established, which cannot be violated with impunity. They dwell much on the working of disease, but do not, as a general rule, arouse the attention to the laws which must be sacredly and intelligently obeyed in such to prevent disease. Especially if the physician has not been correct in his dietetic practices, if his own appetite has not been restricted to a plain, wholesome diet, in a large measure discarding the use of the flesh of dead animals,—he loves meat, he has educated and cultivated a taste for unhealthful food. His ideas are narrow, and he will as soon educate and discipline the taste and appetite of his patients to love the things that he loves, as to give them the sound principles of health reform. He will prescribe for sick patients, flesh-meats, when it is the very worst diet that they can have; it stimulates, but does not give strength. They do not inquire into their former habits of eating and drinking, and take special notice of their erroneous habits which have been for many years laying the foundation of disease. Conscientious physicians should be prepared to enlighten those who are ignorant, and should with wisdom make out their prescriptions, prohibiting those things in their diet which he knows to be erroneous. He should plainly state the things which he regards as detrimental to the laws of health, and leave these suffering ones to work conscientiously to do those things for themselves which they can do, and thus place themselves in the right relation to the laws of life and health. When from an enlightened conscience they do the very best they know how to do, to preserve themselves in health, then in faith they may look to the great Physician, who is a healer of the body as well as of the soul. We are {24} health reformers. Physicians should have wisdom and experience, and be thorough health reformers. Then they will be constantly educating by precept and example their patients from drugs. For they well know that the use of drugs may produce for the time being favorable results, but which will implant in the system that which will cause great difficulties hereafter, which they may never recover from

during their lifetime. Nature must have a chance to do her work. Obstructions must be removed, and opportunity given her to exert her healing forces, which she will surely do, if every abuse is removed from her, and she has a fair chance.

The sick should be educated to have confidence in nature's great blessings which God has provided, and the most effective remedies for disease are pure soft water; the blessed God-given sunshine coming into the rooms of the invalids; living outdoors as much as possible; having healthful exercise; eating and drinking in foods that are prepared in the most healthful manner. To resort to the drugging process lays upon nature a most fearful, merciless burden from which they may never recover. There are many laboring under chronic diseases. They will swallow anything in the line of drugs prescribed by the unbelieving physician, when an intelligent knowledge that they are indulging in unnatural appetites which explains to them the cause of their suffering, if Christians, they would place themselves in a position as health reformers. They would change the cause which produces this sure result.

There are many, many afflicted in our world with tobacco poison, but the physicians who are summoned to treat their patients under painful afflictions brought upon them by tobacco using,—are not instructed by these worldly physicians to let the poisons alone, in order that they may recover health; for many of these physicians use these poisons themselves. How can they, then, consistently enlighten the understanding of those who indulge in the poisonous narcotic, tobacco? The physician, if he is not a novice, can trace the effects back to the true cause, but he dares not forbid its use, because he indulges in it himself. Some will in an undecided, halfway manner advise the tobacco users to take less of this narcotic; but he does not say to them, This habit is killing you. They prescribe drugs to cure a disease which is the result of indulging unnatural appetites, and two evils are produced in the place of removing one.

Thousands need to be educated patiently, kindly, tenderly, but decidedly, that nine-tenths of their complaints are created by their own course of action. The more they introduce drugs into the system, the more certainly do they interfere with the laws of nature and bring about the very difficulties they drug themselves to avoid. Let everyone who contemplates erecting an institution, carefully consider whether they are to make it an institution conducted upon the principles of health reform, or whether they design to copy the popular institutions all through our land. If an institution for health is conducted upon the principles of health reform, it will require for its management a large amount of faith, large amount of patience, a large amount of perseverance, a large amount of moral power, such as they have scarcely dreamed of, to make such an institution a success and to pay its own way. The managers will require moral backbone, as well as superior educated skill. Lectures need to be given in such an institution every day upon some points connected with the custom and habits of the people, of disease and its causes, and the only true course to be taken to prevent disease. All connected with our health institutions as managers and helpers {25} should possess the very best ability, should have abundance of Christian courtesy, should practice universally Christian politeness, should be tender, pitiful, courteous. This is positively essential in order to leave the right impression upon the minds of sick people. While trying to educate them away from the habits and customs of the world, many will be glad to be enlightened, while many who are wedded to their own fashionable, health-destroying indulgences will be offended, and make it very unpleasant for those who wish to do them good; and some have not the moral courage to keep right on in the fear of the Lord. There is even among those who have intelligence in regard to the laws of life and health, a constant selfish indulgence in those things which are injurious to both soul and body. There is intemperance in eating, and in the many varieties of food taken at one meal. In the preparation of food, there are unhealthful mixtures which ferment in the stomach, and cause great distress. And yet these go on, continuing their indulgence, which lays the foundation for numerous difficulties. If these would have self-control, and educate their taste to eat only those things which the abused stomach can and will assimilate, they would save large expense in doctor bills, and avoid great sufferings.

There are many who spend their money for that which is not bread—for tea, coffee, the large use of flesh meats. All of these produce their sure results in painful affliction. Many animals have been butchered, when their blood was in a high state of fever, apparently boiling with madness.

Those who eat of these meats are subject to inflammation and blood-poisoning. Some have distressing spasms, some have great distress of the bowels. It is the work of the physician to educate those who are ignorant in regard to these things. There should be training-schools to educate nurses and prepare the minds to sense the danger and to see the importance of bringing in skill and tact in the preparation of foods which shall be substituted for the meat diet. This kind of education will pay in the end. Wisdom should be used not to remove meat all at once from those who have been in the habit of using it, but educate the mind to see the importance of the use of healthful foods.

We must not go to work in building our institutions, until we shall carefully look the ground over and see whether we can complete that which we have in our mind to undertake. There is danger of making rash moves which will not bear the sanction of heaven, of erecting large buildings, and binding up a large amount of God's means that is needed at the very time in other branches of the work in sustaining our poverty-stricken missions that are directly engaged in the salvation of souls. This means invested in this important work may not bring the greatest honor and flattering praise to the one who invests it; but in the heavenly records every dollar is placed to their account as treasures laid up that they will come into possession of when Christ shall come. Let none flatter themselves that it is an easy way to erect and conduct an institution upon health reform principles. It is not an easy matter to run an institution where the sick of all classes shall be treated. Every such institution should have as its managers and helpers the very best talents that the world can produce. Then they will have an educating school and be thoroughly disciplined and fitted, that representatives shall be sent out to any part of the world to impart their knowledge to those who are ignorant, and who greatly need it. This drill is to be kept up, until men and women are prepared to do the very best kind of work as educators, as well as all the time to be learning themselves, disciplining their powers to obtain increased knowledge, that they may as stewards of God have wisdom {26} and light, that they can impart, too, that they are connected with in any branch of the work.

In all our institutions there are many who are deficient in knowledge, who

might be fitted to do a much better work, if they made the best use of the opportunities and privileges which God has given them. These will boast of their knowledge, when they are very ignorant of the things which they ought to know. If they knew themselves better, they would have a sense of their inefficiency; they would grasp the higher rounds of the ladder, without climbing with painstaking efforts round after round to reach this elevation. It is much easier to boast than to execute. In these institutions we have it (illegible corrections) a most puzzling question how to keep managers and helpers in harmonious working order. The very best kind of material is needed for the upbuilding of institutions for the sick. We have had an experience from the first establishment of the institution in the city of Battle Creek, and in the institution at St. Helena, and we feel compelled to say that it has cost much time and great amount of perplexity, and quite an amount of money, to get these institutions in working order. There have been counsels and painful reproofs given, most earnest entreaties and appeals made; one set of workmen discharged because inefficient, and others have been placed in their place. Step by step a little has been gained here and there. There has been much said in order to keep out licentious practices and improper familiarity between men and women. This has to be met and reproved, and constantly guarded against, and the ones that are corrected become angry; in the place of reforming, they try to work their revenge upon the faithful workers in the institution. My own soul has been weighed down with burdens that are inexpressible, as I have tried in the fear of God to do my duty to all parties and to the institution.

DEAR BROTHER PETER WESSELS

November 6, 1899
(Nov. 9, '99-5- W-182)
Maitland, New South Wales

I HAVE SOME THINGS TO SAY to you which you need. There are places you might fill, places in which you might be a blessing in many ways. But erroneous ideas keep you from filling these places. Your character needs to be pruned; for there is a superfluous growth that needs to be cut away from you. The idea which you hold that no remedies should be used for the sick is an error. God does not heal the sick without the aid of the means of healing which lie within the reach of man; or when men refuse to be benefitted by the simple remedies that God has provided in pure air and water.

There were physicians in Christ's day and in the days of the apostles. Luke is called the beloved physician. He trusted in the Lord to make him skillful in the application of remedies. When the Lord told Hezekiah that He would spare his life for fifteen years, and as a sign that He would fulfill His promise, caused the sun to go back ten degrees, why did He not put His direct, restoring power upon the king? He told him to apply a bunch of figs to his sore, and that natural remedy blessed by God, healed him. The God of nature directs the human agent to use natural remedies now.

I might go to any length in this matter, my brother, but I leave it now with a few instances. A brother was taken sick with inflammation of the {27} bowels and bloody dysentery. The man was not a careful health reformer, but indulged his appetite. We were just preparing to leave Texas, where we had been laboring for several months, and we had carriages prepared to take away this brother and his family, and several others who were suffering from malarial fever. My husband and I thought we would stand this expense rather than have heads of several families die and leave their wives and children unprovided for. Two or three were taken in a spring wagon on spring mattresses. But this man who was suffering from inflammation of the bowels, sent for me to come to him. My husband and I decided that it would not do to move him. Fears were entertained that mortification had set in. Then the thought came to me like a communication from the Lord to take pulverized charcoal, put water upon it, and give this water to the sick man to drink, putting bandages of the charcoal over the bowels and stomach. We were about one mile from the city of Denison, but the sick man's son went to a blacksmith's shop, secured the charcoal, and pulverized it, and then used it according to the directions given. The result was that in half an hour there was a change for the better. We had to go on our journey and leave the family behind, but what was our surprise the following day to see their wagon overtake us. The sick man was lying in a bed in the wagon. The blessing of God had worked with the simple means used.

I still remember another case. At our first camp-meeting here, held in Brighton, a young lady was taken sick on the ground, and remained sick during most of the meeting. She was thought to have typhoid fever, and although many prayers were offered in her behalf, she left the ground sick. Dr. M.G. Kellogg, half-brother to J.H. Kellogg, of Battle Creek, was attending her. He came to me one morning, and said, Sister Price is in great pain. I cannot relieve her. She cannot sleep, and every breath seems as though it would be her last. We prayed for her, and then like a flash of lightning there came to me the thought of the charcoal. "Send to the blacksmith for charcoal, and pulverize it, I said, "and put a poultice of it on her side." He tried this, and in one hour he came to me and said, "That prescription was an inspiration from God. Sister Price could not have lived until now if no change had come. The sick one fell into a restful sleep; the crisis passed, and she began to amend. In a few days she was taken from Melbourne to her home in Melbourne (?), and is alive and well today.

All these things teach us that we are to be very careful lest we receive radical ideas and impressions. Your ideas regarding drug medication, I must respect; but even in this you must not always let the patients know that you discard drugs entirely until they become intelligent on the subject. You often place yourself in positions where you hurt your influence and do no one any good, by expressing all your convictions. Thus you cut yourself away from the people. You should modify your strong prejudice.

I cannot speak as fully on this subject as I would like to, but let me say, "Hide Peter Wessels in Christ." Here I must leave you; for I have not time to write more.

DEAR BROTHER WESSELS,

February 16, 1890
(L.B. #00, P. 255 File W. 35 1890)
Battle Creek, Michigan {28}

I SHALL HAVE TO APOLOGIZE for delaying to answer your letter. It seemed to be my duty to attend the ministerial institute, and to speak to the brethren assembled there. Then I am under the necessity of keeping four workers busy on different kinds of books. This with my much letter writing seems to keep me employed from three o'clock A.M. till seven o'clock P.M. I deeply sympathize with you, my brother, in your perplexities and trials. As to praying for the sick, it is too important a matter to be handled carelessly. I believe we should take everything to the Lord, and make known to God all our weaknesses, and specify all our perplexities. When in sorrow, when uncertain as to what course to pursue, two or three who are accustomed to pray should unite together in asking the Lord to let His light shine upon them, and to impart His special grace; and He will respect their petitions, He will answer their prayers. If we are under infirmities of body it is certainly consistent to trust in the Lord, making supplications to our God in our own case, and if we feel inclined to ask others in whom we have confidence, to unite with us in prayer to Jesus who is the mighty Healer, help will surely come if we ask in faith. I think we are altogether too faithless, too cold and lukewarm.

I understand the text in James is to be carried out when a person is sick upon his bed; if he calls for the elders of the church, and they carry out the directions in James, anointing the sick with oil, in the name of the Lord, praying over him the prayer of faith. We read, "The prayer of faith shall save the sick, and the Lord shall raise him up; and if he hath committed sins, they shall be forgiven him." It cannot be our duty to call for the elders of the church for every little ailment we have, for this would be putting a task upon the elders. If all should do this, their time would be fully employed,—they could do nothing else; but the Lord gives us the privilege of seeking Him individually in earnest prayer, of unburdening our souls to Him, keeping nothing from Him who has invited us, "Come unto me, all ye who are weary and heavy laden, and I will give you rest." O how grateful we should be that Jesus is willing and able to bear all our infirmities and strengthen and heal all our diseases if it will be for our good and for His glory. Some died in the days of Christ and in the days of the apostles because the Lord knew just what was best for them. I would not speak one word to lessen your faith and perplex and worry you. There is never danger of our being too much in earnest and having too much confidence and trust in God. Be of good courage; look to Jesus constantly.

Now in regard to that which we can do for ourselves. There is a point that requires careful, thoughtful consideration. I must become acquainted with myself, I must be a learner always as to how to take care of this building, the body God has given me, that I may preserve it in the very best condition of health. I must eat those things which will be for my very best good physically, and I must take special care to have my clothing such as will conduce to a healthful circulation of the blood. I must not deprive myself of exercise and air. I must get all the sunlight that it is possible for me to obtain. I must have wisdom to be a faithful guardian of my body. I should do a very unwise thing to enter a cool room when in a perspiration; I should show myself an unwise steward to allow myself to sit in a draught, {29} and thus expose myself so as to take cold. I should be unwise to sit with cold feet and limbs and thus drive back the blood from the extremities to the brain or internal organs. I should always protect my feet in damp weather. I should eat regularly of the most healthful food which will make the best quality of blood, and I should not work intemperately if it is in my power to avoid doing so. And when I violate the laws God has established in my being, I am to repent and reform, and place myself in the most favorable condition under the doctors God has provided,—pure air, pure water, and the healing, precious sunlight. Water can be used in many ways to relieve suffering. Draughts of clear, hot water, taken before eating (half a quart, more or less), will never do any harm, but will rather be productive of good. A cup of tea made from catnip herb will quiet the nerves. Hop tea will induce sleep. Hop poultices over the stomach will relieve pain. If the eyes are weak, if there is pain in the eyes, or inflammation, soft flannel clothes wet in hot water and salt, will bring relief quickly. When the head is congested, if the feet and limbs are put in a bath with a little mustard, relief will be obtained. There are many more simple remedies which will do much to restore healthful action to the body. All these simple preparations the Lord expects us to use for ourselves, but man's extremities are God's opportunities. If we neglect to do that which is within the reach of nearly every family, and ask the Lord to relieve pain, when we are too indolent to make use of these remedies within our power, it is simply presumption. The Lord expects us to work in order that we obtain food. He does not propose that we shall gather the harvest unless we break the sod, till the soil, and cultivate the produce. Then God sends the rain and the sunshine and the clouds to cause vegetation to flourish. God works and man cooperates with God. Then there is seed time and harvest. God has caused to grow out of the ground, herbs for the use of man, and if we understand the nature of those roots and herbs, and make a right use of them, there would not be a necessity of running for the doctor, so frequently, and people would be in much better health than they are today. I believe in calling upon the Great Physician when we have used the remedies I have mentioned. In regard to manner of labor, we certainly need to be wise as serpents and harmless as doves. We might be very zealous, but it might be an unwise zeal, and serve to hedge up our way. Then there is danger of being so circumscribed in our work as to do very little good.

EXTRACT FROM MANUSCRIPT

October 22, 1907
(Ms. 115 1907)

THE GREAT REASON WE HAVE sanitariums is that these institutions may be agencies in bringing men and women to a position where they may be numbered among those who shall someday eat of the leaves of the tree of life, which are for the healing of the nations.

"And there shall be no more curse; but the throne of God and of the Lamb shall be in it; and His servants shall serve Him."

Our sanitariums are established as institutions where patients and helpers may serve God. We desire to encourage as many as possible to act their part individually in living healthfully. We desire to encourage the sick to discard the use of drugs, and to substitute the simple remedies {30} provided by God, as they are found in water, in pure air, in exercise, and in general hygiene.

Some have asked me, "Why should we have sanitariums? Why should we not, like Christ, pray for the sick, that they may be healed miraculously?"

I have answered, "Suppose we were able to do this in all cases: how many would appreciate the healing? Would those who were healed become health reformers, or continue to be health destroyers?"

Jesus Christ is the great healer, but He desires that by living in conformity with His laws, we may co-operate with Him in the recovery and the maintenance of health. Combined with the work of healing there must be an imparting of knowledge of how to resist temptation. Those who came to our sanitariums should be aroused to a sense of their own responsibility to work in harmony with the God of truth.

We cannot heal. We cannot change the diseased condition of the body. But it is our part, as medical missionaries, as workers together with God, to use the means that He has provided. Then we should pray that God will bless these agencies. We do believe in God; we believe in a God who hears and answers prayer. He has said, "Ask, and ye shall receive, seek, and ye shall find; knock, and it shall be opened unto you."

EXTRACT FROM MANUSCRIPT

MS. 29, 1911

ANY MAN, BE HE MINISTER or layman, who seeks to compel or control the reason of any other man, becomes an agent of Satan, to do his work, and in the sight of the heavenly universe he bears the mark of Cain.

The Wage Question.—Those engaged in the Master's service are not to wait for a stipulated sum as their wages, as if the great Husbandman-householder would not deal truly with them. Murmurers will obtain no sympathy for their murmuring. A grumbling worker will always find something to grumble at; it is his heart that needs to be changed.

The parable of the householder's dealing with the workers in his vineyard represents God's dealing with the human family. Had the hearts of the first laborers been purified from selfishness, they would have recognized the liberality of the householder in paying those who came at the eleventh hour, the same wages as he paid them who came at an earlier period.

In the parable, the first laborers agreed to work for a stipulated sum, and they received the amount specified, nothing more. Those later hired believed the Master's promise, "Whatsoever is right, that shall ye receive." They showed their confidence in him by asking no question in regard to wages. They trusted his justice and equity. They were rewarded, not according to the amount of their labor, but according to the generosity of his purpose.

So God desires us to trust in him who justifieth the ungodly. He does not deal with his servants after the manner of the world. The standard of men received no recognition. {31}

Those who are ever watching for something to find fault with in their brethren and sisters, show that they have no conception of God's manner of dealing. The spirit of fault-finding and complaining is the spirit of the elder brother, but it finds a place in the hearts of many who rank as followers of Christ. The murmurer may be first in enduring hardships and in bearing burdens, but his unchristlike spirit spoils his service.

EXTRACT FROM LETTER

August 29, 1898
(Letter B. 69 1898) ▪

AS TO DRUGS BEING USED in our institutions, it is contrary to the light which the Lord has been pleased to give. The drugging business has done more harm to our world and killed more than it has helped or cured. The light was first given to me why institutions should be established, that is, sanitariums were to reform the medical practices of physicians. This is God's method. The herbs that grow for the benefit of man, and the little handful of herbs kept and steeped for sudden ailments, have served tenfold, yes, one hundred-fold better purpose, than all the drugs hidden under mysterious names and dealt out to the sick. It is a delusion and farce, and the Lord has revealed to me that this practice would not preserve life, but would introduce into the system those things which should never be there, for they would do a deleterious work on the human organism.

The living connection with the Great Physician is worth more than connection with a world of drugs. The soothing power of pure truth, seen, and maintained in all its bearings, is of a value no language can express, to people who are suffering with disease.

Keep ever before the suffering sick the compassion and tenderness of Christ, and awaken their conscience to a belief in His power to relieve suffering, and lead them to faith and trust in Him, the great Healer, and you have gained a soul and ofttimes a life.

Therefore, personal religion for all physicians in the sickroom is essential to success in giving the simple treatments without drugs. He who is a physician and guardian of the health and body, God would have every way educated to learn lessons of the Great Teacher, how to work in Christ and through Christ to save the souls of the sick. How can any physician know this until the Saviour shall be received as a personal Saviour to him who administers to suffering humanity?

Religion should be made prominent in a most tender, sympathetic, compassionate way. No one of all the parties with whom he is acquainted can do as much for the sick one as a truly converted nurse and physician. Actions of purity, refinement in looks and words, and above all the sweet words of prayer, though few, yet if sincere, will be a sure anchor to the suffering ones.

Of all men, the physician should be the most earnest, and sincere, full of faith and of the Holy Spirit, and then he can accomplish more than the minister in the pulpit. {32}

EXTRACT FROM LETTER

October 9, 1902
(Letter K. 159 1902)

OUR FAITH IN ETERNAL realities is weak, our sense of duty small, in view of the opportunities that we have to point souls to the Saviour as their only hope. We are not to be cold and indifferent in regard to giving efficacious remedies for the healing of the soul. It is our duty to make known the truth, not in our own strength, but in the strong faith, assurance and confidence that God imparts.

In our sanitariums no day should be allowed to pass without something being done for the salvation of souls. We are to offer special prayers for the sick, both when with them and when away from them. Then when they inquire about the remedy for sin, our own souls, softened by the Holy Spirit, will be all aglow with a desire to help them give their hearts to God.

All the nurses and helpers are to give treatments and perform other kinds of service in such a delicate, reverential way, and withal so solidly, thoroughly, and cheerfully, that the Sanitarium will prove a haven of rest.

The individual worker in any line in the treatment of the sick and the afflicted in a medical institution, is to act as a Christian. He is to let his light shine forth in good works. His words are to magnify our Lord Jesus Christ. In the place of waiting for great opportunities to come before doing anything, he is to make the very best use of the talents lent him of God, in order that these talents may be constantly increased. He is not to think that he must be silent on religious subjects.

It is highly important to know how to approach the sick with the comfort of a hope gained through faith in Christ Jesus and acceptance of His promises. When the awakened conscience cries out, "Lord, be merciful to me a sinner; make me thy child," be ready to tell the sufferer, the once indifferent one, that there is hope for him, that in Jesus he will find a refuge.

The Saviour is inviting everyone, "Look unto Me, and live. Come unto Me, and find rest." Those who in meekness and in love present the hope of the gospel to afflicted souls so much in need of this hope, are the mouthpiece of the One who gave Himself for all mankind, that He might become a healer, a tender, sympathetic, compassionate Saviour.

Let every means be devised to bring out the saving of souls in our medical institutions. This is our work. If the spiritual work is left undone, there is no necessity of calling upon our people to build these institutions. Those who have no burning desire to save souls are not the ones who should connect with our sanitariums.

DR. DAVID PAULSON AND ELDER W. S. SADLER

June 14, 1906
(June 14, 1906 -8- B.172—1906)
Sanitarium, California

Dear Brethren:

IHAVE BEEN WORKING HARD, and am weary, and yet I will not give up, for {33} there is much to do. During the dedication of the Loma Linda Sanitarium, I spoke for a short time on the open platform on the lawn, while the wind was blowing. The exercises were very impressive. We also had an excellent meeting at the dedication of the Paradise Valley Sanitarium.

I am glad that these sanitarium properties have come into the possession of our brethren and sisters in the Southern California Conference. For years we have worked at a disadvantage; but now I am so thankful that in the providence of God many facilities have been placed within our reach, and we can encourage our brethren in Southern California to awake to their opportunities. Everyone in that field should be grateful to God; for He has wrought for us in a remarkable manner.

The Sanitarium at Loma Linda, is in need of larger quarters for their treatment-rooms. An addition for this purpose will be built this summer. The Paradise Valley Sanitarium has added a large wing to the main building, and is now provided with excellent treatment-rooms. The second story of the new part is finished for the accommodation of patients, but the third story is not yet finished. However, both institutions are in running order, and are making good use of the facilities they have.

Through circumstances that I could not well control, I have been suffering for some time from the weariness of constant anxiety. I am sensible to the fact that I am mortal, and that I must guard my physical mental and moral powers. The constant changing from place to place necessitated by travel, and the taking hold of public labor wherever I have gone, have been too much for me, in addition to the writings that I have been preparing day and night as the Lord has worked my mind by His Holy Spirit. And when I am meeting with evidences that these communications will be treated by some in accordance with the human judgment of those who shall receive them; when I realize that some are watching keenly for some words which have been traced by my pen and upon which they can place their human interpretations in order to sustain their positions and to justify a wrong course of action,— when I think of these things, it is not very encouraging to continue writing. Some of those who are certainly reproved, strive to make every word vindicate their own statements. The twistings and connivings and misrepresentations of the Word, are marvelous. Persons are linked together in this work. What one does not think of, another mind supplies.

When the true converting power comes home to us as human agents, we see a power in God's plans, and embrace the evidence of the divine remedy for sin. "If I walk in the light, as He is in the light, we have fellowship one with another, and the blood of Jesus Christ His Son cleanseth us from all sin." I can rely wholly and unmistakably upon the sure Word of prophecy.

I am now carrying a very heavy burden for those who are lost in the mysteries of false science. I have had physical suffering of the heart; therefore I could not quickly answer the questions that you and Elder Sadler have presented to me. A severe cold has been upon me ever since the Loma Linda meeting. I assure you it is not because I do not respect you, Brethren Paulson and Sadler, that I do not answer your questions now. Pray for me, and I will pray for you; and as soon as I can, I will clear {34}up, if possible, the misunderstandings regarding the work God has given me to do. Certainly a very great work is before us. I must now watch and pray and wait.

"And every man that hath this hope in him purifieth himself, even as He is pure."

EXTRACT FROM LETTER
January 19, 1904
(Letter F. 35, 1904)

THE LORD HAS GREATLY HELPED me healthwise. Difficulties that I have had for twenty-five years have been removed. I have used no medicine, but for hours during the night season, when I was unable to sleep, I prayed for the healing power of God. I asked the Lord to restore my eyesight, to strengthen my heart, and to relieve the spinal difficulty. I have improved wonderfully. My health is better this winter than it has been for many years. The Great Physician has wrought in my behalf, and I praise His holy name.

FROM DOCUMENT FILE
January 8, 1904
(File No. 111)

MANY ACT AS IF HEALTH and disease were things entirely independent of their conduct, and entirely outside their control. They do not reason from cause to effect, and submit to feebleness and disease as a necessity. Violent attacks of sickness they believe to be special dispensations of Providence, or the result of some overruling, mastering power; and they resort to drugs as a cure for the evil. But the drugs taken to cure the disease weaken the system. If those who are sick would exercise their muscles daily, women as well as men, in outdoor work, using brain, bone, and muscle proportionately, weakness and languor would disappear. Health would take the place of disease, and strength the place of feebleness.

FROM MANUSCRIPT 83
June 25, 1908

I WISH TO MAKE SOME statements regarding our sanitariums which I hope will not be misunderstood. The light given me is that where a sanitarium is established, there should also be a school. This can be placed near enough to the sanitarium so that the medical teachers can meet often with the students, yet it should not be so near that there will be danger of the students disturbing the patients or patrons of the health institution being a means of hindrance to the students.

Education includes the important work of voice culture. The students are to be taught to give their reading and recitations

such expression as will make their work interesting to the hearers. They are to be taught how to use the abdominal muscles in speaking, and this study will prove to be a remedy for many voice and chest difficulties, and the means of prolonging life.

Let the same lessons be given to the patients. The physician should {35} teach the patient how to breathe deeply, and this in many cases will be found to be a means of healing.

Those who desire to become missionaries are to hear instruction from competent physicians, who will teach them how to care for the sick without the use of drugs. Such lessons will be of the highest value to those who go out to labor in foreign countries. And the simple remedies used will save many lives.

DRUGS
1908
(MS No. 49, 1908)
"Lessons from the Experience of Pentecost"

IN OUR SANITARIUMS, we advocate the use of simple remedies. We discourage the use of drugs, for they poison the current of the blood. In these institutions sensible instruction should be given, how to eat, how to drink, how to dress, and how to live so that the health may be preserved.

Before there were any sanitariums amongst us, my husband and I began work in medical missionary lines. We would bring to our house cases that had been given up by the physicians to die. When we knew not what to do for them, we would pray to God most earnestly and He always sent His blessing. He is the mighty Healer, and He worked with us. We never had time or opportunity to take a medical course, but we had success as we moved out in the fear of God, and sought Him for wisdom at every step. This gave us courage in the Lord.

Thus we combined prayer and labor. We used the simple water treatments, and then tried to fasten the eyes of the patient onto the great Healer. We told them what He could do for them. If we can inspire the patients with hope, this is greatly to their advantage. We want all that have any part to act in our sanitariums to have a firm grasp on the power of the Infinite. We believe in Him and in the power of His word. When we do our best for the recovery of the sick, we may then look for Him to be with us, that we may see of His salvation.

We put too little confidence in the power of the hand that rules the world.

EXTRACT FROM LETTER

March 24, 1908
(Letter B.90 1908)

I HAVE BEEN SHOWN that we should have many more women who can deal especially with the diseases of women, many more lady nurses who will treat the sick in a simple way and without the use of drugs.

There are many simple herbs which, if our nurses would learn the value of, they could use in the place of drugs, and find very effective. Many times I have been applied to for advice as to what should be done in cases of sickness or accident, and I have mentioned some of these simple remedies, and they have proved helpful. {36}

On one such occasion a physician came to me in great distress. He had been called to attend a young woman who was dangerously ill. She had contracted fever while on the campground, and was taken to our school building, near Melbourne, Australia. But she became so much worse that it was feared she could not live.

The physician, Dr. Merritt Kellogg, came to me and said, "Sister White, have you any light for me on this case? If relief cannot be given our sister, she can live but a few hours."

I replied, "Send to a blacksmith shop, and get some pulverized charcoal, make a poultice of it, and lay it over her stomach and sides."

The doctor hastened away to follow out my instructions. Soon he returned, saying, "Relief came in less than half an hour after the application of the poultices. She is now having the first natural sleep she has had for days."

I have ordered the same treatment for others who were suffering great pain, and it has brought relief, and been the means of saving life.

My mother told me that snake bites and the sting of reptiles and poisonous insects could often be rendered harmless by the use of charcoal poultices.

When working on the land at Avondale, Australia, the workmen would often bruise their hands and limbs, and this in many cases resulted in such severe inflammation that the worker would have to leave his work for some time. One came to me one day in this condition, with his hand tied in a sling. He was much troubled over the circumstance; for his help was needed in clearing the land. I said to him, "Go to the place where you have been burning the timber, and get me some charcoal from the eucalyptus tree, pulverize it, and I will dress your hand." This was done, and the next morning he reported that the pain was gone. Soon he was ready to return to his work.

I write these things that you may know that the Lord has not left us without the use of simple remedies which when used, will not leave the system in the weakened condition in which the use of drugs so often leaves it. We need well-trained nurses who can understand how to use the simple remedies that nature provides for restoration to health, and who can teach those who are ignorant of the laws of health how to use these simple but effective cures.

EXTRACT FROM LETTER

February 20, 1908
Letter B.82

T HIS BLENDING OF OUR SCHOOLS and sanitariums will prove an advantage in many ways. Through the instruction given by the sanitarium, students will learn how to avoid forming careless, intemperate habits of eating. Let the instruction be given in simple words. We have no need to use the many expressions used by worldly physicians, which are so difficult to understand that they must be interpreted by the physician. These long names are often used to conceal the character of the drugs being used to combat disease. We do not need these. {37}

Nature's simple remedies will aid in recovery without leaving the deadly after-effects so often felt by those who use poisonous drugs. They destroy the power of the patient to help himself. This power the patients are to be taught to exercise by learning to eat simple, healthful foods, by refusing to overload the stomach with a variety of foods at one meal. All these things should be given showing how to preserve health, how to shun sickness, how to rest when rest is needed.

There are many inventions which cost large sums of money, which it is just as well should not come into our work. They are not what our students need. Let the education given be simple in its nature. In giving us His Son the Father gave the most costly gift that heaven could bestow. This gift it is our privilege to use in our ministration to the sick. Let Christ be your dependence. Commit every case to the great Healer; let Him guide in every operation. The prayer offered in sincerity and in faith will be heard. This will give confidence to the physicians and courage to the sufferer.

I have been instructed that we should lead the sick in our institutions to expect large things because of the faith of the physician in the great Healer who, in the years of His earthly ministry, went through the towns and villages of the land, and healed all who came to Him. None were turned empty away; He healed them all. Let the sick realize that, although unseen, Christ is present to bring relief and healing.

FROM LETTER

May 25, 1903
Letter K. 100 1903

B E SURE THAT THE ORCHARD has some means expended on it. It will respond to treatment. Give it the care that will enable it to do its best. I look upon that orchard as of great value to the institution.

Do all that you possibly can to perfect the institution inside and out. Be sure that your premises are in the best of order. Let there be nothing about them that will make a disagreeable impression on the minds of the patients.

Encourage the patients to live healthfully and to take an abundance of exercise. This will do much to restore them to health. Let seats be placed under the shade of the trees, that the patients may be encouraged to spend much time out-of-doors. And a place should be provided, enclosed either with canvas or with glass, where, in cooler weather, the patients can sit in the sun without feeling the wind.

Obtain the best help in the cooking that you can. If food is prepared in such a way that it is a tax on the digestive organs, be sure that investigation is needed. Food can be prepared in such a way as to be both wholesome and palatable.

Fresh air and sunshine, cheerfulness within and without the institution, pleasant words and kindly acts,—these are the remedies that the sick need, and God will crown with success your efforts {38} to provide these remedies for the sick ones who come to the sanitarium. By happiness and cheerfulness and expressions of sympathy and hopefulness for others, your own soul will be filled with light and peace. And never forget that the sunshine of God's blessing is worth everything to us.

Teach nurses and patients the value of those health-restoring agencies that are freely provided by God, and the usefulness of simple things that are easily obtained.

I will tell you a little about my own experience with charcoal as a remedy. For some forms of indigestion it is more efficacious than drugs. A little olive oil into which some of this powder has been stirred tends to cleanse and heal. I find it is excellent. Pulverized charcoal from eucalyptus wood, we have used freely in cases of inflammation...

When we first went to Cooranbong, the men who were clearing in the woods often came in with bruised hands. In these and other cases of inflammation, I advised the trial of a compress of pulverized charcoal. Sometimes the inflammation, which was very high before the compress was applied, would be gone by the next day.

Always study and teach the use of the simplest remedies, and the special blessing of the Lord may be expected to follow the use of these means which are within the reach of the common people...

Do not forget that a worker must not take upon himself so many burdens that his soul will become weary. His first and greatest care should be to keep fresh and fragrant in spirit. In the unfolding of God's plan, we are to be restored to a state corresponding to the perfection of divinity.

FROM DOCUMENT NO. 111

September 4, 1902
(Document File No. 111)
Long Courses of Study

QUESTIONS HAVE ARISEN in regard to the management of sanitariums, and in regard to the plans to be followed in the education of physicians and nurses. We are asked whether a few or many should take a five years' course.

All are to be left perfectly free to follow the dictates of an enlightened conscience. There are those who with a few months' instruction would be prepared to go out and do acceptable medical missionary work. Some cannot feel that it is their duty to give years to one line of study.

Nurses not to be restricted

After the nurses have served the term agreed upon, and have given their services in return for their education, they should be at liberty to take up work where they wish, and to earn what they can. Some may not have been able to save any money while getting their education. Their board

and clothing, with the gifts they have made to the cause of God, may have taken all their earnings. Then if they are taken sick, they have no money to fall back on, and they are helped by the sanitarium as cases of charity. {39}

This is a species of slavery to which some will conscientiously submit, while others will backslide from the truth.

The young men and women who take their medical course of the nurses' course, should not be taught that after their graduation they will ever after be amenable to the association under which they received their education. When nurses go to patients not in the sanitarium, they should not be required to return to the sanitarium all that they earn, except just enough to cover the cost of food and clothing.

There is much to be considered in regard to this matter. From the light I have, I know that these things are not properly adjusted. The nurses give their services in return for the education that they receive. They are not always to be required to pay a portion of their wages to the sanitarium. This is not just.

And when their term of service has expired, the nurses should be left free to work where they please, and to recognize that they are accountable only to God for the use they make of the money they earn. They are not to be required to pay to the sanitarium at which they received their training, a certain part of their earnings. They are to be left free as those who have settled their indebtedness, and are now at liberty to use their earnings as God directs.

Perhaps they have brothers and sisters who need an education in our schools. Perhaps their parents need what they can spare from their earnings. Their duty to their parents comes first. There has been suffering in families for want of the means that nurses have given in donations to our sanitariums. This very money was needed by their parents.

A reformation is needed on this point, for justice has not been done. A hold is not to be retained on the nurses educated in our sanitariums, as if they had sold themselves to the institution for life. This matter has been presented to me as something that needs to be set right.

How much depression and anxiety has been the result of this unwise business arrangement will never be known until the cases of all are seen as they really are. Many of the arrangements made in the name of medical missionary work, need

adjusting by the wisdom of a Physician that is above all human physicians. Men need to understand that equity and justice and mercy are the attributes of the Most High. In no case will the Lord be pleased with a course such as has been followed in dealing with those who are anxious to obtain a knowledge in the treatment of the sick. These nurses and helpers rendered faithful service, but have not received an equivalent.

Practical Instruction to be Given

Great care should be exercised in the training of young people for the medical missionary work; for the mind is molded by that which it receives and retains. Too much incomplete work has been done in the education given. The most useful education is that found in practical work.

Our institutions are not to be so overgrown that the most important {40} points in education do not receive the proper consideration. Instruction should be given in medical missionary work. The teaching given in medical lines should be blended with a study of the Bible. And physical training should not be neglected.

Great care should be exercised in regard to the influences that prevail in the institution. The influences under which the nurses are placed will mold their characters for eternity...

Simplicity in Diet and Treatments

It would have been better if, from the first, all drugs had been kept out our sanitariums, and use had been made of such simple remedies as are found in pure water, pure air, sunlight, and some of the simple herbs growing in the field. These would be just as efficacious as the drugs used under mysterious names and concocted by human science. And they would leave no injurious effects in the system.

Thousands who are afflicted might recover their health if, instead of depending upon the drug-store for their life, they would discard all drugs and live simply, without using tea, coffee, liquor, or spices, which irritate the stomach and leave it weak, unable to digest even simple food without stimulation. The Lord is willing to let His light shine forth in clear, distinct rays to all who are weak and feeble.

Vegetables, fruits, and grains should compose our diet. Not an ounce of flesh-meat should enter our stomachs. The eating of flesh is unnatural. We are to return to God's original purpose in the creation of man.

EXTRACTS FROM LETTER

February 2, 1905
(Letter B. 53 1905)

IF ONLY OUR SOULS WILL be converted from the error of their ways, and seek the Lord, and learn the science of preserving the health of the body and the soul! And where can they learn these much-needed lessons as well as at our sanitarium, which the Lord has said should be established in many places? Lectures might be given to the multitudes, but while the words spoken would enlighten many minds, how can people understand fully without a practical knowledge? One patient, successfully treated, will have a testimony to bear of the virtue of the simple methods of treatment, the simple, healthful remedies that nature has provided, without the use of drugs.

When Christ was upon this earth, He did not direct fisherman to leave their nets and boats, and go to the Jewish teachers to gain a preparation for the gospel ministry. Walking by the Sea of Galilee, He saw "two brothers, Simon, called Peter, and Andrew his brother, casting a net into the sea; for they were fishers. And He said unto them, Follow Me, and I will make you fishers of men. And they straightway left their nets, and followed Him. And going on from thence, He saw two other brethren, James the son of Zebedee, and John his brother, in a ship with Zebedee their father, mending their nets; and He called them. And they immediately left the ship, and their father, and followed Him." {41} This prompt obedience, without any question, without one promise of wages, seems remarkable. But the words of Christ were an invitation that implied all that He meant it should. There was an impelling influence in His words. There was no long explanation, but what He said had a drawing power.

It was at the very beginning of His ministry that Christ began to gather in His helpers. This is a lesson to all ministers. They should constantly be looking for and training those who they think could help them in their work. They should not stand alone, trying to do by themselves all that needs to be done.

Christ would make these humble fishermen, in connection with Himself, the means of taking men out of the service of Satan, and making them believers in Christ; teaching them in regard to the kingdom of God. In this work they would be-come His ministers, fishers of men. They were to be His prime ministers. But He did not tell them to go to worldly schools to obtain the advantages of worldly cultivation. He did not tell them to go to the Jewish synagogues to learn of the rabbis, their customs and traditions, in order that they might be prepared for the work He had for them to do as His evangelists. He said, "Follow Me, and I will make you fishers of men."

FROM LETTER H.

February 23, 1904
(Letter H. 97, 1904)

DO YOU KNOW if any clover tops were gathered and dried for me in Battle Creek? If so, will you please send them to me?

EXTRACTS FROM LETTER K.

July 18, 1905
(Letter K. 203 1905)

WHEN AN OPPORTUNITY presents itself to purchase at a low price buildings in which our work may be carried on, let us take advantage of these opportunities. Had this been done by the leaders of the medical work in Battle Creek, there would now be many, many plants in our cities in America, cities that have not yet been enlightened by the truth upon health reform.

There should be sanitariums in all our large cities. Advantage should be taken of the opportunities to purchase buildings in favorable locations, that the standard of truth may be planted in many places.

Our sanitariums are to be schools in which instruction shall be given in medical missionary lines. They are to bring to sin-sick souls the leaves of the tree of life, which will restore to them peace and hope and faith in Christ Jesus. Forbid not those who have a desire to extend the work. Let the light shine forth. All worthy health productions will create an interest in health reform. Forbid them not. The Lord would have all opportunities to extend the work, taken advantage of. {42}

We shall have to labor under difficulties, but because of this let not our zeal flag. The Bible does not acknowledge a believer who is idle, however high his profession may be. There will be employment in heaven. The redeemed state is not one of idle repose. "There remaineth therefore a rest to the people of God, "But it is a rest found in loving service. Some among the redeemed will have laid hold of Christ in the last hours of life, and in heaven instruction will be given to these who, when they died, did not understand perfectly the plan of salvation. Christ will lead the redeemed ones beside the river of life, and will open to them that which while on this earth they could not understand.

DEAR BROTHER AND SISTER KRESS

July 16, 1910
(August 8, 1910 -6- K. 64)
Sanitarium, California

I HAVE RECEIVED AND READ your letters. I will say that I have not received light that your connection with the Sanitarium at Takoma Park should be broken. This connection may be a special advantage to you in your missionary work in the cities, and you may also be a help to the health institution in Washington. As the Lord's servant, set apart to the gospel ministry, you should be fully qualified to speak the truth, pointing sinners to the great Healer of both soul and body.

I have had no light that you should wholly disconnect from the Sanitarium. But it would not be consistent for you to act as head physician; for your work in the cities will lead to your absence from the institution a large part of the time. Your ministerial labor will not disqualify you for counseling with your brethren regarding the work of the institution, nor for doing the work of a physician in the Sanitarium while you are there.

You are both to be led and taught of God. If you individually seek Him daily, you will have the Holy Spirit's guidance. I can see that you greatly need divine wisdom to enable you to serve in two positions of responsibility,—as a skillful physician, and also as a preacher of the gospel. There must be a daily conversion in order to blend successfully the work for body and soul. I cannot tell you in detail just how this should be done, but I know that you can do an important work in the ministry of the Word, in instructing the souls for whom you labor to believe in Jesus Christ. Encourage the suffering ones to receive treatment from the great Physician, for the healing of both body and soul.

A sanitarium is a most favorable place in which to set forth convincing truths. I would that all our physicians might have a living connection with the great Chief Physician, that they might speak wisely to the suffering sick. Those who minister in our sanitariums need to be sanctified, that they may speak words in season, presenting Christ as the Healer of sin-sick souls, as well as of afflicted and diseased bodies. {43}

Not a poisonous drug should be used. When you have a case that does not respond to the use of simple remedies, take it to the Lord in prayer. Talk to Him as the only one who can help. Quote simple scripture with tenderness and faith. As Christ's chosen physicians, speak His words, sometimes to convince of sin, but always to inspire hope. When laboring for the patients, consider that their sensibilities must be awakened to the fact that Christ came to our world to save perishing souls.

I am pained that there are not more decided efforts put forth to win souls to a belief of the truth. I am pained at the indifference manifested in our institutions established for the care of the sick, by many who know the truth. Many who come to these institutions are ignorant of the great life and death question, and they need to be enlightened. But among those connected with our sanitariums there seems to be a lack of earnest seeking after God, that they may speak words that will exert an influence for the truth. This is a work too often left undone in our churches and in our health institutions. Those connected with these institutions should be representatives of Christ.

In your labors you are acting in Christ's stead. The mind must be kept open to receive impressions from Him. If you understand the gospel message, remember that you are accountable, if, when you come in contact with those who are unsaved, you do not represent the truth in its saving influence.

I am unable to describe to you the impression made upon my mind when I realize that many, even among our brethren who are teachers of the word, are not daily converted. Christ stands ready to impart wisdom and grace; but those in important positions of responsibility cannot guide others in the right paths unless they are converted daily. If they rely upon their own supposed wisdom, they will mislead others who look to them believing that these ministers understand the sacred work entrusted to them. Those who accept responsible charges need to be on their guard, and by humble prayer to be sanctified, refined, and purified. Unless they sense their true condition, and unless they become Christ-

like, they can never reveal the truth as it is in Jesus.

In the night seasons I seem to be addressing large congregations in the words:

"Cry aloud, spare not, lift up thy voice like trumpet, and show My people their transgressions, and the house of Jacob their sins. Yet they seek Me daily, and delight to know My ways, as a nation that did righteousness, and forsook not the ordinances of justice; they take delight in approaching to God."

The Lord has a decided work to be done now. We need ministers of the gospel who are true to the knowledge of the truth. Many fables of every character will be brought in as subjects of discussion. We must have good, sanctified, common sense in dealing with human minds. May the Lord sanctify our hearts and minds that we may lay hold upon the important work to be done. {44}

I am writing to my brethren most earnestly; for I cannot hold my peace. Night after night I am in agony. There is a world to be warned. The neglect to do work that should have been started in various lines many years ago has made the work much harder to plan for and to execute. May the Lord now give wisdom. If the workers make a complete consecration of soul, mind, and body, much may be accomplished.

I have read letters telling of the meetings held in New York City regarding the city work. As you see the magnitude of the work that needs to be done, you can better understand why I have felt so keenly the necessity of having our people arouse that they may sense the situation. May the Lord teach our ministers how to take up the great work that should interest every worker. I have more hope as I see that the situation is being sensed, and that our leading brethren seem determined to take hold of the work earnestly. I shall now feel more courage.

DEAR BROTHER CHAPMAN
November 29, 1898
(L.B. 18, P. 426 C-106)

WE WERE PLEASED TO RECEIVE word from you this week. Your letter was read to me by Willie. Every word of it was of interest.

This morning I sent you copies of the things I said to the people when in Rockhampton. I have a very deep interest in the church in that place. Why should I

feel an interest in them? Because the Lord has an interest in them, an interest much greater than it is possible for me to have. I am praying that the Lord will lead and guide you. I have spoken to the ear, but the Lord alone can speak to the heart. The Lord says, "As many as I love, I rebuke and chasten; be zealous, therefore, and repent." He would have every soul heed His counsel, which is given for their present and eternal good. Again He says: "I know thy works." When these works are not in harmony with the truth, they are against the truth. "Behold, I stand at the door and knock: if any man hear My voice and open the door, I will come in to him, and will sup with him, and he with Me. To him that overcometh will I grant to sit with Me in My throne, even as I also overcame and am set down with my Father in His throne. He that hath an ear, let him hear what the Spirit saith unto the churches."

The Lord is speaking to the church in Rockhampton. O that they would be doers of His word! My brethren and sisters, I call upon you in the name of Christ to hear the word of God and to practice it. Of the Israelites the apostle says, "The word preached did not profit them, not being mixed with faith in them that heard it." This opens before us the secret of this matter, the reason why there is so little accomplished by the many discourses that are preached. The words may be indited by the Holy Spirit, but the result lies with the ones who hear. The oft-repeated charge of the Lord in His word is, "He that hath an ear, let him hear."

It makes every difference whether the word spoken is received {45} into good and honest hearts. The Israelites had the word spoken to them by Jesus Christ from the pillar of cloud, but like many who hear the glad tidings of truth and righteousness in these last days, they did not hear with consecrated ears, and believe. Selfishness and pride, murmuring and unbelief compassed them about as with a garment. They aggravated their guilt by not hearing with faith, and practicing the word spoken.

It was faith that men lacked in the days of Noah, and it was this lack of living faith that brought destruction upon them. How different would have been the result had they heeded Noah's appeal as the voice of God speaking through him. But they were unwilling to hear and to receive the engrafted word which would have saved them. It is faith, an active faith, that will make the gracious promise of any avail.

Again the apostle speaks, "But as we

were allowed of God to be put in trust for the gospel, even so we speak; not as pleasing men, but God which trieth our hearts. For neither at any time used we flattering words, as ye know, nor a cloak of covetousness; God is witness, nor of men sought we glory, neither of you, nor yet of others, when we might have been burdensome, as the apostles of Christ. But we were gentle among you, even as a nurse cherisheth her children: so being affectionately desirous of you, we were willing to have imparted unto you, not the gospel of God only, but also our own souls, because ye were dear unto us. . . For what is our hope, or joy, or crown of rejoicing? Are not even ye in the presence of our Lord Jesus Christ at His coming? For ye are our glory and joy." (1 Thessalonians 2:4-8, 19-20)

We know and understand the deep poverty of many who are striving for the crown of life. We are not ignorant in regard to the deep working of Satan, which our brethren will have to encounter. Brethren, you must bear in mind that Satan is working with all deceivableness of unrighteousness in them that perish. He moves upon men to make it hard and trying for those who strive for the crown of life. He has come down with great power, working his will, carrying out his plans, that he may keep souls under his control.

I write to the church: Be not unbelieving, but have faith. Receive the message sent to you from God. He has sent you light, not because he would afflict you and cause you pain, but because He loves you and would have you escape from the snares of the enemy which would entangle your souls. Let the good work of purification go forward. Meet the standard the Lord has given you. My brethren in Rockhampton, who I love in the Lord, I feel an intense desire that Satan shall not triumph over you, but that you should think soberly and righteously and make thorough work for eternity. Read the third chapter of First Thessalonians. The apostle had a great burden for his brethren in Thessalonica. He writes, "For this cause, when I could no longer forbear, I sent to know your faith, lest by some means the tempter have tempted you, and our labor be in vain." (1 Thessalonians 3:5) {46}

When we read the letter from Brother Chapman, we praised the Lord. We felt somewhat as we supposed Paul felt when he wrote, "But now when Timotheus came from you unto us, and brought us good tidings of your faith and charity, and that ye have good remembrance of us always, greatly desiring to see us, as we also to see you, therefore, brethren, we were comforted over you in all our afflictions and distress by your faith: for now we live, if we stand fast in the Lord. For what thanks we render to God again for you, for all the joy wherewith we joy for your sakes before our God; night and day praying exceedingly that we might see your face, and might perfect that which is lacking in your faith...And the Lord make you to increase and abound in love one toward another and toward all men, even as we do toward you: to the end that He may establish your hearts unblamable in holiness before God, even our Father, at the coming of our Lord Jesus Christ with all His saints." (1 Thessalonians 3:6-10, 12-13)

The same spirit which moved the apostle to write to his brethren has moved me to write to the church in Rockhampton. I feel a tender solicitude for you that the Lord may do for you all that the apostle Paul so greatly desired should be done for his brethren in Thessalonica.

The apostle continues, "Furthermore, then, we beseech you brethren, and exhort you by the Lord Jesus, that as ye have received of us how ye ought to walk and to please God, so ye would abound more and more, for ye know what commandments we gave you by the Lord Jesus. For this is the will of God, even your sanctification, that ye should know how to possess his vessel in sanctification and honor...For God hath not called you unto uncleanness, but unto holiness. He therefore that despiseth, despiseth not man, but God, who hath also given unto us His Holy Spirit. But as touching brotherly love, ye need not that I write unto you: for ye yourselves are taught of God to love one another. And indeed ye do it toward all the brethren which are in all Macedonia: but we beseech you, brethren, that ye increase more and more; and that ye study to be quiet, and to do your own business, and to work with your own hands, as we commanded you; that ye may walk honestly toward them that are without and that ye have lack of nothing." (1 Thessalonians 4:1-4, 7-12)

We must keep the standard uplifted. God is not slack in the fulfillment of His promises. He is jealous for His name's glory. A whole heaven of resources are at His command. Seasons of prayer are essential. We all need to pray more, and to watch unto prayer. Read the first chapter of second Thessalonians. I present this entire chapter as appropriate for your case. I speak to you in love, for my heart is full of tender compassion in your behalf. You will have trial, but ever guard your soul, that you may not dishonor your Lord who has bought you with a price. He will that you should have strong faith and a lively hope. He wants you to improve in order and discipline and courage and fortitude and love for one another, that you may seek to help one another to keep the law of God, and be blessed. {47}

Brother Chapman, be of good courage in the Lord. Have faith. Place yourself in the hands of the great Physician, believing He will restore you to health. Do not doubt for a moment. Did not Christ come to the world as the One testified to in the prophecy of Isaiah?

"The Spirit of the Lord God is upon me; because the Lord hath anointed me to preach good tidings unto the meek; He hath sent Me to bind up the broken hearted, to proclaim liberty to the captives, and the opening of the prison to them that are bound; to proclaim the acceptable year of the Lord, and the day of vengeance of our God; to comfort all that mourn; to appoint unto them that mourn in Zion, to give unto them beauty for ashes, the oil of joy for mourning, the garment of praise for the spirit of heaviness; that they might be called trees of righteousness, the planting of the Lord, that He might be glorified." (Isaiah 61:1-3)

And the very One who gave this prophecy to Isaiah testified to his own work in Luke 4:16-18; therefore we are encouraged to hope largely and receive abundantly of His rich grace. We must come in faith. Take the Lord at His word. He is abundantly able and glad to respond to the faith of his believing ones.

Satan is the destroyer, the Lord is the Restorer.

The Lord has not worked a physician in the way that He desires to work, because He says, Ye will not come to Me, that I may give your life. We look to every source to relieve except to the One who proclaimed over the rent sepulcher of Joseph, "I am the resurrection and the life." (John 11:25) Christ came into our world to seek and to save that which was lost. His work as the one who heals all manner of diseases is unequalled. There are those whom the Lord uses as His co-laborers in the medical missionary work. These He is seeking to illuminate, that they may receive light and knowledge to communicate to others, and thus brighten the dark pathway of those who are oppressed by suffering and disease. If the sufferers would only come in faith to the divine Healer, they would see of the salvation of God.

But instead of co-operating with the mighty Healer, by using the very means He has provided, by educating themselves to use water and fresh air, and to avoid all uncleanness of person and premises, they turn to physicians who are in no way connected with the Lord Jesus, and take their prescriptions of drug medications. These leave their poisonous trail behind, implanting in the system seeds of suffering and death. Why do they not inquire of God? Why do they not seek help from the One who so loved them that He gave His only begotten Son to save all who would believe on Him? Is He not just as well able now to heal disease as when He walked in humanity upon the earth? Where is our faith when we turn to every conceivable resource but to the One who declares that He came to the world to do a special work in healing the sick. Why are not all who accept Christ so illuminated that they can irradiate others, and lift them from groveling in intemperance of all kinds, leading them to let drugs alone. {48}

Christ met one poor soul who had spent all her living in order that she might be cured of a physical malady. The statement is that she had spent all that she had on many physicians, and was nothing better, but rather made worse. But one touch of Christ by faith took away the infirmity of long years. This suffering woman came behind Christ, and touched His garment by faith in the person whom the garment covered, and instantly she was made whole. "Who touched Me," said Christ. Peter was astonished. He answered, "Thou seest the multitude thronging thee, and sayest thou, Who touched Me?"

Christ desired to give a lesson which all present would never forget. He would show the difference between the touch of living faith and a casual touch. He said, "Somebody hath touched Me; for I perceive that virtue hath gone out of Me." When the woman saw that she could not be hid, she came forward trembling, and throwing herself at His feet, told her pitiful story. Christ comforted her. "Daughter," He said, 'thy faith hath made thee whole; go in peace and be whole of thy plague."

Why do we not come to Jesus in faith? Many give Him a casual touch, coming in contact only with His person. The woman did more than this. She put forth her hand in faith, and was healed instantly.

The Lord will heal those who believe, but He has given natural blessings for the benefit of the afflicted, and He would have these used. God could have healed Hezekiah with a word. But He heard Hezekiah's prayer, and gave directions that a bunch of figs be placed upon the diseased parts. This was done, and Hezekiah recovered. But his recovery was not instantaneous. He had not the same faith that the afflicted woman had. We need to exercise faith. To practice the use of drug medication does not harmonize with faith. Appealing to worldly physicians is dishonoring to God. Those who come to God in faith must co-operate with Him in accepting and using His heaven-sent remedies,—water, sunlight, and plenty of air.

It is of no use to have seasons of prayer for the sick, while they refuse to use the simple remedies which God has provided, and which are close by them. If there is an unsanitary condition of things in the house and about the premises, the very first thing is to take up the work that has been neglected, and cleanse and purify the house and premises, making everything sweet, that the atmosphere may not be tainted by the least offensive smell.

The Lord gave certain directions to the children of Israel. They were to gather at the base of Mount Sinai, to hear the voice of God speaking the ten commandments. But first they were to wash their clothes. Again He commanded that no uncleanliness should be tolerated in the encampment, lest the Lord should pass by and see their uncleanness, and because of this refuse to go up with their armies to battle.

Some people ask God to preserve their families from all sickness and disease, while uncleanliness and untidiness are seen in the home, with the very things that create disease. Can God glorify His name by working a miracle to prevent the plague coming nigh the dwelling of those who do not care to act their part to prevent malaria and {49} fevers? The Lord does not work in this way. The human agent must act his part intelligently, keeping his body and his clothing clean, and every room in the house in order. Then the Lord can approach his dwelling. I will be honored, saith the Lord, by them that approach unto Me.

All who claim to love and serve God have a duty to perform. They are to keep themselves from all filthiness of the flesh and of the spirit, and perfect holiness in the fear of the Lord. It is the failure to do these things that makes the religion of those who profess to be Christians vain. Our God is too pure and holy to tolerate any disorder, any uncleanness. The individual who poisons his breath with tobacco is defiling the temple of God, and him will God destroy. The will of God must be done on earth. Ignorance in regard to these things is sin.

The friends of the truth will honor Him who is the Author and Finisher of their faith. Christ will prove Himself a physician in restoring the body as well as the soul. The workers together with God will yoke up with Christ, and place themselves, soul, body, and spirit, in right relation to God. Individuals and households will reveal the character of their faith by their dress, by their purity of speech, by their diligence in educating themselves and their children to be clean in the house, allowing no impurity in the home, no uncleanness on the premises, lest the Lord pass by and see their uncleanness. The Lord would have all things sweet about the home, that angels of God from the heavenly courts may be welcome guests, and not kept away by dirt and uncleanness.

The will of men, women, and children must be trained by cooperation with God. When they uplift themselves, the Lord will set them in desirable places. Then, by precept, and example, they can exert a refining, elevating influence upon their neighbors. The melody of spiritual joy and spiritual as well as physical health will be revealed, and will promote that blessedness which the Lord Jesus came to our world to impart to every individual who will believe. All may not be preachers, but all can minister, showing others how to be tidy and hopeful. This is like medicine to body and soul. Thus we may add grace to grace, and be all the time fitting ourselves for heaven. I send this that you may read it to the church.

THE CHICAGO WORK

March 20, 1906
(MS 33, 1906)
Sanitarium, California

DURING THE GENERAL MEETING held here in June 1902, I attended three meetings in the Sanitarium Chapel. I had a decided message to bear to the people. A heavy burden rested upon me to make a clear statement of the principles that should be followed in our medical missionary work. I was very thankful that Judge Arthur {50} was present to hear the message that the Lord had given me. I asked the Lord to help, and was assured of His presence.

On the third morning Judge Arthur came in a little late. After I had finished speaking, he rose and bore his testimony. He said that he had felt very tired that morning, and had told his wife that he would not attend the morning meeting. But afterward he felt impressed that he must attend, and he did. During his remarks, he said, "I could not rest till I had come to this meeting, and I am so thankful that I did not miss it. This message will be a great blessing to me. I have heard the very things I needed to hear." He bore an excellent testimony, and we were all very much pleased with the words spoken.

Shortly after the meetings closed, Judge Arthur and his wife spent part of a day at my home. We had much pleasant and profitable conversation. Among other things discussed was the matter of the representation that had been given me of an expensive building in the city of Chicago, used for various lines of medical missionary work. I related how that when I was in Australia, I was shown a large building in Chicago, which, in its erection and equipment, cost a large amount of money. And I was shown the error of investing means in any such buildings in our cities.

At the time that I saw this representation, scenes that would soon take place in Chicago, and other large cities also, passed before me. As wickedness increased, and the protecting power of God was withdrawn, there were destructive winds and tempests; buildings were destroyed by fire and shaken down by earthquakes. I saw the expensive building above referred to fall, with many others.

As I related some of these matters, and described the building that had been shown me, Judge Arthur said: "I can tell you something in regard to that building. A plan was drawn up for the erection of just such a building in Chicago. It seemed necessary to our work. It would have cost considerable money. Brother William Loughborough of Battle Creek, drew up the plans, and several men occupying responsible positions in the medical work met together to consider the matter. Various locations were considered. One of the plans discussed was very similar to what you have described."

Sometime after this, I was shown that the vision of buildings in Chicago and the draft upon the means of our people to erect them, and their destruction, was an object lesson for our people, warning them not to invest largely of their means in property in Chicago, or any other city, unless the providence of God should positively open the way and plainly point out duty to build or buy as necessary in giving the note of warning. A similar caution was given in regard to building in Los Angeles. Repeatedly I have been instructed that we must not invest means in the erection of expensive buildings in cities.

In a letter that I wrote to Dr. Kellogg, dated Oct. 28, 1903, I spoke of this matter as follows:}

"Repeatedly it has been shown me that in many cases you have worked upon minds to undermine confidence in the Testimonies. The evil leaven that you have placed in these {51} minds has destroyed their faith in the principles of the truth and in the Testimonies. Since the re-opening of the Sanitarium, you have placed this leaven in many minds, and it will do its work. One thing that can now be done to undo this work is for me to present to our people the Testimonies as they have been given me, that others may not go on undermining the faith of their associates. They must not be left to retain impressions that have been made on their minds, as, after receiving a Testimony of reproof from me, you have said, 'Somebody has told her these things, but they are not so.'

"Over and over again you have told others how I once sent you a testimony reproving you for erecting a large building in Chicago, before any such building had been erected there. In the visions of the night a view of a large building was presented to me. I thought that it had been erected, and wrote you immediately in regard to the matter. I learned afterward that the building which I saw had not been put up.

"When you received my letter, you were perplexed, and you said, 'someone has misinformed Sister White regarding our work.' But no mortal man had ever written to me or told me that this building had been put up. It was presented to me in vision. If this view had not been given me, and if I had not written to you about the matter, an effort would have been made to erect such a building in Chicago, a place in which the Lord has said that we are not to put up large buildings. At the time when the vision was given, influences were working for the erection of such a building. The message was received in time to prevent the development of the plans and the carrying out of the project.

"You should have had discernment to see that the Lord worked in this matter. The very feature of the message that perplexed you should have been received as an evidence that my information came from a higher source than human lips. But instead, you have over and over again related your version of the matter, saying that someone must have told me a falsehood."

When Dr. Paulson showed me the location that had been secured for sanitarium work at Hinsdale, I was thoroughly pleased; for this place answered to the representations that had been given me of places that would be obtained by our people for sanitarium work outside of the large cities. Time will show that such properties as this can be used to a far greater advantage than buildings in Chicago; for the wickedness of Chicago is as the wickedness of Sodom and Gomorrah. It was also represented to me that there were other places near Chicago, but away from the city, which the Lord would have His people secure. There are souls to be reached. The message must be proclaimed. This is the light that has been given to me. {52}

I have been given a representation of the preaching of the word of truth with clearness and power in many places where it has never been heard. The Lord would have the people warned; for a great work will be done in a short time. I have heard the word of God proclaimed in many localities outside the city of Chicago. There were many voices proclaiming the truth with great power. That which they proclaimed was not fanciful theories, but the warning message. While the solid truth of the Bible came from the lips of men who had no fanciful theories or misleading science to present, there were others who labored with all their power to bring in false theories regarding God and Christ. And miracles were wrought, to deceive, if possible, the very elect.

I heard the message proclaimed in power by men who had not been educated in Battle Creek. Among those who were engaged in the work, were young men taken from the plow and from the fields, and sent forth to preach the truth as it is in Jesus. Unquestioning faith in the Lord God of heaven was imparted to those who were called and chosen. "All this," said my Instructor, "is a parable of what should be and what will be."

For the present, some will be obliged to labor in Chicago; but these should be preparing working-centers in rural districts, from which to work the city. The Lord would have His people looking about them, and securing humble, inexpensive places as centers for their work. And from time to time, larger places will come to their notice, which they will be able to secure at a surprisingly low price.

(Signed) Ellen G. White

BASLE, SWITZERLAND
MS 15, 1886

IHAVE BEEN SHOWN THAT in times past men have made grievous mistakes. Some who have stood in positions of sacred trust have sullied their integrity. They have not, in their individual responsibility, stood in moral power before God. Those who were not worthy have been flattered while those who have stood fast for truth and for righteousness, because their ideas did not agree with those of their brethren have been denounced, discredited, and misjudged. Evil has been imagined against them.

Greatness without goodness, is valueless. It is as a tinkling symbol. The man who does not gather about him the rays of light that God has let shine upon his pathway will surely surround himself with the shadows of darkness. God designs that his people shall press closer and still closer to the light. Then they will go forward and upward.

"Light is sown for the righteous, and truth for the upright in heart." There is altogether too little searching, with painstaking effort, for the truth, as for hidden treasure. With hearts softened and subdued by the grace of God, the conscience quickened by habitual prayer and searching of the Scriptures, the whole soul may become familiar with heavenly truth. Such will stand firmly for the right because it is right. Pure and undefiled religion will be interwoven {53} with the life-practice. They will honor God, and God will honor them.

I have been shown that there is a fault with us. We honor and flatter human beings, accepting their ideas and their judgment as the voice of God. We advocate their cause. But they are not always safe to follow. Their judgment is erring.

God would have us ever refuse to plead against the truth. His frown is upon all that is false and unfair. This should be the po-

sition of everyone who stands to minister in the service of their Master. For if one to whom God has entrusted holy responsibilities allows envy, evil surmising, prejudice, and jealousies to find place in the heart, he is guilty of breaking the law of God. And his words, his ideas, and his errors will extend just as far as his sphere of influence extends. God says to every man to whom He entrusts responsibilities, "Put not your trust in man, neither make flesh your arm." Look to God. Trust in his infallible wisdom. Regard as a sin, the practice so common, even among Seventh-day Adventists, of becoming the echo of any man, however lofty his position. Listen to the voice of the great Shepherd, and you will never be led astray. Search the Scriptures for yourself, and be braced for duty and for trial by the truth of God's word. Let no friendship, no influence, no entreaty let not the smiles, the confidence, or the rewards of any man, induce you to swerve from the path in which the Lord would lead you. Let Christlike integrity and consistency control the actions of your life. The man who sits most at the feet of Jesus, and is taught by the Saviour's spirit, will be ready to cry out, "I am weak and unworthy, But Christ is my strength and my righteousness."

Godliness, sobriety, and consistency will characterized the life and example of every true Christian. The work which Christ is doing in the sanctuary above will engage the thoughts, and be the burden of the conversation, because by faith he has entered into the sanctuary. He is on earth, but his sympathies are in harmony with the work that Christ is doing in heaven. Christ is cleansing the heavenly sanctuary from the sins of the people, and it is the work of all who are laborers together with God to be cleansing the sanctuary of the soul from everything that is offensive to him. Everything like evil surmising, envy, jealousy, enmity, and hatred, will be put away; for such things grieve the Holy Spirit of God, and put Christ to an open shame. Love of self will not exist, nor will any engage in this work be puffed up. The example of Christ's life, the consistency of His character, will make his influence far-reaching. He will be a living epistle, known and read of all men.

"Finally, be ye all of one mind, having compassion one of another, love as brethren, be pitiful, be courteous: not rendering evil for evil, or railing for railing, but contrariwise, blessing; knowing that ye are thereunto called, that ye should inherit

a blessing. For he that will love life, and see good days, let him refrain his tongue from evil, and his lips that they speak no guile; let him eschew evil, and do good; let him seek peace, and ensue it. For the eyes of the Lord are over the righteous, and his ears are open unto their prayer but the face of the Lord is against them that do evil." (1 Peter 3:8-12) {54}

It is not safe for us to open our minds and hearts to envy and evil speaking. The fruits of God's Spirit are plainly specified, so that we need not entertain or cherish those attributes that proceed from the enemy of God and man. The false tongue beguiles the unwary, and makes an easy conquest of those who are not strengthened, stablished, and settled, having root in themselves. The atonement of Christ is to be the anchor of our hope, and the word of God a lamp to our feet, and a light to our path. Then our words will not be of self, but of Christ and of the all-essential work for this time.

With many there is but a very limited perusal of the Holy Scriptures. The truth is not dwelt upon, and the result is that it is not made the theme of conversation. It is made evident that Christ is not abiding in the heart. Our tongues should speak more of the matchless love of Jesus.

"If some of the branches were broken off, and thou, being a wild olive tree, wert grafted in among them, and with them partakest of the root and fatness of the olive tree; boast not thyself against the branches. But if thou boast, thou bearest not the root, but the root thee. Thou wilt say then, The branches were broken off, that I might be grafted in. Well; because of unbelief they were broken off, and thou standest by faith. Be not highminded, but fear: for if God spared not the natural branches, take heed lest he also spare not thee. Behold therefore the goodness and severity of God; on them which fell, severity; but toward thee, goodness: otherwise thou shalt also be cut off." (Romans 11:17-22)

The Lord has shown me that as a people we must have a purer morality. There is among us a flippant reproduction of arguments that are the product of other brains than ours, while the man who first uttered them has not spent hours of earnest study each day in order to know the truth. In his self-sufficiency he has turned away from the truth unto fables. He has not poured out before God his earnest prayer that he might know the hidden mysteries of God's word, that he might present to the people things new and old, which painstaking effort he has dug from the mine of truth.

Mysteries which have been hidden for ages are to be revealed in these last days to a humble people, who lean upon the arm of infinite power. Truth will be opened to the humble seeker, whose life is hid with Christ in God.

God calls upon his people to be Christians in thought, in word, in deed. Luther made the statement that religion is never so much in danger as among reverend men. I can say that many who handle the truth are not sanctified through the truth. They have not the faith that works by love, and purifies the soul. They become accustomed to handling sacred things, and because of this, many handle the word of God irreverently. They have not walked in the light, but have closed their eyes to light.

This is an age of signal rejection of the grace God has purposed to bestow upon his people, that in the perils of the last days they may {55} not be overcome by the prevailing iniquity, and unite with the hostility of the world against God's remnant people. Under the cloak of Christianity and sanctification, far-spreading and manifest ungodliness will prevail to a terrible degree, and will continue until Christ comes to be glorified in all them that believe. In the very courts of the temple scenes will be enacted that few realize. God's people will be proved and tested, that he may discern between him that serveth God, and him that serveth him not.

Vengeance will be executed against those who sit in the gate, deciding what the people should have, and what they should not have. These take away the key of knowledge. They refuse to enter in themselves, and those who would enter, they hinder. These bear not the seal of the living God. All who now occupy responsible positions should be solemnly and terribly afraid lest in this time they shall be found as unfaithful stewards.

Satan has come down with great power, knowing that his time is short. The continued apostasy, the abounding iniquity, which chills the faith and constancy of many, should call the faithful ones to the front. Straight, clear, decided testimonies, freighted with light for the time, will be given. Truth, undimmed by the furnace, will shine brighter and brighter until the perfect day. The Spirit and power of the coming One will be imparted in large measure to those who are preparing to stand in the day of God, who are hastening the sec-

ond advent of our Lord and Saviour Jesus Christ. To these faithful ones Christ gives special communications. He talks with them as he talked with his disciples before leaving them. The Spirit of truth will guide them into all truth. God has lines of communication with the world today. Through his appointed agencies, he speaks to the people he is purifying, warning and encouraging them.

There are those who listen with open ears and quickened understanding for the words of reproof and encouragement addressed to them. But Satan is ever on the alert to make these words of counsel of none effect. He seeks to close every avenue through which people receive truth. Unto those that have shall more be given, but from those that have not, shall be taken away, even that which they have. If the ears are dull of hearing, if the eyes are closed to the light which God flashes into the pathway, the light previously received is so mingled with supposition, uncertainty, and darkness, that light cannot be distinguished from darkness. There are those whom we have loved in the faith who have turned from it, and given heed to seducing spirits. "They went out from us, but they were not of us, for if they had been of us, they would no doubt have continued with us. But they went out, that they might be made manifest that they were not all of us. (1 John 2:19)

The love, the tender compassion, the marvelous condescension of Christ for his disciples is without a parallel. He made them the depositaries of sacred truth, as they could comprehend it. But He said to them, "I have many things to say unto you, but ye cannot bear them now." (John 16:12) Although Christ was with them, as their instructor, yet their former teaching had so molded their ideas and opinions that should Christ unfold the many things he longed to communicate, they would have misinterpreted his words. While {56} he was with them, He sought to impress upon them the knowledge there was for them in the mysteries of the kingdom of God. He would have them see that it was an evidence of his love for Him to lift the veil of the future, and make them the depositaries of knowledge concerning events to come. But much He had told them had been dimly comprehended, and much would be forgotten. He told them that after His crucifixion and ascension the Holy Spirit would open many things to them, and give them a better understanding of what He had tried

to tell them. He would still continue to reveal sacred truth to them, and His Spirit would more fully impart truth to them.

While Christ unfolded the iniquity and sorrow that must come to His disciples, the persecutions, and the trials they must bear, and the rejection of their testimony. He did not design that they should cloud their lives by looking on the dark side. He assured them that they would not be left alone, but be sustained by His Holy Spirit, which would guide them into all truth. "The Comforter, which is the Holy Ghost," He said, "whom the Father will send in My name he shall teach you all things, and bring all things to your remembrance, whatsoever I have said unto you." "I have yet many things to say unto you, but ye cannot bear them now. Howbeit when he, the Spirit of truth is come, he will guide you into all truth; for he will not speak of himself, but whatsoever he shall hear, that shall he speak; and he will show you things to come."

Here is a precious promise; the purposes and plans of God are to be opened to his disciples. What is a disciple?—A learner, ever learning. Coming events, of solemn character, are opening before us, and God would not have any one of us think that in these last days there is no more that we need to know. This is a continual snare of Satan. He would have us meet coming events without that special preparation which is essential to guide them through every difficulty. He would have all stumbling their way along in ignorance, making self-conceit, self-esteem, self-confidence, take the place of true knowledge. The more satisfied any one is with himself, and his present knowledge, the less earnestly and humbly will he seek to be guided into all truth. The less of the Holy Spirit of God he has, the more self-satisfied and complacent he will feel. He will not search earnestly and with the deepest interest to know more truth. But unless he keeps pace with the Leader, who is guiding into all truth, he will be left behind, belated, blinded, confused, because he is not walking in the light.

All who follow Christ will walk in the light as He is in the light. They will not then regard light with indifference, nor will they misapply the light, or stumble over it as did the Jews.

A spurious light will be accepted in the place of truth by some who feel called upon to be expositors of the Scriptures, because of their calling or position. Extravagance, dishonesty, fraud, licentiousness, is mingled with sacred things, until no difference is made between the sacred and the common. Many who claim to preach the word contemplate some portions of Scripture truth, but do not apply it to the heart and character. They expatiate upon the plan of redemption, and upon the law of God, and become enthusiastic upon some of these glorious themes, but they take no personal interest in the matter. Christ is not brought into their lives. Can we then be surprised to hear of ministers falling under temptation and sin, disgracing {57} the cause they were professedly advocating? Can we wonder that there are apostasies, when men who urge conversion upon others are not themselves converted; when they commend to others the love of Christ, which does not glow in their own souls, preaching repentance which they themselves have not practiced, and faith which they have no experimental knowledge of, telling of a Saviour whom they have never known except by rumor? They are self-deceived men, not far from destruction. Pitiful indeed is their situation. All may seem peaceful to them, because the palsy of death is upon them.

We are fully aware that dishonest men, immoral men, who preach the word, are not always reproved and warned. They are not unmasked. They learn to hold the truth in unrighteousness, and can tamper with it without a trembling heart and rebuke of conscience. O that with pen and voice we might lead the people who claim to be depositaries of sacred and eternal truth to feel the necessity of enthroning the word of God in their heart, and bringing every thought, word, and action into subjection to Jesus Christ. It is a fearful responsibility to be in daily connection with the truth of God, telling others of eternity, and yet be unsanctified through the truth.

It is not safe to place men in the position God should occupy; for men cannot be trusted. If they do not constantly live as in the presence of God, if they do not walk humbly before God and their brethren, they will diverge almost imperceptibly, and by slight degrees, from the straight line of God's work. Trusting to their own wisdom, they will deceive themselves and their fellow-men. Their ideas become so confused that they offer strange fire before the Lord.

The word of God is to be the man of our counsel. With pen and voice I proclaim to all who bear credentials, to all licenti-ates, to all colporteurs, and all canvassers, that the Bible, and the Bible only, studied on your knees, laid up in your heart, and practiced in your life, attended by the Holy Spirit's power, can be your safeguard. It alone can make you righteous and holy and keep you thus. Every human influence is weak and varying unless the truth of God's word is brought home to the soul, and placed upon the throne. Not till this is done, will the heart be sanctified, purified and made holy, a fountain out of which are the issues of life.

Discourses that have little of Christ and his righteousness in them are given in the desk. They are Christless sermons. To preach in the demonstration of the Spirit is completely beyond the power of those who are without Christ. They are feeble, empty, and without nourishment. They have no Christ to carry with them in private life. They are full of boasting, of pride, of self-esteem, speaking evil of things of which they have no real knowledge. They manifest an impatience of everything that does not follow in their line. They will even scoff and mock at sacred things, because they do not see that spiritual things are spiritually discerned. They degrade themselves by perverting and falsifying truth.

By his Holy Spirit, the Lord will demonstrate that his word is the only thing that can make men right and keep them right. I have been shown that God's revealed truth alone can keep men in the path of humble obedience. Standard bearers are falling round us, not only through death, but through the deceptions of Satan. All heaven is looking upon {58} the remnant people of God, to see if they will make truth alone their shield and buckler. Unless the truth is presented as it is in Jesus, and is planted in the heart by the power of the Spirit of God, even ministers will be found drifting away from Christ, away from piety, away from religious principle. They will become blind leaders of the blind.

Our faith cannot be vested in any man. We need Christ's righteousness. We need Jesus ever by our side. He is our Rock. It is by his might that we conquer, and by his righteousness that we are saved. When I see men exalted and praised, extolled as almost infallible, I know that there must come a terrible shaking. When God's lamp of life shines into the heart with clear and steady ray, darkness will instantly be dispelled. Every idol will be dethroned, and the peace of God which passeth all under-standing will reign in the heart. Truth, precious truth, will be seen, appreciated, and obeyed. The standard will be elevated, and many will rally round it.

(Signed) Ellen G. White

LESSONS FROM THE VISIONS OF EZEKIEL, PART ONE

July 4, 1906
Sanitarium, California {59}

Exhortation to Faithfulness

IN THE VISIONS OF THE NIGHT I seemed to be speaking with great earnestness before an assembly of people. A heavy burden was upon my soul. I was presenting before those gathered together the message of the prophet Ezekiel regarding the duties of the Lord's watchmen.

"Again the word of the Lord came unto me, saying, Son of man, speak to the children of thy people, and say unto them, When I bring the sword upon a land if the people of the land take a man of their coasts, and set him for their watchman; if when he seeth the sword come upon the land, he blow the trumpet and warn the people; then whosoever heareth the sound of the trumpet, and taketh not warning; if the sword come, and take him away, his blood shall be upon his own head. He heard the sound of the trumpet, and took not warning: his blood shall be upon him. But he that taketh warning shall deliver his soul. But if the watchman see the sword come and blow not the trumpet, and the people be not warned; if the sword come, and take any person from among them, he is taken away in his iniquity: but his blood will I require at the watchman's hand."

"So thou, O son of man, I have set thee a watchman unto the house of Israel; therefore thou shalt hear the word at my mouth, and warn them from me. When I say unto the wicked, O wicked man, thou shalt surely die; if thou dost not speak to warn the wicked from his way, that wicked man shall die in his iniquity, but his blood will I require at thine hand. Nevertheless, if thou warn the wicked of his way to turn from it; if he do not turn from his way, he shall die in his iniquity; but thou hast delivered thy soul.

"Therefore, O thou son of man, speak unto the house of Israel: Thus ye speak, saying, If our transgressions and our sins be upon us, and we pine away in them, how should we then live? Say unto them, As I live, saith the Lord God, I have no pleasure in the death of the wicked; but that the wicked turn from his way and live: turn ye, turn ye, from your evil ways; for why will ye die, O house of Israel?" (Ezekiel 33:1-11)

The prophet had by the command of God ceased from prophesying to the Jews just at the time when the news came that Jerusalem was invaded, and siege laid to her. In the twenty-fourth chapter Ezekiel records the representation that was given to him of the punishment that would come upon all who would refuse the word of the Lord. The people were removed from Jerusalem, and punished by death and captivity. No lot was to fall upon it to determine who should be saved and who destroyed.

"Wherefore thus saith the Lord God: Woe to the bloody city, to the pot whose scum is therein, and whose scum is not gone out of it! bring it out piece by piece; let no lot fall upon it. For her blood is in the midst of her. . . . Therefore thus saith the Lord God; Woe to the bloody city! I will even make the pile for fire great. Heap on wood, kindle the fire, consume the flesh, and spice it well, and let the bones be burned. . . . She hath wearied herself with lies, and her great scum went not forth out of her: {60} her scum shall be in the fire. In thy filthiness is lewdness: because I have purged thee, and thou wast not purged, thou shalt not be purged from thy filthiness any more, till I have caused my fury to rest upon thee. I the Lord have spoken it: it shall come to pass, and I will do it; I will not go back; neither will I spare, neither will I repent; according to thy ways and according to thy doings shall they judge thee, saith the Lord God.

"Also the word of the Lord came unto me, saying, Son of man, behold I take away from thee the desire of thine eyes with a stroke; yet neither shalt thou mourn nor weep, neither shall thy tears run down. Forbear to cry; make no mourning for the dead. . . . So I spake unto the people in the morning: and at even my wife died: and I did in the morning what I was commanded.

"And the people said unto me, Wilt thou not tell us what these things are to us, that thou doest so? Then I answered them, The word of the Lord came unto me, saying, Speak unto the house of Israel, Thus saith the Lord God; Behold, I will profane my sanctuary, the excellency of your strength, the desire of your eyes, and that which your soul pitieth; and your sons and your daughters whom ye have left shall fall by the sword. And ye shall do as I have

done; ye shall not cover your lips, nor eat the bread of men. And your tires shall be upon your heads, and your shoes upon your feet; ye shall not mourn nor weep; but ye shall pine away for your iniquities, and mourn one toward another. Thus Ezekiel is unto you a sign: according to all that he hath done shall ye do; and when this cometh, ye shall know that I am the Lord God." (Ezekiel 24:6-24)

I am instructed to present these words before those who have had light and evidence, but who have walked directly contrary to the light. The Lord will make the punishment of those who will not receive his admonitions and warnings as broad as the wrong has been. The purpose of those who have tried to cover their wrong, while they have secretly worked against the purposes of God, will be fully revealed. Truth will be vindicated. God will make manifest that He is God.

There is a spirit of wickedness at work in the church that is striving at every opportunity to make void the law of God. While the Lord may not punish unto death those who have carried their rebellion to great lengths, the light will never again shine with such convincing power upon the stubborn opposers of truth. Sufficient evidence is given to every soul regarding what is truth and what is error. But the deceptive power of evil upon some is so great that they will not receive the evidence and respond to it by repentance.

A long-continued resistance of truth will harden the most impressionable heart. Those who reject the Spirit of truth place themselves under the control of a spirit that is opposed to the word and work of God. For a time they may continue to teach some phases of the truth; but their refusal to accept all the light God sends will after a time place them where they will do the work of a false watchman.

The interests of the cause of present truth demand that those who profess to stand on the Lord's side shall bring into exercise all their {61} powers to vindicate the advent message, the most important message that will ever come to the world. For those who stand as representatives of present truth to use time and energy now in attempting to answer the questions of the doubting ones, will be an unwise use of their time. It will not remove the doubts. The burden of our work now, is not to labor for those who, although they have had abundant light and evidence, still continue on the unbelieving side. God bids us

give our time and strength to the work of preaching to the people the messages that stirred men and women in 1843 and 1844.

We are now to labor unceasingly to get the truth before Jew and Gentile. Instead of going over and over the same ground to establish the faith of those who should never have accepted a doubt regarding the Third Angel's Message, let our efforts be given to making known the truth to those who have never heard it. God calls upon us to make known to all men the truths that have made us what we are, Seventh-Day Adventists.

God is speaking to His people today as He spoke to Israel through Moses, saying, "Who is on the Lord's side?" My brethren, take your position where God bids you. Leave alone those who after light has been repeatedly given them have taken a stand on the opposite side. You are not to spend precious time in repeating to them what they already know, and thus lose your opportunity of entering new fields with the message of present truth. Take up the work which has been given us. With the word of God as your message, stand on the platform of truth and proclaim the soon coming of Christ. Truth, eternal truth, will prevail.

For more than half a century the different points of present truth have been questioned and opposed. New theories have been advanced as truth, which were not truth, and the Spirit of God revealed their error. As the great pillars of our faith have been presented, the Holy Spirit has borne witness to them, and especially is this so regarding the truths of the sanctuary question. Over and over again the Holy Spirit has in a marked manner endorsed the preaching of this doctrine. But today, as in the past, some will be led to form new theories and to deny the truths upon which the Spirit of God has placed His approval.

Any man who seeks to present the theories which would lead us from the light that has come to us on the ministration in the heavenly sanctuary, should not be accepted as a teacher. A true understanding of the sanctuary question means much to us as a people. When we were earnestly seeking the Lord for light on that question light came. In vision I was given such a view of the heavenly sanctuary, and the ministration connected with the holy place, that for many days I could not speak of it.

I know from the light that God has given me that there should be a revival of the messages that have been given in the past, because men will seek to bring in new theories, and will try to prove that those theories are scriptural, whereas they are error which if allowed a place will undermine faith in the truth. We are not to accept these suppositions and pass them along as truth. No, no; we must not move from the platform of truth on which we have been established.

There will always be those who are seeking for something new, and who stretch and strain the word of God to make it support their ideas and {62} theories. Let us, brethren, take the things that God has given us, and which His Spirit has taught us is truth, and believe them, leaving alone those theories which His Spirit has not endorsed.

LESSONS FROM THE VISIONS OF EZEKIEL, PART TWO

July, 4, 1906
Sanitarium, California {63}
Warning Against Rebellion
Ezekiel again writes:

"THE WORD OF THE LORD came again unto me, saying, Son of man, say unto the Prince of Tyrus, Thus saith the Lord God; Because thine heart is lifted up, and thou hast said, I am a God, I sit in the seat of God, in the midst of the seas; yet thou art a man and not God, though thou set thine heart as the heart of God: behold, thou art wiser than Daniel; there is no secret that they can hide from thee; with thy wisdom, and with thine understanding thou hast gotten these riches, and has gotten gold and silver into thy treasures: by thy great wisdom and by thy traffic hast thou increased thy riches, and thine heart is lifted up because of thy riches; therefore thus saith the Lord God; Because thou hast set thine heart as the heart of God; behold, therefore I will bring strangers upon thee, the terrible of the nations; and they shall draw their swords against the beauty of thy wisdom, and they shall defile thy brightness. They shall bring thee down to the pit, and thou shalt die the deaths of them that are slain in the midst of the seas. Wilt thou yet say before him that slayeth thee, I am God? But thou shalt be a man, and not God, in the hand of him that slayeth thee. Thou shalt die the deaths of the uncircumcised by the hand of strangers: for I have spoken it, saith the Lord God.

"Moreover the word of the Lord came unto me saying, Son of man, take up a lamentation upon the king of Tyrus, and say unto him, Thus saith the Lord God; Thou sealest up the sum, full of wisdom, and perfect in beauty. Thou hast been in Eden, the garden of God; every precious stone was thy covering, the sardius, topaz, and the diamond, the beryl, the onyx, and the jasper, the sapphire, the emerald, and the carbuncle, and gold; the workmanship of thy tabrets and of thy pipes was prepared in thee in the day that thou wast created. Thou art the anointed cherub that covereth; and I have set thee so; thou wast upon the holy mountain of God; thou hast walked up and down in the midst of the stones of fire; thou wast perfect in thy ways from the day that thou wast created till iniquity was found in thee. By the multitude of thy merchandise they have filled the midst of thee with violence, and thou hast sinned; therefore I will cast thee as profane out of the mountain of God, and I will destroy thee, O covering cherub, from the midst of the stones of fire. Thine heart was lifted up because of thy beauty, thou hast corrupted thy wisdom by reason of thy brightness: I will cast thee to the ground, I will lay thee before kings, that they may behold thee. Thou hast defiled thy sanctuaries by the multitude of thine iniquities, by the iniquity of thy traffic; therefore will I bring forth a fire from the midst of thee, it shall devour thee, and I will bring thee to ashes upon the earth in the sight of all them that behold thee. All they that know thee among the people shall be astonished at thee: thou shalt be a terror, and never shalt thou be any more.

"Again the word of the Lord came unto me, saying, Son of man, set thy face against Zidon, and prophecy against it. And say, Thus saith the {64} Lord God; Behold, I am against thee, O Zidon; and I will be glorified in the midst of thee and they shall know that I am the Lord, when I have executed judgments in her, and shall be sanctified in her. For I will send into her pestilence, and blood into her streets; and the wounded shall be judged in the midst of her by the sword upon her on every side; and they shall know that I am the Lord.

"And there shall be no more a pricking brier unto the house of Israel, nor any grieving thorn of all that are round about them, that despised them; and they shall know that I am the Lord God. Thus saith the Lord God; When I shall have gathered the house of Israel from the people among whom they are scattered, and shall be sanctified in them in the sight of the heathen, then shall they dwell in their land that I have given to my servant, Jacob. And they shall dwell safely therein, and shall build houses, and plant vineyards; yea, they shall dwell with confidence, when I have executed judgments upon all those that despise them round about them; and they shall know that I am the Lord their God." (Ezekiel 28:1-26)

The first sinner was one whom God had greatly exalted. He is represented under the figure of the prince of Tyrus flourishing in might and magnificence. Little by little Satan came to indulge the desire for self-exaltation. The Scripture says:

"Thine heart was lifted up because of thy beauty; thou hast corrupted thy wisdom by reason of thy brightness." "Thou hast said in thine heart. . . I will exalt my throne above the stars of God; . . .I will be like the Most High."

Though all his glory was from God, this mighty angel came to regard it as pertaining to himself. Not content with his position, though honored above the heavenly host, he ventured to covet homage due to the Creator. Instead of seeking to make God supreme in the affections and allegiance of all created beings, it was his endeavor to secure their service and loyalty to himself. And coveting the glory with which the infinite Father has invested His Son, this Prince of angels aspired to power that was the prerogative of Christ alone.

To the very close of the controversy in heaven, the great usurper continued to justify himself. When it was announced that with all his sympathizers he must be expelled from the abodes of bliss, then the rebel leader boldly avowed his contempt for the Creator's law. He denounced the divine statutes as a restriction of their liberty, and declared that it was his purpose to secure the abolition of law. With one accord, Satan and his host threw the blame of their rebellion wholly upon Christ, declaring that if they had not been reproved, they would never have rebelled.

Satan's rebellion was to be a lesson to the universe through all coming ages, a perpetual testimony to the nature and terrible results of sin. The working out of Satan's rule, its effects upon both men and angels, would show what must be the fruit of setting aside the divine authority. It would testify that with the existence of God's government and His law, is bound up the well-being of all the creatures He has made. Thus the history of this terrible experiment of rebellion was to be a perpetual safeguard to all holy intelligences, to prevent them from being deceived {65} as to the nature of transgression, to save them from committing sin, and suffering its punishment.

At any moment God can withdraw from the impenitent the tokens of His wonderful mercy and love. Oh, that human agencies might consider what will be the sure result of their ingratitude to Him and of their disregard of the infinite Gift of Christ to our world! If they continue to love transgression more than obedience, the present blessings and the great mercy of God that they now enjoy, but do not appreciate, will finally become the occasion of their eternal ruin. When it is too late for them to see and understand that which they have slighted as a thing of naught they will know what it means to be without God, without hope. Then they will realize what they have lost by choosing to be disloyal to God and to stand in rebellion to His commandments.

In His great mercy God has spoken words of encouragement to the children of men. To all who repent and turn to Him, He offers abundant pardon. Repentance for sin is the first fruits of the working of the Holy Spirit in the life. It is the only process by which infinite purity reflects the image of Christ in His redeemed subjects. In Christ all fullness dwells. He teaches us to count all things but loss for the excellency of the knowledge of Christ Jesus our Lord.

This knowledge is the highest science that any man can reach. It is the sum of all true science. "This is life eternal," Christ declared, "that they might know Thee, the only true God, and Jesus Christ whom Thou hast sent."

The time has come when the righteous should understand that God's judgments are to fall on all who transgress His law, and that those who walk humbly with Him will triumph with holy gladness. As Jehovah is holy He requires His people to be holy, pure, undefiled. For without holiness no man shall see the Lord. Those who worship Him in sincerity and truth will be accepted by Him. If church members will put away all self worship, and will receive in their hearts the love for God and for one another that filled Christ's heart, our heavenly Father will constantly manifest His power through them. Let His people be drawn together with the cords of divine love. Then the world will recognize the miracle working power of God, and will acknowledge that He is the Strength and the Helper of His commandment-keeping people.

Hold Fast the Beginning of Your Confidence

June 3, 1906
(MS-61)
Sanitarium, California {66}

FOR MANY MONTHS I HAVE BEEN troubled as I have seen that some of our brethren whom God has used in His cause are now perplexed over the scientific theology which has come in to lead men away from a true faith in God. Sabbath night, a week ago, after I had been prayerfully studying over these things, I had a vision, in which I was speaking before a large company where many questions were asked concerning my work and writings.

I was directed by a messenger from heaven not to take the burden of picking up and answering all the sayings and doubts that are being put into many minds. "Stand as the messenger of God anywhere in any place," I was bidden, "and bear the testimony I shall give you. Be free. Bear the testimonies that the Lord has for you to bear in reproof, in rebuke, in the work of encouraging and lifting up the soul; 'teaching them to observe all things whatsoever I have commanded you: and lo, I am with you always, even unto the end of the world.'"

After the vision I prayed aloud with great fervor and earnestness. My soul was strengthened; for the words had been spoken: "Be strong, yea, be strong. Let none of the misleading words of ministers or physicians distress your mind. Tell them to take the light given them in publications. Truth will always bear away the victory. Go straight forward with your work.

"If the Holy Spirit is rejected, all My words will not help to remove, even for the time being, the false representations that have been made, and Satan stands ready to invent more. If the evidence already given is rejected, all other evidence will be useless until there is seen the converting power of God upon minds. If the convincing impressions of the Holy Spirit made in the past will not be accepted as trustworthy evidence, nothing that can be presented hereafter will reach them, because the bewitching guile of Satan has perverted their discernment."

To those who have been convinced again and again as the Holy Spirit has borne witness, all the words that can now be said cannot be as forcible as the impression made by the Holy Spirit of God.

To my brethren, I say, Go forward.

Be of good courage. Whenever the Spirit of God is entertained in the place of the underworking of evil influences on mind and heart, those who have been working against God will come to their right bearings. A great work is to be done now in convicting souls. The message must in no case be changed from what it has been. As has been foretold in the Scriptures, there will be seducing spirits and doctrines of devils in the midst of the church, and these evil influences will increase; but hold fast the beginning of your confidence firm unto the end.

Let not souls be drawn into Battle Creek. Warnings are to be given. A message similar to that borne by John the Baptist is to be heard. But beware of men; for they will seek to divert the mind from the necessity of heeding the true issues for this time. Carry {67} on the work now for those who need the truth and who have not resisted the evidences of the truth for fallacies and scientific imaginations.

The time is at hand when Satan will work miracles to confirm minds in the belief that he is God. All the people of God are now to stand on the platform of truth as it has been given in the Third Angel's Message. All the pleasant pictures, all the miracles wrought, will be presented in order that if possible the very elect should be deceived. The only hope for any one is to hold fast the evidences that have confirmed the truth in righteousness. Let these be proclaimed over and over again, until the close of this earth's history.

The perils of the last days are upon us. Devote not precious time in trying to convince those who would change the truth of God into a lie. Proclaim the Third Angel's message. Bear a straight-forward, clear-cut message.

Thus I was speaking before a perplexed company just before I called them to take their stand on the right side. If some chose another position, let them alone. Labor for those who have never had the evidence of truth. So long as men hold fast to men, and believe men in the place of the word of God, you can do little to help them. You are working against principalities and powers, as is represented in Ephesians 6:12.

We are to revive the truth; to stand in the truth. Whoever is determined to depart from the faith cannot be helped by you. All your reasoning will be as idle tales.

Take the banner of truth and hold it aloft, higher and still higher. The Lord calls for faithful minute men. Go into the cities that need the message of a soon-coming Saviour. Thousands of unbelievers in our cities need to hear the last message of warning.

It is Satan's plan to produce these variances, to keep our minds on dissensions and unprofitable problems until the last woe shall come upon the world. Time is too precious to be lost through confusion. Proclaim to the world that Christ is soon coming.

Gather not at Battle Creek; spoil not the minds of youth, physicians and ministers. Set at work in the cause of God every soul who has heeded the words of warning given.

I have been instructed that it is not extravagant display which is now required in giving the last message of mercy to our world. We must go forth in the simplicity of true godliness. Our sanitariums, our schools, our publishing houses, are to be God's instrumentalities to represent the humble manner of Christ's teaching. In a marked manner the Lord will be the strength and power of His people. Maintain simplicity; and pray in faith constantly. Wherever you are, your only safety is in prayer. Hold fast the beginning of your confidence firm unto the end.

Beware of the leaven of evil. Talk less; criticize less. Let everyone remember that he is now on test and trial for life, eternal life.

God now calls for all who choose to serve Him, to stand firmly on {68} the platform of eternal truth. Let those who have brought about the present state of confusion by making the division that exists, stop to consider seriously before going any farther. "Choose you this day whom ye will serve." "If the Lord be God, follow Him; but if Baal, then follow Him."

(Signed) Ellen G. White

AN APPEAL FOR LABOR IN THE CITIES

September 16, 1910
Sanitarium, California {69}
To Conference Presidents:

DURING THE NIGHT OF FEBRUARY 27, a representation was given me in which the unworked cities were represented before me as a living reality, and I was plainly instructed that there should be a decided change from past methods of working. For months the situation has been impressed on my mind, and I urge that companies be organized and diligently trained to labor in our important cities.

These workers should labor two and two, and from time to time all should meet together to relate their experiences, to pray, and to plan how to reach the people quickly, and thus if possible redeem the time.

This is no time to colonize. From city to city the work is to be carried quickly. The light that has been placed under a bushel is to be taken out and placed on a candle stick, that it may give forth light to all that are in the house.

Thousands of people in our cities are left in darkness, and Satan is well pleased with the delay; for this delay gives him opportunity to work in these fields with men of influence to further his plans. Can we now depend upon our men in positions of responsibility to act humbly and nobly their part? Let the watchmen arouse. Let no one continue to be indifferent to the situation. There should be a thorough awakening among the brethren and sisters in all our churches.

For years the work in the cities has been presented before me and has been urged upon our people. Instruction has been given to open new fields. There has sometimes been a jealous fear lest someone who wished to enter new fields should receive means from the people that they supposed was wanted for another work. Some in responsible positions have felt that nothing should be done without their personal knowledge and approval. Therefore efficient workers have been sometimes delayed and hindered, and the carriage wheels of progress in entering new fields have been made to move heavily.

In every large city there should have been a strong force of workers laboring earnestly to warn the people. Had this been undertaken in humility and faith, Christ would have gone before the humble workers and the salvation of God would have been revealed.

Let companies now be quickly organized to go out two and two, and labor in the spirit of Christ, following His plans. Even though some Judas may introduce himself into the ranks of the workers, the Lord will care for the work. His angels will go before and prepare the way. Before this time, every large city should have heard the testing message, and thousands should have been brought to a knowledge of the truth. Wake up the churches. Take the light from under the bushel.

Where are the men who will work and study and agonize in prayer as did Christ? We are not to confine our efforts to a few

places. If they shall persecute you in one city, flee ye to another. Let Christ's plan be followed. He was ever watching for opportunity to engage in personal labor, ever ready to interest and draw men to a study of the Scriptures. He labored patiently for men who had not an intelligent knowledge of what is truth. While we are not {70} awake to the situation, and while much time is consumed in planning how to reach perishing souls, Satan is busy devising and blocking the way.

O, if I could but see the depth of experience coming to our people which they must have before they can enter heaven, then would I be filled with grateful thanksgiving to God! I speak to our people, ministers, physicians, and all who profess to believe the truth. A work of thorough conversion needs to be done. Walk in the footsteps of Christ Jesus. Why do we not take heed? The Lord has long waited for us as a people who know the truth, to make that truth known to all possible who will hear and be converted.

(Signed) Ellen G. White

TO THE BATTLE CREEK CHURCH

July 2, 1907
Sanitarium, California {71}

I AM URGED TO SAY TO THOSE who have had the light of the word, but who fail to walk according to the word, your failure to act upon the light is imperiling your eternal welfare.

The Lord knows all about the needs and trials of His people. Through affliction He seeks to point them to heaven. There they will know no disappointment or trial or grief.

In the word of God we are encouraged to study the character of the world's Redeemer. He is the pattern of every man in his work of character-building. The Son of God was tempted in all points like as we are, but He resisted every temptation. Through prayer He obtained the power to become victor in the struggle with the powers of Satan. In the groves and mountains the Saviour spent whole nights in prayer for Himself and His disciples, and for those for whom His disciples would labor. Christ's followers are to find strength where their Master found it.

The world hides a man from himself. It conceals from him his dangers by shutting out the prospect of a future life, and by constantly appealing to his human senses.

By thus keeping in his mind only the interests of this life, it seeks to make him a creature of time. But fixing his eyes upon the eternal world, man sees the cross of Christ and the death of the Son of God to save a perishing world.

Christ left the courts of Heaven, laid aside His kingly crown and royal robe, and came to live the life of the poor. He subjected Himself to all the temptations common to humanity, that man might look upon the Prince of Heaven, and see in Him a perfect exhibition of the conquest of sin. In all trials and temptations and trials Christ sinned not, neither was guile found in His mouth. He clothed His divinity with humanity, but in His teaching and ministry His divinity was clearly manifest.

On one occasion Christ was moved to condemn: "Then began He to upbraid the cities wherein most of His mighty works were done, because they repented not: Woe unto thee, Chorazin! woe unto thee, Bethsaida! for if the mighty works which were done in you, had been done in Tyre and Sidon they would have repented long ago in sackcloth and ashes. But I say unto you, It shall be more tolerable for Tyre and Sidon at the day of judgment, than for you. And thou, Capernaum, which art exalted unto Heaven, shall be brought down to hell: for if the mighty works, which have been done in you, had been done in Sodom, it would have remained unto this day. But I say unto you, That it shall be more tolerable for the land of Sodom and in the day of judgment than for thee." (Matthew 11:21-24)

Here is a wonderful statement. The cities that have had the most done for them, and yet do not yield to the evidences of truth, are rejecting the power of the Holy Spirit. They are refusing the great light shining amid their moral darkness.

I am instructed that one place which will be classed with those {72} where many mighty works have been done, and where the people have turned from light and evidence, is Battle Creek. Battle Creek has been the seat of rebellion among a people to whom the Lord has given great light and special opportunities. But the light has been discarded for the privilege of pleasing self, and of following the unsanctified will. Minds and characters that might have been molded and fashioned after the divine similitude, have been marred and stunted by self-serving. The opportunities that God has given whereby men might secure His help and favor have been neglected.

And every place that has turned from light and evidence falls under the same condemnation. Woe unto those who having received great light, having seen manifestations of the powers of God, and having acknowledged this light and this power as from God, have turned from the light and refused to accept the evidence! To those as to the cities of Chorazin and Bethsaida, the words are spoken, "If the mighty works which were done in thee, had been done in Tyre and Sidon, they would have repented long ago in sackcloth and ashes."

If the people of these cities had accepted the message, exercised themselves unto repentance, and carried the light of truth to other cities, thousands of souls would have been converted as a result. Now Christ will take humble men, and reveal to them the great and precious truths for these last days; these He will use in carrying to completion His work in the earth.

Surrounding every soul there is an influence either for or against truth and righteousness. "He that is not for Me," Christ said, " is against Me; and he that gathereth not with Me, scattereth abroad." Influence is an important talent. Used on the side of Christ, it becomes a power unto life eternal.

The faculty of speech is a precious talent. Like the talent of influence, it conveys either light or darkness to those about us. Sanctified to God, it becomes the means of imparting the grace of Christ.

God designs that our knowledge of the truth shall be to men a savor of life unto life. The highest employment of the powers of speech is that of imparting divine truth. Wherever the audience may be, whoever may compose that audience, Christ's witness is to speak the plain, unvarnished truth. He is to minister grace to his hearers. His words will be in harmony with the teaching of Christ. The soul who is truly converted will have his lips touched with the sacred fire of cleansing. To every individual he meets he will find an opportunity of speaking the good news of salvation. He believes; therefore he utters the sentiments of his heart. He stands as the oracle of God, speaking to men the words of life and salvation. No one will mistake his position; no one will doubt on which side he stands. He stands as Christ's witness, consecrated, set apart, to declare to others the character of the Redeemer.

My brethren and sisters, Lift Him up, the risen Saviour. Lift Him up, as you plead before God in prayer.

(Signed) Ellen G. White

To the Elders of the Battle Creek Church, and to Ministers and Physicians

July 5, 1906
(-7 B.230 1906)
Sanitarium, California, {73}

I HAVE INSTRUCTION TO GIVE from the Lord. The condition of things in Battle Creek is to be clearly outlined and understood. Those who have brought about this condition are sadly deceived, and are misleading others. But the Lord will be glorified. Great spiritual transformations are to take place. All those who would be led of God, should walk very humbly before Him. In no case are they to be diverted from the path of duty that God has marked out for His people. They are not to believe falsehoods, though they be published in abundance.

A voice is to be heard in the Tabernacle giving God's word for this time in clear notes of warning. God has human instrumentalities that will not hold their peace. They are to advocate the word and will and way of Jehovah. In a clear, decided manner they are to proclaim the truth in all its beauty and power. No strange doctrines are to be introduced. There is to be no undermining of the fundamental truths that the Lord has submitted by many miraculous evidences. A voice is to be heard in clear affirmation of the truth, in contradiction to the skepticism and fallacies that have been coming in from the enemy of truth. Reformations will take place, and the working out of the principles of divine truth will reveal growth in grace; for the divine agencies are efficient to enlighten and sanctify the human understanding.

The truth as it is in Jesus, as it was proclaimed by Him when He was enshrouded by the pillowy [billowy] cloud, is verity and truth in this our day, and will just as surely renovate the mind of the receiver as it has renovated minds in the past. Christ has declared, "If they hear not Moses and the Prophets, neither will they be persuaded, though one rose from the dead." (Luke 16:31)

As a people, we must prepare the way of the Lord, under the overruling guidance of the Holy Spirit, for the spread of the gospel in its purity. The stream of living water is to deepen and widen in its course. In all fields, nigh and afar off, men will be called from the plow, and from the more common commercial business vocations that largely occupy the mind, and will become educated in connection with men who have had experience—men who understand the truth. Through most wonderful workings of God, mountains of difficulty will be removed and cast into the sea. Let us labor as those who have experienced the virtue of truth as it is in Jesus.

There is to be, at this period, a series of events which will reveal that God is master of the situation. The truth will be proclaimed in clear, unmistakable language. Those who preach the truth will strive to demonstrate the truth by a well-ordered life and godly conversation. And as they do this, they will become powerful in advocating the truth, and in giving it the sure application that God has given it. {74}

When the men, who have known and taught the truth, turn aside to human understanding, and mete out to deceived minds their own dish of fables, it is high time for those who have once been laborers in evangelistic work, but who have been drawn away into the management of restaurants, food stores, and other commercial lines of work, to come into line, study their Bibles diligently, and with the word of God in hand, dispense the Bible truth, the spiritual food, in cooperation with the heavenly angels. This work now calls loudly for workmen of divine appointment. Omnipotence will then say to the mountains of difficulty, Be thou removed and cast into the sea.

The call is to go forth, "Son, go labor today in My vineyard." As this call is obeyed, the message that means so much to the dwellers on the earth, will be heard and understood. Man will know what is truth. Onward, and still onward, will the work advance. And marked events of Providence will be seen and recognized, in judgments and in blessings. The truth will bear away the victory.

To all students we would say, In the name of the Lord do not permit yourselves to be held where the spiritual atmosphere is poisoned with skepticism and falsehood. Those who have had the evidence of truth, but who for days, weeks, months, and years, have had about them a subtle influence that gives a distorted representation, a false coloring, to the truth of God, are not fit for teachers for our youth. Where falsehoods regarding the word and work of God are reported as truth is no place for students who are preparing for the future, immortal life. We are seeking heaven, wherein can enter none who have changed the truth of God into a lie.

Truth has a spiritual influence. It enters the mind, direct and uncorrupted, from One who is truth. The reception of truth in the inward parts is charged with the greatest results. Truth is to be received into the heart, and developed and expressed in the character.

No lie is of the truth. On every occasion possible, Satan is on hand to introduce the leaven of his deceptive fallacies. Listen not a moment to the interpretations that would loosen one pin, remove one pillar, from the platform of truth.

Human interpretations, the reception of fables, will spoil your faith, confuse your understanding, and make of none effect your faith in Jesus Christ. Study diligently the third chapter of Revelation. In it is pointed out the danger of losing your hold upon the things that you have heard and learned from the Source of all light. "Remember. . .how thou hast received and heard, and hold fast, and repent." Why repent? Because there have come in faults, in the form of theories so subtle that by the influence of mind upon mind, through the agency of those who have departed from the faith, the wily foe will cause you imperceptibly to be imbued with the spirit that will draw you away from the faith.

There are many who are in a perilous position spiritually, many who are "ready to die." The Revelator was bidden to write to the church in Sardis: "These things saith he that hath the seven Spirits of God, and the seven stars; I know thy works, that thou {75} livest, and art dead. Be watchful, and strengthen the things which remain, that are ready to die: for I have not found thy works perfect before God. Remember therefore how thou hast received, and heard, and hold fast, and repent." (Revelation 3:1-3)

There is a censure resting upon those who have heard the truth, received the truth, and who afterward have acted like men spiritually dead. "Remember therefore." In our work we are not to be drawn into any plausible theories that would lead to a denial of our past faith in the truth we have heard and advocated. "If therefore thou shalt not watch, I will come on thee as a thief, and thou shalt not know what hour I will come upon thee." (Revelation 3:3)

"Thou hast a few names even in Sardis which have not defiled their garments; and they shall walk with Me in white: for they are worthy." (Revelation 3:4)

"Moreover I will make a covenant of peace with them; it shall be an everlasting covenant with them; and I will place them, and multiply them, and will set My sanctuary in the midst of them forevermore. My tabernacle also shall be with them: yea, I will be their God, and they shall be My people." (Ezekiel 37:26-27)

This last scripture carries our minds forward to the triumph of Israel and Judah. The accomplishment of the work will be through human instrumentalities charged with divine power. All the glory is ascribed to the great power of God, but it is through unity and cooperation of the human with the divine, that the result is made possible. Humanity, blended with divinity, grasps the divine efficiency, and the work is complete.

We have been filled with pain of heart, which language cannot describe, as we have seen feature after feature of the work that should have been conducted in the purest channels as a means of bringing souls to a knowledge of the truth, corrupted by ambition and commercialism. Thus some features of the health work have proved a snare to capture talents of influence that might have been used in feeding souls with the bread of life. While thousands are perishing without a knowledge of the truth, while multitudes have not the bread of life to feed upon, while God is calling for a quick work to be done to prepare a people for the coming of Christ, shall our hygienic restaurants prove a snare, by being operated merely for commercial advantage, and their influence extend no farther? It was hoped that much good would be done by preparing food for worldlings, that thereby many would be brought to a knowledge of the truth. And this might have been, had the glory of God been kept in view. But these enterprises have been run so largely on a commercial basis, for the temporal advantages to be gained, that they have often become a snare, as it were, to hold men and women of talent, who, by study and diligent effort, could do acceptable service in the winning of souls to Christ. The end of all things is at hand. We must learn to fulfill God's purposes. Let no one delay.

There are those who once were teachers of righteousness, but who have turned from the truth and are wandering in the mists of error. Satan with much persistency is striving for the mastery. {76} Christ calls upon many who are in training for His service, to obtain an education of a character altogether different from that which they have been receiving. The Lord Jesus calls upon us to fulfil His commission given just before His ascension to meet the heavenly armies that escorted Him to the city of God.

We have the battle of tribulation before us, but our commission is, "Go ye therefore, and teach all nations, baptizing them in the name of the Father, and of the Son, and of the Holy Ghost; teaching them to observe all things whatsoever I have commanded you: and, lo, I am with you always, even unto the end of the world." Who will pass this by, and continue in any commercial business that will not bring souls to Christ? Shall this condition change? Will you give the last note of warning to the world?

(Signed) Ellen G. White

TO THE BRETHREN IN BATTLE CREEK

April 17, 1907
Sanitarium, California {77}

I SPEAK TO THE BELIEVERS in Battle Creek: Cling to the Lord with mind and heart. Give heed to the warnings that the Lord has sent, and you will not be overcome by Satan's delusions. You will have trials to meet, but if you will look to the Lord, He will be your strong tower, to which you may run and be safe.

My heart aches when I consider the stubborn resistance on the part of some to the truth we have held for half a century. Night after night I cannot sleep. My soul is bowed down with heavy burdens when I consider that some of my old friends, and some of my own relatives are refusing to walk in the light that God is sending by His Holy Spirit. O that the searcher of hearts would arouse these souls to realize their true condition. I call to mind the trial that Christ was called to endure when He was rejected by the members of His own family. "Neither did His own brethren believe in Him,"—this must have been one of the cruelest of His many trials.

May the Lord open the blind eyes, that the men who have withstood the counsels and warnings of God, and have acted as though it were a virtue to resist the instruction of the Holy Spirit, may discern their true condition. I have written to Frank Belden, and to Russel Hart, but my appeals have not moved them. They continue to reveal what manner of spirit has taken possession of them.

In my dreams I seem to be pleading with the believers in Battle Creek. I am so burdened for these souls who seem determined to fight against the message sent, that I awake in the night pleading with God to open the blind eyes.

I thank the Lord that there are many who can discern now, if not before, the spirit that has taken possession of those who resist the warnings of the Spirit of God. I am bidden to say to the believers in Battle Creek, Press together. Let no words be spoken to irritate or provoke. Stand firmly in the faith in which God has led us for the last fifty years.

Time is passing into eternity. Many who ought to have keen perceptions are blinded by false theories and false influences. They are unready to meet the last great conflict, and they do not realize their unprepared condition. My prayer for them is: "O Thou searcher of hearts, let Thy word, which is quick and powerful and sharper than any two-edged sword, pierce to the dividing asunder of soul and spirit, and discern the thoughts and intents of the heart. Bring these souls who are in so great peril because of their lack of discernment to realize that they must cope with Satanic powers."

Many are closing their hearts against the Holy Spirit of God. Many who once understood the workings of the Spirit of God, Christ does not own today. O that Christ would stir the hearts of those who have once walked in the light, but who now walk in darkness; who have once known what it meant to have the grace of God in their hearts, but who are now destitute of that grace. They have had the light of the Spirit of God, but in their blindness they have quenched {78} that light, and they are now under the condemnation of God.

Who have a realization of the condition of the unbelieving world? Who are preparing their hearts to receive the impressions of the Spirit of God? Those who receive the light and walk in the light, will have increased light.

In these last days God calls for united efforts from His people. Never was there a time when there was greater need of the deep movings of the Spirit of God than now when we are called to contend with men imbued with the spirit of Satan. Those who have departed from the faith will make manifest that they were led away by seducing spirits and doctrines of devils, and that these have taken possession of the soul.

What an account must be rendered to God by those who are placing themselves on Satan's side! I am praying that God will anoint their eyes with eye salve, that they may see their peril and escape from their dangerous position as quickly as possible. When these poor souls realize that they have lost time, lost experience which should have made them wise unto salvation, they will understand that they have been working on the enemy's side. Then they will ask themselves, What have I been teaching to others? What has been my testimony for truth and righteousness? How does my record stand in the books of heaven?

"Then came the word of the Lord unto Jeremiah saying, Thus saith the Lord of hosts, the God of Israel; Go and tell the men of Judah and the inhabitants of Jerusalem, will ye not receive instruction hearken to my words? Saith the Lord. . . I have sent also unto you all My servants the prophets, rising up early and sending them, saying, Return ye now every man from his evil way, and amend your doings, and go not after other gods to serve them, and ye shall dwell in the land which I shall give you and to your fathers, but ye have not inclined your ear, nor hearkened unto Me. . .Therefore thus saith the Lord God of hosts, the God of Israel, Behold, I will bring upon Judah and all the inhabitants of Jerusalem all the evil that I have pronounced against them; because I have spoken unto them and they have not heard; and I have called upon them, but they have not answered.

"And Jeremiah said unto the house of the Rechabites, Thus saith the Lord of hosts, the God of Israel; Because ye have obeyed the commandments of Jonadab your father, and kept all his precepts, and done according unto all that he hath commanded you: therefore thus saith the Lord of hosts, the God of Israel; Jonadab the Son of Rechab shall not want a man to stand before me forever." (Jeremiah 35:12-19)

As a people we need to study this portion of sacred history: for these experiences are being brought into the lives of the people of God in these last days. A people who have had great light and every evidence of truth are turning away from the light, and following their own impulses. The instruction God has given in the record of His people in early days is not regarded. The mistakes and sins of His early people are being repeated in His people today: warnings and admonitions given in that day are not being heeded in this. Notwithstanding all the warnings that have been given, they {79} see not their danger, but join the ranks of the enemy, and fight on his side. They choose to entertain their own ideas and to follow the suggestions of their own minds. The Lord is greatly dishonored by their course, and he is removing His Spirit from them. "Shall I not judge them for these things," saith the Lord, "unless they repent?"

In the thirty-sixth chapter of Jeremiah is recorded an act on the part of Jehoiakim, king of Judah, that our people would do well to study. "And it came to pass in the fourth year of Jehoiakim the son of Josiah king of Judah, that this word came unto Jeremiah from the Lord, saying, Take thee a roll of a book, and write therein all the words that I have spoken unto thee, from the days of Josiah even unto this day. It may be that the house of Judah will hear all the evil which I purpose to do unto them; that they may return every man from his evil way; that I may forgive their iniquity and their sin. Then Jeremiah called Baruch the son of Neriah: and Baruch wrote from the mouth of Jeremiah all the words of the Lord, which he had spoken unto him, upon the roll of a book.

"And Jeremiah commanded Baruch, saying, I am shut up; I cannot go into the house of the Lord: therefore go thou, and read in the roll, which thou hast written from my mouth, the words of the Lord in the ears of the people in the Lord's house upon the fasting day: and also thou shalt read them in the ears of all Judah that come out of their cities. It may be they will present their supplication before the Lord, and will return everyone from his evil way: for great is the anger and the fury that the Lord hath pronounced against this people. And Baruch the son of Neriah did according to all that Jeremiah the prophet commanded him, reading in the book the words of the Lord in the Lord's house. . .

"When Michaiah the son of Gemariah, the son of Shephan, had heard out of the book all the words of the Lord, then he went down into the King's house, into the scribe's chamber: and, lo, all the princes sat there. . . . Then Michaiah declared unto them all the words that he had heard, when Baruch read the book in the ears of the people. Therefore all the princes sent Jehudi. . . unto Baruch saying, Take in thine hand the roll wherein thou hast read in the ears of the people, and come. So Baruch the son of Neriah took the roll in his hand, and came unto them. And they said unto him, Sit down now, and read it in our ears.

So Baruch read it in their ears.

"Now it came to pass, when they had heard all the words, that they were afraid, both one and other, and said unto Baruch, We will surely tell the king all these words. And they asked Baruch, saying, Tell us now, How didst thou write all these words at his mouth? Then Baruch answered them, He pronounced all these words unto me with his mouth, and I wrote them with ink in the book. Then said the princes unto Baruch, Go, hide thee, thou and Jeremiah; and let no man know where ye be.

"And they went into the king into the court, but they laid up the roll in the chamber of Elishama the scribe, and told all the words in the ears of the king. So the king sent Jehudi to fetch the roll: and he took it out of Elishama the scribe's chamber. {80} And Jehudi read it in the ears of the king, and in the ears of all the princes which stood beside the king.

"Now the king sat in the winter house in the ninth month, and there was a fire on the hearth burning before him. And it came to pass when Jehudi had read three or four pages, he cut it with the penknife, and cast it into the fire that was on the hearth, until all the roll was consumed in the fire that was upon the hearth. Yet they were not afraid, nor rent their garments; neither the king, nor any of his servants that heard all these words. Nevertheless Elnathan and Delaiah and Gemariah had made intercession to the king that he would not burn the roll: but he would not hear them." (Jeremiah 36:1-25)

Some in the experience of the past few years have virtually repeated the act of king Jehoiakim in burning the messages of the Spirit of God. But today as of old these messages of warning have been repeated.

"Then the word of the Lord came to Jeremiah, after that the king burned the roll, and the words which Baruch spake at the mouth of Jeremiah, saying, Take thee again another roll, and write in it all the former words that were in the first roll, which Jehoiakim the king of Judah hath burned. And thou shalt say to Jehoiakim king of Judah, Thus saith the Lord; Thou hast burned this roll saying, Why hast thou written therein, saying, The king of Babylon shall certainly come and destroy this land, and shall cause to cease from thence man and beast? Therefore thus saith the Lord of Jehoiakim king of Judah; He shall have none to sit upon the throne of David: and his dead body shall be cast out in the day to the heat, and in

the night to the frost. And I will punish him and his seed and his servants for their iniquity; and I will bring upon them and upon the inhabitants of Jerusalem, and upon the men of Judah, all the evil that I have pronounced against them; but they hearkened not." (Jeremiah 36:27-31)

The Lord has been trifled with by his people. The time that should have been devoted to repentance and reform has been spent in criticism and in following man-formed opinions and ideas. A terrible influence for evil is exerted when men turn from the right way to follow selfish devisings. Satan is playing the game of life for the souls of men, and he is gaining victory. We can learn from a study of King Jehoiakim's example what men will do when they pass the boundary line. We see it in the persecution and suffering that Christ endured at the hands of wicked men. We see it in the treatment that the Lord's faithful servants in every age have received.

(Signed) Ellen G. White

AGGRESSIVE WORK TO BE DONE

July 3, 1906
(-7- B.214, 1906)
Sanitarium, California {81}

To Ministers and Physicians:

THERE IS A HEAVY BURDEN resting on my soul. I pray the Lord to impress the hearts of His people with the solemnity of the time in which they are living, and with the necessity of making straight paths for their feet. Some who have long known the truth, are confused by leaders who have been walking in false paths.

"I am the Way, the Truth, and the Life," Christ declares. "No man cometh unto the Father, but by Me." Those who have a living connection with Christ will reveal it by their works. "Faith, if it hath not works, is dead, being alone."

We have reached an important chapter in our experience. We have advance movements to make. Straightforward work must be done. Faith without works is dead, unproductive of good. Faith works by love, and purifies the soul; faith must be revealed and substantiated by works. There is a spurious faith, which does not work to the point, because the heart is decidedly opposed to the truth. Some may take comfort in the thought that God will number them with His people because they make a profession. We may have a measure of faith, a knowledge of the theory of truth, but unless self dies, unless we live Christ's life of obedience, our profession is worthless.

Nothing can take the place of obedience to a "Thus saith the Lord." Knowledge that does not lead to a practice of self-denial and self-sacrifice, to a daily walk in the foot-steps of Christ, but rather to self-exaltation and self-sufficiency, is opposed to practical godliness. God calls for obedience.

Self-sufficiency, exercised in a family or institution, means great injury to the work of God. It is destructive to the spiritual life of those who cherish it. True faith leads away from selfish plans and from the self-pleasing life. Obedience, in order to be acceptable to God, must be the whole-souled obedience that Christ ever offered to the Father.

In response to the question, Who shall enter the kingdom of heaven? Christ says, "Not everyone that saith unto Me, Lord, Lord, shall enter into the kingdom of heaven, but he that doeth the will of My Father which is in heaven." (Matthew 7:21)

What must we do to inherit eternal life? The answer is, Keep the commandments. To the question, Who are the blessed? Christ answers, "Blessed are they that hear the Word of God, and keep it." "Blessed are they that do His commandments, that they may have right to the tree of life, and may enter in through the gates into the city." "Without are dogs, and sorcerers," "and murderers, and idolaters, and whosoever loveth and maketh a lie."

The theories that lead to unbelief in the Word of God, and to a lack of the faith that works by love and purifies the soul, are {82} theories of the enemy. They may be very pleasing, and very attractive, but they develop into strange doctrines, which unsettle faith in the past experience of God's people, and take away the foundation pillars. These theories have come in amongst us, and have been a seductive power, robbing some of the faith that enables human beings to see where they are living in the history of the world. They are false theories, leading away from the truth into subtle errors.

When physicians are diligent students of the Scriptures, when our ministers live in accordance with the Word of God, making this Word their text-book, then the truth will be proclaimed with power, and souls will be converted.

Christ, our divine Teacher, and the greatest Medical Missionary that ever trod this earth, came to our world at great sacrifice to show human beings that correct light in which to regard God. He has given His life as our example in all things. I have been instructed that those who in the daily life heed not the instructions of the Bible, do not know God or Christ whom He has sent. Those who have not lived the Scriptures will invent sophistries to occupy the mind and absorb the attention, and teach things that the One who owns man—body, soul, and spirit—has not said should be taught.

Just before His ascension, Christ gave His disciples a wonderful presentation, as recorded in the twenty-eighth chapter of Matthew. This chapter contains instruction that our ministers, our physicians, our youth, and all our church members need to study most earnestly. Those who study this instruction as they should will not dare advocate theories that have no foundation in the Word of God. My brethren and sisters, make the Scriptures, which contain the alpha and the omega of knowledge, your study. All through the Old Testament and the New there are things that are not half understood.

"Jesus came and spake unto them, saying, All power is given unto Me in heaven and in earth. Go ye therefore, and teach all nations, baptizing them in the name of the Father, and of the Son, and of the Holy Ghost: teaching them to observe all things whatsoever I have commanded you: and, lo, I am with you always, even unto the end of the world." (Matthew 28:19, 20)

The giving of this message is our work in the world. Those of our people who are living in large centers, would gain a precious experience, if, with their Bibles in their hands, and their hearts open to the impressions of the Holy Spirit, they would go forth to the highways and by-ways of the world with the message they have received. There is aggressive work to be done. Evangelistic work, opening the Scriptures to others, warning men and women of what is coming upon the world, is to occupy more and still more of the time of God's servants.

Regarding the messages he had written out, John the Revelator declared: "I testify unto every man that heareth the words of the prophecy of this book, If any man shall add unto these things,"—to lessen the force of their meaning—"God shall add unto him the plagues that are written in this book." Many will make the words of the Revelation a spiritualistic mystery, robbing them {83} of their solemn import. God declares that His judgments shall fall with increased dreadfulness upon anyone who shall try to change the solemn words written in this book—the Revelation of Jesus Christ. "Blessed is he that readeth, and they that hear the words of this prophecy, and keep those things which are written therein; for the time is at hand." "If any man shall take away from the words of the book of this prophecy, God shall take away his part out of the book of life, and out of the holy city, and from the things which are written in this book. He which testifieth these things saith, Surely I come quickly. Amen. Even so, come, Lord Jesus." (Revelation 22:19, 20)

"Know ye not, that to whom ye yield yourselves servants to obey, his servants ye are to whom ye obey." Study these words. Study the instruction found in Matthew 25:14-46. Compare this instruction with your life-record. Let every man put away his boasting. Self-sufficiency is a fearfully dangerous thing for anyone to entertain. It leads men to make of no effect the words of Christ.

Let us walk in the footsteps of Christ, in all the humility of true faith. Let us put away all self-trust, committing ourselves, day by day and hour by hour, to the Saviour, constantly receiving and imparting His grace. I beg those who profess to believe in Christ to walk humbly before God. Pride and self-exaltation are an offense to Him. "If any man will come after Me," Christ declares, "let him deny himself, and take up his cross, and follow Me." Those only who obey this word will He recognize as His believing ones. "As many as received Him ,to them gave He power to become the sons of God, even to them that believe on His name; which were born, not of blood, nor of the will of the flesh, nor of the will of man, but of God. (John 1:12-14)

"And the Word was made flesh, and dwelt among us." Oh, wonderful condescension! The Prince of heaven, the Commander of the heavenly hosts, stepped down from His high position, laid aside His royal robe and kingly crown, and clothed His divinity with humanity, that He might become the divine Teacher of all classes of men, and live before human beings a life free from all selfishness and sin, setting them an example of what, through His grace, they may become.

"The Word was made flesh, and dwelt among us, (and we beheld His glory, the glory as of the only begotten of the Father,) full of grace and truth." Praise God for this wonderful statement! The possibilities that it presents seem almost too great for us to grasp, and put to shame our weakness and our unbelief. Let us praise God that we can see our Saviour by faith. Let us grasp the great gift. Our only hope in this life is to reach forth the hand of faith, and grasp the hand outstretched to save. Daily we are to "behold the Lamb of God, which taketh away the sin of the world." If we would look away from self to Jesus, making him our guide, the world would see in our churches a power that it does not now see.

(Signed) Ellen G. White

REMARKS MADE BY MRS. E. G. WHITE

May 22, 1904
Berrien Springs, Michigan {84}

WE MAY FIND VALUABLE instruction in the words of Christ: "If thou bring thy gift to the altar, and there rememberest that thy brother hath ought against thee; leave there thy gift before the altar, and go thy way; first be reconciled to thy brother, and then come and offer thy gift." (Matthew 5:23, 24)

In moving the College from Battle Creek and establishing it in Berrien Springs, Brethren Magan and Sutherland have acted in harmony with the light that God gave. They have worked hard under great difficulties. Upon the school there was a heavy burden of debt that they had not created. They labored and toiled and sacrificed in their endeavor to carry out right lines of education. And God has been with them. He has approved of their efforts.

But who has appreciated the work that has been done in this place? Many have taken an attitude of opposition, and have spoken words that have made it hard to carry forward the work. Wicked prejudice and false accusations have been met. With some there has been a settled disposition to complain and to find fault with those who have striven with all their might to carry out the Lord's instruction.

Sister Magan worked with her husband, struggling and praying that he might be sustained. And God did sustain them, as they walked in the light. From her small store of money, Sister Magan gave five hundred dollars, to erect the Memorial Hall. She strove untiringly to maintain a perfect home government, teaching and educating her children in the fear of

God. Twice she had to nurse her husband through an attack of fever.

But it seemed to her as though some of our brethren had not a heart of flesh. After the General Conference in Oakland, a report was circulated that Sister White had turned against Brother Magan. There was not a word of truth to this statement. But his poor wife, who had toiled and sacrificed and prayed with him was informed that Sister White had taken a stand against her husband. O why did anyone ever say such a thing? Sister White never turned against Brother Magan or against Brother Sutherland. But Sister Magan was so weighted down with sorrow that she lost her reason.

I ask, Who, in the day of judgment, will be held responsible for putting out the light of that mind, that should be shining today? Who will be accountable in the day of God for the work that caused the distress which brought on this sickness? She suffered for months, and the husband suffered with her. And now the poor woman has gone, leaving two motherless children. All this, because of the work done by unsanctified tongues.

Her husband has the comfort of the promise, "Blessed are the dead which die in the Lord." Sister Magan was a Christian. She was one of Christ's followers, and He loved her. Her works do follow her.

You see the work that has been established here. You see that {85} advancement has been made, and that the education has been carried forward in right lines. This work of opposition and dissatisfaction has come from the devil. It has cost the life of a wife and mother. But it has not taken away her crown of eternal life, nor hindered her from receiving the commendation, "Well done, good and faithful servant, . . . enter thou into the joy of thy Lord."

I would say to Brethren Magan and Sutherland, God has looked with pleasure upon you as you have struggled through the difficulties you have had to meet here. Now the work has reached a point where you can go to labor elsewhere. You have written to me that you had a burden to work in the Southern field. There is plenty of room for you there. They are in need of more workers. They need school-teachers, they need managers. We have been looking and praying for men to take up the work there, and we are glad that God has opened the way for you to work in that field.

And to our brethren I can say, Brother Sutherland and Brother Magan do not

go out from this place as men who have made a failure, but as men who have made a success. They have taught the students from the Bible, according to the light given through the Testimonies. The students that have been with them need not be ashamed of the education they have received.

To the students I would say, You are to let your teachers go willingly. They have had a hard battle here, but they have made a success, and as they leave, the Lord will go with them. His arms will be beneath them. If they will follow on to know the Lord, they shall know that His going forth is prepared as the morning. Let the teachers and students who remain take hold of the work in the name of the Lord. Do not be discouraged or depressed.

The burdens here have rested heavily upon Brother Magan. He has not yet fully recovered from the effects of the long fever. He should be allowed to rest for at least one year, that he may have opportunity to regain his strength.

Brethren and sisters, has there not been among us enough of this work of criticizing and accusing? Think you that you can carry this spirit with you to the heavenly courts? You might far better have been praying; you might far better have been doing the work of the Lord, than trying to discourage those who were endeavoring to carry out the educational principles that God had presented before them. Now let there be a thorough examination of your past lives. And wherever you see that you have in any way taken advantage of one of your brethren, repent of it, and make it right.

I speak the truth as God has presented it to me. Sister Magan died as a martyr, right among her own brethren. My brethren, this work of hurting one another does not pay. May God help you to cleanse your hearts from this evil thing. Ask pardon of God, and ask pardon of those whom you have wronged. Soon it will be too late for wrongs to be made right, and while we have a little opportunity granted us, let us, O let us right every wrong.

Everyone is to be judged in the courts of heaven according to the deeds that are done in the body. And this work of oppressing {86} souls, of making the work doubly hard for others will make a very poor showing in the books of heaven. Shall we not cease this work? We need sanctified tongues, we need lips touched by a live coal from the altar. Our voices should give forth melody. When you speak to those who are in discouragement, let them know that they have your sympathy. How much better to speak kind and tender and loving words than words that will bruise and wound the soul! Will you remember that these souls are the purchase of the blood of Christ? He says, As ye do these things unto one of the least of these, my brethren, ye do them unto Me. They are Christ's property, and we want to lift them up, that they may be in health, in courage, in faith, in hope.

Let us seek the Lord. Let us seek Him as we go from this meeting. Let us make a covenant with Him by sacrifice. God longs to meet us here. He does not want us to go away as we are now. He wants every soul to melt into tenderness before Him, that He may bestow His rich blessing upon us. Will not you, who have been accusing your brethren, come off Satan's ground? Will you not learn to speak words that will encourage? It will not blister your tongue to speak words of tenderness and kindness. It will do you good. It will encourage in you the spirit that should dwell in you. Gather with Christ, but do not, by word or action, discourage those who are putting to the strain every nerve and muscle to carry out the work that God has directed to be done.

Let us humble ourselves before God, lest He shall punish us for our course of action in these things. We want to walk humbly with God, and let the spirit of kindness reign in our lives. Let affection and love be cultivated. Let the sweet spirit of Christ come in and abide with us. When you sit together with Christ in heavenly places, let me tell you, you will reveal in your countenances the very light of heaven.

If Brethren Sutherland and Magan shall leave Berrien Springs, and I believe it is their duty to go, I beg of you, for Christ's sake, not to follow them with criticism and fault-finding. And take right hold to help and strengthen whoever comes in here to take their place.

Several times, even before they took up the work in Berrien Springs, Brethren Magan and Sutherland expressed to me their burden for the work in the South. Their hearts are there. Do not blame them for going. Do not put any impediments in their way. Let them go, and may God go with them, and may His blessing attend them. They will take with them from this place many pleasant memories of seasons of peace and joy. There have been times of sorrow, but they do not go because of this. They think that they can better glorify God by going to a new field. This is their own choice; I have not persuaded them. They did not know but what Sister White would stand in their way. But when they laid the matter before me this morning, I told them that I would not hinder them for one moment. Anyone who takes up work in the South has before him a hard battle. The work there should be far in advance of what it is now. We should encourage the men who go there, and hold them up by our faith and by our prayers.

In the South also, our brethren have had to work under a spirit {87} of fault-finding and accusing. I say these things to you now, that you may realize that you are not called by God to say depressing things, or to manifest a spirit of coldness and indifference to those who go to carry burdens in the South. We hope that you will remember these words, and that the terrible history of the past may not be repeated.

For over twenty years, the work of the Southern field has been held up before you, but you have not done for the work what should have been done. There is a large field there, and the burden of sustaining the laborers in this field belongs to the people of America.

If any of the students and workers here desire to go with Brother Magan and Brother Sutherland, let them go and help them to carry the light to those who have never heard the truth, to a class of people that has been suffering with neglect and poverty. I know that Brother Haskell and Brother Butler will be glad to have the help of Brethren Magan and Sutherland, and will unite with them in the work of God. They will have a hard time of it at the best, but if God is with them, they may know that He will sustain them.

(Signed) Ellen G. White

EXTRACTS FROM A RECENT COMMUNICATION ON SCHOOL

Received September 17, 1897{88}

WE HAVE LABORED HARD to keep in check everything in the school like favoritism, attachments, and courting. We have told the students that we would not allow the first thread of this to be interwoven with their school work. On this point we were as firm as a rock. I told them that they must dismiss all idea of forming attachments while at school. The young ladies must keep themselves to themselves, and the young gentlemen must do the same. The school was established at a great expense, both of time and labor, to enable students to obtain an all-round education, that they might gain knowledge of agriculture, a knowledge of the common branches of education, and above all, a knowledge of the word of God.

Those whom the Lord has presented to me as not being properly trained in the home life, who have not thought it necessary to use the powers of their mind and their physical strength and ingenuity as members of the home firm, will always look upon order and discipline as needless restraint and severity. Again and again the Lord has presented this matter before me in clear lines. The teachers must be carefully picked. No haphazard work must be done in the appointment of teachers. Those who have devoted years to study, and yet have not gained the education essential to fit them to teach others, in the lines the Lord has marked out, should not be connected with our schools as educators. They need to be taught the first principles of true, all-around education.

We are living in solemn times, and the reason why there are so many failures in our schools is because teachers neglect to keep the way of the Lord. Some teachers feel the burden and carry the load of responsibility. Others do surface work. They fail to see that the woeful influence of this deficiency is seen in the words and deportment of their students. This influence counter-works the influence that God-fearing teachers, who aim to meet the high standard of Christian education, seek.

I would that the teachers in our schools could be of God's selection and appointment. Souls will be lost because of the careless work of professedly Christian teachers, who need to be taught of God day by day, else they are unfit for the position of trust. Teachers are needed who will strive to weed out their inherited and cultivated tendencies to wrong, who will come into line, wearing themselves the yoke of obedience, and thus giving an example to the students. The sense of duty to their God, and to their fellow-beings, with whom they associate, will lead such teachers to become doers of the word, and to heed counsel as to how they should conduct themselves.

God holds everyone responsible for the influence that surrounds his soul, on his own account, and on the account of others. He calls upon young men and young women to be strictly temperate and conscientious in the use of their faculties of mind and body. Their capabilities can be developed only by the diligent use and {89} wise appropriation of their powers to the glory of God and the benefit of their fellow-men.

To know what constitutes purity of mind, soul, and body is the highest class of education. Paul the apostle sums up in his letter to Timothy the attainments possible for him, by saying, "Keep thyself pure." Impurity of thought or action will never be seen in the child of God. The body is represented as the temple of the Holy Spirit. Every encouragement and the richest blessings are held up before the overcomers of evil practices, but the most fearful penalties are laid upon those who profane the body and defile the soul.

Students and teachers, Blessed are the pure in heart—now; not, Blessed will be the pure in heart. "Blessed are the pure in heart: for they shall see God." Yes, as did Moses, they shall endure the seeing of Him who is invisible. They have the assurance of the richest blessings, both in this life and in the life that is to come.

Avoid exciting the brain. Too much study stimulates the brain and increases the flow of blood to it. The sure result of this is depravity. The brain cannot be unduly excited without producing impure thoughts and actions. The whole nervous system is affected, and this leads to impurity. The physical and mental powers are depraved, and the temple of the Holy Spirit is defiled. The evil practices are communicated, and the consequences cannot be estimated. I am compelled to speak plainly on this subject.

The proportionate taxation of the powers of mind and body will prevent the tendency to impure thoughts and actions. Teachers should understand this. They should teach students that pure thoughts and actions are dependent on the way in which they conduct their studies. Conscientious actions are dependent on conscientious thinking. Exercise in agricultural pursuits, and in the various branches of labor is a wonderful safeguard against undue brain taxation. No man, woman, or child who fails to use all the powers God has given him can retain his health. He cannot conscientiously keep the commandments of God. He cannot love God supremely and his neighbor as himself.

Many whom God has qualified to do excellent work by giving them powers to use to his glory, accomplish little because they attempt little. Thousands who come into the world pass through life as though they had no definite object for which to live, no standard to reach. Such will obtain a reward proportionate to their works. Health and a clear conscience will attend those who work faithfully keeping the glory of God in view. There are many who are mere fragments of men. In Christ is seen the perfection of Christian character. He is our Pattern. His life was not a life of indolence or ease. He lived not to please Himself. He was the Son of the infinite God, yet He worked at the carpenter's trade with His father. As a member of the home firm, He faithfully acted His part in helping to support the family.

All are capable of using their talents in God's service. God asks them only to do their best. Those who study the life of {90} Christ and yoke up with Him, will not use the brain only, but will reason from cause to effect, and will use every part of the human machinery. The Lord designs that useful labor shall compose a part of every man's life.

The flood of corruption that is sweeping over our world is the result of the misuse and abuse of the human machinery. Men, women, and children should be educated to labor with their hands. Then the brain will not be overtaxed, to the detriment of the whole organism. Time is a talent, to be wisely employed. The voice is a talent, to be used in communicating knowledge that will make men pure, holy, and refined. The tongue should be educated to speak in such a manner that God will be magnified. "Lord, increase my faith," will be the prayer of the true child of God. "Deliver me from evil thoughts and perverse actions." Thus he is enabled to say with boldness, "Behold, God is my salvation: I will trust and not be afraid. For the Lord Jehovah is my strength and my song; he also is become my salvation." Completeness of Christian character is possible. How?—"We are complete in Him."

MR. G. W. AMADON

September 12, 1910
(A.-74-1910)
Sanitarium, Napa Co., California {91}
Battle Creek, Michigan

Dear Brother Amadon:

WE HAVE HEARD OF THE calamity that overtook you during the Battle Creek camp meeting, in the wrecking of the large tent. This news does not surprise us; for the prince of the power of the air will do strange things in his efforts to hinder God's people; and much more in the future than he has in the past.

I have been surprised that we have seen so little of the working and manifestation of his wrath. I have seen that just such things as have happened at the Battle Creek camp meeting will take place again. As Lucifer sees that we are making efforts to work the cities as if we meant to give the last message, his wrath will be aroused, and he will employ every device in his power to hinder the work.

Lucifer was cast out of heaven because he was fully determined to have a position above that of Christ. He could not obtain what he coveted, and there was war in heaven, and he was cast out.

Satanic agencies have held control at Battle Creek, and as I read the account of your experience, I was not at all surprised; for I realize that many more such things will take place. As the cities are worked by the Lord's messengers, there will be many strange revelations, but we are to go straight forward, heeding them not.

Take the case of Job. See how Satan was permitted to show himself and his indignation against God's servant. In the future we shall see more of the violence described in the Bible. But we must not be surprised, as though some strange thing happened unto us. As special victories are gained in the work of arousing our people to a sense of their true position, Satan will reveal himself.

We were greatly blessed during our camp meeting at Berkeley. We had an exceptionally favorable location, and this I appreciated. Sara and I had rooms in a house just across the road from the campground. My room was opposite the large pavilion. I had only to walk across the street, go a short distance further, and I was in the tent. I was thankful that it was so little trouble for me to get to the speakers' stand.

Brother Crisler and his family and Willie had a cottage in the back yard of the house we occupied. It was very favorable for me to be so near my workers.

The camp meeting was carried through with success, and no accidents occurred. The attendance at the meeting was large. I solicited an opportunity to speak on the last day of the meeting, when I read and explained some writings that will be of great consequence to those who will accept them. These writings I was deeply impressed {92} to present. By faith we must grasp more firmly the words unfailing truth.

About a week after returning from the camp meeting, I visited the Pacific Union College, where a special meeting was then being held by the teachers of the church schools in this conference. Sara and I left our home for the College on Friday morning, taking the longer route, because the short one is rocky, and at this time of the year very dusty. The long road is about ten miles, four miles farther round than the short route, but it is an excellent road, ascending the mountain gradually. We suffered little annoyance from the dust, but it is a drive of two and a half hours, and a continual ascent, and on reaching the school I felt very weary.

Notwithstanding my weariness, I spoke to a full house the following morning. The Lord gave me freedom of speech, and I spoke for about an hour, The following words, which were on my mind. I spoke to the people:

Entering the Cities: Again and again I am instructed to present to our churches in every place the work that should be done, not only where we have churches already established, but in new fields, where the truth has never been fully established. In our cities, as verily as in far-off lands, there are people of all nationalities, whose souls are precious, and who must hear the message. The way must be opened to reach those unworked fields. Decided work must be done, openings must be made.

Those of our ministers who, Sabbath after Sabbath, preach to the same ones, accomplish very little. If they were wide awake, their words would make a decided impression and souls would be enlightened and led to accept the truth.

It is impossible for man to measure the ingenuity shown by Satan in deceiving human minds. As Christ saw the working out of Satan's plans to deceive man in many ways, He gladly came to our world as an infant, to live in this world, to meet the wily foe in every stage of human life, and to counterwork his Satanic wiles. No one could understand as Christ did the enemy's power of deception. He saw that the world was being captivated by the delusive power exercised through commercialism of various kinds. He came to take human nature, and to stay this overwhelming power of deception, which was leading souls to their ruin.

Thus was laid the plan for Christ to act His part as a Saviour. He came to our world to live, and suffer, and die, that He might win to God the souls deceived by Satan. He is wise in an understanding of the tempter's plans, and He can teach men and women how to become wise to discern and to escape the corruption that Satan is constantly inventing.

Christ declared, I have pledged Myself, as the only begotten Son of the Lord God Almighty, to carry out God's plan to win souls from Satan to the Lord's side. Christ alone can defeat the enemy. He works in man's behalf to uncover his plans, that souls may be led to turn from the arch-deceiver.

(Signed) Ellen G. White

DEAR BROTHER AMADON

January 15, 1906
(1906-7)
Sanitarium, California {93}

I HAVE RECEIVED YOUR LETTER. I will send you copies of things taken from my diaries. These articles contain presentations and instructions given me, point by point. For instance, the evening after the Sabbath I retired, and rested well without ache or pain until half past ten. I was unable to sleep. I had received instruction, and I seldom lie in bed after such instruction comes. There was a company assembled in Battle Creek, and instruction was given by One in our midst that I was to repeat and repeat with pen and voice. I left my bed, and wrote for five hours as fast as my pen could trace the lines. Then I rested on the bed for an hour, and slept part of the time.

I placed the matter in the hands of my copyist, and on Monday morning it was waiting for me, placed inside my office door on Sunday evening. There were four articles ready for me to read over, and make any corrections needed. The matter is now prepared, and some of it will go in the mail today.

This is the line of work that I am carrying on. I do most of my writing while the other members of the family are asleep. I build my fire, and then write uninterruptedly, sometimes for hours. I write while others are asleep. Who then has told Sister White? A messenger that is appointed.

If Elder Daniells is in Battle Creek, please place in his hands the manuscripts I send you. I have my work to do, to meet the misconceptions of those who suppose themselves able to say what is testimony from God and what is human production. If those who have done this work continue in this course, Satanic agencies will choose for them. At the Berrien Springs meeting, the richest blessing was proffered them. This blessing they could have had if they had let Christ help them, confessing their wicked obstinacy. But they refused to take the right course. The holy angels turned away, and evil angels have been holding sway over minds. Evil angels obtained the victory at that meeting. But there is no need for me to give the particulars of this.

If Brother Daniells is not in Battle Creek, please read to the church what I am sending you. I have many letters to write, and I cannot add more to this now. There is just one thing the Lord calls for, and that is, for every man, minister, or physician, or lay member, to confess his own sins. Each one will have a hard battle to fight with his own perverse self. Those who have stood directly in the way of the people, having a clear realization of their perilous condition, will have an account to settle with God. Those who have helped souls to feel at liberty to specify what is of God in the Testimonies, and what are the uninspired words of Sister White, will find that they were helping the devil in his work of deception. Please read Testimony No. 33, p. 211, "How to Receive Reproof." (Or, Testimonies, Vol. 5, p. 683).

(Signed) Ellen G. White

MY DEAR BROTHER OLSEN

May 26, 1896
"Sunnyside," Cooranbong, N. S. W. {94}
Elder O. A. Olsen
Review And Herald
Battle Creek, Michigan

I RECEIVED THE AMERICAN MAIL on Monday, the 25th, and today, Tuesday, Sister McEnterfer read me a letter of which I send you a copy. Whether this particular case is correct or incorrect, just such scenes have been presented before me.

I have written to Brother_____ in reference to himself and his responsibilities. He was answered me in a good humble spirit; and I pray the Lord to strengthen him to resist temptation.

Now, my brother, I want you to make it your first business to investigate, in company with some others of a different spiritual experience than that of_____, and every one of like influence, every man in that office, and that you will make it your special business to inquire of the youth who are employed there in regard to their work. Open your eyes wide to see what needs adjustment and correction.

Less long, sweeping journeys across the continent, and more close investigation of the true inward working of the heart is essential. The rooms in the office need inspection, that the things you know not, you may discern and search out. The temple of God must be cleansed, that His name shall not be dishonored by men who are not connected with Him. My heart is pained as, in my dreams, I am visited, and appealed to by different ones, placing the corruptions in the office of publication before me. I awaken to find it a dream; but know it to be the truth. My dear brother, the spirit of severity, of lording it over the ignorant and helpless, is being opened before me. In the place of the office being an educating school to prepare the youth to give their hearts to the Lord, the teachers and overseers, by their course of action, drive them on to Satan's battleground. It is not a place where the Lord Jesus is entertained as a heavenly guest. Some of the overseers, and the workers under their supervision, give little time to thoughts of a high and holy order; the Lord is not glorified.

I wrote some time since in reference to the Oakland office, and then my guide revealed to me that the same spirit, in a more decided manner, leavened the office at Battle Creek; and there were souls lost, eternally lost, through the influence of words of severity and of harshness. Things will transpire in our institutions that will need adjustment, and at once; but let the reformation be made with a spirit to restore, not to destroy. We are fearfully behind in the work of Christ for the saving of souls. We have not that sharp conception of duty required by the truth which we profess to love and to honor. We allow a freezing atmosphere to surround our souls; we withhold words that ought to be spoken from the Scriptures. In order to fulfil our duty as God's faithful watchmen, we should give words of correction in humility of mind, {95} "considering thyself, lest thou also be tempted." Neglect not to bind up, with your reproof, words of encouragement. Be cheerful, but not light and trifling; pray for discernment, for a wholesome, Christ-like spirit. Paul, in his letter to the Philippians, said, "And this I pray, that your love may abound yet more and more in knowledge and in all judgment; that you may approve things that are excellent; that ye may be sincere and without offense till the day of Christ; being filled with the fruits of righteousness, which are by Jesus Christ, unto the praise and glory of God." (1:9-11)

Sincerity means much more than many are inclined to suppose. It means being true to your brother; never allowing yourself to do him wrong, or suffer him to be unfaithful in the discharge of his duty.

Those who are set to keep the rooms in a healthful condition, that the angel of God passing through may approve, must be sincere. There must be no haphazard work. Carry the Spirit of Christ in all your dealings. I would not, under any consideration, send a child of mine to learn the printer's trade under the present discipline and management of the several rooms. All are not managed in exactly the same objectionable manner; but all are much in need of the sanctifying grace of Jesus Christ. Are the men set over others, wise counselors of youth? Are they sincere Christians, or make-believers? Is their submission to divine authority as perfect as that they require of the youth who are being educated under them? Overbearing, harsh words are unprofitable in professors of religion. A harsh, tyrannical spirit has come in, resulting in great and various evils. The temptations to sin come to every youth; and the overseers in every room need to be thoroughly converted men. What are the attributes most prized, and which bring greatest joy to the Saviour who died to save sinners? It is to have men and women cooperating with him to seek and to save the lost. Everyone who is self-denying, self-sacrificing, for the sake of helping poor souls that need help, will have his reward. If we are children of God, we should be, and will be, living channels of light.

Those who have not received Christ as their personal Saviour should never be placed as directors of the youth. If they cannot submit themselves to the control of God, they are not qualified to teach order and law to those brought under them. Those who claim to be Christ's disciples, if themselves under discipline to God, will make tender, loving, wise guides and instructors of the youth; for Christ says, "I will manifest myself unto them."(sic)

If we love one another God dwelleth in us, and His love is perfected in us; and that love cannot be restrained. God is love, and he that dwelleth in love, dwelleth in God, and God in him. Only by becoming a partaker of the divine nature can the law of God be fulfilled by men. Only he who loves God with all the heart, soul, mind, and strength, and his neighbor as himself, can give glory to God in the highest, and peace on earth, good will to men. This was the work of Christ; and when his work is appreciated and represented by his followers, the great result will be achieved in the "joy that was set before him" in the saving of the souls for whom He gave His life. {96}

The Lord has been laboring constantly from age to age to awaken in the souls of men a sense of their divine brotherhood, and thus to establish an order and divine harmony proportionate to the great and eternal deliverance He has wrought out for everyone who will receive Him. The Lord calls upon all who profess to believe in Him to be co-workers with Him, and to use every God-given ability, opportunity, and privilege to lead perishing souls within the sphere of their influence, to Jesus Christ. Here is the only hope for transformation of character; this will give peace and joy in believing, and fit them for the society of the heavenly angels in the kingdom of God. O how earnest, persevering, and untiring should be the efforts of every sin-pardoned soul to seek to bring other souls to Jesus Christ, that their neighbors shall become joint-heirs with Jesus. Whoever is your neighbor is to be sought for, labored for. Is he ignorant? Let your communication, your association, make him more intelligent. The outcast, the youth, full of defects in character, are the very ones God enjoins upon us to help. "I came not to call the righteous," said Christ, "but sinners to repentance."

See what sinners the colored people were, the downtrodden, the poor. These Christ died to save, and they can, through painstaking and judicious management, become trophies of His grace, heirs to God, and joint-heirs with Jesus Christ. Through faith in Jesus Christ they become purified, sanctified; for the religion of Jesus Christ never degrades the receiver, but works with transforming power, refining the taste, sanctifying the judgment, fitting the soul for the entrance of the word that giveth life, that giveth understanding even to the simple. Those who will be humble enough to learn, the very nobility of the world will consider it an honor to go to heaven in their company, and angels of God will cooperate with such as are workers together with God. We need to hunger and thirst after righteousness, that we may have Christ in us as a well of water, springing up into everlasting life.

Right at the head of the work there must be deeper piety, more faithful taking heed to the word of God, a watching for souls as they that must give an account. Each worker should be moved by a living, abiding, converting principle. It is not large establishments where much money is invested to make them more convenient, that will obtain influence and win hearts. The school and the office should be an asylum for the sorely tempted youth. They are God's property. They have hearts to be won; they have souls to save. Instead of spending money in bicycles, in picture-making, in little and great idols to place upon your tables and on your walls, let the means be used to gather in the youth; teach them, and patiently watch over them, in wisdom dealing with their follies. Pray with them alone. Converse with them, with hearts filled with pity and that love which Christ has shown for you. Angels of God will give every true worker a rich experience in doing this work. We are to labor in earnest to break down every barrier that has been built up to keep Christ from entering the citadel of the heart. There is more joy in heaven over one sinner that repenteth than over ninety and nine persons that (think they) need no repentance. Let instructors do their duty patiently, and although they may be often tried, be assured they will not fail {97} nor be discouraged. Be not weary in well-doing; the heavenly intelligences will work with your every effort. A word of love and encouragement will do more to subdue the hasty temper and willful disposition than all the fault-finding and severe censure that you can heap upon the erring ones.

It is those who are in positions of trust, those who have great light, large opportunities, who are not forming characters and carrying into their life practice principles that will stand the test of trial. These need to be rebuked sharply for their influence over the young. The impetuous temper must be eradicated. When provoked do not pour out a torrent of words and commit sin; but talk with your Lord about it. Say to your soul, "Be still, and know that I am God." If the God-given responsibilities of saving souls ready to perish, were understood, old habits, traditional sentiments that clog and hinder reformatory action would be cut away from the heart and life, and a transformation would take place in character. Advice, reproof, and counsel should be given patiently, taking the bitterness of the self-mingling spirit

out of it. The language should not be exaggerated, but should be gentle and humble, The stern, harsh spirit that humiliates and crushes the wrong-doer will seldom work a reformation. "Thy gentleness hath made me great." It sets before the wrong-doer his sins, and helps him to recover himself from the snares of Satan.

God has not set any man on the judgment seat. "Judge not," He said, "that ye be not judged." The grace of humility should be cherished in the heart. It will modify and mold the words that fall from our lips, into expressions of Christ-like tenderness and care. The Master's work is not to be neglected; but it must be done in love, declaring the Master's message in the Master's Spirit.

Wrongs are often in need of being met; and though firmness and decision may be required, it should not be done in an arbitrary overbearing, crushing manner. Not until the heart is cleansed and purified through obedience to the truth can we be laborers together with God, and work with the mind of Christ.

(Signed) Ellen G. White

DEAR BROTHER OLSEN

December 26, 1906
Sanitarium P. O., Napa Co., California {98}

I AM NOT IN THE BEST condition to write to you; for, for the past week I have been suffering from my third attack of influenza this winter. I have been having special treatment for this disease, and am now improving.

We see in our world confusion upon confusion. We hear of accidents by sea and by land. Crime is increasing, this we know from the reports of our daily newspapers. Political developments in San Francisco are of a character to show how little confidence can be placed in the men who occupy official positions. Many of these men, some even who profess to be religious, are being exposed before the public as guilty of various crimes. They are giving evidence that it is time for the Lord of heaven to destroy their property. The last great issue is soon to come. We must see, we must understand, that the spirit of God is being withdrawn from the wicked nations who have long discarded God's work, His holy law, and have formed false theories and false laws, exalting them above the commandments of God.

The signs are certainly fulfilling that show that the end of this earth's history is

near; and we have an individual work to do in fitting ourselves to sound the last message of warning to our world, and prepare it for the closing scenes which according to the word of God, are soon to come. I feel deeply the need of every worker to stand as faithful watchmen to give this last note of warning, to prepare the church that those who have had the light may be awake, realizing the importance of keeping every piece of the armor on.

"This know also, that in the last days perilous times shall come. For men shall be lovers of their own selves, covetous, boasters, proud, blasphemers, disobedient to parents, unthankful, unholy, without natural affection, truce-breakers, false accusers, incontinent, fierce, despisers of those that are good, traitors, heady, highminded, lovers of pleasures more than lovers of God; from such turn away; having a form of godliness, but denying the power thereof. Ever learning (ever presenting some new theory) but never able to come to a knowledge of the truth." (2 Timothy 3:1-7)

This whole chapter is being fulfilled in San Francisco and Oakland at the present time. These cities, through their newspapers, are daily opening to us their true condition, the iniquity of their high officials. The very men who are placed in office to suppress evil are themselves corrupted with all kinds of evil works.

"As Jannes and Jambres withstood Moses, so do these also resist the truth; men of corrupt minds; reprobate concerning the faith. But they shall proceed no farther; for their folly shall be manifest unto all men, as theirs also was." We have been given this example in Bible History to teach us that God will vindicate His word and fulfil His holy purpose. (2 Timothy 3:8, 9)

By way of contrast the apostle presents the opposite condition {99} of morals that will exist among those who are faithful in their service for keeping the law of God. "Thou hast fully known my doctrine, manner of life, purpose, faith, longsuffering, charity, patience, persecutions, afflictions, which came into me at Antioch, at Iconium, at Lystra; what persecutions I endured." Then for our encouragement he sounds the glad word, "Out of them all the Lord delivered me. Yea, and all that will live godly in Christ Jesus shall suffer persecution. But evil men and seducers shall wax worse and worse, deceiving and being deceived. But continue thou in the things which thou hast learned, and hast been assured of, knowing of whom thou hast learned them; and that from a child thou hast known the holy Scriptures, which are able to make thee wise unto salvation through faith which is in Christ Jesus. All scripture is given by inspiration of God, and is profitable for doctrine, for reproof, for correction, for instruction in righteousness, that the man of God may be perfect, thoroughly furnished unto all good works." Read also Paul's solemn charge to Timothy in the fourth chapter of second Timothy.

The time spent by the officials of San Francisco in investigating the frauds of some of their officers has been, in the providence of God, a precious opportunity for Brethren Simpson and Hibbard to present the truth to large congregations in the city of Oakland. Before these brethren began their series of meetings, Elder Haskell and wife were holding meetings in the large tent in Oakland, following up the work of the camp meeting, and instruction (classes) some who wished to learn how to do Bible work. This was a successful meeting. The Lord manifested His power and grace. Elder Hibbard assisted Elder Haskell in his work, speaking at the evening meetings. This brought the truth before the people of Oakland in clear lines; and the work was continued until Elder Simpson commenced his tent effort.

Brother Simpson's meetings were largely attended, and the people listened to his words with spellbound interest; the interest continued from first to last. With his Bible in his hand, and basing all his arguments on the word of God, Brother Simpson traced out before them the prophecies of Daniel and Revelation. His own words were few; he made the Scriptures themselves explain the truth to the people. After giving them the truth, Elder Simpson would draw an expression of opinion from his congregation. "Now," he would say, "those who see the truth of what I am saying, raise your hands;" and in response many hands would be raised. I can only poorly represent to you the interest his work has created.

In his teaching, Elder Simpson showed that the Spirit of prophecy has an important part to act in the establishment of the truth. When binding off his work, he called for me to go to Oakland to speak to the people.

When the call came, I had just begun to recover from an attack of influenza; but I said, I will go. This was the first time for four weeks that I had left my home premises. We left St. Helena on Thursday after-

noon. On Friday I was very ill; nevertheless I spoke on the Sabbath in the Congregational church in which our people usually meet for their Sabbath worship. Between four and five hundred people were assembled. I was feeling weak from my illness; but I prayed that God would help me. As soon as I began {100} to speak, the reviving influence of the Spirit of God came upon me, and I was strengthened. I spoke one hour and fifteen minutes with a clear voice; for the power of His grace was upon me. I was very thankful for this evidence of the power of the Spirit of God.

On Sunday I rode several miles to the Baths, where Elder Simpson baptized thirty-one candidates. The service was beautifully conducted, and everything passed off with perfect order. The songs interspersed through the service seemed to be carrying the joyful news to heaven. As many more persons will be baptized in about four weeks' time; for all were not fully prepared to go forward in this ordinance at that time. My heart is filled with gratitude for this representation of those who have received the truth under the teaching of Elder Simpson.

I have also spoken in the meeting house in San Francisco which James White and I and a few others were the means of establishing there. The house was preserved through the San Francisco fire, and only slightly injured. The chimneys were thrown down, and some of the plaster shaken off.

The work is still being carried forward in San Francisco and Oakland; for souls must be warned. Now is our time and opportunity, while these revelations of dishonesty and fraudulent transactions are being made. While these people have these things brought daily before their notice, the reasonable arguments of the word of God, its predictions that just such practices will be carried on in every city, will appeal to their minds and consciences better than would any language we could use to represent the existing evil and point out their meaning. Elder Simpson will take up his work again in about two weeks' time, and after that he will labor in San Francisco. The truth is being proclaimed in these cities as it has never been before. We feel that now is our time to work, just now. We must unite, be united in the work, and press together.

My workers are now engaged in preparing my diaries of my experience in Europe and Australia. We want to prepare

this matter for book publication, that the people may understand the character of the work the Lord has given me to do for the last half century.

I am of good courage in the Lord, and I praise His holy name for this.

(Signed) Ellen G. White

DEAR CHILDREN
February 6, 1894
George's Terrace {101}
Mr. and Mrs. J. E. White

SINCE THE CAMP MEETING WE have settled down in the school building. We are very pleasantly situated in the second story of terrace no. 3. I have a very large room with three ample windows. I sleep in this room, and have plenty of air. The next apartment is the dining room, pleasant and roomy. May sleeps alone in that room. Sister Tuxford and May do the cooking in still another room. We go down a half-a-dozen steps from the dining room, then up two or three steps; first we come to the bath room, then to the kitchen with a gas stove, then to still another room, where Sister Tuxford and Emily sleep and Emily does her work. Our family consists of Sister Tuxford, Marian, Emily, May, and myself. Here we are, well settled, to remain only six weeks; then we must be emptied out, for the fall term of school begins.

I am getting to be very tired of moving. It worries me out, settling and unsettling, gathering up Manuscripts and scattering them, to be gathered up again. If I should look to my poor, finite self, I should soon become discouraged; but in looking unto Jesus, the Author and Finisher of my faith, I take courage, and press forward with His name on my lips to the mark for the prize of the high calling which is in Christ Jesus. If we at times feel our infirmities encompassing us, and a discouragement comes upon us, we must look away from self unto Jesus, and pray for spiritual eyesight. We need it now, in order to understand His word. A flood of light is poured into the chambers of the mind and the soul temple that we may understand the scriptures. There is truth, precious, sacred truth. "The entrance of thy words giveth light; it giveth understanding to the simple." All who are simple (meek and lowly in heart) will humble self, and seek counsel of the Lord in His Holy word. Feeling is nothing reliable, but the word is solid rock. We can safely study our Bibles, and the Holy Spirit will impress our minds and heart.

The Lord has a work for you to do, and if you listen to His voice, you will not be left in darkness. The Saviour says, "My sheep hear my voice, and I know them, and they follow me." "And a stranger will they not follow; for they know not the voice of strangers." I am sure that the Lord is revealing to you the perfection and fullness of the atoning work, that your whole heart may be filled with love and thanksgiving, and that you may reveal to others that which the Lord is revealing to you. The image of Christ engraved upon the heart is reflected in character, in practical life, day by day, because we represent a personal Saviour. The Holy Spirit is promised to all who will ask for it. When you search the scriptures, the Holy Spirit is by your side, personating Jesus Christ. The truth is a living principle made to shine in precious clearness to the understanding, and then, O then, it is time to speak words from the Living Christ. "Ye are laborers together with God." Christ said to the woman of Samaria, "If thou knowest the gift of God, and who it is that said to thee, Give me to drink; thou wouldest have asked of him, and he would have given thee living water. . . A well of {102} water springing up into everlasting life." Those who have the out pouring of the gospel of Christ which comes from the heart imbued by His Holy Spirit will give light and comfort and hope to hearts that are hungering and thirsting for righteousness. It is not excitement we wish to create, but deep, earnest consideration, that those who hear shall do solid work, real, sound, genuine work that will be enduring as eternity. We hunger not for excitement, for the sensational; the less we have of this, the better. The calm, earnest reasoning from the scriptures is precious and fruitful. Here is the secret of success, in preaching a living, personal Saviour in so simple and earnest a manner that the people may be able to lay hold by faith of the power of the word of life. Present not Anna Phillips' productions, but the truth, substantiated by the authority of the living word, which is the power of God unto salvation.

My dear Son Edson, I am deeply interested in your experience, and I hope you will trust in the Lord continually. I hope you will not allow your feelings to control you. God has given you a work to do; be faithful to your Redeemer. God can open the way before you, he can place your feet in safe paths, and lead you on to victory. We want to understand daily the meaning of these words: "Turned to God." Here are true holiness, rest and peace, grace and glory. Turn not to any living man to be your helper. Tell everything to Jesus. He knows all the bearings, all the results of every purpose and every plan. His wisdom is unerring, and He has given evidence how much He loves His purchased possession, and how willing, how gratified He is to help His children, to guide them in judgment. My God shall supply all your need, according to His riches in glory by Jesus Christ.

Then come to Jesus although you feel your unworthiness. The life of simple dependence upon God is a daily lesson in knowing God and Jesus Christ whom He hath sent. "He that spared not his own Son, but delivered him up for us all, how shall he not with him also freely give us all things?" The voice of invitation is, "Come unto me, all ye that labor and are heavy laden, and I will give you rest. Take my yoke upon you, and learn of me; for I am meek and lowly in heart: and ye shall find rest unto your souls. For my yoke is easy, and my burden is light." To God, only to God, pour out the sorrows, the great needs and troubles of your soul. He will help you. "My soul, wait thou only upon God; for my expectation is from him. He only is my rock and my salvation; he is my defense; I shall not be moved." (Psalms 62:5, 6)

Under the showers of the latter rain the inventions of man, the human machinery, will at times be swept away, the boundary of man's authority will be as broken reeds, and the Holy Spirit will speak through the living, human agent with convincing power. No one then will watch to see if the sentences are well rounded off, if the grammar is faultless. The living water will flow in God's own channels. But let us be careful now not to exalt the men, their sayings and doings; and let not any one consider it a grand point to have a startling experience to relate; for here is a fruitful field where credence will be given to unworthy persons. Young men and women will be lifted up, and will regard themselves as wonderfully favored, called to do some great thing. There will be conversions many, after a peculiar order but they will not bear the divine signature. Immorality will come in and extravagance and {103} many will make shipwreck of faith. Our only safety is in keeping fast hold of Jesus. Never are we to lose sight of Him. He says, "Without me ye can do nothing." We must cultivate an abiding sense of our own inefficiency and helplessness and rely wholly on Jesus. This should keep us individually calm and steadfast in words and deportment. Excitement in the speaker is not power but weakness. Earnestness and energy are essential in presenting Bible truth, the gospel, which is the power of God unto salvation.

March 16, I am unable to sleep this morning, and arise from my bed at two o'clock to write to you, my dear children. In the last letter that I sent you I made suggestions in reference to your coming to this country, but I fear that our course of action will be such that it will not be advisable at present. Your plans in reference to working for the colored people are, I believe, correct. But, Edson, do not gather responsibilities upon yourself. The enemy will seek to get you involved in plans and in inventions that will embarrass you. Take up the work in some line where you can work to a purpose. The talent God has given you in the ability to comprehend the truths of His word is a precious gift. If your opportunities are improved, your mind will be led into fruitful study, to an intelligent understanding of the grand, elevating, sanctifying truths for this time, and you can bless others in your work.

The Lord evidently designs to cut you clear from any earthly dependence and to teach you the precious lessons of entire trust in Him. The Holy Spirit has been grieved that you have not surrendered your will to God's will, and years have passed into eternity, that might have been rich in good works for the saving of souls. I wish I could communicate all that is in my mind upon some points, but today the mail leaves for America, and I have not been able to write as much as I desired. Since I came to Melbourne the work has been pressing urgently upon me. I have spoken in Brighton and in Williams-town, where the interest is excellent, and the field ripe for the harvest. The weather has been very warm, and it has been taxing to speak under the tent, but I have reason to praise my heavenly Father that he grants me so largely of His Holy Spirit, that I can continue to bear the message of His grace and love in demonstration of His Spirit. The congregations listen with profound interest. Should I not praise God for this with heart and soul and voice?

In Brighton several have taken their position on the Sabbath. In Williamstown also some have decided to obey the truth. There was not a Sabbath-keeper in the place when the tent was set up there, but the interest has steadily increased since camp meeting, several are now in the valley of decision. I speak in the hall in that place next Sunday afternoon. O my son, I pray for the Lord to work in His own way upon the minds of the people, that a healthy church may be raised up in Williamstown. Already the matter of erecting a church building in this place is under serious consideration. It can be done, and must be done at once. Besides laboring for these who are just hearing the truth, we find work to do in setting things in order among ourselves, that the machinery may run without friction.

Edson, I feel a deep interest for your prosperity, and I know that your only safe course is to break away from every business transaction, and put your mind and soul into the exposition of the word. Be determined that you will not fail nor be discouraged. If you trust {104} in the Lord moment by moment, if you search the scriptures with earnest prayer, you will have opened to you the richest treasures from the word of God. In humility, as a learner in the school of Christ, you will learn His meekness and lowliness of heart. God is more willing to give the Holy Spirit to them that ask Him than parents are to give good gifts unto their children. I am sure that there is a heaven full of the richest enduring treasures to be freely given to all who will appropriate them to themselves, and becoming enriched thereby will impart freely to others. I know this to be truth. I have many things to say; my heart is full of thankfulness. I often awake in the night season praising the Lord that He has given me the measure of health I now enjoy, and that His hand, in loving, pitying tenderness, has laid hold upon you, my son, and placed your feet upon the Solid Rock. And in this I see how much can be done in saving other poor souls that are ready to perish.

But there are presented to me dangers and quicksands that must be carefully avoided. While those who are obeying the word in Isaiah, "Cry aloud, spare not, lift up thy voice like a trumpet, and show my people their transgression, and the house of Jacob their sins," in this work so essential to be done, things will be encouraged that will result in marring the work of God, unless the messengers are endowed with heavenly wisdom. We must act like men in earnest. We need to obtain a rich daily experience in prayer; we should be like the importunate widow, who, in her con-

scious need, overcame the unjust judge by the bare force of her determined pleading. God will be enquired of to do these things for us; for this is giving depth and solidity to our experience. The soul that seeks God will need to be in earnest. He is a rewarder of all those that seek him diligently.

There are quicksands upon which many are in danger of being swamped. It is always safe to seek for the earnest of the Spirit of God, if we do not mingle with it a force and presumption that is not heaven born. There is need of caution in all our utterances lest some poor souls of ardent temperament shall work themselves up into a zeal not according to knowledge. They will act as though it was their prerogative to use the Holy Spirit instead of letting the Holy Spirit use them, and mold and fashion them after the Pattern of the divine. There is danger of running ahead of Christ. We should honor the Holy Spirit by following where it shall lead. "Lean not to thine own understanding." This is one danger of those who teach the truth to others. To follow where Christ leads is a safe path for our feet. His work will stand. Whatsoever God saith is truth.

But ministers who bear the last message of mercy to fallen men must utter no random words; they must not open doors whereby Satan shall find access to human minds. It is not our work to experiment, to study out something new and startling that will create excitement. Satan is watching his chance to take advantage of anything of this order that he may bring in his deceiving elements. The Holy Spirit moving upon the human agents, will keep the mind well balanced. There will not be a wrought-up excitement, to be followed by reaction. Satan will make use of every extravagant expression to the injury, not only of the speaker but of those who shall catch the same spirit and infuse others {105} to their harm. Calmness and solemnity should be cultivated; the solemn truths we dwell upon will lead us to manifest deep earnestness. How can we do otherwise when weighted with the most sacred message to bear to perishing souls, weighted by the sense of the nearness of our Saviour's coming.

If we are constantly looking unto Jesus and receiving His Spirit, we shall have clear eye sight. Then we shall discern the perils on every side, and shall guard every word we utter, lest Satan find opportunity to weave in his deceptions. We do not want to have the minds of the people wrought

up into an excitement. We should not encourage an expectation to see strange and wonderful things. But teach them to follow Jesus, step by step. Preach Jesus Christ, in whom our hope of eternal life is centered.

The enemy is preparing to deceive the whole world by his miracle working power. He will assume to personate the angels of light, to personate Jesus Christ. Everyone who teaches the truth for this time is to preach the word. Those who cling to the word will not throw open the doors for Satan by making unguarded statements in reference to prophesying or to dreams and visions. To a greater or less degree false manifestations have been coming in, here and there, since 1844, after the time when we looked for the second coming of Christ. We have had them in the Garmire case, in the statements of E. R. Jones, in the Stanton movement. We shall have them more and more, and like faithful sentinels we must be on guard. Letters are coming to me from many persons concerning visions which they have had and feel it their duty to relate. May the Lord help His servants to be cautious.

When the Lord has a genuine channel of light, there are always plenty of counterfeit. Satan will surely enter any door thrown open for him. He will give messages of truth mingling with the truth ideas of his own, prepared to mislead souls, to draw the mind to human beings and their sayings, and prevent it from holding firmly to a Thus saith the Lord. In God's dealing with His people, all is quiet; with those who trust in Him all is calm and unpretending. There will be simple, true, earnest believers in the Bible, and there will be doers of the word as well as hearers. There will be sound, earnest, sensible, waiting upon God. The believer will hang his helpless soul on Jesus Christ. Christ will be exalted. Working and praying, watching and waiting, is our position. We should not desire to be recognized and to have our work appreciated in the fullest measure. Heaven is the best and safest place in which to hear from the lips of our Redeemer the result of our work.

It is not necessary or helpful nor is it pleasing to the spiritual worker, to have the name paraded in the papers with flattering words concerning his talents and efficiency. God knows all about the work accomplished by every laborer in His vineyard. I plead not for less earnestness, for every soul needs now the vitalizing power of God; but if the Holy Spirit works through the human agent it is because he hides self in Jesus, and becomes (he is) in Christ a laborer together with God.

My son, walk humbly with God. Your power and efficiency are in Jesus. The mighty tide of spiritual power will come upon the men {106} who preach the word, uplifting Jesus. This inspires in the hearer a living faith, which brings forth fruit abundantly. We want the truth spoken to human hearts by men that have been baptized with holy love for Christ, and for the purchase of His blood, men who are themselves thoroughly impressed with the truth they are presenting to others; and who are practicing the same in their own life. The word of God is sure, and every speaker should seek to link the hearer to Christ (read John 17:22-24; Ephesians 1:3-8).

Here are presented to us the riches of heaven's blessings. We cannot conceive of anything greater or more blessed. We have here the possibility before the human agent. It is the will of God that we should be so thoroughly identified with His Son that we shall be one with Christ as Christ is one with the Father. Through faith we may be wholly one with Christ; we may have our entire soul, body and spirit bound up with Christ in God, so that we shall share in the very same love wherewith Christ is loved by the Father.

And we are to be sharers in His glory; for Christ says, "The glory which thou givest me I have given them." What is that glory? The character of Christ. Can we ask any greater endowment? To have any place in heaven, to be in the presence of Christ, seems a blessing too great for sinful human beings to enjoy. But the marvelous mercy and goodness and love of God are beyond our comprehension. By accepting Christ as his personal Saviour, man is brought into the same close relation to God, and enjoys His special favor as does His own beloved Son. He is honored and glorified and intimately associated with God, his life being hid with Christ in God. O, what love, what wondrous love! Read the scriptures referred to; copyist left them out for want of time.

This is my teaching—moral purity. The opening up of the blackness of impurity will not be one half as efficacious in uprooting sin as will the presentation of these grand and ennobling themes. The Lord has not given to women a message to assail men, and charge them with their impurity and incontinence. They create sensuality in place of uprooting it. The Bible, and the Bible alone has given the true lessons upon purity. Then preach the word. Such is the grace of God, such the love wherewith He hath loved us, even when we were dead in trespasses and sins, enemies in our minds by wicked works, loving divers lusts and pleasures, the slaves of debase appetites and passions, servants of sin and Satan. What depth of love is manifested in Christ, as He becomes the propitiation for our sins. Through the ministration of the Holy Spirit souls are led to find forgiveness of sins.

The purity, the holiness of the life of Jesus as presented from the word of God, possess more power to reform and transform the character than do all the efforts put forth in picturing the sins and crimes of men and the sure results. One steadfast look to the Saviour uplifted upon the cross will do more to purify the mind and heart from every defilement than will all the scientific explanations by the ablest tongues. Before the cross the sinner sees his unlikeness of character to Christ, he sees the terrible consequences of transgression, he hates the sin that he has practiced, and he lays hold upon Jesus by living faith. He has judged his position of uncleanness in the light of the {107} presence of God and the heavenly intelligence. He has measured it by the standard of the cross; he has weighed it in the balances of the Sanctuary. The purity of Christ has revealed to him his own impurity in its odious colors. He turns from the defiling sin, he looks to Jesus and lives.

He finds an all absorbing, commanding, attractive character in Jesus Christ, the One who died to deliver him from the deformity of sin, and with quivering lip and tearful eye he declares, "He shall not have died for me in vain. Thy gentleness hath made me great." How prone we are on all occasions to look to our fellowmen for sympathy for uplifting, instead of looking to Jesus! How ready is the human agent to forsake the fountain of living waters, the cool snow waters of Lebanon, and drink of the turbid streams of the valley. O, in His mercy and faithfulness, God will cause our fellow-men in whom we place confidence to fail us in order that we may learn the folly of trusting in man, and making flesh our arm. Listen to the words of the prophet: (see Jeremiah 17:5-8). Talk of heavenly things, talk of the eternal weight of glory that will be awarded to the overcomer, and you will have success in your work.

(Signed) (Mother) Ellen G. White

DEAR BROTHER AND SISTER HASKELL

Prior to July, 1915
Sanitarium, Napa Co, California {108}

THANK YOU FOR YOUR letter, telling me about your movements and plans. . . .

That you should receive an invitation to go to Battle Creek, and give Bible lessons to the nurses and medical students, is not a surprise to me. I have been instructed that an effort would be made to obtain your names as teachers to the nurses at Battle Creek, so that the managers of the Sanitarium can say to our people that Elder and Mrs. Haskell are to give a course of lessons to the Battle Creek Sanitarium nurses, and use this as a means of decoying to Battle Creek those who otherwise would heed the cautions about going there for their education.

I warn you against doing anything which would help those who are working directly contrary to the counsels of God, to carry out any of their deceptive plans. I know you would not willingly place yourself in any such position, and I warn you because I know the men and the plans better than you do.

If you should be drawn into such a plan, it would bring much perplexity upon me, and I should have another hard battle to fight. You must take no part in healing "the hurt of the daughter of My people slightly." Should the word to forth that Elder and Mrs. Haskell were to take part in teaching the nurses in the Battle Creek Sanitarium, it would be my duty to send forth testimonies, that I do not wish to be called upon to bear.

Elder and Mrs. Farnsworth have been requested to spend some time in Battle Creek, laboring for the church. I encourage them to do so, and shall counsel them how to labor. It will be well for Elder Farnsworth and Elder A. T. Jones to stand shoulder to shoulder preaching the Word in the tabernacle for a time, and giving the trumpet a certain sound. There are in Battle Creek souls who need bracing up. Many will gladly hear and distinguish the note of warning. But Elder Farnsworth should not remain in Battle Creek long. I write these things to you, because it is important that they should be understood.

God would have men of talent who will not deviate from the principles of righteousness to stand in defense of the truth in the tabernacle at Battle Creek. One man should not be stationed in Battle Creek for a long time. After he has faithfully proclaimed the truth for a time, he should leave to labor elsewhere, and someone else be appointed who will give the trumpet a certain sound.

We should understand by experience word for word the message the Lord gave to Isaiah, and from this message there is to be no deviation. The Holy Spirit's meaning will be understood. This meaning is not to be changed a hair's breadth to harmonize with any new doctrine.

We know that in the past the truth has been demonstrated by the Holy Spirit. Not one word of human devising is to be {109} permitted to subvert minds, or to add unto or to take from the message God has given.

There must be connected with our Sanitariums in various places ample facilities for the training of workers. And great care should be taken in the selection of young people to connect with our Sanitariums. We cannot afford to accept everyone who is willing to come. Great injury is done to our medical institutions when we connect with them inexperienced youth, who do not understand what it means to do faithful service for God.

Every soul connected with our institutions is to be tested and tried. If self is not hid with Christ in God, the workers will blindly do many things that will hinder the precious work of God.

"Sanctify the Lord of hosts Himself; and let him be your fear, and let him be your dread. And he shall be for a sanctuary; but for a stone of stumbling, and for a rock of offense to both the houses of Israel, for a gin and for a snare to the inhabitants of Jerusalem. And many among them shall stumble, and fall, and be broken, and be snared, and be taken. Bind up the testimony, seal the law among my disciples." (Isaiah 8:13-16)

God has a denominated people, who are to wait on and trust in Him. They are to be true to the light He has given them, following closely the sacred landmarks. Their language is to be:

"I will wait upon the Lord, that hideth His face from the house of Jacob, and I will look for Him. Behold, I and the children whom the Lord hath given me, are for signs and for wonders in Israel from the Lord of hosts, which dwelleth in Mt. Zion. (Isaiah 8:17, 18)

"And when they shall say unto you, Seek unto them that have familiar spirits, and unto wizards that peep and that mut-ter: should not a people seek unto their God? for the living to the dead? To the law and to the testimony: if they speak not to this word, it is because there is no light in them." (Isaiah 8:19, 20)

The things mentioned in this scripture will be worked out before us. Some of them we see even now.

Those who have crowded into Battle Creek, and are being held there, see and hear many things that tend to weaken their faith, and engender unbelief. They would gain a more practical knowledge in an effort to impart to others that which they receive of the word of God. They should scatter out, and be working in all our cities, under the training of men who are sound in the faith. If those who teach these workers are true and loyal, a great work will be accomplished.

There is to be a working of our cities as they never have been worked. That which should have been done twenty, yea, more than twenty years ago, is now to be done speedily. The work will be more difficult to do now than it would have been years ago, but it will be done.

Our work is made exceedingly hard because of many false theories {110} that have to be met, and because of the dearth of efficient teachers and willing helpers.

It is not the work of the Lord that so many are gathered in Battle Creek, receiving a mold which unfits them for the work of the Lord till they are thoroughly converted.

The Lord is to do a strange work very soon. A representation has been given me, that I have not yet had strength to trace upon paper. I must know when to speak, and when to keep silent. When the Lord bids me speak, I cannot keep silent.

The Lord will work. Great facts will be revealed in the word. There are rich experiences to be received from the great Medical Missionary. The knowledge of salvation through faith, and a full trust in a personal God and a personal Saviour, will be manifest. Those who have held the beginning of their confidence firm unto the end, will have the proof of the things which they have learned by personal experience.

The gospel will be revealed and verified. The experience of the day of Pentecost will surely be repeated. Some will receive the Holy Spirit of truth; yea, some who are now in uncertainty. The Lord has given His word. For years he has been sending messages of warnings, but by many they have been unheeded. Notwithstanding the repeated urgent warnings God has given, many have been turned away from their original faith, and are lost in the fog of error. They have refused to follow the light that God has given to point out the true path.

Christ is the same Christ that He has ever been. He is our Redeemer. Those who have been striving to quench their thirst at broken cisterns, which can hold no water, need to be born again, that Christ may be formed within, the hope of glory.

There are those who will never receive the gospel message in its fullness; they will never see the greater light and working of the Holy Spirit. There is a depth of depravity in unbelieving human nature, that will never be healed, because the true light has been misinterpreted, and misapplied. The Lord has given His Spirit in abundance of assurance to enable men and women to understand the fallacies and errors of Satan and to guard against them.

Some will soon turn from their deceptive errors and calculations. To those who will be born again, the Bible will become a new book. There is a higher elevation to reach. True faith is to take the place of unbelief. The living springs of the word of God, with all their rich treasure are to flow into the soul. The truth of the Christian religion depends upon the divine authority of the word of God. The authority of the word is yea and amen.

Jesus Christ is the Way, the Truth and the Life. Our great need is to have Him formed within, the hope of glory. He is to come into our individual experience, as a personal Saviour. He is the foundation of our faith, the Rock of Ages. "Blessed is the man to whom the Lord imputeth not iniquity." (Psalms 32:2) {111}

When Christ shall come in His glory and all the holy angels with Him, then will all men be convinced of the truth that God has set apart him that is godly for Himself. But the words of Isaiah will come to many winds. "Cry aloud, spare not, lift up thy voice like a trumpet, and show My people their transgression, and the house of Jacob their sins." The fifty-eight chapter of Isaiah gives a wonderful presentation of truth.

I wish you could make a visit at my home. I should indeed be pleased to see you and talk with you. Do nothing that will lead others to make of no account the long, determined resistance which has been shown to the messages sent by the Lord.

We do not want the impression left on

minds that our nurses should be educated and trained in Battle Creek. You are not to remove the impression that I have been trying to make that our people are to be drawn away from Battle Creek.

I have light regarding the impression that your going to Battle Creek would make on our people who have had placed before them many falsehoods regarding the work and influences there. Your going to Battle Creek in answer to the call you have received, would not be in harmony with the light God has given me.

If you cannot understand this, I can, and I will make every possible effort possible to save our people from being mixed up with the methods followed by some of the Battle Creek Sanitarium managers.

The Lord would have Dr. Morse leave Battle Creek, and labor where the light of truth has not been taught, and that he may break every thread of sophistry. The sophistry that there is no personal God and no personal Christ has been set forth, and still lives, to be brought forth and fastened up human minds. I have seen Satanic agencies leading and controlling the minds of those who have taught these theories. Unless the snare is broken ruin will result as surely as to the house built upon the sand.

Great trials are right upon us, to test every soul. The end of the world is near at hand. We are not to consent to have our workers, God's workers, tied up in Battle Creek. "Out of Battle Creek" is my message. I understand perfectly the meaning of the invitation that has been sent you. You have not a sense of what it means, but I am to tell you that God has not given you the work of teaching nurses in Battle Creek, or in any encouraging our youth to go there for their training. . . .

If we turn unto the Lord with full purpose of heart, teaching in the places He indicates, all things that He has commanded, we may be assured of the promise, "Lo, I am with you always, even unto the end of the world." God is able and waiting to be gracious.

(Signed) Ellen G. White

DEAR CHILDREN, EDSON AND EMMA WHITE

June 16, 1899
Sunnyside, Cooranbong, N. S. W. {112}

I HAVE BEEN WRITING OUT some matters in reference to the South. I have read your letters to Brother Irwin and myself. Prior to this I had written in my di-ary in regard to yourself and Emma. The light that I have is that you should have a change. W. C. White and I have been consulting together, and from the light given me this burden resting upon you cannot be born with the want of cooperation evidenced. There is a spirit cherished among men at Battle Creek, those not standing in the position where they can be worked by the Holy Spirit, that they will think they see something to criticize in you, and then this is made an excuse why they do not feel a burden to do what they would otherwise do in the work in which you are engaged.

And when you are straining every nerve and every muscle to make the work a success, you are yourself led to be sharp in the use of the pen, and it hurts your influence to do the same work they are doing in criticizing. And as this work has been hurting them, and as the enemy sees he can hurt you, weaken your hands, and discourage your heart, he is pleased. You are wearing out too fast, and the Lord does not require that you and Emma should, under the existing state of things, carry the load without the cooperation of those in responsible places. Some would encourage you if there was not such an influence to meet in doing so. Therefore you are sacrificing life and health under a great disadvantage, and must have a respite. Your own spirit is becoming soured and you tempted. Now the Lord would have you come apart and rest awhile, and let the Southern field be worked by men whom they may choose to put into it, and let the responsibility rest upon them, and they carry it.

There is a great work to be done in this (Australian) field, and there are souls just as precious in the sight of God as those for whom you are laboring. They will never have a more devoted worker, or one better adapted to the work than you have been, or that will, under the same circumstances, show better results. The Lord has been your helper.

How much I have needed you connected with my work no one knows or ever will know. I can support you in this field myself, but this will not be necessary. While you work for me I expect to do this. But there is an extensive field you can take, in the islands of the sea. You can visit these islands and see what can be done to help them to do the very work you are doing in the South. The experience you have had will be of value with our American workers.

Willie proposes that you come by the way of England, stopping at different islands and places on the route. He thinks it would be a great help, but in talking with Brother Irwin, he thinks the very best route for you to take is the same as he took, by Vancouver. It is the best and cheapest route for you and Emma to take. You can spend two or three years here and see if you cannot avoid a complete breakdown in health. W. C., yourself, and Emma are malarious subjects, and the Southern field is most taxing {113} on your strength and vitality, and the poison of malaria will obtain a strong hold upon you. This climate, where we are located, among the blue gum trees, seems to be a healthful climate. I wish you could see Willie's children. They are rugged and solid in bone and muscle. All our family are in good health, except Marian, who is not strong, but not down sick.

I will in this letter send you an order on Review and Herald for your passage money. The trying season will have fully opened upon you in the South before this reaches you, and it is important that you should make a change. I therefore invite you to come direct to this place as we need you. I expect we shall have a printing press shipped from Pacific Press if they will make us a donation of such an article. We must now have a press of our own so that we can issue small books and use these books to help us in carrying forward the work here.

We are much pleased with your little paper Gospel Herald. The editing of it is excellent.

I shall not write you a long letter, but I am going to send the copies of letters written. You will see I have had important matters to handle. We are doing all we can, and we desire your help to start our press and set it in operation. We do not propose to confine you to the preparation of books, but you can help us in this. If after two years' trial in this country you recover your health, you can then return, if it is your desire, and take up the work in any line you see fit. If you choose to remain here in this country, and it seems to be the will of the Lord, and if your talent can accomplish more good here than in America, then you follow your own convictions.

I have not been willing to call you from the Southern field, knowing your unwillingness to leave that field. But the Lord has been giving me special light for different men who have been working in different fields, that their lives would be shortened by continuing to remain, although they themselves were reluctant to leave, but the health must be preserved. If the work is too taxing in one locality, or the atmosphere unfavorable, they must try other localities. As there is no dearth of work to be done, and there are places that are in need of workers, no one need, in this country be confined to an unhealthful location. We have therefore changed the location of the workers with the best results. New Zealand has a bracing climate. Tasmania is excellent, more like Colorado. Adelaide has a mild and healthful climate. I am not disposed to recommend Melbourne. But we have the opportunity to select most any climate easy of access.

Here we have plenty of fruit in its season. In August will be our crop of oranges. Our own trees are loaded with oranges and lemons. The sight is beautiful. We can begin to use them in July, but I want all who shall come to our Conference to behold the show. The little trees bear on little branches five or six large oranges in a cluster. The Mandarin trees are loaded with fruit of the largest size, and the frosts are not so severe as to cut them or do them any damage. Come, children, and see them. If you could only come so as to be here at Conference time, how glad I should be, but I have not hope that you will be here then. {114} At this Conference you would see the men who have been laboring in the islands of the sea.

I must now leave the matter with you, for you must consider for yourself; but you could be a great help to me. The Lord would strengthen you in making a change now. I see that W. C. W. is fully in harmony with what I have written you. He thinks that after you have been here two years you will then be settled what is best for you to do. My health is good when I do not have to stand on my feet to speak so often; but I am getting old. What I have to do I wish to do quickly and solidly. I wish now to take the Old Testament history from Solomon to the last chapter of Malachi, and the New Testament from the ascension of Christ to the Revelation; but how can I do it? Brother Colcord is helping me. W. C. White is necessarily called to advise and to attend frequent councils, for with the buildings being erected we need constant help from the Lord to teach us His way and His will.

I now leave this matter with you. Write me at once. I have good help in the three lady workers, Maggie Hare, Minnie Hawkins, and Sarah Peck. But there must be those who have been with me from my earliest experience who understand the workings of the cause and our history from earlier dates. My memory is good. Trusting in the Lord, my writing ability continues, but how long this will be I know not. But I now have to leave this with you and Emma. Certainly if you continue as you have been doing your health will not endure the strain of the Southern climate, and my need of your help is now very great.

If you can get out my books I can then have something to pay you and keep all my workers. You have no need to fear in that matter. There is to be a holding of the four winds a little longer, and when they are let loose there will be no peace any longer upon the earth. The truth is now our only shield and buckler. It is our front guard and rearward. May the Lord work for His people is my prayer. I am now writing to our people on important subjects. But I must close this letter. I am up at half past two o'clock in the morning. June 21, 1899.

The mail leaves today. Brother Irwin goes to Sydney today to spend the Sabbath, and from there to Melbourne and Adelaide and will then return to the Conference here at Cooranbong. He will then return by direct route to America, spend one Sabbath in California, and pass on to the center of the work at Battle Creek.

Brother Ballenger has sent me a letter in regard to his plans for the South, but, Edson, I cannot encourage such plans. He will calculate to have all things move smoothly. A community to settle in the South in accordance with the plans he has thought would prove a success, would prove a failure. What is the prospect for feeding and clothing this community? Where is the money to be pledged for building homes for families? The outlay would be greater than the income. There would be a gathering of good and bad, there would be the need of men of clear conception, baptized with the Holy Spirit of God, to {115} run such an enterprise. I might present many things that make it objectionable. There cannot be any colonizing without Satan's stirring up the Southern element to look with suspicion on the Northern people, and the least provocation would awaken up the Southern Whites to produce a state of things they do not now imagine.

There must be laborers in the South who possess caution. They must be as wise as serpents and harmless as doves. All who engage in this work should be men who have their pen and tongues dipped in the Holy oil of Zechariah 4:11-14. An unadvised word will stir the most violent passions of the human heart and set in operation a state of things that will close the way for the truth to find access to the fields now in such great need of workers.

It is not ministers that can preach that are needed so much as men and women who understand how to teach the truth to poor, ignorant, needy, and oppressed people. And as to making it appear that there is not need of caution, it is because those who say such things do not know what they are talking about. It needs men and women who will not be sent to the Southern field by our people, but who will feel the burden to go into this neglected portion of the vineyard of the Lord; men while their hearts burn with indignation as they see the attitude of the white people toward the black, will learn of the Master, Jesus Christ, that silence in expression regarding these things is eloquence. They all need the intelligence that they may learn of Jesus Christ and the simplicity of how to work.

The cultivation of the soil is an excellent arrangement, but it is not by Northern people grouping together in a community that will accomplish the work they imagine will be a success. Hot tempered men better remain in the North. Men and women who possess the true Christ-like spirit of ministry may do excellent work among the Southern colored people. Make no masterly efforts to break down the prejudices of the Southern people, but just live and talk the love of Jesus Christ. There cannot be any greater harm done to the Southern colored people than to dilate on the harm and wrong done them by the white Southerners. Just keep the lips closed although there cannot but be the burning indignation that longs to express itself.

There is need of level-headed men and women who love the Lord Jesus, and who will love the blacks for Christ's sake, who have the deepest pity for them. But the methods of Sister S—— are not the methods that will be wise to practice. They cannot be petted and treated just as if they were on a level with the whites without ruining them for all missionary work in the Southern field. There is a difference among the blacks as there is among the whites. Some possess keen and superior talents, that if the possessor is not made too much of, and is treated from a Bible standpoint, as humble men to do a Christ-like missionary work, not exalting them, but teaching them religious love, and Christ-like love for the souls of their own colored race, and keep before them that they are not called into the field to labor for the whites, but to learn {116} how to labor in the love of God to restore the moral image of God in those of their own race, then a good work can be done.

There is a work to be done in opening schools to teach the colored people alone, unmixed with whites, and there will be a successful work done in this way. The Lord will work through the whites to reach the black race, many of them through white teachers, but it needs the man and his wife to stand together in the work. More than one family of white teachers should locate in a place. Two or three families should locate near each other, not huddle together, but at a little distance apart, where they can consult together, and unite in worship of God together, and work to strengthen each others' hands to raise up colored laborers to work in the South.

There is a mistake often made by those who labor in Southern fields expecting that their brethren in the Northern fields of labor can advise them what to do. Those who have had no experience in the Southern field are not prepared to give reliable advice. It is those who are engaged in the work that must understand that when emergencies arise they must not depend upon men who have not any experience to advise them. They will often obtain advice that if followed would be ruinous to the work. Therefore it is not good policy for one family alone to settle in a locality. Men and women who have not children are best qualified for the Southern field, and if the Southern field is too taxing or debilitating, one family from the two or three who have settled in a locality can be spared. But let none feel that it is their bounded duty to remain in the Southern field after their health has testified that they cannot do this safely. Some persons can endure the climate and do well. But let our brethren in a more favorable climate consider all these things and provide every facility possible to make the conditions of workers in these unfavorable locations as pleasant as possible.

In places where money has been expended on buildings, and a start has been made, it is the duty of the men in responsible positions to give attention to that locality, so that workers shall be sustained in accomplishing the work designed when the plant was made. There is to be a work done in the South, and it needs men and women who will not need to be preachers so much as the teachers, humble men who are not afraid to work as farmers to educate the Southerners how to till the soil, for whites and blacks need to be educated in this line. But when perplexities arise in the South, spread out your wants to the Master of the vineyard. And those who know nothing of the Southern field, let them be sparing and cautious what advice they give. But sympathy, kind words, and encouragement are always in place.

Your mother,
(Signed) Ellen G. White

ELDER M. N. CAMPBELL AND G. A. AMADON

May 6, 1907
Paradise Valley Sanitarium,
National City, California {117}

Dear Brethren,

I AM NOW VISITING THE Paradise Valley Sanitarium. Since I came here last Wednesday I have spoken twice to the workers in the institution, and to the church in San Diego Sabbath morning and Sunday afternoon.

Wherever I go I try to emphasize the fact that our success in missionary effort is dependent upon the character we manifest. The truth of the word of God, obeyed, and carried out in earnest action, after the divine pattern, will bring sure results. But if we yield to worldly influences, there will be a decline of Christian zeal and devotion, and a corresponding failure to win souls to the truth.

The church is to increase in activity and to enlarge her bounds. Our missionary efforts are to be expansive; we must enlarge our borders. There must be action and reaction. The work of educating our youth must be maintained and increased. They are to be taught to reach higher and still higher, pressing toward the standard of genuine Christian education.

While there have been fierce contentions in the effort to maintain our distinctive character, yet we have as Bible Christians ever been on gaining ground. Remembering that the fear of the Lord is the beginning of wisdom, we are to labor earnestly ever praying that the saving grace of God will instruct us at every step. We must ever seek to ascertain the will of the Lord, and to walk in harmony with it. Let us follow on to know the Lord, whom to know aright is life eternal.

The Lord is giving me strength for my labors in Southern California. I am trusting Him for strength to speak to our people in Redlands and Riverside and San Bernardino. Never have I felt more deeply the necessity of keeping the way of the Lord, and of doing His will at all times. Wherever I speak to our people, I tell them that now is the time to do a thorough work for eternity. We must be humble, yet trustful. We must make use of every talent the Lord gives us.

We have been blessed with great and precious light from the word of God, and we should study how we can make the very best use of this light. Individually we are on test and trial. God is watching to see how we use His great blessings.

What can we say to arouse our people to use their entrusted talents to honor and glorify God. Property is of real value only as it is used in the carrying forward of the Lord's work The world's greatest need is consecrated effort in labor for the conversion of souls. Thousands upon thousands are perishing without a knowledge of the truth. My soul is sometimes stirred to its very depths, as I see the terrible picture. I prize {118} the truth that we now hold sacred, and I would urge upon all our people that they seek to bring every thought into subjection to Christ, that all their powers may be employed in the work of saving souls.

There should be no sleeping now. It is time to awake, and to watch for souls as they that must give an account. As members of the church of Christ, we must do His will on earth.

Let those who desire to be refreshed in mind and instructed in the truth, study the history of the early church during and immediately following the day of Pentecost. Study carefully in the book of Acts the experiences of Paul and the other apostles; for God's people in our day must pass through similar experiences.

Those who have held the beginning of their confidence firm unto the end are to bear their living testimony, and their words will have a convincing power upon the people, and many will turn to the Lord. Some will be imprisoned because they refuse to desecrate the Sabbath of the Lord. As the world becomes more imbued with the spirit of the enemy, there will be a very much more vehement opposition to the Word.

Will our churches now arise, and awake to the situation? The representatives of Christ are to carry a burden for souls. Every nation, and kindred, and tongue, and people, is to hear the last message of mercy to a fallen world. When our churches shall arouse from their drowsy stupor they will have a better understanding of Bible truth, and they will be ready to devote their money to the cause of God, and to give themselves in earnest labor under the guidance of the Holy Spirit. God's people are His agents, appointed to proclaim the truth in all parts of the world. The heavenly agencies will act their part, and we must cooperate with them. Behold Christ, our Pattern, how He travailed in soul for the salvation of men.

By their indifference many church members have grieved the Holy Spirit of God. In Christ's stead they are to beseech others to become reconciled to God. Heavenly agencies stand ready to cooperate with those who engage in the work of the Lord. The Holy Spirit is waiting to unite in sympathy with every true believer, and to make him a laborer together with God. Let no means be neglected that will advance the work to be done. There must be no self-exaltation, and far more prayer.

Make Christ all in all, and He will give dignity to your work; His mind will guide you, and you will be sanctified by His truth. Acknowledge Him as your Redeemer, and you become one with Him, even as He is one with the Father.

Christ has taught us to pray, "Thy kingdom come. Thy will be done in earth as it is in heaven." This opens to us a height to which we are to attain by steady progression and continual advancement. If all would do unto others as they would that others should do to them, it would be an indication of a converted world. Upon this principle the Christian is to {119} build. We are to ascend a ladder of progress whose top reaches unto heaven.

Every church member is to be engaged in active service for the Master. "Why stand ye here all the day idle?" asks the Master. "Go work today in My vineyard. Work while it is day; for the night cometh in which no man can work." "Ye are My witnesses, saith the Lord." Can we comprehend it? We are Christ's property, bought with a price even the precious blood of Christ. (Matthew 21:28; John 9:4; Isaiah 43:10)

Now is our period of stewardship. We are training on our Lord's goods. Our means, our speech, our influence, all are talents to be used in the Master's service, to be multiplied by wise investment. We must increase our capabilities. If God has entrusted us with three talents, He will not accept of two in return. If we have but one talent, but with it gain yet another, we shall have a position and a place in Christ's service, and will finally hear the blessed words of commendation and approval from the lips of our Saviour.

What a terrible mistake for a professed Christian to devote to himself all his time and means and energies! All are to deny themselves, that they may follow Christ. Many souls have not refrained from accepting martyrdom for the sake of Christ. For them is the blessed promise, "He that loseth his life for My sake shall save it unto life eternal." (Matthew 10:39)

(Signed) Ellen G. White

ELDER M. N. CAMPBELL

March 23, 1907
Sanitarium, Napa Co., California
(April 3, 1907-6- C. 116)
Battle Creek, Michigan

Dear Brother:

WE HAVE RECEIVED AND READ the interesting letters from you and Brother Amadon. We feel deeply grieved at the course that Frank Belden has pursued. That my nephew should urge his unsanctified opinions in such a persistent manner causes me much sorrow of heart. This is a repetition of the way in which he conducted himself when he had plans of his own to carry at the Review and Herald office. His actions reveal the spirit that controls him. I feel sorry for him beyond anything that I can express, and I ask you to pity him and to pray for him. His mother was my sister, and a sincere, devoted Christian.

There have been presented before me scenes that often occurred in the Review and Herald office when Frank Belden had some plan {120} that he desired to carry out. He would determinedly stand up and with a loud voice continue to talk until he had fully presented his ambitious plans before his brethren; and I am sorry to say that very often these plans were adopted. He did more than any other one man in the office to bring in wrong sentiments and carry out his own plans. These plans, when afterward brought to bear upon himself, he did not find so agreeable. I feel sad when I think of the record he must meet of impetuous action and the surrender of those principles that his uncle James White and I have ever striven to maintain. Frank Belden has excellent talent, and had he walked humbly with his God, the Lord would have used him to His name's glory.

In the Saviour's life is given us a pat-tern of the character we are to attain. He met the severest temptations of an obstinate foe, and in spite of powerful and sorcerous delusions, made His path plain.

The simplicity of the work of the Messiah gave unmistakable evidence of His mission. He swept away the errors that existed in the religious world with a confidence and tact that could not be gainsaid. He would have truth stand out clear and free from every error with which Satan would try to enshroud it. He presented heaven-born principles so clearly before the minds of the people, that the way to heaven was made clear and plain, and he who missed the way had no excuse.

To the forerunner of Christ was given the message, "Repent ye for the kingdom of heaven is at hand." The work of the herald of Christ was a continuous effort to destroy the popular delusion concerning the coming Messiah, and to show that repentance and forsaking of sin are necessary preparations for the coming kingdom. This work constituted the preparation for the establishment of the true church.

On coming to the temple at the opening of His ministry, Christ repaired to the temple, and found His Father's house desecrated by worldly traffic. He drove out from the temple courts the buyers and the sellers, and the priests and rulers. He "poured out the changers' money, and overthrew the tables, and said unto them that sold doves, Take these things hence; make not my Father's house a house of merchandise." The money taken by the dealers for the sacrificial offerings was robbery of the people; and they had made the house of God a den of thieves, and with a stern rebuke Christ exposed their extortionate traffic.

By expelling the worldly traffickers who were profaning sacred things, Christ would impress upon those who were to compose His church on earth that name and position weigh as nothing in the scale with virtue and purity of character, with honesty and righteous dealing.

What excuse will be rendered to God by those who, having had every advantage of the knowledge of the precious truth for this time, disregard the word of God and go contrary to His expressed will, violating the principles of the divine law {121} so definitely stated?

I feel more sorry than I can express that my own nephew should so boldly place himself in opposition to all the light that has been given. He has steadily pursued his own way for so long, and has expressed his own opinions so often, that he now ridicules truth, and discards that which once he respected. I have had presented distinctly before me the past, present, and future of those who have thus departed from the faith.

I was instructed to write out the truth as it was revealed to me, and point by point give it to the people. I have done this, and still there is much to present that the truth may be made simple and plain. The work God has given me to do is to stand firmly and intelligently for that which I know to be truth. That which I have given to the people was given in the purpose of God, to strengthen the believers, that they might not be led away by seducing spirits and doctrines of devils.

I have no appeals to make to those who have once stood firmly for the truth, but who have now departed from the faith and refuse a "Thus saith the Lord." My books contain the light that God has given me, and they are my argument. Those who having believed their testimony in the past, now cast it aside, will have no excuse to render for their course; for today as then the light shines clearly, declaring what is truth.

There is much more that I wish to write to our people, but what I shall write will only be a confirmation of the messages given in the past. I shall be called once more to give the light to those who are departing from the faith, giving heed to seducing spirits, and moving in strange paths. But the Lord has shown me that all that can be given to these souls is but a repetition and confirmation of the truths that have already been placed impressively before them. Not one principle of the truths we have held in the past can be denied.

The men in Battle Creek who are taking their position against the warnings of the Spirit of God, have received message after message, but with some there has been no change. O that they would make a covenant with God, and humble their hearts before Him! O that they would repent of the time they have lost in taking up a work that God has not given them to do! O that Frank Belden would see his mistakes and repent!

Who will give evidence that they want to know the will of God concerning them? Who are willing to receive the message of the Lord which has been coming to them through His servant to point out their errors? O that these men would see them-

selves as the Lord sees them. They have an earnest work to do in repenting before God of the harm they have done to themselves and others. {122}

The prophet Isaiah in the fifty-eighth chapter of that book delineates the case of these men. They need to repent and afflict their souls before God. Now is their time to contemplate the Saviour's life of humiliation and His death of suffering. The cross of Christ was needed to bring salvation within our reach, and to make our redemption certain. "God so loved the world, that He gave His only begotten Son, that whosoever believeth in Him should not perish but have everlasting life." (John 3:16)

(Signed) Ellen G. White

DEAR BROTHER AND SISTER FARNSWORTH

March 12, 1906
Sanitarium, California

I FEEL THE DEEPEST INTEREST in you both. I hope that Brother Farnsworth will not leave Battle Creek just now.

Let us say nothing to provoke men to anger, but ever present the affirmative of truth, Bible truth. This is to be our position.

I feel no surprise in regard to the course of _____. Last night my mind was called out upon many subjects. In the visions of the night I was reading the Scriptures, and the power and Spirit of God was upon me. Many things were presented to me in vision, which I may give at the right time.

I was saying with great power: "Isaiah 49:8-17; 52:5." (See those references). Hear and understand this matter. The time is now short. We must remember that we are not to be conquered by discouragement. No power can conquer Satanic agencies but the power of Him who gave His life to redeem man, dying in the sinner's place, that all who will may repent and be converted. Christ is the propitiation for the sins of all who repent and believe in Him as their personal Saviour.

"I gave my back to the smiters, and my cheeks to them that plucked off the hair." Do you understand that it was the Lord our Saviour who went through these scenes of humiliation? Hear ye, and understand, and let every soul take in the situation. Christ suffered all this that is written of Him. Who prompted this cruel treatment? The one who was once the most exalted of the angels in the heavenly courts. He was imbuing minds with his own attributes. It was Satan who led men to treat Christ

thus. See Isaiah 50:7-11. {123}

My brother and sister, be of good courage. Let your hearts be glad and rejoice. There is no need for us to complain; for the Lord is the strength of His people. You may be surprised to hear words that you have heard from _____, but I am not at all surprised. This is the development of the man when the spirit that is counter to the Spirit of God comes upon him. In him as he is at the present time, you have a representation of a man who is not under the molding influence of the Spirit of God. The Lord accepts no such demonstrations of bitterness. They do not become the man, when the Lord has been so gracious to him, helping him in the time of his distress.

Read in my books, "Patriarchs and Prophets," and "Great Controversy," the story of the first great apostasy. History is being repeated and will be repeated. Read then, and understand. The time is drawing to a close when power of influence, of intellect, of knowledge in science, can cover the least departure from the Lord's way. He has pledged His word that He will humble every oppressor of His ministers, or the appointed agencies engaged in His work. Persecuting powers will be brought to judgment; for all the resources of heaven and earth are to be called at God's command to do His work. God sees and knows those who are proud and self-sufficient, and He will bring them into judgment. Before the flood men cast off the fear of God, and trampled underfoot His holy law, but judgment overtook them. Read Isaiah 47:10.

Say to our brethren and sisters who have known and understood the voice of God in His word, Let nothing interpose between you and eternal interests. Think of this representation given of Christ in the Scriptures I have quoted. The Saviour, in His supreme power, could have palsied the hands that smote Him, challenging Him, the Prince of life, to prophesy.

When men refuse the counsels of God, and walk directly contrary to them, they make very strange speeches, but do not be the least concerned or surprised. The Lord is watching every movement. There are straight messages to be given, and in no case are we to fear the face of man. If Christ endured so much, can we not endure something for His sake? Who was He? The Prince of heaven. (Read Isaiah 9:6; Matthew 28:18-20).

These words outline our appointed work, and we are to engage in this work as never before. Soul-saving is to be our object; Christ's words are our commission; and we are to lay hold of the Saviour by faith, and put all our capabilities to the task of learning the science of soul-saving. The fields that have been neglected call now for repentance on the part of those who have heard the truth; they call upon them to take up their appointed work.

(Signed) Ellen G. White

ALONZO T. JONES, C. H. JONES, AND M. C. WILCOX

January 27, 1903
"Elmshaven," Sanitarium, California
(1903-8- J. -27) {124}

My dear Brethren in Positions of Trust:

I RECEIVED YOUR LETTER THIS morning, and will respond at once.

Brother Harper came to St. Helena last week especially to lay before me the question of the location of the General Conference soon to be held. He told me that the brethren and sisters of the Healdsburg church offered to entertain the delegates free of cost, if the General Conference would be held there. He asked if I had any preference to express. I told him that if the Healdsburg church proposed to entertain the delegates free, the Conference would be held at Healdsburg, if I had any voice in deciding this matter; for to hold it there would be much more in accordance with the light given to leave the cities as much as possible, than holding it in Oakland would be.

I thought that if the brethren and sisters at Healdsburg would do what I was told they were so desirous of doing, to hold the Conference there would be much more desirable than to hold it in Oakland at this time of the year. I knew that accommodations in Oakland for entertaining to large a company were very limited, and expensive.

I desire my personal preferences to have no special influence in determining where the Conference shall be held; for unless specially convinced by the Spirit of the Lord that it is my duty to be present, I will not attend, no matter where the meeting may be held. If I knew that I should have to attend the Conference, I might express my preference for Healdsburg as the location; for I could drive over, and have my horse and carriage there to use at any time, and to return when necessary.

At present, I most decidedly dread to attend either camp meetings or Confer-

ences. When present at such meetings, I am reigned up to speak plainly and strongly in regard to matters; for I dare not do otherwise than to tell the truth. The burden that comes upon me at such times is very heavy. The experiences I have passed through in attending meetings since returning to America, have been most afflicting; for it seems as if my efforts are of none effect. The testimonies borne bring upon me a great burden of soul, and seem to accomplish so little to change the order of things. The testimonies are speculated upon, and do not reform existing evils.

Just now my courage is not the best. Since the Fresno camp meeting, I have carried the burden of the Southern field in direct opposition to the plans of leading brethren. I have {125} lost confidence in some of these men as being taught and directed of God. If they are thus taught and directed, I am not teaching the way of the Lord. Therefore I am convinced that my place is at home. I can continue to write, if I avoid the crushing burdens that overwhelm me. And these burdens come upon me whenever I attend a meeting where there are men whom I know are not walking in the counsel of God. I care not to face such matters any longer; for it seems useless. I long for retirement, and I mean to have it, if it be the Lord's will to give it to me.

(Signed) Ellen G. White

BROTHER AND SISTER AMADON

June 26, 1906
Sanitarium, California
(1906-7- A. -200-)

I HAVE READ YOUR LETTERS, but have not had time to answer them. I have been permitted to view the case of Elder A. T. Jones. His bitterness is as gall, though he has been warned. At Washington, during the General Conference, I conversed with him for about three hours, but he would not receive my warnings. He seemed very self-confident, and when he spoke of his work at Battle Creek, his boastings were a surprise to many. All that I could say to him at Washington, seemed to make no impression on his mind.

A. T. Jones has had precious opportunities to see and feel the power of the messages of warning sent by the Lord to His people. He himself has been admonished to be constantly on guard, else the power of other minds would be exercised

on his mind, and he was cautioned regarding the subtle working of spiritual science upon human minds. He had eyes, but he saw not; ears, but he heard not, and he has done the very work that he was warned to avoid doing. I am very sorry for the man, for all these chapters in his experience are bringing him over a road that will have to be retraced step by step, if he ever comes to an understanding of the work he is now doing, and turns his feet to follow the precious Saviour, our Leader.

We must walk circumspectly before God. We cannot afford to make mistakes now. Truth will bear away the victory. I am not angry as I read statement after statement of falsehood, regarding my writings and my work. I am sure that the Lord {126} has helped you to stand for and vindicate the truth. Brother Farnsworth made a wise decision when he said, I will keep to the affirmative. We are to show the people that the truth of heavenly origin is sufficient to keep every soul. It is our duty to rebuke sin, for with Satanic energy, men will do all in their power to overcome the testimony of the righteous, with falsehoods and misstatements.

One time when we were in Healdsburg, we heard reports that cast a shadow on the integrity of Brother Cady. I met these with the remark that I had confidence in Brother Cady, and it must be that they were mistaken in the matter of the report. There was another matter regarding his relation to the school that had troubled me much. I thought a mistake had been made in proposing that he should work in the interest of all the schools in general. I felt that his place in the Healdsburg school could not then be properly supplied. I felt that the Healdsburg school should have the continual influence that Brother and Sister Cady would exert. I considered that he had done a good work in this school, and I greatly feared that the school would not succeed as it had done, were he separated from it.

When I was about to leave for Washington, I left in his care a young man whom I wished him to see and to take into Healdsburg College. What was lacking in his expenses, I promised to pay.

In a recent letter I wrote:

"In response to the enemy's work on human minds, I am to sow the good seed. When questions suggested by Satan arise, I will remove them if I can. But those who are picking at straws had better be educating mind and heart to take hold of the grand and soul-saving truths that God has given through the humble messenger, in the place of becoming channels through whom Satan can communicate doubt and questioning.

"To allow images of straw to be created as something to attack is one of the most unprofitable things that one can engage in. It is possible for one to educate himself to become Satan's agent in passing along his suggestions. As fast as one is cleared away, another will be proffered.

"I have been instructed to say, The Lord would not have my mind thus employed. I have written something on the meaning of the words, "I", "we", and "us" in the Testimonies. This point is, as it were, a man of straw, set up in the imagination of some who have been sowing tares."

(Signed) Ellen G. White

DEAR BRETHREN AND SISTERS

March 15, 1894
George's Terrace, St. Kilda Road,
Melbourne {127}

AS THE REPORT HAS BEEN quite widely circulated that Sister White has endorsed what has been written and circulated as revelations from God through Miss Anna Phillips, I feel that it is my duty to speak. I have not endorsed these productions. Warnings have been given to me in reference to them, that they will most certainly mislead. Woven in them will be statements that will lead to extremes and to wrong action on the part of those who accept them. It would be well for our brethren and sisters to move more cautiously, in accordance with the light given them. They should test these so-called visions before accepting them and presenting them in connection with the light God has given me. I see that our people are in danger of making grave blunders and premature movements. God says of these prophets that are springing up, "I have not sent them, yet they ran. Believe them not."

But that which grieves me is that some of our brethren have associated the exercises of Annie Phillips with the testimonies of Sister White, and have presented the two to the people as one and the same thing. Many have accepted the whole as proceeding from me. And when the result of such productions shall be seen in the true character, when falsehoods are presented as truths from God, and individuals act upon these things, believing them to be a message from the Lord, movements will

be made that bear not the divine credentials, doubt will be cast on the true work of the Spirit of prophecy, and the testimonies that God sends to the people will bear the stigma of these false utterances. These revelations are largely a repetition of that which has been before the people in publications for years; and yet mingled with this are some things that will lead astray.

I cannot endorse the course Brother_____ has pursued. He has not written one word to me, to see if God has given any light in these matters; yet he has presented them in public, making manifest his confidence in them. The fact that Brother _____ has been presenting precious light to the people, leads them to regard all he says as if inspired of God, else Brother_____ would not present them as he has done, I cannot see wisdom in this course. More clearly than do my Brethren I discern the inwardness of this thing, and the results that will follow. I have already made decided statements in reference to this matter, and I am sorry it has been brought in as it has, to do a work which will cast reflections upon the testimonies God has given. Where these so-called revelations are accepted, they will surely lead many into erroneous, precipitate action. I am burdened over these things.

Recently a letter was published in the Melbourne Age, from a New York correspondent, giving an account of the wonderful meeting held in Battle Creek on the occasion when so much jewelry was donated. And the work was said to have been done {128} after the reading of a vision given by Mrs. White, a prophetess, urging the people to sell and give away their property. How can you think I feel, to be at work here in this new field, and just as the interest is ripening off, souls deciding for the truth, to have some of the productions of Anna Phillips brought in, to be received and to go out as my testimony? Will my brethren please make no reference to the testimonies of Sister White in connection with Anna Phillips? In the name of the Lord I protest against this mixing up work, for it will result in making the testimonies God has given me responsible for the influence and effect of Anna Phillips' words. I beg my brethren just to come to the people with the evidence from the Bible, and not strengthen the opposition which is so strong against us, and is intensified by the falsehoods of Grant and Canright.

From time to time reports come to me concerning statements that Sister White is

said to have made, but which are entirely new to me, and which cannot fail to mislead the people as to my real views and teaching. A sister, in a letter to her friends, speaks with much enthusiasm of a statement by Brother _____, that Sister White had seen that the time had come when, if we hold the right relation to God, all can have the gift of prophecy to the same extent as do those who are now having visions. Where is the authority for this statement? I must believe that the sister failed to understand Brother _____, for I cannot think that he made the statement. The writer continues: "Brother_____ said last night that is the case, not that God will speak to all for the benefit of everyone else, but to each for his own benefit, and this will fulfil the prophecy of Joel. He stated that this is already being developed in numerous instances. He spoke as if he thought none would hold such a leading position as Sister White had done, and will still do. Referred to Moses as a parallel. He was a leader, but many others are referred to as prophesying, though their prophecies are not published. He, (Brother _____), will not give permission to have the matter copied for general circulation that has been read here from some sister. I wonder if you have seen one of these visions? They represent us as in the closing moments of time, with hours all in the past, and it is moments now. How solemn!"

These statements, interwoven with other matter that professes to be from God, are misleading; many minds will eagerly seize upon them, and through false impressions will misapprehend our true position and work. With much that is truth, there is mingled error that is accepted in its extreme meaning, and acted upon by persons of excitable temperament. Thus fanaticism will take the place of well-regulated, well-disciplined, heaven ordained efforts to carry forward the work to its completion.

These ideas in relation to prophesying, I do not hesitate to say, might better never have been expressed. Such statements prepare the way for a state of things that Satan will surely take advantage of to bring in spurious exercises. There is danger, not only that unbalanced minds will be led into {129} fanaticism, but that designing persons will take advantage of this excitement to further their own selfish purposes. Jesus has raised His voice in warning: "Beware of false prophets, which come to you in sheep's clothing, but inwardly they are ravening wolves. Ye shall know them by their fruits." "Thus saith the Lord of hosts, hearken not unto the words of the prophets that prophesy unto you: they make you vain. They speak a vision of their own heart, and not out of the mouth of the Lord." "If any man shall say to you, Lo, here is Christ; or, lo, He is there; believe him not: for false christs and false prophets shall arise, and shall show signs and wonders, to seduce, if it were possible, even the elect. But take ye heed: behold, I have foretold you all these things."

I have a warning to give to our brethren, that they shall follow their Leader, and not to run ahead of Christ. Let there be no haphazard work in these times. Beware of making strong expressions, which will lead unbalanced minds to think that they have wonderful light from God. The one who bears a message to the people from God must exercise perfect self-control. He should ever bear in mind that the path of presumption lies close beside the path of faith. In no case should he make use of extravagant expressions, for a certain class are sure to be affected, and influences are set in motion that can no more be controlled than can an impetuous horse. Once let impulse and emotion get the mastery over calm judgment, and there may be altogether too much speed, even in traveling a right road. He that travels too fast will find it perilous in more ways than one. It may not be long before he will branch off from the right road into a wrong path.

Not once should feeling be allowed to get the mastery over our judgment. There is danger of excess in that which is lawful, and that which is not lawful will surely lead into false paths. If there is not careful, earnest, sensible work, solid as a rock in the advancement of every idea and principle, in every representation given, souls will be ruined. Truth is mighty, and it will prevail. It will do its own work upon human hearts. We need not resort to the use of strong expressions that lead to over action. The truth stated calmly, clearly, will enter into the mind of the receiver, and become a part of their very nature. The Comforter, the Holy Spirit, remolds the character, making a new man in Christ Jesus. The thoughts, the ideas, the principles, are sound, sensible, bearing with them a weight of influence that flows in the new and divine channel. The heart and the soul are enlisted. The yea and amen of heaven must bring up the rear of every movement, else the worker will lose the reward of success. But he should weed out from every effort all extravagant

expressions. This caution will make his work far more efficient and commendable, even to those who do not believe the truth. There is danger, even in reproof, of cunning minds to dwell upon topics that lead to sensuality. Even the subject of moral purity may be so treated as to produce the very results it is desired to guard against.

The greatest care should be exercised concerning those who {130} claim to receive revelations from God. There needs to be much close watching and much praying. Those who are acting a part in the great work for these last days need to counsel together in regard to every new thing that shall be introduced, for no one man's mind is to be left to judge of, or to place before the public, important matters which have a relation to the cause of God. At this very time we are suffering from the reproach that was brought on the cause in the first message by unwise, ill-balanced minds, who thought they were obtaining a wonderful experience which should receive the credence of all men. In our early experience we had to encounter their over-strained humility and false notions. The first labor given me to do was to reprove their man-made tests. The testimony which I bore against fanaticism gained for me the envy, jealousy, evil-surmising, and criticism of those who participated in those movements. We know full well what it cost us personally because we would not receive the visions, dreams, and testimonies of those fanatics. We were compelled to know something of their cruel influence upon the cause of God. The truth had to bear the reproach of the error and fanaticism which we were everywhere called to condemn and reprove. And now that fanaticism I labored faithfully to repress, bearing the testimony given me of God to counteract its baleful influence is by Grant and Canright charged upon me. I have been shown that whenever and wherever God works, we must watch; every man and woman must stand as a faithful sentinel, for the arch-deceiver is waiting and ready to set in operation various devices for misleading souls. If possible he will mingle the counterfeit with the genuine, so that, in the effort to separate the two, souls will be imperiled. Whenever and wherever God works, Satan and his angels are on the ground. (Please read "Life Sketches," pages 92-94.)

The Lord has not commissioned Brother _____ to present Anna Phillips' revelations to our people. The truth of the word

of God is of sufficient authority and power. It bears its own credentials. The testimonies given me from God are designed to call the attention of the people to a "Thus saith the Lord." Brother _____ is in positive danger, and his brethren do not see that danger. They are placing the servant where God should be. The Lord has given Brother _____ a message to prepare a people to stand in the day of God; but when the people shall look to Elder _____ as to God they will become weak instead of being strong. It is no time now to be careless and ignorant of Satan's masterly devices to draw the people into deceptions and delusions.

(Signed) Ellen G. White

_____

WAGGONER AND A. T. JONES

February 18, 1887
Basle, Switzerland {131}

Dear Brethren

I HAVE SOME THINGS TO SAY to you that I should withhold no longer. I have been looking in vain as yet to get an article that was written nearly twenty years ago in reference to the added law. I read this to Elder Waggoner; I stated then to him that I had been shown his position in regard to the law was incorrect, and from the statements I made to him he has been silent upon the subject for many years.

I have not been in the habit of reading any doctrinal articles in the paper, that my mind should not have an understanding of anyone's ideas and views; and that not a mold of any man's theories should have any connection with that which I write.

I have sent repeatedly for my writings on the law, but that special article has not yet appeared. There is such an article in Healdsburg. I am well aware, but it has not come as yet. I have much writing many years old on the law; but the special article that I read to Elder Waggoner has not come to me yet.

Letters came to me from some attending the Healdsburg College in regard to Brother E. J. W.'s teachings in regard to the two laws I wrote immediately protesting against their doing contrary to the light which God had given us in regard to all differences of opinion, and I heard nothing in response to the letter. It may never have reached you.

If you, my brethren, had the experience that my husband and myself have had in regard to this known difference being published in articles in our papers, you would never have pursued the courses you have, either in your ideas advanced before our students at the College, neither would it have appeared in the Signs.

Especially at this time should everything like differences be repressed. These young men are more self-confident and less cautious than they should be. You must, as far as difference is concerned, be wise as serpents and harmless as doves. Even if you are fully convinced that your ideas of doctrines are sound, you do not show wisdom that that difference should be made apparent. I have no hesitancy in saying you have made a mistake here. You have departed from the positive directions God has given upon this matter, and only harm will be the result.

This is not in God's order. You have now set the example for others to do as you have done, to feel at liberty to put in their various ideas and theories and bring them before the public, because you have done this. This will bring in a state of things that you have not dreamed of.

I have wanted to get out articles in regard to the law, but I have been moving about so much my writings are where I cannot have the advantage of them. It is no small matter for you to come out in the Signs as you have done, and God has plainly revealed that such things should not be done. We must keep {132} before the world a united front. Satan will triumph to see differences among Seventh-day Adventists. These questions are not vital points.

I have not read Elder Butler's pamphlet, or any articles written by any of our writers, and do not mean to; but I did see years ago that Elder Waggoner's views were not correct, and read to him matter which I had written. The matter does not lie clear and distinct in my mind yet. I cannot grasp the matter, and for this reason I am fully convinced that presenting it has been not only untimely but deleterious.

Elder Butler has had such an account of burdens he was not prepared to do this subject justice. Brother E. J. W. has had his mind exercised on this subject, but to bring these differences into our General Conferences is a mistake. It should not be done.

There are those who do not go deep, who are not Bible students, who will take positions decidedly for or against, grasping at apparent evidence, yet it may not be truth. And to take differences into our Conferences where the differences become widespread, and sending forth all through the fields various ideas, one in opposition to the other, is not God's plan; but at once arise questionings, doubts, whether we have the truth, whether after all we are not mistaken and in error.

The Reformation was greatly retarded by making prominent differences on some points of faith, and each party holding tenaciously to these things where they differed. We shall see eye to eye ere long. But to become firm, and consider it your duty to present your views in decided opposition to the faith or truth as it has been taught by us as a people, is a mistake, and will result in harm, and only harm, as in the days of Martin Luther.

Begin to draw apart, and feel at liberty to express your ideas without reference to the views of your brethren, and a state of things will be introduced that you do not dream of.

My husband had some ideas on some points, differing from the views taken by his brethren. I was shown that however true his views were, God did not call for him to put them in front before his brethren, and create differences of ideas. While he might hold these views, subordinate himself, if they were once made public other minds would seize upon them, and just because others believed differently would make these differences the whole burden of this message, and get up contention and variance.

There are the main pillars of our faith, subjects which are of vital interest. The Sabbath, the keeping of the commandments of God, and speculative ideas should not be agitated, for there are peculiar minds that love to get some point that others do not believe, and argue and attract everything to that one point, and urge that point, magnifying that point when it is really a matter which is not of vital importance, and will be understood differently. {133}

Twice I have been shown that everything of a character to cause our brethren to be diverted from the very points now essential for this time, should be kept in the background. Christ did not reveal many things that were truth because it would create a difference of opinion and get up disputations. But young men, who have not passed through this experience we have had, would have as soon a brush as not. Nothing would suit them better than a sharp discussion.

If these things come into our Conference, I would refuse to attend one of them for I have had so much light upon this subject that I know that unconsecrated and unsanctified hearts would enjoy this kind of exercise.

Too late in the day, brethren; too late in the day. We are in the great day of atonement, a time when a man must be afflicting his soul; confessing his sins, humbling his heart before God and getting ready for the great conflict.

When these contentions come in before the people they will think one has the argument, and then that another directly opposed has the argument. Thus the poor people become confused, and the Conference will be a dead loss, worse than if they had had no Conference.

Now when everything is dissension and strife there must be decided efforts to publish with pen and voice these things that will reveal only harmony.

Elder Waggoner has loved discussions and contention. I fear that E. J. W. has cultivated a love for the same. We need now good humble religion. E. J. W. needs humility and meekness, and Brother Jones can be a power for good if he will constantly cultivate practical Godliness that he may teach this to the people. But how do you think I feel to see our two leading papers in contention? I know how these papers came into existence. I know what God has said about them,—that they are one, that no variance should be seen in these two instrumentalities for God. They are one, and they must remain one, breathing the same spirit exercised in the same work to prepare a people to stand in the day of the Lord,—one in faith and one in purpose.

(Then follows remarks concerning the Gospel, Sickle, etc., but nothing further on this.)

(Signed) E. G. White

EXTRACTS FROM LETTER TO H. W. K.

August 3, 1894
Norfolk Villa, Prospect St., Granville, N. S. W., {134}

WHEN WE CAME to Australia, our people had not a meeting house in the whole country. Since that time a church has been erected in Parramatta, but there is a heavy debt upon it. There is a church in Kellyville, in an orange grove; the building is small, plain and neat, and is free from debt. At Seven Hills there is a little company of twenty who have accepted the truth. Including the children, there are about forty who meet on the Sabbath. They have no dwelling house large enough to hold meetings in. Some weeks ago it became too cold for the tent, for it is now mid-winter here. We decided that a simple, neat church must be erected, that should cost about three hundred dollars. The Sabbath keepers at Seven Hills are intelligent, excellent people, but they are all poor. They have lifted the cross, separating from opposing friends and relatives, and have taken their stand under the blood stained banner of Christ, to be loyal to all the commandments of God. We could not leave this little company without a place where they could assemble to worship God, lest our labor should prove in vain. It has cost much steady, earnest, persevering effort to secure the result we now see. Brother Hickox labored alone for many weeks after the camp meeting; then he married one who could be his helper, and she has stood nobly by his side. We have done what we could to help him in speaking to the people, and in labor for them; if there is joy in the presence of the angels over one sinner that repenteth, we know that there is joy over these twenty precious souls, whom, one after another, have had the moral courage to decide to obey the truth. Now this little flock are babes in Christ, and need to be taught and led along, step by step, into faith and assurance; they need to be educated and trained to do the work of soldiers in the army of the Lord, and to bear hardness, that is, trials and opposition, contempt and scorn, as good soldiers of Jesus Christ.

Last Sabbath, Elder Corliss, Emily Campbell, and I rode out to Seven Hills to attend the service. I could not venture to enter the private house where so many men, women and children were assembled; I had been very ill with affection of the heart for one week, with difficulty of breathing. I sat in the carriage, in the grove outside, while Elder Corliss opened the Scriptures to feed the little company in the house. They had Sabbath School, followed by a Bible reading, which was interesting and instructive to all.

Then I stood in the door of the cottage and spoke to them nearly half an hour. The Lord strengthened me, and put words in my mouth, presenting the love of God as expressed to the world in giving Jesus to a life of shame, reproach, and suffering, and a cruel death to save sinners. Just prior to His crucifixion, the Lord Jesus prayed for His disciples, "Father, keep them in thy name." None can be kept in His name, if they are careless and inattentive in regard to keeping themselves. They have something to do, if their souls are to {135} be kept in the love of God; they must cooperate with God in the grand work. Their faith is to lay hold upon the divine nature, that they may be kept by the power of God, through faith, unto salvation.

The question is asked, "Who shall separate us from the love of Christ? Shall tribulation, or distress, or persecution, or famine, or nakedness, or peril, or sword?" Hear the triumphant cry of victory from the apostle Paul, that hero of faith: "I am persuaded, that neither death, nor life, nor angels, nor principalities, nor powers, nor things present, nor things to come, nor height, nor death, nor any other creature, shall be able to separate us from the love of God, which is in Christ Jesus our Lord." "I know in whom I have believed," We are not to be ignorant as to whose precious blood was shed for us, that we may rejoice in a personal Saviour. Satan desires to sift us, everyone, as wheat; but thank God, our Advocate is praying for us.

I tried to lead these dear souls to have sense of their responsibility as light bearers to the world. We encouraged all to feel that individually they had a part to act in every meeting when assembled to worship God. The Lord has given us rich promises. "Then they that feared the Lord spake often one to another: and the Lord hearkened, and heard it, and a book of remembrance was written before him for them that feared the Lord, and that thought upon his name. And they shall be mine, saith the Lord of hosts, in that day when I make up my jewels; and I will spare them, as a man spareth his own son that serveth him." All but one of the company testified for the Lord, giving evidence of the power of truth on the human heart. We felt that the meeting was a success because of the presence of Jesus. All seemed cheered and comforted and blest. We then rode eight miles to our home in Granville, and as the horse climbed the hilly road, we ate our lunch with cheerfulness and gladness of heart. Thank God, the meeting-house is going up; it is small, as cheap as possible, but it will be a precious place, dedicated to the service of God. O, how carefully we considered the question of means. What a hunting there was to see if we could not find some hidden treasure which we could appropriate; how we prayed and studied and planned! Our family did what they could. I engaged to be responsible for five pounds, brethren Starr and Hickox united in giving five pounds stg., Willie gave two pounds, and some other members of the family gave one pound. Well, the amount was still insufficient to make a start. The little company in their poverty did all they possibly could, each giving one pound; one brother gave five pounds; yet the amount was so small; then I doubled my subscription, making it ten pounds, but I saw that discouragement was upon the minds of the brethren as to the possibility of reaching the sum required. Again I doubled my subscription, and then added still five pounds more, making twenty-five in all. The meeting house must not have a debt hanging upon it.

In every place where churches are raised up, just such a work must be done. If there are twelve believers, there must {136} be a house of worship where they can assemble for the service of God. This part of the work is a positive necessity. During my illness two years ago I received from my brethren in California donations amounting to nearly forty dollars for my own personal benefit. I have added to it enough to swell it to fifty, and have given it toward lifting the debt from the church in Parramatta. These three little meeting houses in New South Wales are the only ones we own in all Australia, one at Kellyville, eleven miles from Granville, one in Parramatta under a heavy debt, and one in process of building at Seven Hills, in a farming district. This church we will not dedicate until the last dollar is paid, not if I have to increase my donation.

I tell you all this that you may be enlightened, and may enlighten others, in regard to the character of the work in these missions. It is very difficult for those so far distant to lift their eyes to see far off. If they desire to build as they have done in Battle Creek, they will do so, adding building to building, when God has cautioned them not to do it. Battle Creek will not escape the dragon's wrath; there will be stormy times, perilous times. The interests that have been centered and accumulating in this modern Jerusalem will be a mark for the arrows of Satan. It becomes those who are connected with our institutions to move as God shall direct, and not follow the imagination of their own heart. If they choose their own way, they will become entangled in perplexities, and lose the favor of God because they do not move aright. They have absorbed the means which the Lord desired to have placed in missionary fields where the believers have nothing of their own to give character to the work. As this has been laid out before me, I have tried to present it to my brethren in Battle Creek, and at the Pacific Press, and I still cry aloud, and spare not. Your counselors need to be under the inspiration of the Spirit of God, they need to be converted and transformed, need to look and labor more decidedly for regions beyond.

Though I may fail to make an impression on the minds of some of my brethren, I shall not keep silent; I will begin to plead with another class. I have said quite enough to those who ought to have taken heed. I have endured agony of soul because of the disregard of the warnings God has given, because of the want of consecration on the part of men who should be in touch with God, living channels of light, faithful sentinels with eyes keen to see and discern the needs for this time. God has given me relief. I have spoken the word of the Lord, and now I will wait and let God bear me up. I will trust in Him, and Him alone. I feel shaken off from every human being. I shall look to God, and to Him alone, to learn my duty, for I dare not trust in man or make flesh my arm. My work will be to cry aloud and spare not, whether men will bear or forbear.

I am writing this letter by lamp light, sitting upon my bed. I could not sleep longer than half past two A.M. The Lord lives and reigns. There is to be such a time of trouble as there never was since there was a nation. Already nations are angry, already Satan is working with signs and lying {137} wonders, and this will increase until the end. God will use his enemies as instruments to punish those who have followed their own pernicious ways whereby the truth God has been misrepresented, misjudged, and dishonored. These enemies of God are living evidences of the truth of His word; they are fulfilling that which holy men of old spake as they were moved by the Holy Ghost. God does not forewarn His people of trifles; the repetition of caution and warnings shows that there is importance in that which was spoken. Do those who claim to want light, treat the light with the respect which is due?

O, the solemnity of the day of God is upon us. The Lord cometh out of His place to punish the inhabitants of the world for their iniquity, and the earth shall disclose her blood, and shall no more cover her slain. A great work is to be done in God's moral vineyard. I can say from the heart, I have done all I could to help the work in this new field; I have borne agony of soul because there has been so little perception of the work to be done in these far off regions. If God has seen fit to send the truth to these countries, it is not that it shall be hindered, but the responses shall be made to our appeals for this field because there is an intelligent understanding of the whole field and an appreciation of the work done by the workers in these fields. It becomes those who act a part as Christ's representatives at this time not to dwell upon one portion of the work or of the vineyard, to the neglect of others portions of the field. All should share equally in attention, cultivation, and development. The great saving truths, vital with interest for this time, are to be proclaimed. These truths are to be the woof and warp of every discourse given, every plan devised, and every effort made, the sum, the substance, the core, the life of every appeal. The converting power of God must come to our people, not in spasmodic waves, but as a holy breathing from heaven, making known God's hidden treasure, the unsearchable riches of the Scriptures.

I am told that before finishing the life of Christ I ought to visit Jerusalem, the holy land. What made it holy? The Majesty of heaven clothed His divinity with humanity, and dwelt upon our earth. He was despised and rejected of men; in Jerusalem He was crucified by wicked hands. I have not the slightest inclination to visit Jerusalem, to see where it is thought probable that Jesus trod, where He may have labored, and where He may have been crucified. The means which might be expended thus I would prefer to treasure, that I may point souls to the Saviour risen from Joseph's tomb, and proclaiming, "I am the resurrection and the life." I can trace His footprints in the sure word of prophecy, and can obtain a better idea of His works and of His ways, than I could by visiting Jerusalem, defiled with unholy feet and unholy deeds. I could not expend money to visit these places when the living interests of Christ's kingdom are to be presented to the people. We are to teach the word of God, and to be doers of that word, which is represented as building upon the rock; the structure thus built will withstand the storm and the tempest, because it is founded on the eternal Rock. {138}

I wish to see Jerusalem when the fires of the last great day shall have cleansed it from all sinful defilement. Jerusalem is now no more sacred to me than any other place on the globe. Wherever by his Holy Spirit Jesus makes known His presence, wherever his righteousness shines forth in bright and glorious beams, wherever his divine love illuminates the humble places of the earth, wherever his honor dwells, there I am pleased to be. Christ looks with sadness upon the delusions that ensnare human minds who are so eager to behold the place where His feet are supposed once to have trodden, and yet who do not heed His command, "Follow me," who do not walk in the light as He is in the light. A shadow is resting over Jerusalem, a terrible shadow, which I have no desire to come under. Everywhere a curse is visible, which I have no desire to look upon. I can see marks of the curse everywhere. To be able to say I have visited Jerusalem would not shed a distinct ray of light upon one soul. It would not enable me better to tell men and women what they must do to be saved. I present the word of God in truth. I listen to the precious lessons which Christ gave His disciples. In my mind the scenes of His ministry, the places where He taught by the lake side, and clothed with the solemnity and beauty which nature and the word of God have given them. I am content: I would not have darker pictures. I do not wish to look upon the desecrated shrines, with all the repulsive features that would meet my view. I would not be hired to behold the traces of the curse so evidently resting upon Jerusalem. I hope to see this spot when the earth shall be made new, when I shall behold Him whom my soul loveth, in His majesty and glory crowned as King of kings and Lord of lords.

I have not one word of encouragement for any person, neither have I money to impart to any person, to visit Jerusalem. As it now is, it would be a picture I would never wish to hang in memory's hall. Brethren, do you believe that you will soon see Jesus? Then do not needlessly expend means that is of so great value to save precious souls; they need never get a sight of Jerusalem under the curse, but with inspired words you can point them to the New Jerusalem, to Jesus the Mediator of the better covenant, whoever liveth to make intercession for us, and whose intercession is wholly efficacious in our behalf. I know that Christ looks with sadness upon those who are searching for the places He passed over while in the flesh, but who fail to recognize Him as a living Saviour, on any ground, in any place. He says, "Lo, I am with you always, even to the end of the world." Men may search in vain for the foot-prints of Christ in Jerusalem. I care more for where He is now, in heaven, and for what He is doing in my behalf.

Give to Jesus your devotion where He is in the heavenly sanctuary; seek for the holy Spirit as His representative wherever His people bow to worship Him. It becomes us to know Jesus by an experimental knowledge, as a personal Saviour. We should be gathering up every ray of divine light, not looking to old Jerusalem where Christ was once, but to the New Jerusalem where He is now. Let us be gathering from the {139} tree of life that God has planted, leaves that shall be for the healing of the nations, and fruit, precious, life-giving fruit as food to the soul.

O, search with prayer, most earnest prayer, to know what God has written; and to trace the foot-prints of Jesus in His life of perfect obedience to His Father's commandments. Endeavor to catch the inspiration in expounding the word, the sure word of prophecy, that it shall not be as dead letter, but a living, burning, shining light from the throne of God, preparing a people to endure the trails, the sufferings and persecution which Christ endured.

Who can be made to understand that the inner life must be hid with Christ in God? Such are in the habit of praying, for Christ prayed. Such are in the habit of searching the Scriptures for themselves, and more earnestly as they see the day approaching. Such ones, who love God supremely and their neighbors as themselves, will give themselves to God as a free will offering, and that gift will include all they have. None can give themselves without reserve unless their possessions also are included, and they are dispensing their God-given trust of means as the Lord's goods. They produce fruit in good works. "Blessed are they that do his commandments, that they may have right to the tree of life, and may enter in through the gates into the city."

(Signed) Ellen G. White

TESTIMONY TO MEMBERS OF THE B. C. CHURCH
October 24, 1907

SOME ARE ACTING THE PART of Aaron, to help on the work of apostasy. They have been weighed in the balances, and have been found wanting. Men are spoiling their record, and are proving

that they are not to be trusted, but that they will betray the interests of the cause of God, making them the sport of sinners. The messages of heavenly origin that God has sent to his people, to prepare them to stand in the last days, they have sneered at and scorned. But the evidence we have had for the past fifty years of the presence of the Spirit of God with us as a people, will stand the test of those who are now arraying themselves on the side of the enemy and bracing themselves against the message of God.

DOCTOR PAULSON'S COLLECTION
August 3, 1894
{140}

GREAT PRINCIPLES AND minute practice cannot be disconnected in a symmetrical life.

Mrs. E. G. White

A. O. TAIT
August 27, 1896

O HOW LITTLE MEN, even presidents of conferences, know of the power and helpful strength that God gives to the earnest, humble seeker who puts his trust in God, and does not place men as counselors, in the place where God alone should be. There are thousands upon thousands and ten thousand times ten thousand angels that minister unto those who shall be heirs of salvation.

J. N. LOUGHBOROUGH
February 19, 1899

JUST AT THAT TIME THE devil was influencing minds to hold back my books published at Review and Herald. Those at the head of the work there discouraged the agents about handling "Patriarchs and Prophets" and "Great Controversy," the very books which the people should have had at once, and concentrated their efforts on "Bible Readings," promising that at a certain time they would concentrate their efforts on my books. But this promise they never kept. At the very time when "G. C." should have been circulated everywhere, it was lying idle on the shelves of the Review and Herald and Pacific Press. . . .

The light given by God for the people was hidden away in the publishing houses. The inner working of this matter was presented to me, and I saw that the very men

who said that the canvassers would not handle my books, were themselves arranging matters so that they should not handle them. They told me falsehoods.

THE WORK IN OAKLAND AND SAN FRANCISCO
December 26, 1906
{141}

THE LORD JESUS SENT a mighty angel to make plain to John, by the use of symbols, the things that were to come to pass until the coming of Christ. He was bidden to write the instruction in a book for the benefit of the seven churches. This writing we now have preserved in the book of Revelation, but this book is understood by only a few. It contains the message for the last days, and we are to dwell much upon these prophecies.

UNITY AND HUMILITY AMONG THE WORKERS
January 5, 1892
North Fitzroy

THE STEWARDS OF GOD HAVE not done their duty. If they had, the work would be far in advance of what it is today. But we labor under far less difficulty than the world's Redeemer had to encounter. We should feel that we are stewards of His grace, trusted with our Masters goods. If we do our best, exercise our entrusted capabilities with the sole purpose of doing our Master's work and promoting His glory, the smallest talent, the humblest service, may become a consecrated gift, made acceptable by the fragrance of His own merit.

We have grant [great] and mighty truths, and in presenting these truths to the world there is a field for the exercise of the highest capabilities. But the Lord will scorn your unwilling service. The truth is grand, eternal, because it proceeds from Him who is truth, and righteousness. And He will not accept the half-hearted, reluctant service of one of you. Unless you have a love for Jesus, unless you receive in your heart the Bible truth, and Christ as your personal Saviour, He will not accept your worthless sacrifice or your service.

When it is evident that those who are engaged in the Lord's work have made mistakes in some things, Satan is jubilant; he taunts Jesus and the angels of God with the sins he tempts men to commit. He presents these mistakes in all their discouraging features, clothing the erring ones with filthy garments. As the accuser of the brethren he presents these errors and wrong-doings in the worst light possible, and parades them before those who will help him in his work. Then the murmurers and those who are far from God think they have an excuse to be stubborn and sullen. They do not see that hell is triumphing, and that if they had a sense of their responsibility they would like faithful soldiers seek to retrieve the disgrace of defeat, not by leaving the ranks, but by closing up the ranks and pressing to the charge against the enemy, that God might not be dishonored and His cause languish.

The time when the work goes the hardest is the very time to test the spiritual strength and wisdom of every worker. When difficulties arise in any branch of the cause, as they will, for the church militant is not the church triumphant, all heaven is watching to see what will be the course of those who are entrusted with sacred responsibilities.

Like their Master, those who are abiding in Christ will not fail nor be discouraged. (See Isaiah 42:4-6)

The Lord requires our undivided affection. If men are not whole hearted, they will fail in the day of trial. When the enemy shall put his forces in array against them, and the battle seems to go hard, at the very time when all the strength of intellect, all the tact of wise-generalship, is needed to repulse the enemy, those who are half-hearted will turn their weapons against their own soldiers; they weaken the hands that should be strong for warfare. God is testing all {142} who have a knowledge of the truth to see if they can be depended on to fight the battles of the Lord when hard pressed by principalities and powers and the rulers of the darkness of the world and wicked spirits in high places. Perilous times are before us, and our only safety is in having the converting power of God every day, yielding ourselves fully to Him to do His will, and walk in the light of His countenance. (See 1 Peter 2;9)

Now when we are just on the borders of the promised land, let none repeat the sin of the unfaithful spies. They acknowledged that the land they went up to see was a good land, but they declared that the inhabitants were strong, the giants were there, and they themselves were in comparison as grasshoppers in the sight of the people and in their own sight. All the difficulties were magnified into insurmountable obstacles. They made it appear as fol-

ly and presumption to think of going up to possess the land. Thus they leavened the whole congregation with their unbelief. The people broke forth into lamentations and loud outcries. But Caleb stilled them before Moses, and said, "Let us go up at once, and possess it; for we are well able to overcome it."

This was the language of faith; but the men who had spoken discouragingly were not to be baffled in their attempts to prevent the people from going forward in doing the word of the Lord. They tried to cry down the voice of Caleb, saying, "We be not able to go up against the people; for they are stronger than we." And they exaggerated the difficulties until all the congregation were crazed with discouragement and fear. The people wept all night, and murmured against the very men in whom they should have had confidence. Then in their exasperation they cast reflections upon God, wishing that they had died in Egypt or in the wilderness; they planned rebellion, proposing to thrust aside their God-appointed leaders. "Let us make a captain," they said, "and let us return into Egypt." What sorrow can be brought upon the ones whose hearts are in the work, by those who are unconsecrated, stubborn, and rebellious. Amid all the lamentations and bitterness of feeling, Caleb and Joshua spoke to the congregation, "The land which we passed through to search it is an exceeding good land." (See Numbers 14:8-10) but the people wished to believe the worst, and while the ringing voice of Caleb was heard above the tumult they stood with stones in their hands to batter down the men who bore the right testimony. Then "the glory of the Lord appeared in the tabernacle of the congregation before the children of Israel. (See Nos. 14:1, 12)

While the people were cherishing doubts, and believing the unfaithful spies, the golden opportunity for Israel passed by. The inhabitants of the land were aroused to make a determined resistance, and the work which the Lord had prepared to do, for them to manifest His greatness and His favor to His people could not be done because of their wicked unbelief and rebellion.

Shall it be thus in these last days, just before we enter into the heavenly Canaan, that God's people shall indulge the spirit that was revealed by ancient Israel? Men full of doubts {143} and criticisms and complaints can sow seeds of unbelief and distrust that will yield an abundant harvest.

The history of Israel was written for our admonition, upon whom the ends of the world are come. (See Hebrews 3:7-14) (Hebrews 4:1, 2)

Our only safety is in a diligent searching of the Scriptures. If we waste our precious opportunities to become familiar with the word of God, we are losers in every respect. "All Scripture is given by inspiration of God, and is profitable for doctrine, for reproof, for correction, for instruction in righteousness; that the man of God may be perfect, thoroughly furnished unto all good works."

(Signed) Ellen G. White

SISTER FANNIE

February 6, 1894
George's Terrace, St. Kilda Road

I HAVE SO OFTEN TOLD you that your words and ideas must not take the place of the words and ideas given me, that the repetition of this is utterly useless. You have chosen your own way, and mingled self with your work, and have become less and less sensible of the danger to your own self and to the work. You have come to think that you were the one to whom credit should be given for the matter that comes from your hands. I have had warnings concerning this, but could not see how I could come to the very point. . . .

Ellen G. White

MR. AND MRS. J. E. WHITE

February 6, 1894
George's Terrace

Dear Children:

U NDER THE SHOWERS OF THE latter rain the inventions of man, the human machinery, will at times be swept away, the boundary of man's authority will be as broken reeds, and the Holy Spirit will speak through the living, human agent with convincing power. No one then will watch to see if the sentences are well rounded off, if the grammar is faultless. The living water will flow in God's own channels. But let us be careful now not to exalt the men, their sayings and doings; and let not anyone consider it a grand point to have a startling experience to relate; for here is a fruitful field where credence will be given to unworthy persons. Young men and women will be lifted up, and will regard themselves as wonderfully favored, called to do {144} some great thing. There will be conversions many, after a peculiar order but they will not bear the divine signature.

Immorality will come in and extravagance and many will make ship-wreck of faith. Our only safety is in keeping fast hold of Jesus. Never are we to lose sight of Him. He says, "Without Me you can do nothing." We must cultivate an abiding sense of our own inefficiency and helplessness and rely wholly on Jesus. This should keep us individually calm and steadfast in words and deportment. Excitement in the speaker is not power but weakness. Earnestness and energy are essential in presenting Bible truth, the gospel, which is the power of God unto salvation. . . .

There are quicksands upon which many are in danger of being swamped. It is always safe to seek for the earnest of the Spirit of God, if we do not mingle with it a force and presumption that is not heaven born. There is need of caution in all our utterances lest some poor souls of ardent temperament shall work themselves up into a zeal not according to knowledge. They will act as though it was their prerogative to use the Holy Spirit instead of letting the Holy Spirit use them, and mold and fashion them after the Pattern of the divine. There is danger of running ahead of Christ. We should honor the Holy Spirit by following where it shall lead. "Lean not to thine own understanding." This one danger of those who teach the truth to others. To follow where Christ leads is a safe path for our feet. His work will stand. Whatsoever God saith is truth.

But ministers who bear the last message of mercy to fallen men must utter no random words; they must not open doors where by Satan shall find access to human minds. It is not our work to experiment, to study out something new and startling that will create excitement. Satan is watching his chance to take advantage of anything of this order that he may bring in his deceiving elements. The Holy Spirit moving upon the human agents, will keep the mind well balanced. There will not be a wrought up excitement, to be followed by re-action. Satan will make use of every extravagant expression to the injury, not only of the speaker but of those who shall catch the same spirit and infuse others to their harm. Calmness and solemnity should be cultivated; the solemn truths we dwell upon will lead us to manifest deep earnestness. How can we do otherwise when weighed with the most sacred message to bear to perishing souls, weighted by the sense of the nearness of our Saviour's coming.

If we are constantly looking unto Jesus and receiving His Spirit, we shall have clear eye sight. Then we shall discern the perils on every side, and shall guard every word we utter, lest Satan find opportunity to weave in his deceptions. We do not want to have the minds of the people wrought up into excitement. We shall not encourage an expectation to see strange and wonderful things. But teach them to follow Jesus, step by step. Preach Jesus Christ, in whom our hope of eternal life is centered.

The enemy is preparing to deceive the whole world by his miracle-working power. He will assume to personate the angels {145} of light, to personate Jesus Christ. Everyone who teaches the truth for this time is to preach the word. Those who cling to the word, will not throw open the doors for Satan by making unguarded statements in reference to prophesying or to dreams and visions. To a greater or lesser degree false manifestations have been coming in, here and there, since 1844, after the time when we looked for the second coming of Christ. We have had them in the Garmire case, in the statements of E. R. Jones, in the Stanton movement. We shall have them more and more, and like faithful sentinels we must be on guard. Letters are coming to me from many persons concerning visions which they have had and feel it their duty to relate. May the Lord help His servants to be cautious.

When the Lord has a genuine channel of light, there are always plenty of counterfeit. Satan will surely enter any door thrown open to him. He will give messages of truth mingled with the truth ideas of his own, prepared to mislead souls, to draw the mind to human beings and their sayings, and prevent it from holding firmly to a Thus saith the Lord. In God's dealing with His people, all is quiet; with those who trust in Him all is calm and unpretending. There will be simple, true, earnest believers in the Bible, and there will be doers of the word as well as hearers. There will be sound, earnest, sensible, waiting upon God. The believer will hang his helpless soul on Jesus Christ. Christ will be exalted. Working and praying, watching and waiting, is our position. We should not desire to be recognized and to have our work appreciated in the fullest measure. Heaven is the best and safest place in which to hear from the lips of our Redeemer the result of our work. . . .

(Signed) Mother
Ellen G. White

ELDER URIAH SMITH

August 30, 1892
North Fitzroy
Battle Creek, Michigan

Dear Brother:

I AM DEEPLY INTERESTED THAT in every move you make, you should have the Lord with you. God bestows upon His people great blessings in giving them faithful, upright ministers. In all ages He has wrought through human instrumentalities to give decided messages of warning to His people, that they may be aroused and convicted of their sins, and be led to repent and reform. But at the very time when He is thus empowering men by His Holy Spirit to cry aloud, to spare not, to lift up the voice like a trumpet, and to show His people their transgressions and the house of Jacob their sins, there are {146} other influences at work to counteract the work of God through His appointed agencies. There are those to whom this Scripture is applicable, "They have healed the hurt of the daughter of My people slightly, saying, Peace, peace; when there is no peace." . . .

It is sin in some form that brings variance and disunion. The affections need transforming, a personal experience of the renewing power of Christ must be obtained. "In whom we have redemption through His blood, the forgiveness of sins, according to the riches of His grace;" The apostle speaking to Christian believers, called by God's grace says, "If we walk in the light, as He is in the light, we have fellowship one with another, and the blood of Jesus Christ His Son cleanseth us from all sins." Here are conditions plainly stated, If we walk in the light as He is in the light, the sure result will follow; We have fellowship one with another. . . .

True Christianity will always be aggressive, and wherever it exists, it will arouse enmity. All who live a conscientious life, who bear testimony of the claims of God, of the evil of sin, of the judgment to come, will be called the disturbers of Israel.

Those whose testimony awaken the apprehension of the soul, offend pride, and arouse opposition. The hatred of evil against good exists as surely now as in the days of Christ, when the multitude cried, "Away with Him!" "Release unto us Barabbas." There is no kind of evil in our world, but that some have an interest in maintaining it. Evil is ever warring against good. And since we know that the conflict with the prince of darkness is constant, and must be severe, let us be united in the warfare. Cease to war against those of your own faith. Let no one help Satan in his work. . . .

The first thing recorded in Scripture history after the fall was the persecution of Abel. And the last thing in Scripture prophecy is the persecution against those who refuse to receive the mark of the beast. We should be the last people on the earth to indulge in the slightest degree the spirit of persecution against those who are bearing the message of God to the world. This is the most terrible feature of unchristlikeness that has manifested itself among us since the Minneapolis meeting. Sometime it will be seen in its true bearing, with all the burden of woe that has resulted from it.

A passive piety will not answer for this time; let the passiveness be manifested where it is needed, in patience, kindness, and forbearance. But we must bear a decided message of warning to the world. The Prince of Peace thus proclaimed His work, "I come not to send peace on earth but a sword." Evil must be assailed; falsehood and error must be made to appear in their true character; sin must be denounced; and the testimony of every believer in the truth must be as one. All your little differences, which arouse the combative spirit among brethren, are devices of Satan to divert minds from the great and fearful issue before us. The true peace will come among God's people when through united zeal and {147} earnest prayer the false peace that exists to a large degree is disturbed. Now there is earnest work to do. Now is the time [to] manifest your soldierly qualities; let the Lord's people present a united front to the foes of God and truth and righteousness. . . .

When the Holy Spirit was poured out upon the early church, "The whole multitude of them that believed were of one heart and of one soul." The spirit of Christ made them one. This is the fruit of abiding in Christ. But if dissensions, envy, jealousy, and strife are the fruit we bear, it is not possible that we are abiding in Christ. To draw nourishment from the Living Vine is the same that Christ represents as eating His flesh and drinking His blood. And if we are feeding upon Him, we shall manifest His spirit.

Jesus longs to bestow the heavenly endowment in large measure upon His people. Prayers are ascending to God daily for the fulfillment of the promise, and not one of the prayers put up in faith is lost.

Christ ascended on high, leading captivity captive, and gave gifts unto men. When after Christ's ascension the Spirit came down as promised, like a rushing, mighty wind, filling the whole place where the disciples were assembled, what was the effect? Thousands were converted in a day. We have taught, we have expected that an angel is to come down from heaven, that the earth will be lighted with his glory. Then we shall behold an ingathering of souls similar to that witnessed on the day of Pentecost.

But this [mighty] angel comes bearing no soft, smooth, message, but words that are calculated to stir the hearts of men to their very depths. That angel is represented as crying mightily with a strong voice, saying, "Babylon the great is fallen, is fallen, and is become the habitation of devils, and the hold of every foul spirit, and a cage of every unclean and hateful bird." "Come out of her, My people that ye be not partakers of her sins, and that ye receive not of her plagues." Are we indeed as the human agencies, to cooperate with the divine instrumentalities in sounding the message of this mighty angel who is to lighten the earth with his glory? . . .

(Signed) Ellen G. White

CAPTAIN C. ELDRIDGE

January 9, 1893
George's Terrace, St. Kilda Road
Melbourne

Battle Creek, Michigan

Dear Brother:

THE WORD OF THE LORD HAS come to me in clear lines in reference to the principles and practices of those connected with the {148} Review Office. There has been need of self-examination on the part of the workers. Every man who has to do with sacred things should perform his work in a Christ like manner. There must be no sharp practice. "A false balance is abomination to the Lord." A false balance is a symbol of all unfair dealings, all devices to conceal selfishness and injustice under an appearance of fairness and equity. God will not in the slightest degree favor such practices. He hates every false way. He abhors all the selfishness and covetousness. Unmerciful dealing He will not tolerate, but will repay in kind. God can give prosperity to the working man whose means are acquired honestly. But His curse rests upon all that is gained by selfish practices. When one indulges in

selfishness or sharp dealing he knows that he does not fear the Lord or reverence His name. Those who are connected with God will not only shun all injustice, but will manifest His mercy and goodness toward all with whom they have to do. The Lord will sanction no respect of persons; but He will not, approve the course of those who make no difference in favor of the poor, the widow, and the orphan. . . .

The Lord is looking upon men in the different spheres in which they move, and the character is tested under the different circumstances in which they are placed. The truth, pure, refined, elevating, is a continual test, to measure the man. If truth controls the conscience and is an abiding principle in the heart, it becomes an active, working agent; it works by love, and purifies the soul. But if the knowledge of the truth produces no beauty in the soul, if it does not, subdue, soften, and recreate the man after God's own image, it is of no benefit to the receiver; it is as sounding brass or tinkling cymbal. The truth as it is in Jesus, planted in the heart by the Holy Spirit, always works from within outward; it will be revealed in our words and spirit and actions toward everyone with whom we are connected.

The wave of truth flowing from the infinitely wise God to His frail human agents, is not subject to the will of man. God prescribes the terms, and specifies every condition upon which we may receive His gifts. With the one party there is infinite power, wisdom, mercy, and goodness; with the other party is weakness, and ignorance, and helplessness, and sin. Even the faculties and resources of men, which God will accept in cooperation with the divine, are ours only in trust. In the great condescension of God to admit finite beings as co-laborers in the saving of the world, He makes it a condition that the human agent shall receive counsel from God, diligently obeying every word that proceedeth out of the mouth of God. And our success in the religious life will be according to the integrity and thoroughness with which these conditions are fulfilled. . . .

God designs that all who are laborers together with Him should have a rich experience in His love and His power to save. Never should we say, "I have no experience;" for that God who gave Paul an experience will reveal Himself to everyone who will earnestly seek Him. What said God of Abraham? "I know him," saith the heart-searching God, "that He will command His children and His household after Him; and they shall keep the way of the Lord, to do justice and judgment." Abraham would cultivate home religion, and the fear of the Lord would lead to integrity {149} of life. He who blesses the habitation of the righteous says, "I know Him, that He will command." There is no betraying of sacred trusts, no hesitating between right and wrong. The Holy One has given rules for the guidance of all, the standard of character from which none can swerve and be guiltless. God's will is to be diligently and conscientiously studied, and it must be made paramount in all the affairs of life. The laws which every human agent is to obey flows from the heart of infinite love.

That same holy Watcher who says, "I know Abraham," knew Cornelius also, and sent His angel with a message to the man who had received and improved all the light God had given him. The angel said, "Thy prayers and thine alms are come up for a memorial before God. And now send men to Joppa, and call for one Simon, whose surname is Peter." Then the specific directions are given, "He lodgeth with one Simon a tanner, whose house is by the seaside; he shall tell thee what thou oughtest to do." Thus the angel of the Lord works to bring Cornelius in connection with the human agent through whom he might receive greater light. Study the whole chapter carefully, and see the simplicity of the whole transaction. Then consider that the Lord knows every one of us by name, and just where we live, and the spirit we possess, and every act of our life. The ministering angels are passing through the churches, noting our faithfulness in our individual line of duty. . . .

BROTHER FOSTER AND DOCTRINAL DIVISION

January 9, 1893
George's Terrace, St. Kilda Road,
Melbourne

THIS AFTERNOON I HAD A LONG conversation with Brother Foster a member of the Prahran Church, who is in perplexity and trial. He is a tailor by trade, and is a first class workman. Before accepting the truth he had a position that commanded $30.00 a week. When he began to keep the Sabbath, he was permitted to retain his position, losing only the day's wages for the Sabbath. He is a man of good address, and has good ability to teach the truth. He left his position, and went into the field as a laborer, but was sent alone into a hard field, and became discouraged and confused, and almost fell under the delusive power of Satan. At the conference one year ago he had a conversation with me. He became free, the meeting did him good. He has since moved to Melbourne, and works at his trade and leads the meetings in Prahran. But in the present depression of business, he is in close circumstances; and being in poor health, with a large family, he has become much discouraged, and in this state of mind Satan has pressed temptation and darkness upon him. For weeks he has been in sore trial, and today he came to tell me his troubles.

He says he knew so little of the testimonies, he did not understand the relation they sustained to the cause. Some time since, while he was in perplexity, asking the Lord for light, he had a very striking dream. He saw Sister White in a boat riding on the billows, which were sending the spray like light {150} in every direction. It came into the room where he was with many others; he moved to get beyond its reach, when a hand stretched out to him gave him a paper. The paper was on fire, and a voice said, "Read quickly." He put out the fire, and opened the paper. There was a testimony, and a key lying upon the testimony. The interpretation came to his mind with great force, "The key to the testimonies is the testimonies themselves." He woke with the blessing of God upon him. Then he prayed, "Lord direct me to the testimony I should read to help my case." He took up testimony 31 and opened at the article, "The testimonies rejected." He read it through with intense interest and was deeply impressed that the testimonies were from God.

After this he saw in the Review the article of Brother A. T. Jones in regard to the image of the beast, and then the one from Elder Smith presenting the opposite view. He was perplexed and troubled. He had received much light and comfort in reading articles from Brethren Jones and Waggoner; but here was one of the old laborers, one who had written many of our standard books, and whom we had believed to be taught of God, who seemed to be in conflict with Brother Jones. What could all this mean? Was Brother Jones in the wrong? Was Brother Smith in error? Which was right? He became confused. When the important laborers in the cause of God take opposite positions in the same paper, whom can we depend upon? Who can we believe has the true position?

Brother Foster was in such perplexity, that he sent word by letter that he could not lead in the meetings. Since the beginning of the week of prayer, temptations have pressed so strongly upon him that he has received no benefit. These differences among our leading men have absorbed all his thoughts and he is much distressed over the matter. I told him I expected that others who should read these articles would have the same experience. These differences should not have been made public, for some who are weak in the faith would be caused to stumble, and as the result might lose their souls. I felt keen regret and deep sorrow of heart, for I knew that the Lord was displeased.

But I said, "Brother Foster, you have the Bible. Search its pages with a prayerful heart; your Redeemer has promised that the Holy Spirit shall lead you into all truth. You have an Instructor that is full of wisdom, one who never errs. I charge you before God to cease worrying, receive the precious rays of light that come to you, feast upon the truth as it in Jesus, walk in the light while you have the light, and more light will shine upon you from the Source of all light. Do not suffer your mind to dwell upon the differences you think you discern. If our leading Brethren are so unwise as to allow their conflicting views to appear in the paper published to go to the world; if they present these differences before the large gatherings that assemble to worship God in the tabernacle or elsewhere, they are doing the very things the Lord Jesus told them not to do, and going directly contrary to the light given them through the testimonies." {151}

Now, brethren, the zeal that leads to this kind of work is not inspired of God; Christ never prompts any man to work against Christ. He will not lead us to counteract His own instruction, or to act contrary to the spirit of the prayer He offered for His disciples just before He left them. He knew they would be exposed to trials from the opposition of the world, and He said, "While I was with them in the world, I kept them in Thy name: Those that Thou gavest Me I have kept, and none of them is lost, but the son of perdition; that the Scripture might be fulfilled. And now I come to Thee; and these things I speak in the world, that they might have My joy fulfilled in themselves and I have given them Thy word; and the world hath hated them, because they are not of the world, even as I am not of the world, but that Thou shouldst keep them from the evil."

Our work is clearly aggressive. Our warfare is to be directed against error and sin, not against one another. God requires us to be a strength to one another, to heal, not to destroy. We are to be constantly receiving light; and we are not to spurn the message or the messengers by whom God shall send light to His people.

If before publishing Elder Jones' article concerning the image of the beast, Elder Smith had conferred with him, plainly stating that his own view differed from that of Brother Jones, and that if the article appeared in the Review, he himself must present the opposite position, then the matter would appear in a different light from what it now does. But the course pursued in this case was the same as that taken at Minneapolis. Those who opposed Brethren Jones and Waggoner manifested no disposition to meet them like brethren, and with the Bible in hand consider prayerfully and in a Christ-like spirit the points of difference. This is the only course that would meet the approval of God, and His rebuke was upon those who would not do this at Minneapolis. Yet this blind warfare is continued; men of the same faith, in the same city, turn their weapons against each other. It is an astonishment to the heavenly universe. I feel deeply grieved, and if these things are a grief to me, how do they appear to Jesus, who suffered untold agony upon the cross to redeem men from the power of Satan and make them one in Christ? "All ye are brethren." What can lead brethren to present before the world opposite opinions, without first coming together in love, and comparing views to see if they cannot come into harmony? Will my brethren tell me what spirit is moving them to action?

We know that Brother Jones has been giving the message for this time, meat in due season to the starving flock of God. Those who do not allow prejudice to bar the heart against the heaven sent message, cannot but feel the spirit and force of the truth. Brother Jones has borne the message from church to church, and from state to state; and light and freedom and the out-pouring of the Spirit of God has attended the work. As events of a most startling nature in the fulfillment of prophecy has shown that the great crisis in rapidly approaching, Brother Jones seeks to arouse the professed people of God from their death-like slumber, to see the importance of giving the warning {152} to the world. But he advances some ideas with which all do not agree, and instantly Brother Gage is aroused; he harnesses for the battle, and before the congregation in the tabernacle he takes his position in opposition to Brother Jones. Was this in the order of God? Did the Spirit of the Lord go before Brother Jones and inspire Brother Gage to do this work? Suppose that Brother Jones' statement concerning the formation of the image was premature; did the case demand such demonstrations? I answer No, no; not if God has ever spoken by me.

The Bible rules must be strictly followed. The matter concerning which difference of opinion prevails should be calmly considered, with much prayer, with hearts yearning for unity, and with perfect love for one another's souls. Examine every point as if you could see the whole heavenly universe looking upon you. If there is positive evidence that one of the brethren is in error, try to convince him from the work of God. If success should not crown your efforts, even then the world has no business with the matter; for it would only dishonor the God of truth, and Jesus Christ whom He hath sent.

I have received letters from different points telling the sad, discouraging results of these things. We have opposition enough from our foes, and we shall have conflicts fierce and strong; let us not now cause Satan to glory because of the pitched battles within our own ranks. The unity for which our Saviour prayed should be brought into our practical life. Peace, the peace of Christ, inspired by truth, and sustained by righteousness, we must each cultivate. God so loved the world, that He manifested His love by giving His only begotten Son, that whosoever believeth in Him should not perish, but have everlasting life. Jesus said, A new commandment I give unto you that ye love one another; as I have loved you, that ye also love one another. By this shall all men know that ye are My disciples, if ye have love one for another, as I have loved you." Let your zeal be manifest, not in exposing your variances but in cultivating the precious plant of love, just as Jesus has told us to do.

"Hereby perceive we the love of God, because He laid down His life for us: and we ought to lay down our lives for the brethren. . . My little children, let us not love in word, neither in tongue; but indeed and in truth. And hereby we know that we are of the truth, and shall assure our hearts before Him. . . And this is His commandment, That we should believe in the name of His Son Jesus Christ, and love one another; for love is of God; and every one that loveth is born of God, and knoweth God. He that loveth not, knoweth not God; for God is love. In this was manifested the love of God toward us, because God sent His only begotten Son into the world, that we might live through Him. Herein is love, not that we loved God, but that He loved us, and sent His Son to be the propitiation for our sins.

"Beloved, if God so loved us, we ought to love one another. No man hath seen God at any time. If we love one another, God dwelleth in us, and His love is perfected in us. Hereby know we that we dwell in Him, and He in us, because He hath {153} given us of His Spirit." "If a man say, I love God, and hateth his brother, he is a liar; for he that loveth not his brother whom he hath seen, how can he love God whom he hath not seen? And this commandment have we from Him, that he who loveth God loveth his brother also."

I have quoted only a few passages, but the Bible abounds in just such lessons. If it is not possible to love God unless we love our brother, the case will certainly go against us in the courts of heaven if we do not cherish Christ like love for one another. The word is very explicit. I am pained beyond measure when I see how little love is cherished and manifested among brethren. How long shall Satan use his arguments against us and weaken our influence by revealing to others how little love and deference and respect are shown for one another? Is it not time we were doers of the word, and not hearers only? Shall we not closely examine our own hearts, and see whether we are in possession of the love of God? Jesus came in the likeness of sinful flesh, by a pure and holy life to condemn sin in the flesh. He came to our world to represent the character of God, and it is our work to represent the character of Christ. If we have lost His love out of our hearts, our work is to seek the Lord, that our hearts may be renewed by His Holy Spirit.

"I beseech you, brethren, by the name of our Lord Jesus Christ, that ye all speak the same things and that there be no divisions among you; but that ye be perfectly joined together in the same mind and in the same judgment." For it has been declared unto you, my brethren, by them which are of the house of Chloe, that there are contentions among you. Now this I say, That every one of you saith, I am of Paul; and I am of Apollos; and I of Cephas; and I of Christ. Is Christ divided? Was Paul crucified for you? Or were you baptized in the name of Paul?

The cause of divisions or discord in the church is separation from Christ. The secret of unity is union with Christ. Christ is the great center. We shall approach one another just in proportion as we approach the center. United with Christ, we shall surely be united with our brethren in the faith. To be a Christian means a great deal more than is supposed. A Christian is Christ-like. Membership in the church does not make us Christians. Has the light from Christ penetrated the heart? Are justice and purity and truth abiding in the soul temple? We may know; for the fruits will appear. "The fruit of the Spirit is love, joy, peace long-suffering, gentleness, goodness, faith, meekness, temperance; against such there is no law. And they that are Christ's have crucified the flesh with the affections and lusts. If we live in the Spirit, let us also walk in the Spirit. Let us not be desirous of vain glory, provoking one another, envying one another. Brethren, if a man be overtaken in a fault, ye which are spiritual, restore such an one in the Spirit of meekness, considering thyself, lest thou also be tempted. Bear ye one another's burdens, and so fulfil the law of Christ. For if a man think himself to be something, when he is nothing, he deceiveth himself. This is not a time for brother to cherish prejudice against brother. Put not into our enemies' hands anything that {154} bears the least suggestions of differences among us, even in opinion.

The conference at Minneapolis was the golden opportunity for all present to humble the heart before God, and to welcome Jesus as the great Instructor; but the stand taken by some at that meeting proved their ruin. They have never seen clearly since, and they never will; for they persistently cherish the spirit that prevailed there, a wicked criticizing, denunciatory spirit. Yet since that meeting, abundant light and evidence has been graciously given, that all might understand the truth. Those who were then deceived might since have come to the light. They might rejoice in the truth as it is in Jesus, were it not for the pride of their own rebellious hearts. They will be asked in the Judgment, "Who required this at your hand, to rise up against the message and the messengers I sent to My people with light, with grace and power? Why have you lifted up your souls against God? Why did you block the way with your own perverse spirit? And afterward when evidence was piled upon evidence, why did you not humble your hearts before God, and repent of your rejection of the message of mercy He has sent you? The Lord has not inspired these brethren to resist the truth. He designed that they should be baptized with the Holy Spirit, and be living channels of light to communicate the light to our world, in clear, bright rays.

"The Lord hath from the beginning chosen you to salvation through sanctification of the Spirit and belief of the truth." Here, according to the appointment of God, are the two agencies in man's salvation,—the divine influences, and a strong, living, working faith, a faith that receives the truth. God requires no man to cast aside his reason, and yield to the control of blind credulity. But we are to search the Scriptures in the spirit of learners. In the meekness of Christ canvas every point of difference. Search for the truth as for hidden treasures. It will not do to ignore these questions of vital interest. Human assertions are as valueless as straw. Many will miss the path to heaven because they rest their faith upon men. They resist the message of mercy because someone in whom they have confidence is indifferent to it. But the soul is of too great value to rest its faith on man. No one but Christ can ransom the soul. We have the word of God, and this alone can we trust unwaveringly. Let brethren seek God together. Let them fall upon the Rock and be broken. "Ye are laborers together with God." We must understand the obligations imposed upon us by this co-operation, or we shall never stand approved in the Judgment. Laborers together with God means fellow-laborers with those of our own fallen race, but co-operating with divine agencies. It is the work of salvation to accomplish this union of the human with the divine.

The time of peril is now upon us. It can no longer be spoken of as in the future. And the power of every mind, sanctified to the Master's work, it to be employed, not to hedge up the way before the messages God sends to His people, but to labor unitedly in preparing a people to stand in the great day of God. It is not the inspiration from heaven that leads one to be suspicious, watching for a chance and greedily seizing upon {155} it to prove that those brethren who differ from us in some interpretation of Scripture are not sound in the faith. There is danger that this course of action will produce the very result assumed; and to a great degree the guilt will rest upon those who are watching for evil. Had our brethren been free from prejudice, and walking in humility, they would have been ready to receive light from whatever source; recognizing the Spirit of God and the grace of Christ, they would be indeed channels of light, and their long experience would make them safe counselors, men of sound judgment.

God would have His people love one another and help one another, thus strengthening every good work. We should counsel with one another, the old, experienced laborers with those whom God shall raise up to advance His work as we approach the great consummation. But if such men as Elder Smith, Elder Van Horn, and Elder Butler shall stand aloof, not blending with the elements God sees essential to carry forward the work in these perilous times, they will be left behind. God will complete His work in righteousness. These brethren have had every opportunity to stand in the ranks that are pressing on to victory; but if they refuse, the work will advance without them. God will send by whom He will; His message will not return unto Him void, but will accomplish that whereunto it is sent. And if they refuse the message, the men whom God designed should hold the same relation to the younger workers as did Moses to Joshua, will fail of doing the work the Lord designed they should do. They will be a hindrance in the place of a blessing. The work will go forward; but these brethren, who might have received the richest blessings, will meet with eternal loss; for though they should repent and be saved at last, they can never regain that which they have lost through their wrong course of action. They might have been God's instruments to carry the work forward with power; but their influence was exerted to counteract the Lord's message, to make the work appear questionable. Every jot and tittle of this will have to be repented of.

The opposition in our own ranks has imposed upon the Lord's messengers a laborious and soul trying task; for they have had to meet difficulties and obstacles which need not have existed. While this labor had to be performed among our own people, to make them willing that God should work in the day of his power, the light of the glory of God has not been shining in clear, concentrated rays to our world. Thousand who are now in darkness of error, might have been added to our numbers. All the time and thought and labor required to counteract the influence of our brethren who oppose the message has been just as much taken from the work of warning the world of the swift coming judgments of God. The Spirit of God has been present in power among His people, but it could not be bestowed upon them, because they did not open their hearts to receive it.

It is not the opposition of the world that we have to fear; but it is the elements that work among ourselves that have hindered the message. The efficiency of the movements for extending the truth depends upon the harmonious action of those who profess to believe it. Love and confidence {156} constitute a moral force that would have united our churches, and insure harmony of action, but coldness and distrust have brought disunion that has shorn us of our strengths.

The Lord designed that the messages of warning and instruction given through the Spirit to His people should go everywhere. But the influence that grew out of the resistance of light and truth at Minneapolis tended to make of no effect the light God had given to His people through the Testimonies. Great Controversy Vol. IV, has not had the circulation it should have had, because some of those who occupy responsible positions were leavened with the spirit that prevailed at Minneapolis, a spirit that clouded the discernment of the people of God.

The work of opponents to the truth has been steadily advancing, while we have been compelled to devote our energies in a great degree to counteracting the work of the enemy through those who were in our own ranks. The dullness of some and the opposition of others have confined our strength and means largely among those who knew the truth but did not practice its principles. If every soldier of Christ had done his duty, if every watchman on the walls of Zion had given the trumpet a certain sound, the world might ere this have heard the message of warning. What account will be rendered to God for thus retarding the work?

While the angels were holding the four winds that they should not blow, giving opportunity for everyone who had light to let it shine to the world, there have been influences at work among us to cry peace and safety. Many did not understand that we had not time or strength or influence to be lost through dilatory action. While men slept, Satan has been stealing a march upon us, working up the advantages given him to have things after his own order.

The Lord has revealed to us that the Laodicean message applies to the church at this time, and yet how few make a practical application of it to themselves. God has wrought for us; we have no complaint to make of Heaven, for the richest blessings have been proffered us, but our people have been very reluctant to accept them. Those who have been so stubborn and rebellious that they would not humble themselves to receive the light God sent in mercy to their souls, became so destitute of the Holy Spirit that the Lord could not use them. Unless they are converted, these men will never enter the mansions of the blest. Some have been preaching the word whose labors are tainted with impurity and licentiousness. They have done far more harm than good. Unless they shall turn from their evil ways, they will perish with the wicked. Others have carried the truth in a very indifferent manner; they have had no real burden for the work; they have gone backward rather than forward. It is high time for these to retrace their steps; for they have lost their first love. The Lord's injunction to them is, "Remember therefore from whence thou art fallen, and repent, and do the first works; Or else I will come unto thee quickly, and will remove they candlestick out of thy place, except thou repent." {157}

A great work is before us. There are a few who carry the heavy burden of responsibility. They feel that God has committed to our American churches a solemn trust in the messages of truth to be given to the world. From all nations the Macedonian cry is heard, "Come over and help us." God in His providence has opened fields before us, and if the human agents co-operate with the divine agencies, many souls may be made partakers of a pure and saving faith. For years the appeal has been made, but the Lord's professed people have been sleeping over their allotted work, and it remains almost untouched. God has sent message after message to arouse our churches to do something, and to do it now. But to the call of God, "Whom shall I send?" There has been few voices to respond, "Here am I, send me." Through this neglect, many souls will lose the opportunity the Lord desires to give them.

"A certain man made a great supper, and bade many: and sent his servant at supper time to say to them that were bidden, Come; for all things are now ready. And they all with one consent began to make excuse. The first said unto him, I have bought a piece of ground, and I must needs go and see it: I pray thee have me excused. And another said, I have bought five yoke of oxen, and I go to prove them, I pray thee have me excused. And another said, I have married a wife, and therefore I cannot come. So that servant came, and showed his lord these things. Then the master of the house being angry said to his servant, Go out quickly into the streets and lanes of the city, and bring in hither the poor, and maimed, and the halt, and the blind. And the servant said, Lord, it is done as thou hast commanded, and yet there is room. And the lord said unto the servant, Go out into the highways and hedges, and compel them to come in, that my house may be filled. For I say unto you, That none of those which were bidden shall taste of my supper."

When the message of God is brought to them, many will thus excuse themselves. But the work must be pressed wherever there is an opening. Men and money are needed to carry the work forward. Still there is opportunity for us to share the Saviour's self-denial and sacrifice for the salvation of souls. The necessities of the work now demand a far greater outlay than ever before. The Lord calls upon His people to make every effort to curtail their expenses. Again I plead that instead of spending money for pictures of yourselves and your friends, you should turn it into another channel. Let the money that has been devoted to the gratification of self flow into the Lord's treasury to sustain those who are working to save perishing souls. Let those who have houses and lands give heed to the message, "Sell that ye have, and give alms." "Bring ye all the tithes into the storehouse, that there may be meat in mine house, and prove Me now herewith, saith the Lord of hosts, if I will not open you the windows of heaven, and pour you out a blessing, that there shall not be room enough to receive it."

The Lord is soon to come. We must work while the day lasts; for the night is coming, in which no man can work. Many, many have lost the spirit of self-denial and sacrifice. They have been burying their money in temporal possessions. There are {158} men whom God has blessed, whom He is testing to see what response they will make to His benefits. They have with-held their tithes and offerings until their debt to the Lord God of hosts has become so great that they grow pale as the thought of rendering to the Lord His own, a just tithe. Make haste, brethren, you have now opportunity to be honest with God; delay not. For your souls' sake no longer rob God in tithes and offerings.

The Lord calls for every talent of means and ability to be put to use. When the reproach of indolence and slothfulness shall have been wiped away from the church, the Spirit of the Lord will be graciously manifested. Divine power will combine with human effort, the church will see the providential interpositions of the Lord God of hosts, the light of truth will be diffused, the knowledge of God and of Jesus Christ whom He hath sent. As in the apostles' time many souls will turn unto the Lord. The earth will be lightened with the glory of the angel from heaven.

If the world are to be convinced of sin as transgressors of God's law, the agency must be the Holy Spirit working through human instrumentalities. The church needs now to shake off her death-like slumber; for the Lord is waiting to bless His people who will recognize His blessing when it comes, and diffuse it in clear, strong rays of light. "Then will I sprinkle clear water upon you, and ye shall be clean. . . .And I will put My Spirit upon you, and cause you to walk in My statutes." If the wilderness of the church is to become as a fruitful field, and the fruitful field to be as a forest, it is through the Holy Spirit of God poured out upon His people. The heavenly agencies have long been waiting for the human agents, the members of the church, to cooperate with them in the great work to be done. They are waiting for you. So vast is the field, so comprehensive the design, that every sanctified heart will be pressed into service as an agent of divine power.

At the same time there will be a power stirring everything from beneath. The working of evil angels will be manifest in deceptions, delusions, in calamities, and casualties, and crimes of no ordinary character. While God employs the angels of mercy to work through His human agents, Satan sets his agencies in operation, laying under tribute all the powers that submit to his control. There will be lords many and gods many. The cry will be heard, "Lo, here is Christ, and Lo, He is there." The deep plotting of Satan will reveal its working everywhere for the purpose of distracting attention from present duty. The appearance of a false Christ will awaken delusive hopes in the minds of those who allow themselves to be deceived. The church members that are awake will rise to the emergency, manifesting greater diligence as iniquity abounds. The very manifestations of Satanic power are to be presented in their true light before the people. There will be signs and wonders in the world of nature. The powers of earth and heaven will manifest a terrifying, destructive activity. But the eye of faith will discern in all these manifestations harbingers of the grand and awful future, and the triumphs that will surely come to God's people.

Let all who believe the truth for this time put away their {159} differences; put away envy and evil speaking and evil thinking. Press together, press together. "Seeing ye have purified your souls in obeying the truth through the Spirit unto unfeigned love of the brethren, see that ye love one another with a pure heart fervently."

Work, O work, keeping eternity in view. Bear in mind that every power must be sanctified. In yourselves you are powerless to do anything good. Christ declares, "Without Me ye can do nothing." Becoming partakers of the divine nature you can do all things. Through Christ you can have power with God and with men. A great work is to be done. Let the prayer go forth from unfeigned lips, "God be merciful unto us, and bless us; and cause His face to shine upon us; that Thy way may be known upon the earth, Thy saving health among all nations." Our God is waiting to be gracious. "And this is life eternal, that they might know Thee, the only true God, and Jesus Christ whom Thou hast sent." Will the church give to the world the light of the knowledge of Jesus Christ? Shall the light shine forth to all nations, kindreds, tongues and peoples?

"There is no difference between the Jew and the Greek: for the same Lord over all is rich unto all that call upon Him. For whosoever shall call upon the name of the Lord shall be saved. How then shall they call on Him in whom they have not believed? and how shall they believe in Him of whom they have no heard? and how shall they hear without a preacher? and how shall they preach, except they be sent? as it is written, How beautiful are the feet of them that preach the gospel of peace, and bring glad tidings of good things." "For so hath the Lord commanded us, saying, I have set thee to be a light of the Gentiles, that thou shouldst be for salvation unto the ends of the earth."

"But when He saw the multitudes, He was moved with compassion because they fainted, and were scattered abroad, as sheep having no shepherd. Then saith He unto His disciples, The harvest truly is plentious, but the laborers are few; pray ye therefore the Lord of the harvest, that He will send forth laborers into His harvest." Our work is plainly laid down in the word of God. Christian is to be united to Christian, church to church, the human instrumentalities cooperating with the divine, every agency to be subordinate to the Holy Spirit, and all to be combined in giving to the world the good tidings of the grace of God.

(Signed) Ellen G. White

HEALTH REFORM

January 11, 1897
"Sunnyside," Cooranbong, N. S. W.
Ms-3- '97 {160}

I WAS AWAKENED AT 11:30 last night, and commenced writing. We were in a meeting where important instruction in many lines was being given. Among those assembled were physicians, editors, publishers, ministers, and a large number of other persons. We were considering many things in regard to health reform. The matters of exercise and reformatory methods in regard to the foods we eat were under discussion. Some were advocating a flesh meat diet. Speaking in support of this diet they said that without it they were weak in physical strength.

But the words of our Teacher to us were, "As a man thinketh, so is he." The flesh of dead animals was not the original food for man. Man was permitted to eat it after the flood because all vegetation had been destroyed. But the curse pronounced upon man and the earth and every living thing has made strange and wonderful changes. Since the flood the human race has been shortening its period of existence. Physical, mental and moral degeneracy is rapidly increasing in these latter days.

The educational work in the medical missionary line is a great advance step toward awakening man to his moral responsibilities. Had the ministers taken hold of this work in accordance with the light that God has given them in various lines, there would have been a most decided reformation in eating, in drinking, and in dressing.

But there are those who have stood directly in the way of the advance of Health Reform. They have held the people back by their indifferent or depreciatory remarks, and their supposed pleasantries and jokes. They themselves and a large number of others have been sufferers, even unto death, but all have not yet learned wisdom.

The Lord would vindicate the word He has given to His servants. Had all united to walk in the light, from the time the light was first given on this subject, there would have been an army of sensible arguments employed to vindicate the work of God. But it has been by most aggressive warfare that any advancement has been made. The souls and bodies of the people have been the case, if those who claimed to believe the truth had lived out its sacred principles in their lives. But these were unwilling to deny self, unwilling to yield their mind and will to the will of God; they were determined to have their own way, and they have realized in their own sufferings the sure results of such a course.

God has claims upon all who are engaged in his service. He desires that every power and endowment shall be under the divine control, and that they shall be as healthy as careful, strictly temperate habits can make them. We are under obligation to God to make an unreserved consecration of ourselves to him, body and soul, with all the faculties appreciated as God's entrusted gifts, to be employed in his service. All our energies and capabilities {161} are to be constantly strengthened and improved during this period of probationary time.

But those who have occupied positions of influence have not appreciated the work which has been so long neglected. They have not become interested and diligent students of the building which God has made for his habitation. They consider it far more important to become learners upon subjects of less consequence to the human agent. Thousands upon thousands know nothing of the body, and how to care for it. David declared, "I am fearfully and wonderfully made." And when God has given us such a habitation, why should not every apartment be critically examined. The chambers of the mind and the heart apartment are the most important. Why should men and women continue in ignorance, and live in the basement of the house, enjoying sensual and debasing pleasures?

Great care should be taken when the change is made from a flesh meat to a veg-

etarian diet to supply the table with wisely prepared, well-cooked articles of food. So much porridge eating is a mistake. The dry food, that requires mastication is far preferable. The health food preparations are a blessing in this respect. Good brown bread and rolls, prepared in a simple manner yet with painstaking effort will be healthful. Bread should never have the slightest taint of sourness. It should be cooked until it is most thoroughly done. Thus all softness and stickiness will be avoided.

For those who can use them, good vegetables, prepared in a healthful manner are better than soft mushes or porridge. Fruits used with thoroughly cooked bread two or three days old will be more healthful than fresh bread. This with slow and thorough mastication, will furnish all that the system requires.

"As a man thinketh so is he." If the appetite is allowed to rule, then the mind will be brought under its control. When the stomach is educated to discard that which will prove only an injury to it, the simplest kinds of food will satisfy its hunger.

It is not well to take a great variety of foods at one meal. When fruit and bread, together with a variety of other foods that do not agree, are crowded into the stomach at one meal, what can we expect but that a disturbance will be created?

The mixing largely of white or brown flour bread with milk in the place of water is not a healthful preparation. If the bread thus cooked is allowed to stand over, and is then broken open, there will frequently be seen long strings like cobwebs, and this, in warm weather, soon causes fermentation to take place in the stomach. Milk should not be used in place of water in bread making. All this is extra expense, and is not wholesome. The taste may be educated so that it will prefer bread prepared in this way; but the more simply it is made, the better it will satisfy hunger, and the more natural will be the appetite to enjoy the plainest diet.

We had a large family to cook for, and the ten quarts of milk which our cow gave each day was not sufficient for our family {162} use. At times three extra quarts had to be purchased to give us enough to mix the bread with milk. This was a most extravagant business, and wholly unnecessary. I had this order of things changed, and the testimony of nearly all was that the bread was more appetizing than when mixed with milk.

Every housekeeper should feel it her

duty to educate herself to make good sweet bread, and in the most inexpensive manner; and the family should refuse to have upon the table bread that is heavy and sour; for it is injurious. There are a large number of poor families who buy the common baker's bread which is often sour, and is not healthful for the stomach. In every line of cooking the questions that should be considered is, "How shall the food be prepared in the most natural and inexpensive manner?" And there should be careful study that the fragments of food left over from the table be not wasted. Study how, that in some way these fragments of food shall not be lost. This skill, economy, and tact is a fortune. In the warmer part of the season, prepare less food. Use more dry substance. There are many poor families, who, although they have scarcely enough to eat, can often be enlightened as to why they are poor, there are so many jots and tittles wasted.

The meat diet is the serious question. Shall human beings live on the flesh of dead animals? The answer, from the light that God has given is, No; decidedly no. Health Reform institutions should educate on this question. Physicians who claim to understand the human organism ought not to encourage their patients to subsist on the flesh of dead animals. They should point out the increase of disease in the animal kingdom. The testimony of examiners is that very few animals are free from disease, and that the practice of eating largely of meat is contracting diseases of all kinds,—cancers, tumors, scrofula, tuberculosis, and numbers of other like affections. If men will subsist on the food that God has so abundantly provided without having it first pass into the animal organism and become sinew and muscle, and then take it second hand by eating of the corpse, his health would be much better insured.

The ministers in our land should become intelligent upon Health Reform. They need to become acquainted with the science of physiology. They will be intelligent in regard to the laws that govern physical life, and their bearings upon the health of mind and soul. Then they will be able to speak correctly upon this subject. In their obedience to physical laws that are to hold forth the word of life to the people, and lead up higher and still higher in the work of reform. "I beseech you therefore brethren, by the mercies of God, that ye present your bodies a living sacrifice, holy, acceptable unto God, which is your reasonable service." "Dearly beloved, I beseech you as strangers and pilgrims, abstain from fleshly lusts, which war against the soul; having your conversation honest amongst the Gentiles: that, whereas they speak against you as evil doers, they may by your good works, which they shall behold, glorify God in the day of visitation. All who claim to be teachers should urge, both by precept and example the necessity of abstaining from fleshly lusts, which war against the soul. {163}

What shall arouse those who claim to be walking in the light that is shining upon the people of God in these last days? A lethargy of unconscious sensualism through indulgence of perverted appetite, a constant submitting of soul and body and spirit to moral defilement is upon the people. Under the marriage vow, which our Creator has instituted, appetite has been perverted and indulged. And these lustful appetites, with their destroying power, have been transmitted from parents to children, and so intensified that their names are recorded in the books of heaven as transgressors of God's law. Upon their very countenances is imprinted the sin of Sodom. And continuance in these sins will bring the sure and terrible results. They will suddenly be destroyed, and that without remedy. They will receive the sentence, "He that is unjust, let him be unjust still: and he which is filthy, let him be filthy still: and he that is righteous, let him be righteous still: and he that is holy, let him be holy still. And, behold, I come quickly; and my reward is with me, to give every man according, as his work shall be. I am Alpha and Omega, the beginning and the end, the first and the last. Blessed are they that do his commandments, that they may have right to the tree of life, and enter in through the gates into the city. For without are dogs, and sorcerers, and whoremongers, and murderers, and idolaters, and whosoever loveth and maketh a lie."

This is the final judgment. Let the senses of all be aroused; for many whose names now appear on the church books are not the children of God. In the books of heaven it is recorded of them, "Thou art weighed in the balances, and found wanting." Let every church in our land arouse to the importance of studying the word of God, and with much earnest prayer, not stand afar off, but "draw nigh unto God." The promise is, "He will draw nigh unto you." Then you may keep life in your souls, and obtain

a sound experience. Then you will not be of that class of whom it is written, "And because iniquity shall abound, the love of many shall wax cold."

Let the Lord Jesus come into your houses and into your hearts. Every talent entrusted to us is to be used and improved in accordance with the will of the Giver. Days, months, and years are added to our existence that we may improve our opportunities and advantages for working out our own individual salvation, and promoting the well-being of others by our unselfish life. Thus may we build up the kingdom of Christ, and make manifest the glory of God.

Human exertion, physical and intellectual ability, will be taxed to the utmost to keep the feet of the youth in the path where we can trace the footprints of Jesus. The young men have not had all the attention that they should have had in order to develop their talents. The arrangements made in the missionary line of work are far in the rear. Councils have been corrupted, and board meetings been conducted by inefficient members who felt not the necessity of having the constraining power of the Holy Spirit upon the youth, to help them to choose the illumination from above. The youth need sanctified example, an acknowledgment of Omnipotence in the grand work of becoming home and foreign missionaries. They need to behold in the cross of Christ the only {164} true power to sustain the human agent in his continuous struggle against temptations, amid disappointments and reverses. How many of the General Conference have said to the workers "Go," but have left many to make brick without straw, have given them no facilities or help.

The malarious, poisonous atmosphere, which surrounds the souls of those who are dead in trespasses and sins, is causing them to become like the inhabitants of the Noatic world, who, because they chose to follow the imaginations of their own corrupt minds, and dishonor God by their wicked inventions, they became corrupt in body and soul, and hated the God who made them. God sent them a message that they should not live, but should be destroyed because of their wicked works. And whole families today are in need of being terribly alarmed. They have been, and still are, corrupting their way before God. They are so steeped in licentiousness that they do not discern the difference between the pure affections given them of

God, the attributes of human nature, and the destructive lusts which by indulgence and wicked inventions make them as sinful as were those before the flood and the inhabitants of Sodom.

In assuming human nature that He might reach to the very depths of human woe and misery, and lift man up, Christ has shown what estimate He places upon the human race. In this work everything was at stake. Satan claimed to be the lawful owner of the fallen race; and with what persistent efforts did he seek to overthrow Christ through his subtlety! It was only by most desperate conflict with the powers of Satan that Christ could accomplish his purpose of restoring the almost obliterated image of God in man, and place his own signature upon his forehead. It was a desperate battle; for Satan had so long worked in league with human intelligences as to about completely intercept every ray of light shining from the throne of God upon the human mind. The cross of Calvary alone could destroy the works of the devil. In that wondrous sacrifice all eyes were called to "behold the Lamb of God, that taketh away the sin of the world." The love of Christ kindles in the heart of all who continue to behold him.

Satan's ear caught the words spoken by John the Baptist, "Behold the Lamb of God, that taketh away the sin of the world," and he determined to unite all the power of his army and of human beings with himself to accomplish the ruin of the race. He would commence with the appetite. He could bring his temptations to bear upon this point, and by a perverted appetite destroy the mental and physical force, and make man appear a revolting, polluted being before his Maker. And Satan has carried out his purpose.

All nature makes manifest the work of God. Man is fearfully and wonderfully made, and if man had obeyed the laws of Jehovah in his natural laws, the image of God would have been revealed in him. But by sinning against his own body, by indulging his unnatural appetite and disturbing the action of the human machinery; by the use of alcoholic drinks, narcotics, and the flesh of diseased animals, man has dis-ordered and crippled the Lord's divine arrangements. Nature does her best to expel the poisonous drug tobacco, but frequently she is overborne. She gives up the struggles to expel the intruder, and the life is sacrificed in {165} the conflict. Every pernicious drug placed in the human stomach, whether by prescription of physicians, or by man himself doing violence to the human organism, injures the whole machinery. Every intemperate indulgence of lustful appetite is at war with natural instinct and the healthful condition of every nerve and muscle and organ of the wonderful human machinery which through the Creator's powers possesses organic life.

Nature would do her work wisely and well if the human agent would, in his treatment of the body, co-operate with the divine purpose. But how Satan and his whole confederacy rejoice to see how easily his powers of deception and art can persuade men to form an appetite for most unpleasant stimulants and narcotics. And then when nature has been overborne, enfeebled in all her working force, there is the drug medication to come from the physicians, to kill the remaining vital force and leave men miserable wrecks of suffering, of imbecility, of insanity, and of loathsome disease. God is hidden from the human observation by the hellish shadow of Satan.

In Luke 4:16-19, Christ announces his mission and work for the world: "And he came to Nazareth, where he had been brought up, and, as his custom was, he went into the synagogue on the Sabbath day, and stood up for to read. And there was delivered unto him the book of the prophet Esaias. And when he had opened the book, he found the place where it was written, The Spirit of the Lord is upon me, because he hath anointed me to preach the gospel to the poor: he hath sent me to heal the broken hearted, to preach deliverance to the captives, and recovering of sight to the blind, to set at liberty them that are bruised, to preach the acceptable year of the Lord." Jesus himself became man's ransom, his liberator from the oppressive power of Satan. "Ye are not your own," he says, "for ye are bought with a price." We are bought from a power whose slaves we were. And the price our ransom cost was the only begotten Son of God. His blood alone could ransom guilty man. "For God so loved the world that he gave his only begotten Son that whosoever believeth in him should not perish, but have everlasting life."

O, if everyone could discern these matters as they have been presented to me those who are now so careless, so indifferent in regard to their character building; those who plead for indulgence in a flesh meat diet, would never open their lips in justification of an appetite for the flesh of dead animals. Such a diet contaminates the blood of their veins, and stimulates the lower animal passions. It enfeebles keen perception and vigor of thought to the understanding of God and the truth, and a knowledge of themselves.

Christ gave his life a ransom for many. Christ was to come under the cruel power of Satan. Satan hoped if he could once gain the supremacy he would overcome Christ. He had obtained mastery over the human family, and through disobedience to God's holy law, had brought them under his jurisdiction. He unjustly claimed them as his own subjects. But Christ takes the prey from the enemy. Satan was to be overcome by the Son of man. {166}

Christ removed every obstruction that man might return to his allegiance to God. Christ became subject to suffering in behalf of man. And yet man by his selfish indulgence, is willing to place himself in slippery places, and through unnatural appetite obliterate the image of God. Man, who has been endowed with physical, mental, and moral power, has placed himself where he is a weakling. Satan knows that he cannot overcome man unless he can control his will. He can do this by deceiving man so that he will co-operate with him in transgressing the laws of nature in eating and drinking, which is transgression of the law of God.

Here is where the subject on intemperance grows into importance. Here is where Satan works to so confuse minds by a perverted appetite that man cannot discern sacred things from common. Cheap things are placed on a level with the sacred. Animalism is strengthened, the higher powers weakened.

The physical and mental condition of the parents is perpetuated in their offspring. This is a matter that is not duly considered. Wherever the habits of the parents are contrary to physical law, the injury to themselves will be repeated in the future generations. Satan knows this very well, and he is perpetuating his work through transmission. Let the husband and wife in their married life prove a help and a blessing to one another. Let them consider the cost of every indulgence in intemperance and sensualism. These indulgences do not increase love, not ennoble and elevate. Those who will indulge the animal passions and gratify lust will surely stamp upon their offspring the debasing practices, and grossness of their own physical and moral defilement. By physical, mental, and moral culture all may become co-workers with Christ. Very much depends upon the parents. It lies with them whether they shall bring into the world children who will prove a blessing or curse.

There is a much higher standard to be reached in every family. All can rise. By drawing nigh to God, they may receive power to resist the devil; for the Spirit of God lifts up a standard for them against the enemy. The father and the mother who know no higher rule of life than selfish indulgence of lustful passions are not Christians. They are lowering the standard of intellectual and moral character, and are descending down toward the brute creation, rather than upward to work in harmony with Jesus Christ to restore the moral image of God in man. Appetites are cherished that are low and debasing, and entirely unnatural.

God calls for reform in our churches. Satan is playing the game of life for every soul. He is seeking to brutify humanity whom God values. But when the appetite is held under the control of an intelligent, God-fearing mind, there will be a cultivation of pure, spiritual attributes. There will be a refusal to be led into a slavery that kills both physical, mental, and moral worth, and leaves the human agent, for whom Christ has paid so high a price, crippled, worthless, and tossed about with temptation.

Benumb not by intemperate habits, the faculties that God has given for wise improvement. Touch not, taste not, handle not, {167} spirituous liquors in any form. But intemperance does not stop here. There are manufactured appetites which the author of our being has never created, and every departure from the simple natural laws which he has established in our being, is a departure from the law of God. This law embraces the treatment of the entire being. Every nerve and fiber and muscle of the body has been constructed by God, and so arranged as to minister happiness to the human agent. But man has sought out many inventions. He has treated his body as if its laws had no such thing as penalty, and in this sin against his body he has dishonored his Maker.

Satan has carried out his plans in this respect. Man's appetite has become perverted, his organs and powers enfeebled, crippled, and diseased. And these results which he has through his specious temptations brought about he uses to taunt God with. He presents before God the appearance of the human being whom Christ has purchased as his property. And what an unsightly representation he is of his Maker! God is dishonored, because man has corrupted his ways before the Lord.

The Creator of man has arranged the living machinery of our bodies. Every function is wonderfully and wisely made. And God pledged himself to keep this human machinery in healthful action if the human agent will obey his laws and co-operate with God. Every law governing the human machinery is to be considered just as truly divine in origin, in character and in importance as the Word of God. Every careless, inattentive action, any abuse put upon the Lord's wonderful mechanism, by disregarding his specified laws in the human habitation, is a violation of God's law. We may behold and admire the work of God in the natural world, but the human habitation is the most wonderful.

From the first dawn of reason, the human mind should become intelligent in regard to the physical structure. Here Jehovah has given a specimen of himself for man was made in the image of God. It is Satan's determined work to destroy the moral image of God in man. He would make the intelligence of man, his highest, noblest gift, the most destructive agent, to pollute with sin everything he touches.

Not only the human, but the brute creation are made to suffer through Satan's attributes wrought out through the human agent. One human being becomes Satan's co-partner to tempt, allure, and deceive his fellow-men by vicious practices. And the sure result is diseased bodies, because of the violation of moral law; "Because iniquity shall abound the love of many shall wax cold." It is Satan's determined purpose to deceive the human family to such an extent that he can bring them as a mass on his side to work with him in making man believe that the law of God is no longer obligatory upon the human race. Then he will find agencies which will multiply his efficiency in leading man to ignore the law of God. When they do this, then he rules them with a rod of iron.

The only definition of sin given in God's Word is transgression of the law. It is not excusable, and has no defense or justification. It will be the final and eternal condemnation of the originator of sin and all the angels who united with him in the heavenly courts, who joined the confederacy of evil, identifying {168} themselves with the great apostate. When the question

comes, "Why have ye done thus?" every tongue will be silent; the rebellious world will stand speechless before God. Of Satan God had said, "Thou was perfect in all thy ways from the day that thou wast created, until iniquity was found in thee."

Sin entered the world by the defection of one who stood at the head of the holy angels. What was it that wrought so great a change, transforming a loyal, honored subject into an apostate? The answer is given, "Thine heart was lifted up because of thy beauty; thou hast corrupted thy wisdom by reason of thy brightness." Had not the Lord made the covering cherub so beautiful, so closely resembling his own image; had not God awarded him special honor; had anything been left undone in the gifts of beauty and power and honor, then Satan might have had some excuse. But God declares, "Thou sealest up the sum, full of wisdom, and perfect in beauty. Thou hast been in Eden the garden of God; every precious stone was thy covering. . . .Thou art the anointed cherub that covereth; and I have set thee so; thou wast upon the holy mountain of God: thou hast walked up and down in the midst of the stones of fire. Thou wast perfect in all thy ways from the day that thou wast created until iniquity was found in thee. By the multitude of thy merchandise they have filled the midst of thee with violence, and thou hast sinned; therefore I will cast thee as profane out of the mountain of God; and I will destroy thee, O covering cherub, from the midst of the stones of fire. Thine heart was lifted up because of thy beauty, thou hast corrupted thy wisdom by reason of thy brightness; I will cast thee to the ground, I will lay thee before kings, that they may behold thee. Thou hast defiled thy sanctuary by the multitude of thine iniquities, by the iniquity of thy traffic; therefore will I bring forth a fire from the midst of thee, it shall devour thee, and I will bring thee to ashes upon the earth in the sight of all them that behold thee. All that know thee among the people shall be astonished at thee; thou shalt be a terror, and never shalt thou be any more."

Why O why cannot the world see where they are drifting, and the sure result. The Lord has wrought in sending the living preacher with the word of life. It is the word of God to a people who through Satan's devices know him not. When the Lord's ministers in sincerity hold forth the word of life, there should be those connected with him to help him in the work.

The sowing of the gospel seed will not

be a success unless the seed is quickened into life by the dew of heaven. Before one book of the New Testament was written, the Holy Spirit came upon the praying apostles, and the testimony of their enemies was, "Ye have filled all Jerusalem with your doctrine."

The teacher himself must be the living embodiment of truth. His self-denial and charity is his witness that he bears the message of heaven. He has himself eaten of the flesh and drank of the blood of the Son of God, and this is eternal life. Taught by the Spirit, he will not be satisfied with less than the salvation of souls.

REMARKS OF MRS. E. G. WHITE REGARDING AGGRESSIVE MOVES AT LOMA LINDA

April 20, 1911
At a meeting in the Chapel
(MS -9-1911) {169}

(Thursday afternoon, April 20, there was a council meeting called in the Loma Linda Chapel, to consider the opportunity that had just been presented to purchase from Mr. Kelly a tract of land west of the Pepper Drive and south of the Colton Road, consisting of about eighty-four acres.

After very brief remarks about the Vine and the branches, and the benefits resulting from the disciplinary process of pruning, Sister White spoke of various phases of the work.)

TODAY WITH SISTER MCENTERFER, and again with my son, I rode around the Loma Linda grounds, and took more particular notice of them than ever before; and I feel very thankful that we have such a place. Surely we ought to be a grateful people because God has brought us into possession of this beautiful place.

In our meetings during this council, we have been speaking of the higher education. What is the higher education? It is to understand Christ's words and teachings, and to follow on to know the Lord. It is to know that His going forth is prepared as the morning.

Today, as I looked over the place more thoroughly than ever before, and saw the grounds, the drives, and the cottages that were standing before we came here, I felt gratitude in my heart toward God, that through His providence we had been brought into possession of Loma Linda. I felt thankful also to see the improvements that have been made since we have had the place. And I thought how important it is that we make every move in accordance with the will of God.

As the Lord prospers us, we should manifest our gratitude by a willingness to advance. We should see the advantage of adding to that which we already have. I feel a burden regarding the danger of letting anybody come into the neighborhood to spoil the place.

There is a piece of land across the railroad, lying next to a piece already purchased, which should be secured. One day we drove over it, and all around it. We wanted to see all about it. And I am sure from the representations that have been made to me, that this piece of land ought to come into our possession. If you are wise, the next time I come here, you will have that land. I will try to help you all I can. Let us work intelligently.

There are several reasons why you should have this land. You need the produce from it for your cattle to subsist upon; this piece is close at hand, and joins that which you already have. {170}

Here we have our school, and here many important interests are centered. We must not permit elements to come in that will tend to hinder and retard the work. It will be pleasing to the Lord if we keep our eyes wide open, and are fully awake, ready to take advantage of every circumstance, that will place us in right relation to the work we have to do. It would be a grievous error for us to allow to pass an opportunity to secure this property, for we might never again have such an opportunity. I advise you to secure it before it becomes so expensive that you could not afford to buy it.

There is danger of our becoming too narrow. These many little houses close together across the railroad do not look well. If we can get land, and have room, so as not to build any more in that way, it will be better.

You need the land, and it will be a matter of regret bye and bye if it is not secured. Do not make any delay to take steps that will prevent it being taken up by those who would plan for unbelievers to crowd into it. We should keep them out. If we do this, we shall have reasons to rejoice.

The Lord is well pleased with what you have already done here at Loma Linda. When one sees the prosperity that has attended the work, and the spirit of consecration that prevails, the conviction deepens that you are working in harmony with God.

I desire that all the work of this place shall be a correct representation of what our health institutions should be. Let everything that we lay our hands to show the result of the moving of the Spirit of God upon the human hearts. This will be evidence that we have the higher education. Workers whose hearts are in obedience to the movings of the Spirit of God will make this place what God desires it to be. I am surprised, happily surprised to see everything looking so well. It is beyond my expectations. And now let everyone strive to keep it so, and labor for improvement.

I am highly gratified as I look upon the land we already have. This will be one of the greatest blessings to us in the future, one that we do not fully appreciate now, but which we shall appreciate bye and bye. I hope that you will get the other land that I have spoken of, and join it to that which you already have. It will pay you to do this. As I have carried the burden of this place from the very beginning, I wanted to say this much to you. Now I leave the matter with you; and let us work in harmony.

Our Duty to Reach Out

Individually we should stand in freedom before God, serving Him intelligently. The Lord will work through every soul who is consecrated to Him. He will give them knowledge and spiritual understanding; and He will direct their steps. How shall we know that He is leading us? Because we act in accordance with the Holy Spirit, and are in harmony with Christ. {171}

You know how hard the enemy worked that we should not get this place. Now it is in our possession, and you have been working to the point of occupying and using and improving the place for the benefit of the sick and the honor of Christ's name. The Lord is pleased with this. He wants you to work His vineyard faithfully; and your faithful service appeals to the understanding of the patients and visitors. If it were not for this faithfulness, you never would have secured the favor and gained the advantages that you enjoy today in regard to the educational work taken up here. You stand in favor before the people. This advantageous position you could not have gotten if there had been a laxness in the work and a leaving things at loose ends. "Wherefore, gird up the loins of your mind; be sober, and hope to the end for the grace that is to be brought unto you at the revelation of Jesus Christ."

Those who stand here are to be an example in humility, in steadfastness, in high standing, showing to the world what is the higher education, showing what it means to be linked up with Christ. If your will is united with Jesus Christ, we shall see the work of God advance steadily in this place. It will reach to Riverside; it will reach to other places that are all around. There is a work to be done in many little settlements round about here. There is no virtue in settling down in one place, and spending all your time and energies there. There are many towns and settlements where earnest work needs to be done for the saving of souls. You are to have an arm of strength in all these places. The word comes to you: Be wise; be vigilant.

We should feel a deep interest in those souls who are brought into connection with us. We are to labor for them, leaving unused no means that God has put in His world for our use in the behalf of others. It was thus that Christ labored. Going from place to place, He preached the precious gospel, sowing the seeds of truth in the hearts of the men and women who would listen to His testimony. And He wants every soul of us to appreciate the work that He has given us, and the example He has set.

Unity Among the Workers

Do not let division come in to destroy the spirit of unity. We want unity; and when we pray together, let faith lay hold upon the Mighty One. Christ is looking upon us in love. If we will walk in His footsteps, following on to know the Lord, we shall know that His going forth is prepared as the morning.

The blessed Saviour did not refuse to die for men, but for their sakes submitted to abuse and mockery from His enemies. His life was taken away in cruelty. As He hung upon the cross, His enemies, standing at the foot, divided His garments among them. Consider how much Christ endured that we might believe that no experience can come to us that He does not fully understand. We are to be led by a spirit entirely opposite to that which inspired the enemies of Christ. It is our privilege to help one another and sustain one another, thus showing that the Spirit of God is working in heart and mind and character.

I am glad there are sensible men and women here. I am pleased that there is a strong force of physicians and teachers. And I {172} want to say to you all: Work in harmony. "I beseech you, brethren, by the name of our Lord Jesus Christ, that ye all speak the same thing, and that there be no division among you; but that ye be perfectly joined together in the same mind, and in the same judgment." The Lord wants you to do this, and I believe you will. If you cannot possibly do it here, just go away where you can. We need to draw steadily with Christ, and to labor to glorify His holy name. And the responsible men and women in this place should give thanks to God for His manifold mercies. But do not complain, or indulge in criticism, because this is all out of place. It will spoil the work.

Not Amusements, but Consecrated Work

There are some who feel that if there is prosperity here it will be necessary to get up some amusement. Let us not cherish such thoughts as this. Rather let the people see that you have a mind for usefulness and duty, and that to the saving of the soul. The amusements that consume time, just to gratify self, do not pay.

I have felt so thankful regarding the improvements that I see here. God has prospered you, and He will continue to prosper. And we must give ourselves to the education of those who do not appreciate these things. We must keep it before them in the living light. Regarding the securing of means for the development of the work, you must exercise that living faith that takes hold from above. Some here know what a battle we have had in order to secure harmonious action; and we thank the Lord that when the enemy comes in like a flood, then the Spirit of the Lord lifts up for us a standard against the enemy.

Some will think that by having amusements here we will gain more influence. But what we want is to go steadily forward, with our hands firmly holding the divine promises, believing that Christ will lead and guide and bless, and place a heavenly stamp upon our work. Do not feel that there is not enough in all that we have to do in this place for Christ and heaven, and that you must reach out for some amusement outside of your God-given work. Do not do it; for this will not harmonize with Christ's example. Stand solidly for God. Tell the students, Here we have Riverside and other places. If you want to do a good work, take our publications, and carry them to these places. Hold meetings, and let the people see that you have a living connection with heaven.

If you are a child of God, your prayers, and your work to strengthen and build up will have an influence, and God will bestow His blessing upon you. We need not feel that we must provide amusements to gratify the desires of some who come in here hoping to attract attention to themselves. It would be better that such ones should go elsewhere. We are here to give the last message of warning to a perishing world, and every jot of our influence is to be consecrated to God. It is not His will that frivolous, unsanctified amusements shall be instituted here. We have a heaven to win, a hell to shun; let us work solidly in behalf of ourselves and others for eternal life in the kingdom of God. {173}

At Paradise Valley I told the workers that they must do all in their power to honor and glorify God. God makes the impression upon hearts; it is not we who make it. If we work faithfully to glorify God, He makes the impression upon the people. He will lift up and strengthen every soul that seeks Him in sincerity. He will teach us how to lay hold of His promises, so that His grace shall abound in the soul.

It is our privilege to be co-workers with God. Let no one feel that he must secure the highest place in order that he may do the greatest amount of acceptable service. Do not fear that you will lose patronage unless you enter into some of the world's fashions and amusements. Your eyes must be fixed on the pattern Christ Jesus. Imitate Him, in works, in conversation, in your deportment before the people. If you will follow in the footsteps of Jesus, you will have an everlasting reward. The way is open for you to work in unison with Christ; and He who gave His precious life for you will help and strengthen you, and guide you step by step, if you desire to be led.

Ellen G. White

"Be of Good Cheer"

November 9, 1912

Talk by Mrs. E. G. White at the time of the Board meeting of the, College of Medical Evangelists, Loma Linda, California.

I FEEL VERY THANKFUL THAT IT is our privilege to believe in God and to walk carefully in accordance with the instruction He has given us in His Word. If we do this, our hearts will respond to the impressions of the Spirit of God, and we shall follow on to know the Lord, whose going forth is prepared as the morning. And let us always remember that just as His going forth is prepared as the morning, so we are to expect the revelations of His grace as we advance. But if we keep silent, if we do not feel the importance of moving in harmony with His will, we shall not have His blessing attending us. We cannot afford, brethren and sisters, to be without His help and guidance. We need to be in a position where we can talk with God. We are to commune with Him. He who is our sanctification, our righteousness, has given us the privilege of being in a position where we may have a continually increasing faith. We must ever live by faith, and follow on to know the Lord.

God's promises to us are so rich, so full, that we need never hesitate or doubt; we need never waver or backslide. In view of the encouragements that are found all through the Word of God, we have no right to be gloomy or despondent. We may have weakness of body; but the compassionate Saviour says: "Ask, and it shall be given you, seek, and ye shall find; knock, and it shall be opened unto you: for every one that asketh receiveth; and he that seeketh findeth; and to him that knocketh it shall be opened."

Will you believe these assurances? Will you say, "Yes, Lord, I take Thee at Thy word. I will begin where I am to talk an increase {174} of faith; I will take hold of the promises; they are for me." Oh, brethren and sisters, what we want is a living, striving, growing faith in the promises of God, which are indeed for you and for me.

Many, many times I have been instructed by the Lord to speak words of courage to His people. We are to put our trust in God, and believe in Him, and act in accordance with His will. We must ever remain in a position where we can praise the Lord and magnify His name. Then we shall see light in His Word, and follow on to know Him, whose going forth is prepared as the morning.

In the first Epistle of Peter we read: "Peter, an apostle of Jesus Christ, to the strangers scattered throughout Pontus, Galatia, Cappadocia, Asia, and Bithynia, elect according to the foreknowledge of God the Father, through sanctification of the spirit, unto obedience and sprinkling of the blood of Jesus Christ: Grace to you, and peace, be multiplied. Blessed be the God and Father of our Lord Jesus Christ, which according to His abundant mercy hath begotten us again unto a lively hope by the resurrection of Jesus Christ from the dead, to an inheritance incorruptible, and undefiled, and that fadeth not away, reserved in heaven for you, who are kept by the power of God through faith unto salvation ready to be revealed in the last time."

These words are all-sufficient evidence that God desires us to receive great blessings. His promises are so clearly stated that there is no cause for uncertainty. He desires us to take Him at His word At times we shall be in great perplexity and not know just what to do. But at such times it is our privilege to take our Bibles, and read the messages He has given us; and then get down on our knees, and ask Him to help us. Over and over again He has given evidence that He is a prayer-hearing and prayer-answering God. He fulfills His promises in far greater measure than we expect to receive help.

So long as Satan continues to live, we shall have perplexity; and if we choose to follow the counsel of the enemy, we shall have constant difficulty; but if we refuse to yield to Satanic influences, choosing rather to lay hold on God and on the promises of His Word, we shall be able to help and strengthen and uphold one another. Thus we shall bring into the work with which we are connected a spirit of courage. Never are we to utter a word that would arouse doubt or fear, or that would cast shadows over the minds of others. I am determined not to permit myself to speak discouraging words; and when I hear criticism and complaint, or an expression of doubt and fear, I know that he who thus speaks has his eyes turned away from the Saviour. I know every such person does not appreciate Him who at infinite sacrifice left the royal courts and came down into the world that was lost, and lived among the children of men in order that He might speak words of hope and good cheer to the discouraged and the desponding. {175}

Wherever we are, we are under obligation, as disciples of our Lord and Master, to anchor our faith in the promises of God. Individually we are to believe. We are not to cast about for a possible doubt, or imagine that sometime we may have to stand beneath the shadow of a cloud that seems to be gathering. We are chosen of God to be His children. We have been bought with an infinite price, and we have no occasion for placing the suggestions of the enemy before the assurances of the Lord Jesus Christ.

The Lord desires us to act sensibly. We shall have trials; we need never expect anything else; for the time has not yet come when Satan is to be bound. Wherever we may be, we shall continue to have trials.

But if we give up to the suggestions of the enemy, we lose the battle. Can we afford to yield to the arch-deceiver? Oh, no! We are to turn for help and deliverance to Him who "according to His abundant mercy hath begotten us again unto a lively hope by the resurrection of Jesus Christ," even the hope of an eternal inheritance reserved for those "who are kept by the power of God through faith unto salvation."

I was here at Loma Linda when this place was purchased. As I spoke to the people, the power of God came into our midst again and again. On the occasion of my first visit to look over the property, I knelt right down with our brethren and the representatives of the owners of the place who were here, I knelt right down in the midst of them and prayed to God about the work that should be undertaken and carried forward in Loma Linda. When I got up, some of those who were not of our faith seemed to be deeply moved. From that time I have ever felt under bounden duty to God to make this place just what it should be. I know that there are men here who have wrestled in the cause of God, and I know that they have passed through an experience that they never would have had if Satan had not had the power to oppress them.

Let us all strive to make of Loma Linda just what God means it should be. This is the principal thing I have to say— make this place what God would have you make of it. Every one of you is under bounden duty to God to labor in harmony, and to press the battle to the gate. If unbelievers come in and talk their doubts and fears, remember that Satan is not dead. He has agencies through whom he works; but shall we become discouraged because of this? Oh, no! Christ, our Saviour, lives and reigns. Let us not look on the dark side . As soon as we yield to the temptation to do this, we shall have plenty of company. But there is nothing to be gained by looking on the dark side. What we want is courage in the Lord; and we want to follow on to know the Lord, that we may know that His going forth is prepared as the morning. This is not going back into darkness. You know how the morning is prepared. If you follow on to know the Lord every day, you will increase in brightness, in courage, in faith, and the Lord Jesus will be to you a present help in every time of need.

Ellen G. White

_____

TALK TO STUDENTS AND HELPERS

April 16, 1912
Mrs. E.G. White in Chapel {176}
Matthew 6:

"TAKE HEED THAT YE DO not your alms before men, to be seen of them; otherwise ye have no reward of your Father which is in heaven." Now there is a point we want to mark of these points: that if we expect that which Heaven is ready to bestow upon us, we must comply with the condition. "Therefore when thou doest thine alms, do not sound a trumpet before thee, as the hypocrites do in the synagogues and in the streets, that they may have glory of men. Verily I say unto you, They have their reward. But when thou doest alms, let not thy left hand know what thy right hand doeth: That thine alms may be in secret: and thy Father which seeth in secret himself shall reward thee openly." Now we want to understand every word, for it belongs just as much to this company as in the days when Christ was upon the earth to speak the words that he spoke.

"And when thou prayest, thou shalt not be as the hypocrites are: for they love to pray standing in the synagogues and in the corners of the streets, that they may be seen of men. Verily I say unto you, They have their reward. But thou, when thou prayest, enter into thy closet, and when thou hast shut thy door, pray to thy Father which is in secret; and thy Father which seeth in secret shall reward thee openly. But when ye pray, use not vain repetitions, as the heathen do; for they think that they shall be heard for their much speaking. Be not ye therefore like unto them: for your Father knoweth what things ye have need of, before ye ask him." Now how particular is the marking out of this matter:

"After this manner therefore pray ye: Our Father which art in Heaven, hallowed be thy name. Thy kingdom come. Thy will be done in earth as it is in heaven. Give us this day our daily bread. And forgive us our debts, as we forgive our debtors." Now there is a point that is of great advantage to us not to forget. You see we want all these things that are presented before us, we want them decidedly in our minds. "And lead us not into temptation, but deliver us from evil: For thine is the kingdom, and the power, and the glory forever, Amen." Now here is one lesson, and we want to understand this lesson; we want to study it out and we want to see how much force

of Ellen G. White Letters

and power that there is given us that we may understand how to conduct ourselves. "Thy kingdom come. Thy will be done in earth, as it is in heaven. Give us this day our daily bread. And forgive us our debts, as we forgive our debtors. And lead us not into temptation, but deliver us from evil: For thine is the kingdom, and the power, and the glory, forever. Amen." Now here is the prayer for our daily bread, and we want to understand that we are to recognize the gifts of God to us. And then again, "After this manner pray ye: Our Father which art in heaven. Hallowed be thy name. Thy kingdom come." Are we ready for it? Do we want it to come? Have we done all that God has specified that we should do in order that we may take this in completely and entirely? "Give us this day our daily bread. And forgive us our debts as we forgive our debtors." This is especially for us to practice, to learn. "For give us our debts as we forgive our debtors. And lead us not {177} into temptation, but deliver us from evil; for thine is the kingdom, and the power, and the glory, forever, Amen."

Here is a positive agreement with God to us, and we want to understand this perfectly and intelligently, to carry it out. "And lead us not into temptation, but deliver us from evil: for thine is the kingdom, and the power, and the glory, forever. Amen. For if ye forgive men their trespasses"—now let your ears be wide open—"if ye forgive men their trespasses, your heavenly Father will also forgive you: but if ye forgive not men their trespasses, neither will your Father forgive your trespasses.

"Moreover when ye fast"—now here is special directions for us: "Moreover when ye fast, be not, as the hypocrites, of a sad countenance, for they disfigure their faces, that they may appear unto men to fast. Verily, I say unto you, They have their reward." It is all they will get. They won't get anything more. What they want is the very spirit of the prayer that they offer, to take it in and let that prayer be carried out in their daily life. "But thou, when thou fastest, anoint thine head, and wash thy face: That thou appear not unto men to fast, but unto thy Father which is in secret: and thy Father, which seeth in secret, shall reward thee openly." What does Sister White read all this for? you say. Because we have lessons to learn that we have not yet learned. "Lay not up for yourselves treasures upon earth, where moth and rust doth corrupt, and where thieves break through and steal: But lay up for yourselves treasures in heaven where neither moth nor rust doth corrupt, and where thieves do not break through nor steal: for where your treasure is, there will your heart be also." These are lessons that every one of us want to understand and become intelligently upon.

"The light of the body is the eye: if therefore thine eye be single, thy whole body shall be full of light." What a promise! How broad! It could not be broader! "But if thine eye be evil, thy whole body shall be full of darkness. If therefore the light that is in thee be darkness, how great is that darkness!

"No man can serve two masters: for either he will hate the one and love the other; or else he will hold to the one and despise the other. Ye cannot serve God and mammon. Therefore I say unto you, Take no thought"—that is, anxious thought, unbelieving thought—"for your life, what ye shall eat, or what ye shall drink nor yet for your body, what ye shall put on. Is not the life more than meat, and the body than raiment?" Can you answer that question? We want and God wants us to recognize that every gift that we receive, to be a help and strength to us, it cometh from God. And we should be grateful and we are to carry the gratitude in our individual hearts. And if we carry that gratitude into our individual hearts, let me tell you there will be a different atmosphere surrounding our souls from what we now have. Try to live closely—take the truth of God just as it is given in his word.

"No man can serve two masters: for either he will hate the {178} one, and love the other; or else he will hold to the one, and despise the other. Ye cannot serve God and mammon. Therefore I say unto you, Take no thought"—that is, anxious thought—"for your life, what ye shall eat, or what ye shall drink; nor yet for your body, what ye shall put on. Is not the life more than meat, and the body than raiment?" Now that is what we want to understand. We want to understand the Word intelligently, and we do not want to make any makeup or make believe story about it, but we want to know that we are planning for an eternal inheritance in the kingdom of heaven. I want that understood. "Therefore I say unto you, Take no"—what?—anxious thought "for your body what ye shall eat, or what ye shall drink: nor yet for your body, what ye shall put on. Is not the life more than meat, and the body than raiment? Behold the fowls of the air: for they sow not, neither do they reap, nor gather into barns; yet your heavenly Father feedeth them. Are you not much better than they? Which of you by taking thought can add one cubit unto his stature? And why take ye thought (anxious thought) for raiment? Consider the lilies of the field, how they grow; they toil not, neither do they spin; and yet I say unto you, That even Solomon in all his glory was not arrayed like one of these. Wherefore, If God so clothes the grass of the field, which today is, and tomorrow is cast into the oven, shall he not much more clothe you, O ye of little faith? Therefore take no thought, saying, What shall we eat? or, What shall we drink? or, Wherewithal shall we be clothed? (For after all these things do the Gentiles seek:) for your heavenly Father knoweth that ye have need of all these things. But seek ye first the kingdom of God, and his righteousness; and all these things shall be added unto you. Take therefore no thought for the morrow: for the morrow shall take thought for the things itself. Sufficient unto the day is the evil thereof."

Now, I want to bring before you some things that have been presented to me, where many are making a mistake; and that is, their mind is more upon eating and drinking and dressing themselves than in feeling humble and prayerfully to serve God. And from the light the Lord has given me there is a decided change to take place in every family that has not this scripture unfolded in its meaning to them. We want to know what shall I do to be saved? individually. And when you begin to know the word in this way, you will find that God looks upon you and he will impart to you the understanding of his word that you shall not be covetous, after this thing and that thing and the other thing that is in the world. That is what this lesson is given for. And we want to be in that position that we can take our lessons, and that we can learn our lesson faithfully and put on Christ; put on the very elements of Christ's character in all our actions, in all our doings. That is what I felt intensely anxious that you should understand; that there is a work that you are to do in unity with Christ, and if you do that work in unity with Christ, the Holy Spirit will give you representations to the world that you are a man that is following on to know the Lord and to be taught of God. "Therefore I say unto you, Take no thought for your life, what ye shall eat, or what ye shall drink; nor yet for your body, what ye shall put on. Is not the life more than meat, and the body raiment?"

Will you weary your body, and will you worry and will you fret and will you spoil your religious experience, {179} because you do not trust in the Lord Jesus Christ to work for you when you are doing your best on your part? "Nor yet for your body, what shall ye put on. Is not the life more than meat, and the body than raiment? Behold the fowls of the air: for they sow not, neither do they reap, nor gather into barns; yet your heavenly Father feedeth them. Are ye not much better than they? Which of you by taking thought can add one cubit unto his stature? And why take ye thought for raiment? Consider the lilies of the field, how they grow; they toil not, neither do they spin"—excellent opportunity you have to study that—"and yet I say unto you that even Solomon in all his glory was not arrayed like one of these." What a wonderful speech that is! "Wherefore, etc." Now we want to understand this. As it was presented to me, there is so much thinking and worrying and trouble of mind about things that you cannot help if you should think a week upon them. You cannot change it, but the Lord would help you to put your trust in Him, to look to Him, and his Holy Spirit will come upon you and you will have—not a disposition to quarrel because you do not have everything you want—but you will have a disposition to thank God from the heart for what you have. That is what we need. And unless you have that Spirit, and unless you carry it out, you will never enter the kingdom of Heaven.

I wanted to talk this morning, and I want you to see and understand that our Lord is a just and righteous God. We do not want the constant worry and fretting and complaining, we do not want to encourage it at all. We want to just stand in a position that we can see the goodness of God. Then we will have a pleasant disposition, and your company will be that which is pleasant, and the angels of God will see that you are copying the example that they have presented before you. We want, every one of us, to have an amiable disposition, and unless you have a sanctified, amiable disposition, you will lose heaven entirely. So that the care, anxiety, instead of worrying all the time for fear you shall not have something good and nice to eat or some dresses to put on,—now it is the most foolish thing, because you want to stand in a correct position before God. There is a mighty work to be done for every one of us. And we are to understand it, and we cannot afford to lose the lessons that are

brought in. We must know what God wants to work out through us. There is a great deal of mischief done in the imagination of our own hearts and minds that we want our individual way. But God wants us to come into right relation to him. And if we will consent to learn, why then we shall see of the salvation of God.

"Wherefore, if God so clothe the grass of the field, which today is, and tomorrow is cast into the oven, shall he not much more clothe you, O ye of little faith? Therefore take no thought saying, What shall we eat? or, What shall we drink? or, Wherewithal shall we be clothed? (For after all these things do the Gentiles seek:) for your heavenly Father knoweth that ye have need of all these things. But seek ye first the kingdom of God and his righteousness"—now there is where our lack is. We do not study and contemplate that disposition that calls us to help everyone that we possibly can, but we want that everything should come in an easy way to us. Now everyone will have the Holy Spirit of God upon them if they will seek for it in the right way, if they will {180} come to him as little children, and if they will ask him for his Grace and his power and his salvation that they can be lifted up?—No, that isn't it. But that they may have all these advantages to present to be a blessing to those that are around them. What we want is to study the Bible and to find out the way that may take hold of the promises of God and claim them as ours. And we will be happy in that. The devil cannot get a chance either to come in and to tempt you and to destroy your peace. We must bring ourselves in right relation to God.

We want the blessing of God to rest upon every scholar and every teacher and these teachers should be converted daily to God. Angels of God will help them, and the ugly disposition that comes in like a flash—it isn't there. There is no place for it. We do not give it room. We aren't studying how we can get above our brother, or those that are around us, or our Sister. We must not do that. But we want to prepare to meet Christ every day. He came to this earth to give his life for us, that we might gain the precious victory of eternal life in the kingdom of glory. And he wants to encircle every one of you in his precious care, that you shall not reveal to the world a disposition that will not tend to elevate the religion of Jesus Christ, but lower it. You cannot afford it. And the great work that has been presented to me for our peo-

ple is now—We have the great advantages here, and none has worked for them harder than I have tried to work in order that I might every step honor Christ, in our work here in this world. We are not to have a hasty temper; that is the devil's work, and we are not to have a wicked speech and unhappy thoughts of this one and that one and the other. No, indeed. We are not to try and excel this one and excel that one, but let our own fruit, in words, proper words, right words, words that will bless someone—let these words be spoken. But the converting power of God needs to be in all our schools, and we want to act for Christ. We want to serve him. We want to glorify him. We want to honor him, who made it possible by coming into our world and giving himself, giving himself a sacrifice to make it possible for us to be saved. That is what we want to appreciate, and we want to work it out in our life. We do not want to be a careless people here. We want every one of us to be in the path that leads heavenward. And you read in the precious Book that "if you will follow on to know the Lord ye shall know his going forth is prepared as the morning." You know what that is. We need not give you any explanation at all. We want the saving grace of God. We do not want to try—and there is in every place, as it is presented to me, always all this striving to be first, for fear you shall not have the first honor and that you shall not have the glory of this and that and the other thing.

There is a great work to do. The Lord has a very special work to do for every soul of us, if we ever see the kingdom of heaven. Here are the young people. You are to have just that education that can win souls to Christ. It is not yourselves, merely, that are to be saved, but you are winning by giving an example to those that are around you, what the power of truth can be upon the individual mind. We want Christ within, the hope of glory. And when we make up our minds to be right, you just read this and keep it in your life, and you will be the most {181} contented person, and not striving for the best place. No such thing. You want just the place that God would desire for you, where the Lord can look upon you with pleasure, and if you "follow on to know the Lord, you shall know that his going forth is prepared as the morning." Now, I do not need to describe the morning to you. You know all about that. You are right here where you can see it, and we have not had very pleasant days for a few days, but we haven't heard anyone going around and complaining about the sun not shining. No indeed. You just go and try to help some soul that cannot get out of doors and see if you can encourage them, and it will be a blessing to them, but a much larger one to you.

What we want is to get what that as a people we shall reveal the sanctification of the Holy Spirit in our words and in our looks, and thus overcome by the blood of the Lamb and the word of our testimony. Now here is the point that will bring us into right relations to God. And when we begin to think that somebody else is getting ahead of us, just ask the Lord to put his Holy Spirit upon our mind and upon our heart and upon our character. What we want is pure and undefiled religion, and when we get that, let me tell you, three will be such a spirit seen here—Why, I remember how hard we work for fear that we would not get this place. There was a good many standing in our way, that did not want us to have it. They said that they could not carry the debt. They did not want us to have it. But we made our prayers to God, and came right where the men were and said, Not the first thing we will do is to present this case to God, and if he wants us to have this place, and we act in a righteous manner to get it, I have no question but we shall have it. The fears were started from a tall man that was in possession of the house, and dropping, dropping.

Well, now these words are precious in the sight of God, and he wants every one of us to educate ourselves in the faculty of the Spirit that is to circulate in the heavenly court when we shall enter there. And we must circulate that spirit here, or we will never enter there. What we want is righteousness and truth and the glory that God will bestow upon the ones that are diligently seeking in the right way to serve God that they may obtain Christ's righteousness. And in that way we shall find that our homes will be pleasant. Why, fathers and mothers have no right to be scolding and fretting with their children in their homes. It is a sin. We are fitting up—what for? The heavenly mansions. And we can teach it to our children that we can have no words, no crossness, we can have no quarreling in our house because that will send the angels of God away. We want the angels of God to fit us up that we may inherit the kingdom prepared for us from the foundation of the world.

Seek to practice the life that Christ has presented to us, that is a righteous life. That is what I wanted to say to my brethren here. There is to be no quarreling at all. There is room enough in our world, and there is a chance for every one of us to perfect a Christian character in the name of Jesus Christ of Nazareth; and let us take hold of the work intelligently and then when there is any change to take place in the working of {182} the cause here, if there is that sweetness and sanctification of the Holy Spirit of God there will be no such thing as this striving for the mastery. And when I said how here we have worked from place to place in order to obtain the health institutions I have felt it my duty to set before them the only claims they have of eternal life is to speak and act righteously. All this striving for the mastery is of the devil.

We want a place in the kingdom of God, and we cannot afford to speak an unrighteous word. Christ gave his life for us. What have we given him?

When I saw this place I knelt right down before the man and prayed that God would give it to us if it was right that we should have it. And when we got up from praying, he just took us around the premises and in every place and explained things to us, and showed us the greatest courtesy. Said, he, I would rather you would have it than any others. We can't keep it. And said he, we feel perfectly free that you should have this place. We gave him a price that we thought he would accept, and he did accept it, so that it was brought into our possession.

Well now we had three seasons of prayer, perhaps more than that, right in his presence, asking the Lord to have an influence upon our people, a sanctifying influence, because that Satan was going about like a roaring lion seeking whom he could devour; and we could not afford to be devoured. We were trying with all our might to obtain this place in such a manner that it would be perfectly harmonious with the one that wanted to sell it to us. And it was, from the beginning to the end.

Well, I want to tell you that I would not have this place enlarged one step unless there is a different atmosphere that shall circulate all through the premises here, and not one striving to get a place, and another striving to get a place, but that we should take everything into reasonable consideration. And every soul will have to be striving to do that every day. We want the light of heaven to decide our questions.

And when we went around with him from place to place, and he making his remarks about he was glad to have us have it, he thought we ought to have it, why, it pleased me very much. Well, here we have it, and the additions we have, and we are very grateful to God. But I want to tell you that it has been presented to me unless there is a decided change in some of the dispositions that are here, that they can never enter the kingdom of heaven. It is self, self, self. And you can't afford it. We can't any of us afford to serve ourselves. We want to work intelligently, and do that which will bring glory to God. That is what we want. And that spirit must come in here and abide here. It has not been here in all times and in all places; and when there is a striving the enemy comes in and suggests things to the mind. You don't want that. You don't want his companionship nor his advice. Not at all. You want to work like intelligent Christians, and we tried to work that way in obtaining this place. I do not know that there has been one word of disagreement spoken since we have come to purchase the place. But whenever we met the men {183} we would tell them how thankful we were that we had this place, that we needed so very much and didn't know how that we should get along without it. "Well," said he, "I am just as glad as you are that you have got it. I am just as glad that you are the ones that have got the place." Well, now, I would a great deal rather than he would say that then for him to be complaining because we have it.

And I want to say that there is a lot to be done for your children in your homes. No crossness; they are God's children. It is the Lord's heritage, and you have no right to speak to them in a way which will create an unhappy disposition and spoil their tempers. You want to speak to your children kindly. I have felt it my duty, notwithstanding all my trials and these things, to bring up some children. They say, Why, you are bringing up so many children! I want them right in my home. I see the mothers do not know how to discipline them, and they are very glad to have me take them. And so I take them, and I have now three or four children that I have taken and trained in the very way I told you, never to speak a cross word. I would tell them, We will give you a ride every day, and we will try in all our words that there is nothing that shall deserve a tod [a brushy switch?]. That is what we are going to try for. Well now, we accomplish what we try for.

Now there is an additional property that has come to us. Of course we have not purchased it, but we are glad of the addition. Why? Because we shall need it—every foot of it. I know how the matter has been presented to me. And I want to say that the Lord wants us to represent the Christian character. That is what he wants us to do. And it has not been represented here, not by all. But what did Christ do? When they tell me, "Why do you with all your work bring this child and that child and the other child?" Why, I said, "They would lose their souls if I did not." They have got to be educated kindly and brought up in the nurture and admonition of the Lord. And I want to say that the Lord wants every soul of us to be in a position not to strive for the greatest place or the greatest honor. He wants us to work out the disposition that he may work in if you will let him. And we want the truth, and we want you to stand in that position that we will feel that we have not taken all these responsibilities for naught. We want to realize it. Why, I have tried with all my might to work at this and that and the other that would be a blessing, and we must be where we can cooperate with Heaven. And may the Lord give us grace and his Holy Spirit.

I have more to say on this subject. I was going away today, but I told them I must tell them something here; that the converting power of God must come through the congregations of those that settle here in this place if we give honor and glory to God. And this disposition to strive to get the highest place, and to strive for this and that and the other—let us put a stop to it. It does not please Jesus. And instead of laying the rod upon them, I take them in my chamber. {184} Now, children, you have a character to form, I tell them, and unless you overcome the evil of your character, why, the Lord cannot receive you. But the Lord loves you, and he wants to have you. Now, you are younger than I. We will take you out every day, and we will go out into the woods and groves and we will talk together and we will pray together. And this we do.

And God wants us to be converted. O, how my heart aches for our children. We want them saved, but we must save them in God's appointed way. And I want you to understand that we have a Heaven to win, a heaven to win. And when I think of it, that so many children are not prepared nor getting prepared to enter heaven, I want to give every place something of this that we have got. We want heaven, and we want every one of these children should enter the courts of heaven and enjoy that life. What is it? Eternal life in the kingdom of glory. One child saved; one child taken from the clutches of the enemy, and we want you to walk in this direction to save the children. We have got a people that are watching us. And we are to conduct ourselves in such a way that they will be convinced we have got something that they have not got. And we are seeking for heaven, and we want every soul here to gain heaven.

We can be here only now and then. We have got more souls that are watching and waiting and begging for us to come, and we shall go as soon as we get through here, I expect. But I want to tell you we have a heaven to win, and a hell to shun! And it becomes us to be laborers together with Christ to redeem our souls in such a way that Christ shall say, Well done, thou good and faithful servant. Enter thou in to the joy of thy Lord. We are helping the Lord, and we want in all our schools to educate and train the youth, and we want the help of every soul that is in the place. The Son of God gave his life to redeem us, and what can we do for this? What can we do for all that are around us. We have got to act out the principles of heaven. We have got to try with all our might. And the Lord will help us, surely he will help us.

I do not want to weary you; I think I have talked about enough now. But I want you to understand that I appreciate everything that is to the advantage of this place, because I hope there will be an army that will be raised up here to glorify Jesus Christ, who gave his life for us. What can we do, only to show that we appreciate that gift? We are to show it in word, and show it in action; and may God bless every one of us, is my prayer. Amen.

GLENDALE, LOS ANGELES, CALIFORNIA

September 4, 1905

{185}

WE HAVE RECENTLY purchased another sanitarium property, known as Loma Linda. I am most grateful to the Lord for making it possible for us to secure this property. It lies sixty miles east of Los Angeles, on the main line of the Southern Pacific Railway. Its name, Loma Linda,—Beautiful Hill—describes the place. Of the seventy-six acres comprised in the property, about thirty-four form a beautiful hill, which rises one hundred and twenty-five feet above the valley. Upon this hill the sanitarium building is situated.

The main building is an imposing structure of sixty-four rooms, having three stories and a basement. It is completely furnished, heated, by steam and lighted with electricity It is surrounded with large pepperwood trees and other shade trees.

The entrance steps broaden as one ascends, and from them is entered the glass parlor, a large, beautiful room three sides of which are glass. In this room there are ten rocking chairs, and more can be supplied if necessary. At appropriate distances, there are two decorative pillars, which look something like bowls turned upside down, and round these pillars are seats. This room opens into another large parlor, carpeted with excellent body brussels. In this room there are three lounges, ten rockers, and some upholstered chairs.

The second parlor opens into a spacious hall, which is furnished with easy chairs. At the right of the hall, double doors open into a large dining room. Ascending a few steps, one enters an office room, this room opens onto a beautiful grove of pepperwood trees.

About ten rods away, on what is known as Summit Hill, there is a group of fine cottages. The central cottage has nine beautiful rooms and two bathrooms. In the basement is the heating plant for the five cottages. Prettily grouped around this large cottage are four small ones, having four rooms each, with bath and toilet. An interesting feature of these cottages is that each room has its verandah, with broad windows running to the floor, so that the beds can be wheeled right out on to the verandah, and the patients can sleep in the open air.

There is another building, which was known as the Recreation building. In this is a billiard table, which must have cost several hundred dollars. This, of course, will be disposed of. A partition runs through this building, and we have thought that one side could be used for meetings, and the other side for class rooms.

The land is well cultivated, and will furnish much fruit and vegetables for the institution. Fifteen acres of the valley land is in alfalfa hay. Eight acres of the hill are {186} in apricots, plums, and lemons. Ten acres are in good bearing orchard. Many acres of land round the cottages and the main building are laid out in lawns, drives, walks.

There are horses and carriages, cows and poultry, farming implements and wagons. The building and grounds are abundantly supplied with water.

This property is now in our possession. It cost the company from whom we purchased it about one hundred and forty thousand dollars. They erected the buildings, and ran the place for a time as a sanitarium. Then they tried to operate it as a tourist hotel, but this plan did not succeed, and they decided to sell. It was closed last April, and as the stockholders became more anxious to sell, it was offered to us for forty thousand dollars, and for this amount our brethren have purchased it.

O, how I long to see the sick and suffering coming to this institution. It is one of the most perfect places for a sanitarium that I have ever seen. I thank our heavenly Father for giving us such a place. It is provided with almost everything necessary for sanitarium work, and it is the very place in which sanitarium work can be carried forward by faithful workers.

The buildings are all ready, and work must be begun in them as soon as we can secure the necessary physicians and nurses. For some time I have been looking for just such a place as this, with good buildings, all ready for occupancy, surrounded by shade trees and orchards. When I saw Loma Linda, I said, Thank the Lord, This is the very place that I have been hoping to find.

Ellen G. White

DR. JULIA A. WHITE

September 15, 1905

Paradise Valley Sanitarium,
National City, California

Dear Sister:

IWRITE TO URGE YOU to connect with our sanitarium work at Loma Linda. In the providence of God, this property has passed into our hands. The securing of this sanitarium, thoroughly equipped and furnished, is one of the most wonderful providences that the Lord has opened before us. It is difficult to comprehend all that this transaction means to us.

The Lord has signified that the time has come for us to work Redlands, San Bernardino, Riverside, and the neighboring towns. I am filled with a solemn joy at the thought that {187} these places are soon to be entered by our workers.

We need your services, my sister, just as soon as you can come. We are hoping that we may secure the services also of Dr. Holden. Sister Sarah Peck may undertake some of the lines of educational work. We are now anxious to see the work started and we hope to see you just as soon as you can come.

I have recently spent two weeks at Loma Linda. I am sending you a booklet that will give you some idea of the property. The large main building is furnished in an expensive manner. There are also five cottages, one having nine rooms, and others four each. In some of these, the verandahs are so arranged that beds can be rolled out from the rooms. The grounds are beautifully laid out. There are concrete walks between all the buildings. These walks are bordered with flowers. There is a good orchard, and ample grounds for garden. There are many eucalyptus, peppertrees, and many other varieties of ornamental trees and shrubbery. Meeting can be held in the open air on the beautiful lawns. There is also another building that has been used as a bowling alley and billiard hall. This can be utilized as a meeting house.

We hope that you can see your way clear to connect with this sanitarium as lady physician. Your services will be greatly appreciated, and I hope that you may soon be on the grounds.

Ellen G. White

DEAR BROTHER AND SISTER BURDEN

September 27, 1905

Sanitarium, California

ICANNOT EXPRESS THE RELIEF that your recent letter has brought to us. I thank the Lord that you are able to secure the services of Dr. Julia White. I believe she will do well. I think it well for you to ask Dr. Abbott to connect with the Loma Linda Sanitarium for the present.

White I was in Los Angeles, I spoke to you of inviting Dr. Gibbs to connect with the work in our sanitariums. What I said should not lead you to understand that he is to act as chief physician, but he can come in on trial. I hardly feel clear before God in giving him no further opportunity to be proved.

Have you learned how much Dr. Holden proposes to charge for his services? If a physician does his work skillfully, his talents should be recognized, but there is danger of our being brought into perplexity. If we introduce a new system of paying our surgeons high wages, there may be a hard {188} problem to settle after a time. Other physicians will demand high wages, and our ministers will require consideration also.

I very much wish that Brother and Sister Haskell might be with the faculty at Loma Linda, and inaugurate in Redlands, Riverside, and San Bernardino a work similar to the work they conducted in Avondale and in Nashville.

I am glad that you are taking steps to have the water supply at Loma Linda pure and good. Very much depends upon having good water. We must be sure that the representations given in the books descriptive of this place are true in every sense of the word.

Last week we had an important gathering at the sanitarium here of our health food workers. I spoke to them on Sabbath, and on Sunday I addressed them for about an hour on the subject of our restaurant work. I told them that there must be a thorough reformation in the health food business. It is not to be regarded so much as a commercial enterprise. At present but little is seen as the result of this work to lead us to recommend the establishment of more places to be conducted as our restaurants have been in the past. But few have been converted by this work in Los Angeles and in San Francisco. Many of the workers have lost the science of soul saving.

Please read carefully what is published in Testimonies, Vol. 7, regarding the health food work and the evangelical work. I feel more and more impressed that we must make diligent efforts to present the truth. I need not write much now regarding these lines of work, for the light has been in print for some time. But since these testimonies were published, circumstances have arisen that reveal the necessity for the cautions that have been given. Health reform needs a reformation, before it shall stand as God designs it should. We need to practice true godliness in every undertaking. In all the restaurants in our cities there is danger that the combination of many foods in the dishes served, shall be carried too far. The stomach suffers when so many kinds of food are placed in it at one meal. Simplicity is a part of health reform. There is danger that our work shall cease to merit the name which it has borne.

If we would work for the restoration of health, it is necessary to restrain the appetite, to eat slowly, and only a limited variety at one time. This instruction needs to be repeated frequently. It is not in harmony with the principle of health reform to have so many different dishes at one meal. We must never forget that it is the religious part of the work, the work of providing food for the soul, that is more essential than anything else.

Our young men and young women should be encouraged to attend schools away from the cities, that under intelligent teachers, they may receive a training that will fit them to stand on vantage ground. How can our young people advance {189} spiritually, while working as servants simply to prepare food for and serve worldlings? They often do unnecessary work in the preparation of foods that are not even wholesome. Shall our youth be encouraged to rest satisfied with such an education?

The Lord does not design that His denominated people shall exhaust their strength to carry on restaurants in the manner in which they are now conducted. The many complicated combinations of food that are not wholesome tend to make of the health reform a health deform.

There is great necessity for decided reform to be made in regard to our dealings with the workers in our sanitariums. Faithful, conscientious workers should be employed, and when they have performed a reasonable amount of work in a day, they should be relieved that they may secure needed rest.

Only a reasonable amount of labor should be required, and for this the worker should receive a reasonable wage. If helpers are not given proper periods for rest from their taxing labor, they will lose their strength and vitality. They cannot possibly do justice to the work, nor can they represent what a sanitarium employee should be. More helpers should be employed if necessary, and the work should be so arranged that when one has performed a day's labor, he may be freed to take the rest necessary to the maintenance of his strength.

Let no man consider it his place to judge of the amount of labor a woman should perform. A competent woman should be employed as matron, and if any one does not perform her work faithfully, the matron should deal with the matter. Just wages should be paid, and every woman should be treated kindly and courteously, without reproach.

And let those who have charge of the men's work be careful lest they be too exacting. The men should have regular hours for service, and when they have worked full time, they are not to be begrudged their periods of rest. A Sanitarium is to be all that the name indicates.

Every worker should seek to educate himself to perform his work expeditiously. The matron should teach those under her charge how to make quick, careful movements. Train the young to perform the work with tact and thoroughness. Then when the hours of work are over, all will feel that the time has been faithfully spent, and the workers are rightfully entitled to a period of rest.

Educational advantages should be provided for the workers in every sanitarium. The workers should be given every possible advantage consistent with the work assigned them.

Ellen G. White

SANITARIUM WORK

October 27, 1905
Sanitarium, California {190}

SANITARIUM WORK IS ONE OF the most successful means of reaching all classes of people. Our sanitariums are the right hand of the gospel, opening ways whereby suffering humanity may be reached with the glad tidings of healing through Christ. In these institutions the sick may be taught to commit their cases to the great Physician, who will co-operate with their earnest efforts to regain health, bringing to them healing of soul as well as healing of body.

Christ is no longer in this world in person, to go through our cities and towns and villages healing the sick. He has commissioned us to carry forward the medical missionary work that He began; and in this work we are to do our very best. Institutions for the care of the sick are to be established, where men and women suffering from disease may be placed under the care of God-fearing physicians and nurses, and be treated without drugs.

BROTHER AND SISTER BURDEN

November 1, 1905
"Elmshaven," St. Helena, California

I THANK THE LORD WITH HEART and soul and voice that he has brought Loma Linda to our notice, that we might obtain it. I thank the Lord that he has sent you to help me carry out in determined effort that which he designed should be a great blessing to us. Redlands will be a center, and so also will Loma Linda. A school will be established as soon as possible, and the Lord will open the way. I could not but think, as I read the notice of the people flocking into Los Angeles, if Loma Linda had not been sold to us, there would now be a ready sale for it. With all the buildings in connection with the main building, we have large advantages. If we will walk humbly with God, and do according to that which he has prospered us, we will have Christ as our friend and helper. "If any man will come after me, let him deny himself, and take up his cross, and follow me." These are the terms of our discipleship. Will we comply with them?

Christ was the Prince of heaven, but he made an infinite sacrifice, and came to a world all marred with the curse brought upon it by the fallen foe. He lays hold of the fallen race. He invites us, "Come unto me, all ye that labor and are heavy laden, and I will give you rest. Take my yoke upon you, and learn of me; for I am meek and lowly in heart, and ye shall find rest unto your souls. For my yoke is easy and my burden is light." The offer is ours, and every advantage is ours if we will accept the terms. I am trying to do this most earnestly. {191} We can be an example to others by our cheerful obedience to the will of God. Let us comply with the conditions, and in complying we shall find the rest we crave.

In regard to the proposition made by Brother Holden, I look at the matter as you do. We cannot afford to start out on the high wage plan. This was the misfortune of the people in Battle Creek, and I have something to say on this point. We have before us a large field of missionary work. We are to be sure to heed the requirements of Christ, who made himself a donation to our world. Nothing that we can possibly do should be left undone. There is to be neatness and order, and everything possible is to be done to show thoroughness in every line. But when it comes to paying twenty-five dollars a week, and giving a large percentage on the surgical work done, light was given me in Australia that this could never be, because our record is at stake. The matter was presented to me that many sanitariums would have to be established in Southern California; for there would be a great inflowing of people there. Many would seek that climate.

We must stand in the counsel of God, every one of us prepared to follow the example of Jesus Christ. We cannot consent to pay extravagant wages. God requires of

His under-physicians a compliance with the invitation, "Take my yoke upon you, and learn of me; for I am meek and lowly in heart, and ye shall find rest unto your souls. For my yoke is easy and my burden is light."

We see so much help to be given to our ministers laboring in the gospel in every country where messengers are sent. In every place there needs to be a school, and in very many places a sanitarium. In Jesus Christ is our help and our sufficiency to carry the work forward intelligently. God has looked upon the great display made by some who have labored in New York; but He does not harmonize with that way of preaching the gospel. The solemn message becomes mingled with a large amount of chaff, which makes upon minds an impressions that is not in harmony with our work. The good news of saving grace is to be carried to every place; the warning must be given to the world, but economy must be practiced if we move in the spirit of which Christ has given us an example in his life-service. He would have nothing of such outlay to represent health reform in any place.

The gospel is associated with light and life. If there were no sunlight, all vegetation would perish, and human life could not exist. All animal life would die. We are all to consider that there is to be no extravagance in any line. We must be satisfied with pure, simple food, prepared in a simple manner. This should be the diet of high and low. Adulterated substances are to be avoided. We are preparing for the future, immortal life in the kingdom of heaven. We expect to do our work in the light and in the power of the great, mighty Healer. All are to act the self-sacrificing part. Every one of us is to learn of Christ. "Learn of me," he says; "for I am meek and lowly in heart, and ye shall find rest unto your souls." {192}

All the great displays that have been made in the medical missionary work, or in buildings, or in dress, or in any line of adornment, are contrary to the will of God. Our work is to be carefully studied, and is to be in accordance with our Saviour's plan. He might have had armies of angels to display his true, princely character, but he laid all that aside, and came to our world in the garb of humanity, to suffer with humanity all the temptations wherewith man is tempted. He was tempted in all points as human beings are tempted, that he might reveal that it is possible for us to be victori-

ous overcomers, one with Christ as Christ is one with the Father. He came unto his own, and his own received him not; but as many as received him, to them gave he power to become the sons of God, even to them that believed on his name.

God calls upon Seventh-Day Adventists to reveal to the world that we are preparing for those mansions that Christ has gone to prepare for those who will purify their souls by obeying the truth as it is in Jesus. Let every soul who will come after Christ, deny himself, and take up his cross, and follow him. Thus saith the great Teacher.

Love to all the family,

Ellen G. White (stamp)

THE LOMA LINDA SANITARIUM
1905
(SpTBo3b, 12-17)

I WISH TO PRESENT BEFORE our people the blessings that the Lord has placed within our reach by enabling us to obtain possession of the beautiful sanitarium property known as Loma Linda. This property lies sixty miles east of Los Angeles, on the main line of the Southern Pacific Railway. Its name, Loma Linda,—beautiful hill—describes the place. Of the seventy-six acres comprised in the property, about thirty-five form a beautiful hill, which rises one hundred and twenty-five feet above the valley. Upon this hill the sanitarium building is situated.

The main building is a well-planned structure of sixty-four rooms, having three stories and a basement. It is completely furnished, heated by steam, and lighted by electricity. It is surrounded by large pepper trees and other shade trees.

About ten rods away and on the highest part of the hill, there is a group of five cottages. The central cottage has nine beautiful living-rooms and two bathrooms. In the basement is a heating plant for the five cottages.

Prettily grouped around this larger cottage are four smaller {193} ones, having four rooms each, with bath and toilet. An interesting feature of three of these cottages is that each room has its verandah, with broad windows running to the floor, so that the beds can be wheeled right out onto the verandah, and the patients can sleep in the open air.

Between these cottages and the main

building, there is a recreation building, which can be used as a gymnasium, and for classrooms and meetings.

In all there are ninety rooms, The buildings are furnished throughout, and are ready for use.

There is a post office in the main building, and most of the trains stop at the railway station, about forty rods from the sanitarium.

The seventy-six acres of hill and valley land is well cultivated and will furnish much fruit and many vegetables for the institution. Fifteen acres of the valley land is in alfalfa hay. Eight acres of the hill are in apricots, plums, and almonds. Ten acres are in good bearing orange orchard. Many acres of land round the cottages and the main building are laid out in lawns, drives, and walks.

There are horses and carriages, cows and poultry, farming implements and wagons. The buildings and grounds are abundantly supplied with excellent water.

This property is now in our possession. It cost the company from whom we purchased it about $140,000.00. They erected the buildings, and ran the place for a time as a sanitarium. Then they tried to operate it as a tourist hotel. But this plan did not succeed, and they decided to sell. It was closed last April, and as the stockholders became more anxious to sell, it was offered to us for $40,000.00, and for this amount our brethren have purchased it.

We must now secure money with which to complete the payments. Ten thousand dollars have already been paid. Ten thousand more must be paid in September and December, and the remaining twenty thousand at the end of two years.

Until our recent visit, I had never before seen such a place as this with my natural eyes, but four years ago just such a place was presented before me as one of those that would come into our possession if we moved wisely. It is a wonderful place in which to work for the sick, and in which to begin our work for Redlands and Riverside. We must make decided efforts to secure helpers who will do most faithful medical missionary work. If Christ will bless the treatment given, and let His healing power be felt, a great work will be accomplished. We shall need to secure competent physicians and nurses,—men and women who are true and faithful; and who can be relied on; men and women who live in constant dependence upon the great Healer; men and women who humble their hearts before God and believe His word, keeping their eyes fixed on their Leader and Counselor, the Lord Jesus Christ. {194}

O, how I long to see the sick and suffering coming to this institution! It is one of the most perfect places for a sanitarium that I have ever seen, and I thank our heavenly Father for giving us such a place. It is provided with almost everything necessary for sanitarium work, and it is the very place in which sanitarium work can be carried forward on right lines by faithful physicians and managers.

The buildings are all ready, and work must be begun in them as soon as we can secure the necessary physicians and nurses. I am anxious to see the work started. For some time I have been looking for just such a place as this, with good buildings, all ready for occupancy, surrounded by shade-trees and orchards. When I saw Loma Linda, I said, Thank the Lord. This is the very place we have been hoping to find.

The character of the buildings, the terraced hill, covered by graceful pepper-trees, the profusion of flowers and shrubs, the tall shade trees, and the orchards and fields,—all combine to make this place meet fully the descriptions that I have given in the past of the place presented to me as the most perfect for sanitarium work. Everything at Loma Linda is fresh and wholesome and attractive. The patients could live out of doors a large part of the time. The land will serve as a school for the education of patients. By outdoor exercise and working in the soil, men and women will regain their health. Rational methods for the cure of disease will be used in a variety of ways. Drugs will be discarded.

Out of the cities, has been my constant advice. But it has taken years for our people to become aroused to an understanding of the situation. It has taken years for them to realize that the Lord would have them leave the cities and do their work in the quiet of the country, away from the turmoil and noise and confusion. We are thankful to God for Loma Linda. It is one of the best locations for sanitarium work that I have ever seen. At this place the sick can be given every natural advantage for regaining health and strength.

Forty years ago the Lord began to give us instruction in regard to the establishment of sanitariums, as one of His chosen ways for proclaiming the third angel's message. Men and women bring disease upon themselves by transgressing the laws of God. The laws of nature, as truly as the precepts of the Decalogue, are divine, and only in obedience to them can health be recovered or preserved. Many are suffering as the result of hurtful practices, who might be restored to health if they would do what they might for their own restoration. They need to be taught that every practice which destroys the physical, mental or moral energies is sin, and that health is to be secured through obedience to the laws that God has established for the good of all mankind.

Our sanitariums are to be schools in which people of all classes shall be taught the way of salvation. In them the sick are to be taught to overcome the appetite for tea, coffee, flesh-meat, tobacco, and intoxicating liquor of all kinds. {195}

In every one of our medical institutions the sick and suffering are to be pointed to the Saviour as their only hope. In the Christian life there is strength and joy and courage. Turning away from the injurious fashions of this degenerate age brings peace of mind and the assurance of the love and friendship of the heavenly Father. Receiving the Lord in simplicity places men and women where they know the meaning of the words, "As many as received Him, to them gave He power to become the sons of God."

Out of the cities, is my message. Those who have had the light, but have neglected to follow the instruction that the Lord has given regarding the location of our health institutions and our schools, will one day see the folly of clinging to the cities. They will realize how kind the Lord was to point out the right way.

Let your schools, the high and the lowly, be out of the cities. If you desire to live a heavenly life in this world, place yourselves in right relation to God. Let your aspirations be Christlike. Christ lived much in contact with nature. God's missionaries are to form their lives after the divine similitude. They are to have a close connection with Christ. His life is to be their example.

For the past twenty years, the Lord has been giving the message that plants are to be made in many places. He will greatly bless us as we endeavor to carry out His will. Out of the city into the country is the word that has been given, and this word is to be obeyed. Our sanitariums are to be established in the most healthful surroundings. We have tried to follow closely the Lord's directions in this matter, and He has let light shine on our pathway, as we have endeavored to establish sanitariums where sin-sick souls may be led to the great Healer. God declared that we should find buildings suitable for our work, and that these buildings would be offered to us at a very low price. Has not our recent experience in Southern California proved this true?

I could not but weep for joy as I saw how plainly the providence of God had been revealed in our selection of places for sanitarium work in San Diego, Los Angeles, and the Redlands and Riverside districts.

Money is needed with which to establish the work in places outside of the cities, from which the cities can be worked. We must have means with which to meet the payments on Loma Linda. I ask our brethren who have means to awake to the responsibilities resting on them, and to do what they can to help us. Those who have the Lord's money in trust should regard it as a privilege to give of their means to help to pay for a place so well adapted for sanitarium work. Gifts, and loans at a low rate of interest, will be gladly received. My brethren it is the Lord's money that you are handling, and you cannot invest it better than by putting it into the Lord's work. Thus you will lay up treasure in heaven. I beseech you, by the mercies of God, "that ye present your bodies a living sacrifice, holy, acceptable unto {196} God, which is your reasonable service. And be not conformed to this world, but be ye transformed by the renewing of your mind, that ye may prove what is that good and acceptable and perfect will of God."

I have had much to write in regard to the shortness of time. Our work is soon to close, and we are now to place ourselves in working order in God's way. We are not to link ourselves up with those who are not wise to discern what is the will of God. We are to come out from among them and be separate. The end of all things is at hand, and the message of warning must be given. A spirit of anger is stirring the nations, and it will soon be too late to work for the Lord. Every conceivable deception will be brought in, and the enemy will work with masterly power. Stronger and stronger will be his efforts, until in heaven it is said, "It is finished."

Ellen G. White

DR. W. B. HOLDEN

H.-245-1905
Glendale, Los Angeles County,
California

Portland, Oregon

Dear Brother and Sister Holden:

I HAVE BEEN DISAPPOINTED and sorry that you did not feel that you could unite with us in our sanitarium work. If you knew how much we need you, I think you would change your mind. I know you have the ability to act a part in the work in more than one line of work. You can do good work as a teacher and as a surgeon. I ask you to come and help us here in Southern California. Sister Sarah Peck, who has been connected with my work for several years, has been telling me a little of your experience. We are sorry that you have been so disappointed. If you will come to Southern California, I can assure you that you will receive a hearty welcome. We are in great need of a thoroughly trained man to act as surgeon and teacher. Come, and we will treat you as the son of the Prince of life, your wife as the daughter of the King, and your little one as the Lord's child.

I will send you a booklet describing Loma Linda, the institution with which we wish you to connect. For sanitarium work, this place is in advance of any other place that I have yet seen.

Dr. Abbie Winegar-Simpson, with whom you were associated in Battle Creek, is here in the Glendale Sanitarium. I have been talking with her about our work at Loma Linda. She holds you and your wife in the highest esteem, and is anxious that you should come to our help here in Southern California. We need the aid of your talents. We need the help that you {197} can give as a physician and teacher.

I highly esteem your wife's mother, Sister Harris. She was one of our best and truest friends.

I think that Dr. Patience Bourdeau will come to Loma Linda to act as lady physician. I am told that she is an excellent physician.

Brother and Sister Burden, my dear and faithful friends, will be connected with the institution. Brother Burden will be general manager. He is well qualified for the position. His wife will act as accountant. We hope to carry forward the work of the institution in accordance with the will of the Lord.

Dr. Holden, I write you to come and see Loma Linda. It is a grand place for sanitar-ium work. It is the Lord's doing that this place has come into our possession, and we praise His holy name. We realize that we are highly favored in having been able to obtain possession of this property. We are greatly pleased with it.

Right around the Loma Linda Sanitarium there is a wide field for missionary effort. Redlands is only five miles from the institution, San Bernardino about the same distance, and Riverside a little farther away. These cities are all important places. Elder Simpson has done some work in Redlands and Riverside, and in each a neat little meeting house has been erected. But the Lord has a larger work to be done in these places. In the future I expect to spend a portion of my time at Loma Linda.

By placing Loma Linda in our hands, the Lord has opened the way for us to work these places. We are to regard the district in which these towns are situated as our special field of missionary work. We are anxious to become known to the people living in these places, and especially to those whom we can help in spiritual and physical lines. Through the power of Jesus Christ our Lord, we may lift them out of suffering; and bring them to health of body and soul. You know what joy there is in taking the weak and suffering by the hand and raising them up. You have rejoiced in this work in the past, and there is much for you to do in the future. It will bring you lasting joy and satisfaction.

A great battle must be fought. Time is short. Let us keep step with Christ. Let us by faith clasp His hand, and hold it fast. He will never repulse us.

My brother, turn your mind away from your disappointment, and believe that the Lord is leading you. Trust in the Lord God, and let Him be your helper. Use your talents in advancing the most important interests. Let it be your one desire to please God and do His will. Then you will have courage in the Lord. We must all be determined to make a success of our life work, even though some have no {198} appreciation of our efforts. If any man love God, the same is known of Him. Then make the Lord Jesus your trust always.

God sees our dangers, and knows the weight of our burdens. He remembers that we are in need of His strength, and those who make Him their trust will be enabled to resist every temptation. We shall have enemies who will plot against us because they know not the value that God places on those whom He has chosen. But the Lord God knoweth them that are His. However misrepresented and misjudged these may be, if they walk humbly before Him, He will give them help in time of need. They may be compassed with discouragements, but He who knows what is the mind of the Spirit knows all who love Him, and He will honor them.

In the work in Southern California, we need men of earnest, determined faith, and unshaken courage in the Lord. Our time to work is short, and we are to labor with unflagging zeal. I earnestly hope that you will decide to come to our assistance. Please consider this matter carefully, because we need your help. Please respond to this letter, addressing me at Sanitarium, Napa County, California.

Ellen G. White

DEAR BROTHER AND SISTER HASKELL

H.-277, 1905
Sanitarium, Napa County, California

I THANK YOU FOR YOUR LETTER telling me about your movements and plans.

I think I have kept before you my expectation that you would spend a part of the winter in California. By unmistakable representations, the Lord has given evidence that a great work is to be done in Southern California.

Elder Simpson has been holding tent meetings in Los Angeles with good results. Many souls have been converted to the truth. We thank the Lord that we have a good sanitarium at Paradise Valley, seven miles from San Diego; a sanitarium at Glendale, eight miles from Los Angeles; and a large and beautiful place at Loma Linda, sixty-two miles east from Los Angeles, and close to Redlands, Riverside, and San Bernardino. The Loma Linda property is one of the most beautiful sanitarium sites I have ever seen. There has been expended on the place more than one hundred and fifty thousand dollars, and it was purchased by our people for forty thousand. Of the seventy-six acres of land comprised in the property, about one half forms a hill which stands one hundred and twenty-five feet above the valley. On this hill the buildings are situated. {199}

Loma Linda is about five miles from Redlands, five miles from San Bernardino, four miles from Colton, and nine miles from Riverside.

Redlands and Riverside are places

which the Lord has shown me should be thoroughly worked. Elder Simpson has done some evangelical work in these places, and in each of them a company of believers has been raised up, and a meeting house built. But more work must be done there, and a work must be done in San Bernardino.

I have wished that you and your wife could come to Loma Linda, and carry on a work similar to that which you have done in other places. You could make your home at the sanitarium, and drive back and forth to Redlands and Riverside and other surrounding places. The roads are level and well oiled.

By the securing of Loma Linda, the Lord has opened the way for a work to be done in the neighboring cities and towns. The securing of this property at such a price as we paid for it, is a miracle that should open the eyes of our understanding. If such manifest workings of God do not give us a new experience, what will? If we cannot read the evidence that the time has come to work in the surrounding cities, what could be done to arouse us to action?

That you should receive an invitation to go to Battle Creek, and give Bible lessons to the nurses and medical students, is not a surprise to me. I have been instructed that an effort would be made to obtain your names as teachers to the nurses at Battle Creek, so that the managers of the sanitarium can say to our people that Elder and Mrs. Haskell are to give a course of lessons to the Battle Creek Sanitarium nurses, and this as a means of decoying to Battle Creek those who would otherwise heed the cautions about going there for their education.

I warn you against doing anything which would help those who are working directly contrary to the counsels of God, to carry out any of their deceptive plans. I know you would not willingly place yourself in any such position, and I warn you because I know the men and the plans better than you do.

If you should be drawn into such a plan, it would bring much perplexity upon me, and I should have another hard battle to fight. You must take no part in healing "the hurt of the daughter of my people slightly." Should the word go forth that Elder and Mrs. Haskell were to take part in teaching the nurses in the Battle Creek Sanitarium, it would be my duty to send forth testimonies that I do not wish to be called upon to bear.

Elder and Mrs. Farnsworth have been requested to spend some time in Battle Creek laboring for the church. I encouraged them to do so, and shall counsel them how to labor. It will be well for Elder Farnsworth and Elder A. T. Jones {200} to stand shoulder to shoulder, preaching the word in the tabernacle for a time, and giving the trumpet a certain sound. There are in Battle Creek precious souls who need bracing up. Many will gladly hear and distinguish the note of warning. But Elder Farnsworth should not remain in Battle Creek long. I write these things to you because it is important that they should be understood.

God would have men of talent, who will not deviate from the principles of righteousness, to stand in defense of the truth, in the Tabernacle at Battle Creek. One man should not be stationed in Battle Creek for long at a time. After he has faithfully proclaimed the truth for a time, he should leave to labor elsewhere, and someone else be appointed who will give the trumpet a certain sound.

We should understand by experience word for word the message the Lord gave to Isaiah, and from this message there is to be no deviation. The Holy Spirit's meaning will be understood. This meaning is not to be changed a hair's breadth to harmonize with any new doctrine.

We know that in the past the truth has been demonstrated by the Holy Spirit. Not one word of human devising is to be permitted to subvert minds or to add unto or to take from the message that God has given.

There must be connected with our sanitariums in various places ample facilities for the training of workers and great care should be taken in the selection of young people to connect with our sanitariums. We cannot afford to accept everyone who is willing to come. Great injury is done to our medical institutions when we connect with them inexperienced youth, who do not understand what it means to do faithful service for God.

Every soul connected with our institutions is to be tested and tried. If self is not hid with Christ in God, the workers will blindly do many things that will hinder the precious work of God.

"Sanctify the Lord of hosts Himself; and let Him be your fear, and let Him be your dread. And He shall be for a sanctuary; but for a stone of stumbling, and for a rock of offence to both the houses of Israel, for a gin and for a share to the inhabitants of Jerusalem. And many among them shall stumble, and fall, and be broken, and be snared, and be taken." "Bind up the testimony, seal the law among my disciples."

Those who have crowded into Battle Creek, and are being held there, see and hear many things that tend to weaken their faith and engender unbelief. They would gain a more practical knowledge in an effort to impart to others that which they receive of the word of God. They should scatter out, and be working in all our cities under the training of men who are sound in the faith. If those who teach these {201} workers are true and loyal, a great work will be accomplished.

There is to be a working of our cities as they never have been worked. That which should have been done twenty, yes, more than twenty years ago, is now to be done speedily. The work will be more difficult to do now than it would have been years ago; but it will be done.

Our work is made exceedingly hard because of many false theories that have to be met, and because of a dearth of efficient teachers and willing helpers.

It is not the work of the Lord that so many are gathered in Battle Creek, receiving a mold which unfits them for the work of the Lord, till they are thoroughly converted.

The Lord is to do a strange work very soon. A representation has been given me that I have not yet had strength to trace upon paper. I must know when to speak and when to keep silent. When the Lord bids me speak, I cannot keep silent.

The Lord will work. Great facts will be revealed in the Word. There are rich experiences to be received from the great Medical Missionary. The knowledge of salvation through faith and a full trust in a personal God and a personal Saviour, will be manifest. Those who have held the beginning of their confidence firm unto the end will have the proof of the things which they have learned by personal experience.

The gospel will be revealed and verified. The experience of the day of Pentecost will surely be repeated. Some will receive the Holy Spirit of truth; yea, some who are now in uncertainty. The Lord has given His word. For years He has been sending messages of warning, but by many they have been unheeded. Notwithstanding the repeated urgent warnings God has given, many have been turned away from their original faith, and are lost in the fog of error. They have refused to follow the light that God has given to point out the true path.

Christ is the same Christ that He has ever been. He is our Redeemer. Those who have been striving to quench their thirst at broken cisterns, which can hold no water, need to be born again, that Christ may be formed within, the hope of glory.

There are those who will never receive the gospel message in its fullness; they will never see the greater light and working of the Holy Spirit. There is a depth of depravity in unbelieving human nature that will never be healed, because the true light has been misinterpreted and misapplied. The Lord has given His spirit in abundance of assurance to enable men and women to understand the fallacies and errors of Satan, and to guard against them.

Some will soon turn from their deceptive errors and {202} calculations. To those who will be born again, the Bible will become a new book. There is a higher elevation to reach. True faith is to take the place of unbelief. The living springs of the word of God, with all their rich treasure, are to flow into the soul. The truth of the Christian religion depends upon the divine authority of the word of God. The authority of the word is Yea and Amen.

Jesus Christ is the way, the truth, and the life. Our great need is to have Him formed within, the hope of glory. He is to come into our individual experience, as a personal Saviour. He is the foundation of our faith, the Rock of Ages. "Blessed is the man to whom the Lord imputeth not iniquity."

When Christ shall come in His glory and all the holy angels with Him, then will all men be convinced of the truth that God hath set apart him that is godly for Himself. But the words of Isaiah will come to many minds. "Cry aloud, spare not, lift up thy voice like a trumpet, and show my people their transgression, and the house of Jacob their sins." The fifty-eighth chapter of Isaiah gives a wonderful presentation of truth.

I wish you could make me a visit at my home. I should indeed be pleased to see you and talk with you. Do nothing that will lead others to make of no account the long, determined resistance which has been shown to the messages sent by the Lord.

We do not want the impression left on minds that our nurses should be educated and trained at Battle Creek. You are not to remove the impression that I have been trying to make, that our people are to be drawn away from Battle Creek.

I have light regarding the impression that your going to Battle Creek would make on our people who have had placed before them many falsehoods regarding the work and influences there. Your going to Battle Creek in answer to the call you have received, would not be in harmony with the light God has given me.

If you cannot understand this, I can, and I will make every possible effort to save our people from being mixed up with the methods followed by some of the Battle Creek sanitarium managers.

The Lord would have Dr. Morse leave Battle Creek, and labor where the light of truth has not been taught, and that he may break every thread of sophistry. The sophistry that there is no personal God and no personal Christ has been set forth, and still lives, to be brought forth and fastened upon human minds. I have seen satanic agencies leading and controlling minds of those who have taught these theories. Unless the snare is broken, ruin will result as surely as to the house built upon the sand. {203}

Great trials are right upon us, to test every soul. The end of the world is near at hand. We are not to consent to have our workers, God's workers, tied up in Battle Creek. "Out of Battle Creek" is my message. I understand perfectly the meaning of the invitation that has been sent you. You have not a sense of what it means, but I am to tell you that God has not given you the work of teaching nurses in Battle Creek, or in any way encouraging our youth to go there for their training.

We must soon start a nurses' training school at Loma Linda. This place will become an important educational center, and we need the efforts of yourself and your wife to give the right mold to the work in this new educational center, and in Los Angeles, where there are many converts.

If you see your way clear to labor a portion of this winter in Southern California, I think I could be with you, and I will help you all I can to open up the work. If you will gather about you a group of workers, and do for a time in Southern California a work similar to that which you have done in New York and Nashville, praying and working and doing the will of the Lord, God will not fail to show Himself your helper; for you will be following where He has marked out the way.

I do not propose that you divorce yourself permanently from the work in the cities of the Southern States, but I ask you to come and help us start the work of training true medical missionaries in this very fruitful field, Southern California.

If we turn unto the Lord with full purpose of heart, teaching in the places He indicates, all things that He has commanded, we may be assured of the promise, "Lo, I am with you always, even unto the end of the world." God is able and waiting to be gracious.

DEAR BROTHER AND SISTER BURDEN

December 10, 1905
St. Helena Sanitarium, California

I HAVE RECEIVED A LETTER from each of you. I was glad to hear the good news of $5000 being raised, and the interest amounting to $300 being cut out. This is very favorable. I am so much pleased that Sister Burden is in the very place that will be beneficial to her healthwise. I am continually thankful to our heavenly Father that in His providence we have been favored to secure this beautiful location for a health resort. It answers perfectly to the representation that was given me, a main building and cottages to well fitted with windows. The surroundings are very attractive. Praise the Lord for His goodness and mercy expressed to us amidst {204} the difficulties we have to meet. The Lord is our helper, our keeper, and our constant guide. We may expect that everything will not move as encouragingly as we could wish in our connection with the work of God, but we will praise the Lord with heart and soul and voice. I say to you, my brother and sister, Jesus will be to us a present help in every time of need. . . .

I think Elder Haskell is on his way to Loma Linda. I have received a letter from Sister Haskell, stating that they would leave South Lancaster December 7. They are precious help in Bible lines. Loma Linda is just the climate for them, and the whole place will be a delight to their senses.

Do not be disappointed if we do not come just now. I do not know of a place where I should be more pleased to be for a time than in Loma Linda. I could enjoy every bit of the scenery and all the advantages. The reason my coming may be doubtful is that I do not wish to leave my workers just at this stage of my work. I am in good health for me; better than I have been in for years, and while my mind is clear, I want nothing to interpose as an extra burden. I want every jot and tittle of my strength to reproduce the representations the Lord has given me, and to make them as vivid as possible while I can do so. This is the only reason I plead not to leave my workers. We have all the multitudinous productions of the pen to be placed in the best order to handle, and I am more than pleased with the care that is manifested in arranging everything so that it may be well prepared for me to use.

In regard to the school, I would say, make it all you possibly can in the education of nurses and physicians. What about Dr. Holden? Will he not become an education force in the Sanitarium? Brother and Sister Haskell are versed in the Scriptures; and after a few weeks I may meet my son at Loma Linda. But at present I wish to advance a little more decidedly in the writings I am preparing.

We are having beautiful weather. It is almost like summer.

Ellen G. White

DEAR BROTHER BURDEN

December 11, 1905
Sanitarium, Napa County, California

I HAVE BEEN CONVERSING with you in the night season in regard to some matters that I will write you about. We were conversing in reference to Brother Hansen and his manufacturing health foods. In regard to the family, you understand that Sister Hansen must be carefully cared for, because {205} she has had lung trouble. It would be well for them to be provided with a home by themselves. They can be so located that burdens shall not come upon Sister Hansen too heavily, and where she can care for their own family. She may entirely recover from her lung difficulty, but it will be well to take every precaution. Matters can be managed so that those who need to be connected with the institution may not in any way be exposed. You and your wife may be wise on this subject, and a word to the wise is sufficient.

Brother Hansen is fully as severe in his family as is required. He needs the softening, subduing influence of the Spirit of God. He is not hard-hearted, but he needs more of the softening grace of Christ. You will help him on these points. It will be well for those of his children who are old enough to be in school.

We were conversing in regard to erecting a store, and One of authority who was in our midst, speaking to several present, suggested the propriety of erecting such a building at a distance from the main building and all other buildings that are now standing there, so that there will be no danger to them from fire. He suggested that changes would need to be made after thorough study, and that the building should be placed where the wind would not carry the smoke and sparks to the main building. Great care is to be exercised in regard to this matter, and intelligence is to be shown in the movements made.

Although Brother Hansen is an outspoken man, his children and all who associate with him can be so managed that there will be no need of roughness. All can be educators of themselves, placing themselves under God's discipline. Let their criticizing propensities be exercised upon themselves; then no one will suppose that he must place himself on the judgment seat to condemn others.

The Speaker said, "You can all be a blessing to one another, if you open your hearts to receive the precious love of Christ. Let all keep diligent guard over their own disposition, and then pleasant words will be spoken. Let not those who are connected with the Sanitarium as helpers think that they have liberty to exercise authority over others. God will help the ones who are chosen to act a part in the duties connected with the Sanitarium, to labor as workers together with God. Let them be sure to take charge of their own individual selves. Those who come to the Sanitarium as patients are to see that Christian love and kindness are shown to all who are connected with the institution. Let everyone stand in his lot and place, refusing to go out of his way to assume authority as a dictator. The Lord calls upon every man to be courteous and to discipline himself. He is not to exercise authority that is not given him. Let everyone learn daily his lesson of preparing his own heart for the heavenly inspection, for the record is written in the books of heaven. Let souls be emptied of self. Then invite Christ to come in, and open the door of the heart to his knock. He says, "If any man hear my voice, I will come in and will sup with him, and he with me." This divine companionship {206} is what is needed in every home, in every church, in every sanitarium. There is need of strong, spirited men, men who will be sure to do special honor to the Lord Jesus Christ. We must be preparing to become members of the royal family in the heavenly mansions Christ is preparing for everyone who through the grace received will wear his yoke.

Christ invites us, "Learn of me; for I am meek and lowly in heart, and ye shall find rest unto your souls. For my yoke is easy and my burden is light." In our character-building give encouragement to every divine, sacred influence. The blessing from Jesus makes everything good and profitable. Have his praise in your heart and in your voice and in your words, and your hearts will become fit temples for the Holy Spirit of God. Your success depends upon constant watchfulness and earnest prayer. "Ye are my friends, if ye do whatsoever I have commanded you." Depending upon the Lord, you can do the very things that are to be done, without murmuring and without disputing.

Satan is watching to secure every soul possible, to do him service by careless work and careless words. He desires to impress the minds of the converted and the unconverted that those connected with the Sanitarium are lacking in piety and the meekness of Christ, that they are not Christians. Jesus will help you to prevent this impression being made.

Christ would have everyone possess in abundance the grace of heaven. He desires that his joy may be in you, and that your joy may be full. Every soul is to discipline himself in strict, faithful service, just as verily out of meeting as in meeting. You are in full view of the heavenly angels, and every faithful disciple may be, if he will, as was Ezra before the king. The hand of God is upon all those for good who seek Him, but his power and his wrath are against those who forsake him, and who trust in the help and friendship of the world, going to the god of Ekron to inquire, and heeding not the counsel of the living God.

The children of God will know who is their helper. They will know in whom they can trust implicitly, and with Christ's help, they may, without presumption, have a holy confidence. Yes, his servants may safely trust in him alone, without fear, looking unto Jesus, pressing on in obedience to his requirements, leaving everything that is joined to the world, whether the world opposes or favors. Their success comes from God, and they will not fail because they have not the wealth and influence of wicked men. If they fail, it will be because they do not obey the Lord's requirements, and the Holy Spirit is not with them.

I am determined that our only safety is

in being joined to the Lord Jesus Christ. We can afford to lose the friendship of worldly men. Those who join themselves to worldly men, that they may carry out their unsanctified purpose, make a fearful mistake; for they forfeit the favor and blessing of God. I am to urge upon the attention of our people that {207} the Lord Himself has placed a wall of separation between the world and that which He has established on the earth. God's people are to serve Him; for Christ has called them out of the world, and sanctified and refined them, that they may do his service. He has been given all power in heaven and in earth.

There is no such thing as maintaining concord between the profane and the holy. There can be no concord between Christ and Belial. But "the Lord hath set apart him that is godly for himself." And this consecration to the Lord, this separation from the world, is plainly declared and positively enjoined in both the Old and the New Testaments.

Brother Burden, before closing my letter, I will finish what I intended to say about the building of the food factory. This work requires much wisdom and genuine good sense. If you can bring it about, do so. Make the best possible use of "Ministry of Healing" to aid you in your work. I believe that you can accomplish that which seems to be a necessity. I think that if we all walk humbly with God, we shall always have grateful hearts.

There will be those who will invest their means in our sanitariums, with the understanding that they shall be given a home there as long as they shall live. These should receive kind, Christian treatment. I have in mind a Brother Merrel, with whom we stayed while attending the San Jose camp-meeting. He has no family and lives alone. While I was at his house, he questioned me in regard to our sanitariums. Not long ago I sent him a copy of "Ministry of Healing," and asked him to communicate with you if he had means that he could lend to the Sanitarium. Have you received any word from him? I asked him for a loan of five thousand dollars. If such a man could invest his means in the Sanitarium, and make the institution his home, I think it would be a wise move. He is a business man, and I think is pretty careful as to how he invests his means. I thought that if I asked him to lend me some money, he might respond, but as yet I have received no word from him.

Later. This morning, December 14, I could not sleep after one o'clock, so I rose and dressed, and have come to my office to complete the letter that I began writing to you two or three days ago. We are interested in every movement made at Loma Linda.

Did not the Lord have oversight, I should not care to live another day. But his is a question settled in my mind,—that we are under a power which is beyond human control, and in that power we can trust. The Lord is good to us, and if we will walk carefully before him, he will ever reveal his power in our behalf. He will save to the uttermost all who love and obey him.

I long daily to be able to do double duty. I have been pleading with the Lord for strength and wisdom to reproduce the writings of the witnesses who were confirmed in the faith in the early {208 history of the message. After the passing of the time in 1844, they received the light and walked in the light, and when the men claiming to have new light would come in with their wonderful messages regarding various points of Scripture, we had, through the moving of the Holy Spirit, testimonies right to the point, which cut off the influence of such messages as Elder A. F. Ballenger has been devoting his time to presenting. This poor man has been working decidedly against the truth that the Holy Spirit has confirmed. When the power of God testifies as to what is truth, that truth is to stand forever as the truth. No after-suppositions contrary to the light God has given are to be entertained.

Men will arise with interpretations of scripture which are to them truth, but which are not truth. The truth for this time, God has given us as a foundation for our faith. He himself has taught us what is truth. One will arise, and still another with new light, which contradicts the light that God has given under the demonstration of His Holy Spirit. A few are still alive who passed through the experience gained in the establishment of this truth. God has graciously spared their lives to repeat and repeat, till the close of their lives, the experience through which they passed, even as did John the apostle till the very close of his life. And the standard-bearers who have fallen in death are to speak through the re-printing of their writings. I am instructed that thus their voices are to be heard. They are to bear their testimony as to what constitutes the truth for this time.

We are not to receive the words of those who come with a message that contradicts the special points of our faith. They gather together a mass of scripture, and pile it as proof around their asserted theories. This has been done over and over again during the past fifty years. And while the Scriptures are God's word, and are to be respected, the application of them, if such application moves one pillar of the foundation that God has sustained these fifty years, is a great mistake. He who makes such an application knows not the wonderful demonstrations of the Holy Spirit that gave power and force to the past messages that have come to the people of God.

Elder Ballenger's proofs are not reliable. If received they would destroy the faith of God's people in the truth that has made us what we are. We must be decided on this subject; for the points that he is trying to prove by scripture are not sound. They do not prove that the past experience of God's people was a fallacy. We had the truth; we were directed by the angels of God. It was under the guidance of the Holy Spirit that the presentation of the sanctuary question was given. It is eloquence of everyone to keep silent in regard to the features of our faith in which they acted no part.

God never contradicts himself. Scripture proofs are misapplied if forced to testify to that which is not true. Another and still another will arise, and bring in supposedly {209} great light, and make their assertions. But we stand by the old landmarks.

"That which was from the beginning, which we have heard, which we have seen with our eyes, which we have looked upon, and our hands have handled of the word of life; (for the life was manifested, and we have seen it, and bear witness, and show unto you that eternal life, which was with the Father, and was manifested unto us;) that which we have seen and heard declare we unto you, that ye also may have fellowship with us; and truly our fellowship is with the Father, and with his son Jesus Christ. And these things write we unto you, that your joy may be full. This then is the message which we have heard of him, and declare unto you, that God is light, and in him is no darkness at all.

"If we say that we have fellowship with him, and walk in darkness, we lie, and do not the truth: but if we walk in the light, as he is in the light, we have fellowship one with another, and the blood of Jesus Christ his son cleanseth us from all sin. If we say that we have no sin, we deceive ourselves, and the truth is not in us. If we confess our sins, he is faithful and just to forgive us our sins, and to cleanse us from all unrighteousness. If we say that we have not sinned, we make him a liar, and his word is not in us."

I am instructed to say that these words we may use as appropriate for this time; for the time has come when sin must be called by its right name. We are hindered in our work by men who are not converted, who seek their own glory. They wish to be thought originators of new theories, which they present, claiming that they are truth. But if these theories are received, they will lead to a denial of the truth that for the past fifty years, God has been giving to his people, substantiating it by the demonstration of the Holy Spirit.

Let all men beware what is the character of their work. They would better be falling into line; for their own soul's sake and for the sake of the souls of others. "If ye walk in the light as he is in the light, the blood of Jesus Christ his son cleanseth us from all sin." It is nothing to the credit of any man to start on a new track, using scripture to substantiate theories of error, leading minds into confusion, away from the truths that are to be indelibly impressed on the minds of God's people, that they may hold fast to the faith.

(Stamp) Ellen G. White

Mrs. Jessie Christiansen

December 19, 1905
Sanitarium, California {210}
Sebastapol, California
My Dear Sister:

I AM TRYING TO DO ALL I possibly can to urge the work forward in new places. The Lord has signified that in different places there are buildings which would be offered to us at a very low price, which we could use in our work. His word to us regarding this has been verified in our experience in opening up medical missionary work in Southern California. Recently the Lord has placed a great blessing within our reach by enabling us to obtain a beautiful sanitarium property known as Loma Linda. This property is sixty miles from Los Angeles, and it is a wonderful place in which to work for the sick, and in which to begin work for Redlands and Riverside.

Its name—Loma Linda, "beautiful hill,"—describes the place. Of the sixty-six acres comprised in the property, about thir-ty-five form a beautiful hill, which rises one hundred and twenty-five feet above the valley. Upon this hill the sanitarium building is situated.

The main building is a well-planned structure of sixty-four rooms, having three stories and a basement. It is completely furnished, heated by steam, and lighted by electricity. It is surrounded by large pepper trees and other shade trees.

About ten rods away and on the highest part of the hill there is a group of five cottages. The central cottage has nine beautiful living-rooms and two bath-rooms. In the basement is the heating plant for the five cottages.

Prettily grouped around this larger cottage are four smaller ones, having four rooms each, with bath and toilet. In all there are ninety rooms. The buildings are furnished throughout, and are ready for use.

The seventy-six acres of hill and valley land are well cultivated and will furnish much fruit and many vegetables for the institution. Fifteen acres of the valley land are in alfalfa hay. Eight acres of the hill are in apricots, plums, and almonds. Ten acres are in good bearing orange orchard. Many acres of land round the cottages and main building are laid out in lawns, drives, and walks.

This property cost the company from whom we purchased it, about one hundred and forty thousand dollars. They erected the buildings, and ran the place for a while as a sanitarium. They tried to operate it as a tourist hotel. But this plan did not succeed, and they decided to sell. It was closed last April, and as the stockholders became more anxious to sell, it was offered to us for forty thousand dollars, and for this amount our people purchased it.

This property came into our possession in such a way that we knew the hand of the Lord was in the matter. Loma Linda is one of the most perfect places for a sanitarium that I have ever seen, and I thank our heavenly Father for giving us such a place. It is provided with almost everything necessary for sanitarium work, and it is the very place in which sanitarium {211} work can be carried forward on right lines by faithful physicians and managers.

Not far away are the cities of Redlands and Riverside and San Bernardino. These places are to be thoroughly worked. Something has already been done in Redlands and Riverside, and a neat house of worship has been erected in each place. But as soon as possible a thorough evangelistic effort must be made.

Ellen G. White

My Dear Niece Addie

March 1, 1906
Sanitarium, California

LOMA LINDA HAS A LARGE, beautiful lawn, which is encircled with pepper-trees; and on it there are comfortable benches. I once spoke on this lawn to quite an audience, a number not of our faith being present. But the tops of the pepper-trees met over the stand, and the odor of these trees, which I thought would be most beneficial to me, was too strong, I find that we must live to learn. . .

Soon we shall begin evangelistic work in Redlands, a town about four miles from Loma Linda. Elder Haskell and his wife have come from the East to help us start this work. They spent a month with us here, and then visited Sister Haskell's sister at Armona. They are now at Loma Linda. . .

A few miles from Redlands, there are cities that have never been worked. Riverside is eight miles from Loma Linda. We have treatment-rooms there. They are not extensive, but are large enough to accommodate the people of that city. While we were in Redlands last year, we drove to Riverside, a distance of eleven miles, and I spoke to our church there. At this place our people have a very nice meeting-house. We drove over in order to see the country. We passed through acres of orange groves. It was a beautiful and interesting sight; for the trees were loaded with fruit. I never saw anything like it before. We returned to Redlands on the train, and again we passed through miles of orange land, the trees laden with their beautiful, golden fruit. We saw also large groves of grape fruit and lemon trees.

Our future effort must be to reach the people of these cities with the truth. At Fernando, . . . we have a school . . . This school is not far from Loma Linda and Redlands.

President Roosevelt, on a journey through Southern California when he first got a view of the city of Redlands and its surroundings, took off his hat, and said, "This is glorious. I never imagined such a sight." The scenery is indeed charming. {212}

In Redlands we have a splendid opening for work. Some time ago Elder Simpson held a series of tent meetings here, and a company of believers was raised up. They built a small but very neat house of worship, and in this church I spoke when I was in Redlands, a year ago.

It was in the providence of God that we obtained possession of Loma Linda. This property comprises one large building, five cottages, and a seventy-six acres of land, in a most beautiful location. The land was purchased and the building erected and equipped by a company of one hundred and fifty physicians, at a cost of one hundred and fifty thousand dollars. Under their management the institution did not succeed financially, and not long ago we bought it, furnished throughout with durable, high-grade furniture, for forty thousand dollars. Twenty thousand dollars of the purchase price was to be paid in several payments at stated times, with the balance in two years. But the former owners found themselves in need of money, and agreed to take off two hundred dollars interest, were a certain payment made at a date before the time agreed upon. Brother Burden raised the money, and thus saved two hundred dollars.

Once more these men found themselves in a strait place, and they said that if we would pay the remaining amount of indebtedness, they would throw off nine hundred dollars. Brother Burden paid the whole amount, some of our people taking stock in the institution, and some making gifts. This means to the institution a saving of eleven hundred dollars, which otherwise would have had to be paid. This was a great advantage.

In enabling us to obtain possession of this property, the Lord has certainly brought to the cause a most wonderful opportunity. We praise God with heart and soul and voice. There are five cottages, well fitted up, besides the large building. These are all furnished in the best of style. The smaller cottages are made with wide piazzas running round the four sides, and the windows are so arranged that the beds can be wheeled out on to the verandah. In each cottage there is a bathroom. The larger cottage has two stories, and is furnished throughout with solid red and black mahogany furniture.

All the mattresses, blankets, sheets, pillow slips, couch pillows, and bedding in general were in excellent condition when we took over the property. There are about eighty towels besides those in the bathrooms, and about one hundred and thirty-five small linen towels. There are table napkins in abundance, and silverware of all description, as well as chinaware.

There is one room in which sun baths may be taken, and a large parlor, two sides of which are of glass. This is the most beautiful room I was ever in in my life. There is also another large, well-furnished parlor. Two rooms above this have in them twenty rocking chairs and reclining chairs, which are very comfortable. {213}

Besides these buildings, there is another building, which was used as a recreation building. This will serve for a time as a meeting house. Both lower and upper stories are fitted up with rocking chairs. Those in charge seemed to have a passion for rocking chairs.

There are two barns and some carriages, somewhat worn, several horses, four cows, and a large calf, a good number of chickens and some turkeys. There were some hogs, but those have been disposed of.

Ten acres of the land is in oranges and apricots. The apricots are the largest I have ever seen. We only tasted the oranges when we were there, but Brother Burden has recently sent us several boxes of oranges and grape-fruit, which we find most excellent. The apples grown there do not amount to much. We secured the place last summer before the fruit was ripe, and more was put up during the season than they will be able to use this summer. We had to buy peaches for canning. I helped to pick some of them. We bought the fruit on the trees, and it was delicious. They are now setting out more grape vines and orange trees and other kinds of fruit, but these will not come into bearing for some time.

The main building stands on an eminence, and one must climb a long flight of steps to reach the front door. About two hundred rods from the building there is a little railway station. From here there is a drive of easy and gradual ascent, which encircles the rise of ground upon which stand the main building, the nine-roomed cottage, and the four smaller cottages. The hill is set out to ornamental and fruit trees. On it there is still another cottage, which has been used for the laborers.

The Loma Linda Sanitarium will be dedicated in four or five weeks. I hear that the institution is filled with patients. Everyone who has gone there is delighted with the place.

Now I have written you the fullest description of Loma Linda that I have written to anyone, as I thought you would like to hear about the place. I have never lost my interest in you; for you are one of my children, a member of my family. If you will love and serve the Lord I shall be grateful that in your childhood I consented to take charge of you. You are the purchase of the blood of Christ, and I do want you to find entrance into the city whose builder and maker is God. Let us all strive together to secure the immortal inheritance. . . .

Ellen G. White

To Ministers and Physicians

May 1, 1906
Loma Linda, California {214}

I AM NOW CHARGED to write out the straight testimony which was given me Monday night. I am to withhold none of it. I am to say to ministers and physicians, We must have a work done among us which will bear the gospel message. We need the power of the truth in the soul. The close of this earth's history is drawing near, and our work has not extended into the highways and byways as it should have done. In very many places the gospel message must be given in all its power, and in such a way that souls will be aroused. A spirit of self-sacrifice must take possession of ministers and physicians; everyone must do a self-denying work. Souls are perishing in their sins.

Sanitariums must be established in various places away from the cities. Schools must be established in connection with the sanitariums. As far as possible, these organizations must be blended, each helping the other, and yet each doing its special work.

No longer should our people go to Battle Creek as they have been doing. Infidelity has been sown there in words, in false statements, in unsanctified influence of mind over mind. God is dishonored, and we are to prepare to accept the situations God may prepare for us. Never before did the matter appear as the Lord presents it today. False theories, repeated again and again, appear as falsely inviting today as did the fruit of the forbidden tree in the garden of Eden. The fruit was very beautiful, and apparently desirable for food. Through false doctrines many souls have already been destroyed. Some will never see the light and come to their senses. The Lord God of Israel now declares, "If the Lord be God, serve Him; and if Baal, serve him. Choose ye this day whom ye will serve."

The light of truth must be held up in Battle Creek. Faithful watchman must be stationed there. The truth must go forth by the exposition of the Word, to saints and to sinners. Laborers are now needed there, who will distinguish the difference between eating of the fruit of the forbidden tree, and the eating of the fruit of the tree bearing the gospel message.

I am instructed to say, Prepare places where will be given true education free from deceptive theories. Let the plain words of Christ, uncontaminated by false science, be taught. It will require no elaborate preparations to engage sincerely, humbly, prayerfully in this work.

Will we now make thorough work for eternity? We have no time to criticize another soul. Do not consider it your duty to chastise another. See that your own soul is right with God.

Ellen G. White

ABOUT HER TRAVELS

May 28, 1906
Sanitarium, California{215}

MELROSE AND LOMA LINDA are both very beautiful places. Each has excellent advantages, and these two places near cities will open the way for the truth to find access to many people who have never heard it.

Elder Haskell and wife have begun work at San Bernardino, and they are sparing no pains. They are doing their best. They labor earnestly to keep the workers all alive and interested to sell the literature, and the work is certainly taking hold. Some souls have already taken their stand.

We feel deeply interested to see our cities worked. We hope that our workers in Boston will have courage in the Lord. The Lord is soon to come, and there is need that every talent shall be improved.

I have seen the city of San Francisco, and what a scene of devastation it presents. We were an hour and a half riding through the ruins. As we looked at such complete destruction, we could hardly realize that the largest city in California was in ruins.

We shall do all we possibly can to get the truth before the people now. The special number of the "Signs of the Times" is a medium through which much good will be accomplished.

If I were twenty-five years younger, I would certainly take up labor in the cities. But I must reach them with the pen.

Looking at the tall buildings in San Francisco, some of them having one side still standing, it seemed to say, The touch of the Lord's finger will lay in ruins the most costly and the highest of buildings. One of the standing walls of these high structures came down with a crash as we were looking at it. The completeness of the ruin cannot be described. . . .

We know not what may come next to arouse the people to investigate Bible truth. The day of the Lord will come unlooked for, as a thief in the night. If these awful calamities do not make an impression on our minds, what will?

"Be ye also ready, for in such a day as ye think not, the Son of man cometh."

Ellen G. White

DEAR BROTHER AND SISTER HASKELL

June 8, 1906
Elmshaven, Sanitarium, California {216}

I AM GLAD THAT YOU ARE carrying forward the work you have undertaken in San Bernardino. I believe that you are working in harmony with the light that has been given to me. In your work you come in contact with people who need to feel a hunger and thirst after righteousness. The Lord's blessing will be with all who work in harmony with His plans.

It has often been presented to me that there should be less sermonizing by ministers acting merely as local pastors of churches, and that greater personal efforts should be put forth. Our people should not be made to think that they need to listen to a sermon every Sabbath. Many who listen frequently to sermons, even though the truth be presented in clear lines, learn but little. Often it would be more profitable if the Sabbath meetings were of the nature of a Bible class study. Bible truth should be presented in such a simple, interesting manner that all can easily understand and grasp the principles of salvation.

We should seek to follow more closely the example of Christ, the great Shepherd, as He worked with his little company of disciples, studying with them and with the people the Old Testament Scriptures. His active ministry consisted not merely in sermonizing, but in educating the people. As he passed through villages, He came in personal contact with the people in their homes, teaching, and ministering to their necessities. As the crowds that followed Him increased, when He came to a favor-

able place, He would speak to them, simplifying His discourse by the use of parables and symbols.

DEAR BROTHER BURDEN

June 17, 1906
Elmshaven, Sanitarium, California

FOR SEVERAL DAYS I HAVE thought of writing to you, but could not because of so many things demanding immediate attention have come in. I may have written to you regarding the equipment of your treatment rooms, but fearing that I have not, I will come right to the point.

When we were at Paradise Valley Sanitarium, we were conducted through the new treatment rooms. One room was elaborately fitted up with electrical appliances for giving the patients treatment. That night I was instructed that some connected with the institution were introducing things for the treatment of the sick that were not safe. The application of some of these electrical treatments would involve the patient in serious difficulties, imperiling life. {217}

One was conversing with the doctors, and with great earnestness was saying, "Never, never carry out your wonderful plans. There have been various mechanical devices brought into the treatment rooms that are expensive, and the men who make a specialty of treating certain cases are liable to make grave mistakes."

There are men who make a specialty of treating the rectum, and some feel that they have been greatly benefited. But I have been instructed that this treatment, as well as many surgical operations leave many with many a serious weakness.

Several things were mentioned that have been brought into the Paradise Valley Sanitarium, which were not necessary and which should not have been purchased without consultation with other physicians. The amount of money which some of these machines cost, and the salary which must be paid to the one who operates them, should be taken into consideration. I felt impelled to talk with Brother Robinson in reference to these matters, although we were driving with a number of people, and it was not a favorable place to converse about such matters.

Now I am certain that great care should be taken in purchasing electrical instruments and costly mechanical fixtures. Move slowly, Brother Burden, and do not trust to men who suppose that they understand what is essential, and who launch out in spending money for many things that require experts to handle them.

Several times I have been instructed that much of the elaborate, costly machinery used in giving treatments, did not help in the work as much as is supposed. With it we do not get so good results as with the simple appliances we used in our earlier experiences. The application of water in various simple ways is a great blessing.

I have been instructed that the X-ray is not the great blessing that some suppose it to be. If used unwisely, it may do much harm. The results of some of the electrical treatments are similar to the results of using stimulants. There is a weakness that follows. . . .

Keep the patients out of doors as much as possible, and give them cheering, happy talks in the parlor, with simple reading and Bible lessons easy to be understood, which will be an encouragement to the soul. Talk on health reform, and do not you, my brother, become burden bearer in so many lines that you cannot teach the simple lessons of health reform. Those who go from the sanitarium should go so well instructed that they can teach others the methods of treating their families.

There is danger of spending far too much money on machinery and appliances which the patients can never use in their home lessons. They should rather be taught how to regulate the diet, so that the living machinery of the whole being will work in harmony. Let them become intelligent in regard to the importance of laying aside corsets and shortening their skirts. {218

Such lessons will be to the women more valuable than they can estimate.

Ellen G. White

TO ELDERS REASER, BURDEN, AND THE EXECUTIVE COMMITTEE OF THE SOUTHERN CALIFORNIA CONFERENCE

August 19, 1906
Oakland, California

Dear Brethren:

I AM VERY ANXIOUS THAT Brethren Reaser and Burden and their associates shall see all things clearly. God has given to every man a certain work to do, and He will give to each the wisdom necessary to perform his own appointed work.

To Brethren Reaser and Burden I would say, In all your counsels together, be careful to show kindness and courtesy toward each other. Guard against anything that has the semblance of a domineering spirit.

Be very careful not to do anything that would restrict the work at Loma Linda. It is in the order of God that this property has been secured, and He has given instruction that a school should be connected with the sanitarium. A special work is to be done there in qualifying young men and young women to be efficient medical missionary workers. They are to be taught how to treat the sick without the use of drugs. Such an education requires an experience in practical work.

The work at Loma Linda demands immediate consideration. Preparations must be made for the school to be opened as soon as possible. Our young men and young women are to find in Loma Linda a school where they can receive a medical missionary training, and where they will not be brought under the influence of some who are seeking to undermine the truth. The students are to unite faithfully in the medical work, keeping their physical powers in the most perfect condition possible, and laboring under the instruction of the great Medical Missionary. The healing of the sick and the ministry of the Word are to go hand in hand.

There is to be a thorough education in Bible truth. The word of God is spirit and life. We need constantly to look to Jesus. The efficiency of every worker is largely determined by the education and training he receives. In our educational institutions there is to be a higher class of education than can be found elsewhere. The students are to be treated kindly, tenderly, and interestedly.

In order to properly fit the sanitarium and the school at Loma Linda to carry on the work that the Lord has plainly {219} directed should be carried on, means must be raised. And let no one act a part in influencing our brethren and sisters in Southern California not to do that which needs to be done.

The Lord has blessed Elder Burden, and He will continue to bless him, as he continues to move in the fear of God, and plans wisely and economically with his associates for the fitting up and management of the institution. If any of his brethren act arbitrarily in an effort to restrain him in this, they would be found hindering the very work that the Lord has signified should be done. He is not to be forced to turn aside from his convictions as to the way in which the work under his charge shall be carried on.

In the carrying forward of the educational work at Loma Linda, our brethren must certainly guard against the efforts of the enemy to bring in a spirit of criticism and of alienation between brethren.

There are times when certain sanitariums will have to pass through a close, severe struggle for means in order to do a special work which the Lord has particularly designed should be done. In such emergencies, they are to be free to receive gifts and donations from our churches. Some who receive the truth have means, and they will aid in sustaining the good work which should be done in our sanitariums.

My brethren, I am praying that the Lord will guide you in the very best methods of reaching hearts. Let no one, whatever his official position, decide matters fully on his own judgment, or he may make mistakes that will have to be corrected. One thing is certain, we have a short work before us. We are living very near the end of this earth's history.

For years we have wrestled to see the work of God advanced in Southern California. At one time we found such narrow, prescribed plans that the work could not move forward. Then when an effort was made to advance, it resulted in large outlay, and in extravagant plans that were altogether out of order. Then followed a pressure for money, and the work was held back.

Still the light kept coming to me that the work should be conducted after a different order, that many plans and devisings of men needed to be changed. Of late some moves have been made. The Lord has wrought in the securing of properties at Fernando, at Paradise Valley, and at Glendale.

A sanitarium has been established at Loma Linda, and this is in the providence of God. Some know how difficult it has been to accomplish the work that has been done. But the work at Loma Linda is not yet perfected. More money must be raised in order to make this place a center for the training of medical missionary evangelists.

As the president and executive committee of the Southern California Conference unite with Brother Burden and his {220} associates in planning for the thorough accomplishment of the sanitarium and school work at Loma Linda, they will find strength and blessing. Brother Burden is not to be bound about in his work.

Pray to the Lord, my brethren, counsel together, and then labor unitedly to help in establishing the work which we all so greatly desire shall not be hindered.

The work of higher education has been greatly hindered because men and women have not discerned spiritual things as they should. We should know the facts that are of weight in making decisions.

All our brethren are to be sober-minded and cautious. Those who hold office need the ability to view every matter wisely. We are all to be workers together with God.

Ellen G. White

ROY LOGAN

September 3, 1906

Dear Brother:

SISTER KING HAS SPOKEN TO ME of you as a young man desiring advice in regard to entering a school of Osteopathy, conducted by unbelievers.

I would caution you to be on your guard. You cannot be too careful how you place yourself in a position where you will be surrounded by students who are unbelievers, and receive instruction from teachers who are not taught by the great Teacher, the Lord Jesus Christ.

It has frequently been seen that what seemed to be favorable opportunities for obtaining an education in worldly institutions, were snares of the enemy. The time of the students has been fully occupied, to the exclusion of the study of God's word. They have completed the course of study, but they were not fitted to take up the study of the work of the Lord.

It is not necessary for you to go to a worldly school to obtain an education; for there are excellent opportunities before you in schools conducted by those who understand the truth, and where you can receive an education in Bible knowledge. If you desire to fit yourself for medical missionary work, you can find at Loma Linda the very best opening. If you need preliminary work, this you can obtain at the college in Healdsburg. Would it not be wisdom for you to attend one of these schools, rather than to place yourself in the company of those who neither teach nor obey the commandments of God? {221}

You will have severe enough battles to fight, even when you place yourself under the best influences possible. Would it not be presumption to place yourself unnecessarily in school where the teachers do not have respect to the Lord's commandments, where the Sabbath is not recognized as His sign?. . . .

Our young men need above all else, to be thoroughly instructed that they may teach the way of the Lord to perishing souls. "The words that I speak unto you," says Christ, "they are spirit, and they are life." Study the word. The strictest fidelity is to be cherished. The love of the truth, and a genuine desire for improvement in the understanding of the Word, will make you that ye shall neither be barren nor unfruitful in the service of God. As you learn, you should seek for opportunities to explain the truth to others.

The tempter is watching you, in your uncertainty. He will make a determined effort to secure you to serve his purposes. How few understand Satan's great power to deceive! Close every door where he might enter. Surrender yourself, body, soul, and spirit, to God.

Place yourself under those who teach and obey the truth, and learn all you can from them. When you place yourself under the influence of the Holy Spirit, then you can see light in God's light, and you will rejoice in His truth. Keep yourself in the circle of His light, where His light is cherished, and then "let your light so shine before men that they, by seeing your good works, may glorify your Father which is in heaven.". . . .

FROM A SERMON BY MRS. E. G. WHITE

September 9, 1905
Los Angeles, California

WE ARE SO THANKFUL THAT GOD has opened the way for us to secure such favorable locations for our institutions in Southern California. He brought first to our notice the buildings now occupied by the Fernando school. When someone wrote and told me of the buildings that were offered for sale at such reasonable prices, I replied, "Lose no time in securing the property." The instruction given was obeyed, and for two or three years a school has been conducted there. God calls upon you to take a greater interest in this school than you have taken in the past.

The Lord has wonderfully opened up the way for us to establish sanitariums. These institutions should be centers of education. They should be conducted by men and women who have the fear of God in their hearts, and who can speak words in season, bringing to troubled souls the comfort of the grace of God. This is the work that should be done in every sanitarium.

For a long time we have desired to see a work begun in Redlands. Now, in the providence of God, we have come into {222} possession of Loma Linda. This will give you an influence in Redlands and Riverside, enabling us to find openings for the proclamation of present truth. This beautiful property was offered to us at a very low price. It is completely furnished. We have only to take possession. We trust that our people will rally to the support of this institution, that it may not be burdened with a large interest-bearing debt.

A Reform Needed

At this time when Satan is rallying his forces, shall the people of God lay off the armor, and go to sleep? Shall we do nothing, or shall we remember that there is One who says, "All power is given unto Me in heaven and in earth. Go ye therefore, and teach all nations, baptizing them in the name of the Father, and of the Son, and of the Holy Ghost; teaching them to observe all things whatsoever I have commanded you; and, lo, I am with you always, even unto the end of the world."

Many have so little faith in God that He is unable to work for them. Elder Simpson has labored diligently and faithfully in Los Angeles, and the Lord has given him success. But his success would have been far greater had the church rallied to his support, had every member been consecrated to God. Some have thought that Elder Simpson should labor for the church. The church-members should rather have assisted Elder Simpson by going to their neighbors and telling them of the truth, inviting them to attend the meetings.

There is now a large number of believers in Los Angeles. Many of these should be fitting themselves to work for the Master, that the truth may go forth as a lamp that burneth. Read the fifty-eighth chapter of Isaiah. Read it over many times, and you will receive a deeper impression each time.

I have always felt a deep interest in the work in Southern California. For more than twenty years this part of the State has been represented to me as an important field. Our people should be ready to meet those who come and go, and speak to them the words of life. They should scatter the publications containing present truth. The Lord will do great things for those who co-operate with Him.

DEAR BROTHER AND SISTER BURDEN

September 14, 1906
Sanitarium, California

THE WORK OF THE SCHOOL and the sanitarium (Loma Linda) will be a blessing, the one to the other. Each must act its individual part, but both must blend together; then the interests of both will be advanced. If there is co-operation {223} between the educational work and the work of the sanitarium, we can heartily recommend that the higher education be carried on in the sanitarium grounds; for this is the Lord's plan. If the men at the head of this enterprise plan for the usefulness of these institutions, each helping the other, there is nothing to hinder the operations of the school. As the work grows, buildings may have to be prepared.

Ellen G. White

ELDER J. A. BURDEN

November 2, 1906
Sanitarium, California

Dear Brother:

I HAVE WORDS TO SPEAK to you. The Lord has laid upon you responsibilities of no ordinary nature. At the time of the meeting held before you were settled at Loma Linda, when I was so sick, the Lord showed me what was to be your work as director of the Sanitarium, and that if you would connect yourself with divine wisdom, you would be taught of God. You need a clear mind in order to settle wisely the many questions that come to you for decision. The Lord would have you taught of Him.

My brother, do not allow men of limited experience to come in, as Elder Reaser has done, and assume a controlling power. Brother Reaser has placed himself as teacher and adviser and ruler in many matters, and unless you work and watch carefully, such an influence will retard the work. Brother Reaser should learn that he is not qualified to do the work he supposes he is to do.

Brother Reaser supposes that if it was not for his watching of the finances, there would be serious losses; whereas if he had nothing to do and say in these matters, it would save many perplexities. He has taken upon himself burdens that the Lord has not laid upon him. He has learned some of his lessons of Elder Healey, who has done much to retard the work in the South. If he would attend to his work of ministry, and

keep his hands off the work of directing, he would save himself and others many burdens. From the light that has been given me, I know that it is a mistake for him to be connected with our sanitariums; he should not be a manager.

In regard to the health food business, I would urge you to move slowly. Dr. Kellogg's proposition to sell the corn flake rights to our people for twenty years has just been considered by our brethren here; and I fear, if I had not been on the ground, this matter would have been carried through to the loss of our food business. When a thing is exalted, {224} as the corn flakes has been, it would be unwise for our people to have anything to do with it. It is not necessary that we make the corn flakes an article of good.

I would advise you, my brother, to keep away from the influence of Dr. Kellogg's ingenious plans. Let us use our own ingenuity to invent the best kinds of food possible. We are living in the closing days of this earth's history; souls are starving for a knowledge of the word of God and of healthful living. Let us seek to carry our work solidly, giving all possible instruction regarding the principles of health reform, praying with the sick, and teaching the people how to care for themselves in sickness and health.

The Lord has sent us valuable help in Dr. White, who is studying to know how to follow the way of the Lord. Let there be much earnest prayer on the part of the workers, each depending on the great Physician to carry the work according to His purposes. "For we are laborers together with God: ye are God's husbandry; ye are God's building." In our efforts to build up the cause of God in the earth, we are to make sure work for eternity.

Many workers who are bearing responsibilities are embracing too much authority; and they will certainly confuse the human judgment by their dictatorial authority. I must warn my brethren to be on their guard against this. The cause of God is imperiled when the workers become self-confident, and seek to embrace more than the Lord has laid upon them. Hindrance instead of advancement is the result of such a spirit.

Brother Burden, carry your work intelligently, even consulting the word of God; for this word is very precious to the worker in the cause. Study the messages that God has sent to His people for the last sixty years through the Spirit of Prophe-

cy. Do not seek the counsel of men, but by earnest prayer seek the wisdom of God. A mistake has been made in the past by leaning upon the guidance of men. Seek to correct this mistake.

LETTER TO BROTHER BURDEN

November 25, 1906
Sanitarium, California

YESTERDAY WAS A STRANGE DAY for me. I was compelled to leave letters and other writings unfinished.

The Lord has been working with Elder Simpson, teaching him how to give to the people this last warning message. His method of making the words of the Bible prove the truth for this time, and his use of the symbols presented in Revelation and Daniel, are effective. Let the young men learn as for their lives what is truth, and how it should be presented. We are living in the last days of the great conflict; the truth alone will hold us securely in this time of trouble. The {225} way should be prepared for Elder Simpson to give the message, and our young men should attend his evening meetings.

Those who have considered themselves qualified to bear responsibilities in the churches, should seek to obtain light and a knowledge of how to prosecute their work at this time in the cities, north and south, east and west, that are calling for a knowledge of the truth for this time. Our camp meetings should do a more thorough work in preparing the laborers for the work that is to be done in every place.

The camp meetings which my husband attended were made special seasons of seeking the Lord. Every morning at an early hour the ministers assembled in the large tent, where we wrought to become of one mind. The question would be asked, Have we any personal difficulties to settle? If so, let us settle them. Let us not pass one day on this ground cherishing hard feelings against a brother. Let there be no evil speaking one of another; for this will greatly dishonor God. Let us by every means in our power seek to remove the alienation and differences that exist.

Then we would have a season of prayer, and these were times of confession and breaking of heart before God. Often the workers, and especially the ministers, would state their true feelings, relating their temptations, and confessing their loss of confidence in their brethren. These confessions tended to clear away any ill feeling that existed, and brought in a very different atmosphere.

At these camp meetings no one man carried the burden of deciding who should speak, but those were chosen who were experienced in the message and in conducting camp meetings. We used then the very arguments that are now given why the young men should not be brought to the front while the aged workers were passed by.

God speaks through the men who understand the guiding of the Holy Spirit. When thousands come out to attend our meetings, they desire to get the greatest possible benefit, and it is poor policy to place as speakers men who are not fully adapted to meet the needs of the situation. The word should be spoken by men who have felt the deep moving of the Spirit upon their hearts, and who feel the burden of the message that God has given them for the people. The old soldiers of the cross are not to be passed by.

Men who have been placed in office for the first time, and who are just gaining their experience, need to move carefully and in humility of mind; for often they are not able to judge wisely. When Elder Reaser was placed in a position of responsibility, he did not see his need to learn all that he could from the experience of others who had a knowledge of the history of the work in Southern California, and who had burdens laid upon them for that work by the Lord. At the first assuming of his new responsibilities, Elder Reaser should have considered that these persons understood {226} the situation better than he did. By his officious attitude, he has made the work much more perplexing than it otherwise would have been. If he will be taught, the Lord will teach Elder Reaser that he has men on the ground who are fully as capable of planning and devising for the interests of the work as himself.

The Lord has given you your work, Brother Burden. He has not appointed Elder Reaser to tell you what your duty is. As superintendent of the sanitarium, your work is an important one. Elder Reaser is not to intrude himself upon that which God has given you to do. That there shall be no more money in the sanitarium until the institution shall have earned that amount required, is not for Elder Reaser to decide. Hire money, if this is necessary in order to perfect the work.

———

To the Workers in the Paradise Valley Sanitarium

———

February 12, 1907
Sanitarium Post Office, Napa County, California

Dear Brethren and Sisters:

THE PAST NIGHT HAS BEEN one of wakefulness and prayer. I am anxious to understand the ways of the Lord, and to know what words I should speak to those who are in charge of the Paradise Valley Sanitarium.

I heard One of authority speaking to a company of workers, including everyone who has a part to act in the sanitarium. These were the words he said:

"Let not your hearts be troubled; ye believe in God believe also in Me. In my Father's house are many mansions: if it were not so I would have told you. I go to prepare a place for you. And if I go and prepare a place for you, I will come again, and receive you unto Myself, that where I am there ye may be also."

When Jesus spoke these words to His disciples, he was about to leave them. He had just given them a portion of His parting address, and in that he had foretold the work of Judas in betraying his Lord for thirty pieces of silver. When Judas left the presence of Christ to perform this terrible work, Jesus said to His disciples, "Now is the Son of Man glorified, and God is glorified in Him. If God be glorified in Him, God shall also glorify Him in Himself, and shall straightaway glorify Him. Little children, yet a little while I am with you. Ye shall seek me, and as I said unto the Jews, Whither I go ye cannot come; so now I say to you. A new commandment I give unto you, That ye love one another; as I have loved you, that ye also love one another. By this shall all men know that ye are my disciples, if ye have love one for another." {227}

"Simon Peter said unto Him, Lord, whither goest Thou? Jesus answered him, Whither I go thou canst not follow Me now; but thou shalt follow Me afterwards. Peter said unto Him, Lord, why cannot I follow Thee now? I will lay down my life for Thy sake. Jesus answered him, Wilt thou lay down thy life for My sake? Verily, verily I say unto thee, The cock shall not crow, till thou hast denied Me thrice."

The workers in our sanitariums should understand that each has an individual work. Each should realize his duty to keep

his soul and body under discipline to the great Physician, who gave His life to rescue us from the control of a powerful foe. After He had burst the fetters of the tomb, He said to His disciples, "I am the resurrection and the life." And before he ascended to heaven, He declared, "All power is given unto Me in heaven and in earth. Go ye therefore and teach all nations, baptizing them in the name of the Father, and of the Son, and of the Holy Ghost, teaching them to observe all things whatsoever I have commanded you; and, lo, I am with you always, even unto the end of the world."

Here is your work. Teach the sick. Proclaim the gospel to them, persuading them to become Christ's disciples. The Father, the Son, and the Holy Spirit are pledged to be with you in every emergency. Act as Christians, having divine orders. God is to be trusted, believed, obeyed. His character is to be represented in every household.

A wonderful responsibility rests upon those connected with the sanitariums established in His name for the treatment of the sick. This is to be done without the use of poisonous drugs. Those who become workers in the sanitarium are to believe the words of Christ, "Lo I am with you always, even unto the end of the world." Those who have the fear of God in the heart will cultivate a sweet disposition. Forbearance and courtesy will be manifested in the life. Duties will be faithfully discharged and in a way that will not leave a disagreeable impression on the minds of the sick of the well.

In order to maintain a right influence, the workers must reveal that they are one in sentiment. Do not let it be seen that there is disunion among the helpers.

If you have any care of the sick, act tenderly, kindly, faithfully, that you may have a converting influence upon them. You have need of the grade of Christ in order to properly represent the service of Christ. And as you present the grace of truth in true, disinterested service, angels will be present to sustain you. The Comforter will be with you to fulfill the promise of the Saviour, "Lo, I am with you always, even unto the end of the world."

I have a charge to give, a message to bear to our sanitarium workers. Keep your souls in purity. Do a work that will have a winning influence on those placed in your charge. You can speak often to the sick of the great Physician, who can heal the diseases of the body as verily as He heals {228} the sickness of the soul.

Pray with the sick, and try to lead them to see in Christ, their Healer. Tell them that if they will look to Him in faith, He will say to them, "Thy sins be forgiven thee." It means very much to the sick to learn this lesson.

ELDER J. E. WHITE

May 7, 1907
National City, California

Dear Son Edson:

IN MANY PLACES I SEE great need for the investment of means in the cause of God. Next week I expect to return to Loma Linda, and while there I will do what I can to help forward the work in the surrounding cities. I desire to invest some means in the work in these places. I hope to find opportunity to speak to our people in that locality, and to arouse them to a sense of their responsibility to hold up the light of truth. If, before I leave Loma Linda, I can see the right work begun, I shall not feel pressed as a cart beneath sheaves, after I return home.

Mrs. Dr. Starr has been doing a good work in San Bernardino. She has been giving education in health principles, and has found access to many fine homes. I hope to strengthen her hands, and give her encouragement to continue the work in Redlands and Riverside.

AN OPEN LETTER

May 19, 1907
Loma Linda, California

Dear Brethren and Sisters:

THE LORD HAS GREATLY BLESSED our people in Southern California, in enabling them to secure at very low cost valuable sanitarium properties. Through the institutions that are established here, the Lord desires to reach a class that can be reached in no other way. Therefore I would urge upon our people to whom the Lord has entrusted the talent of means, that they make loans and gifts to place these institutions in a position where they can do without embarrassment the work that will be to the honor and glory of God.

For forty thousand dollars our brethren secured at Loma Linda buildings and land that cost originally one hundred and fifty thousand dollars. These buildings were furnished completely, far more elegantly than we would have furnished them. {229}

The Lord has worked wonderfully in bringing us into possession of this place. Here is a center from which light is to shine into the surrounding cities of Redlands, Riverside, San Bernardino, Colton, and other places nearby.

It has been found necessary to provide additional bathroom facilities at Loma Linda, and to make some changes to adapt the building to sanitarium work. An elevator is greatly needed, and a small bakery should be added. We are in need of means to accomplish that which must be done, and we pray the Lord to put it into the heart of our brethren and sisters to help in this time of necessity.

For years the Lord has instructed us that we should have a sanitarium in the vicinity of San Diego, where many thousands of tourists come every year. A valuable property was secured at National City at a very small part of its original cost. There is an important work to be done in caring for the sick, and in reaching many with the light of truth. At the Paradise Valley Sanitarium also it was found necessary to add to the original building, and obligation have been made that must soon be met. The Lord has blessed this institution, and some have been converted to the truth as the result of the work already done.

At Glendale, a few miles from Los Angeles, we purchased a sanitarium at about one fourth its real value. This institution is at the present time full of patients. It is well-equipped for work, and is in a position of influence. Its need is not so pressing as that of the sanitariums at Loma Linda and National City.

The establishment of these three institutions has brought a heavy financial burden to our people in Southern California. Yet they have cheerfully responded to the calls for means that have been made. Brother Burden, Dr. White, and others connected with these sanitariums have invested all they could spare, that the work might not be hindered.

We have none too many sanitariums. There is need for every one that has been established. In these institutions we are endeavoring to carry the work earnestly and solidly. in harmony with the instruction the Lord has given in regard to sanitarium work. They are to stand as a means of teaching the truth in these great centers of tourist resort.

At our request, Brother Burden is going East to attend some of our camp meetings, where he may come in contact with many of our brethren and sisters, and lay before them the opportunities for assisting these important branches of the Lord's work. We unite in asking those who have means to spare, to consider the matter of investing some of their money in these institutions, thus helping to provide necessary facilities, that a thorough work may be done in caring for the sick who are coming to Southern California in search of health. {230}

May the Lord give ability to help, and a willing mind.

DEAR BROTHER AND SISTER HASKELL

May 20, 1907
Sanitarium, Glendale, California

WE LEFT HOME ON OUR VISIT to Southern California April 18. On our way to San Diego, we stopped off at Fernando, and we spent a few days at Loma Linda. At the Paradise Valley Sanitarium we found a very small patronage. Twice I spoke to the helpers and guests. On Sabbath and Sunday, May 4 and 5, I spoke to the church in San Diego. I bore a very plain testimony. Sunday afternoon, I followed an earnest appeal with a prayer. This was followed by a social meeting at which some confessions were made. . . .

I remained at Loma Linda nearly a week, during which time I spoke to the students twice. Sabbath afternoon I spoke to a large number who had assembled from the surrounding churches. The meeting was held on the lawn. Among those present were some who have recently begun the observance of the Sabbath in Redlands, where Elder Hare and Elder Whitehead have been conducting a series of meetings.

Seats were arranged under the pepper trees at the back of the sanitarium. It was an interesting occasion. The Lord blessed me in speaking from the fifty-eighth chapter of Isaiah. Before I closed, I made a strong appeal to those who had means to help in the Lord's work, and I presented the needs of the Loma Linda Sanitarium. I urged them not to spend all their efforts merely in commercial lines, but to lay up treasure beside the throne of God.

In the evening, Brother Nichols came to my room, his face aglow with happiness, and said, "I want to tell you what your words today have accomplished. A sister came to Brother Burden, and gave him ten dollars, and a gentleman has offered to lend him a thousand dollars for a year without interest." I thank the Lord for this response.

From Brother Burden I learned that the

one who had offered to lend him a thousand dollars is a patient who had been in the sanitarium for some time. He had a serious stomach difficulty, and for some time his life was hanging in the balance. The crisis safely passed, he has begun to study the truth, and is deeply interested.

After the morning service, a lunch was provided by the sanitarium, on the lawn, for the visitors. Brother Burden felt that the sanitarium would not be a loser by doing this, and I agreed with him; for I remember the experiences we have had in the past in making similar provision. Such actions are sometimes the means of sowing seed in the hearts of those {231} who are inquiring after truth.

In the afternoon, Elder Luther Warren gave an excellent discourse. Brother Warren is an able worker, and we hope he may labor for a time in this needy field. Now is a favorable time to work Redlands. The Woman's Christian Temperance Union recently held an important convention in Redlands, and Dr. Starr attended their meetings. She was introduced to the convention, and by invitation spoke to them on the subject of healthful dress. She was well received, and has received many invitations to give lectures at various places. We trust that the Lord will open the way before her, that she may be a help in removing the prejudice of some, that they may be willing to listen to the truth.

DEAR BROTHER BURDEN

April 12, 1905
Sanitarium, California

I HEAR THAT PLANS ARE being laid for Elder W. W. Simpson to leave Southern California to labor elsewhere. If Elder Simpson feels it his duty to go, I have nothing to say against it. But I had hoped to see him extend his work from Los Angeles to Redlands and Riverside. The condition of Brother Simpson's health is such that great care must be exercised in regard to the location of his field of labor. He should have suitable help, that he may be relieved from the burden of speaking so frequently. Would it not be well if Elder Corliss and Elder Simpson could labor together?

Redlands and Riverside have been presented to me as places that should be worked. These two places should no longer be neglected. I hope soon to see an earnest effort put forth in their behalf. Will you please consider the advisability of establishing a sanitarium in the vicinity of these towns, with treatment rooms in each place to act as feeders to the institution?

We cannot afford to allow these places to go unwarned. Instead of Elder Simpson's going somewhere else to work, would it not be better to let a determined effort be put forth to make a success of the work in these places. There are other cities in Southern California in which a work similar to that carried on by Elder Simpson in Los Angeles should be conducted. The Lord would have His ministers working zealously for those who have never heard the truth. But Elder Simpson should have someone connected with him to help him in the work.

Our people in the churches of Southern California need to arouse to do a work that is necessary within their own borders. Let them awake to prayer and labor. They need {232} more spiritual vitality. They need to be converted, that they may labor for souls. Wherever there is spiritual life, there will be an imparting as well as a receiving of light and blessing. The nourishment from God's word will be received and earnest work will be done. The act of imparting keeps open the channel for receiving. This truth our Saviour ever sought to keep before the people.

I have a message to bear to the church members in Southern California: Arouse, and avail yourselves of the opportunities open to you. While Christ pleads in your behalf, plead for yourselves, that you may be purified from every unrighteous thought, every unholy action. Make an entire surrender to God of body, soul, and spirit. Be determined to do all in your power to learn the true science of soul-saving. While the light of God's mercy still shines, gather up every divine ray.

Are you prepared to sell all, that you may purchase the field that contains the treasure? Said the apostle Paul, "I count all things but loss for the excellency of the knowledge of Christ Jesus my Lord. . . that I may win Christ, and be found in him."

Give up the self-righteousness that you have been cherishing. If the Lord permits you to behold such work as has been done in Los Angeles, seek with all humility to act your part. Not in your own strength, but in the strength of Christ, you are to ascend the ladder heavenward, round by round. Make diligent, thorough work in humbling yourselves, that the old habits and practices and all evil speaking may be put away. Draw nigh to God, and He will draw nigh to you. Die to self; live to God.

Brother Burden, say to the church that the Lord will manifest Himself to all who seek him with humble hearts. The end of all things is at hand. Let your eyes be fixed upon Christ. As the called and chosen of God, we must represent truth in its purity. Our lives are to be such that the world will take knowledge of us that we have been with Christ, and that truth may seem to them more desirable than error.

If rightly conducted, our sanitariums may exert a refining, ennobling influence, and lead many souls to Christ. The religious principles maintained in these institutions will demonstrate that there is relief for the soul, weary and sick with sin. Many are weak and sick because of disease of the soul. Let Christ be held up before them as the great Healer, who invites them to come to Him and find rest. Tell them that the heart of Christ is drawn out in compassion and love for His blood-bought heritage. He will heal the troubled heart that looks to him in faith.

To the poor, sin-sick soul repeat the Saviour's invitation: "Come to me, all ye that labor and are heavy laden, and I will give you rest. Take my yoke upon you, and learn of me; {233} for I am meek and lowly in heart, and ye shall find rest unto your souls. For my yoke is easy, and my burden is light." There is true joy in learning of Christ.

Tell the suffering ones of a compassionate Saviour. He is the only physician who can heal both body and soul. He has given Him life for the world, that men should not perish, but have everlasting life. He looks with compassion upon those who regard their case as hopeless.

While the soul is filled with fear and terror, the mind cannot see the tender compassion of Christ. Our sanitariums are to be an agency for bringing peace and rest to the troubled minds. If you can inspire the despondent with hopeful, saving faith, contentment and cheerfulness will take the place of discouragement and unrest. Wonderful changes can then be wrought in their physical condition. Christ will restore both body and soul, and, realizing His compassion and love, they will rest in Him. He is the bright and morning star, shining amid the moral darkness of this sinful, corrupt world. He is the light of the world, and all who give their hearts to Him will find peace, rest, and joy.

The world is filled with sickness. Sin is increasing, especially in the large cities. Death is taking away large numbers.

But the great Medical Missionary invites men to come to Him. "Come unto me," He says, "and I will give you rest." "Ask, and ye shall receive; seek, and ye shall find; knock, and it shall be opened unto you."

Our part is, by believing His word, to find rest in Christ Jesus. His words are spirit and life. In believing them there is rest and peace. "Knock, and it shall be opened unto you."

Our prayers will reach the ear of Christ, and He will open unto us the rich treasures of His grace. Through prayer we are brought into communion with the high and holy One who inhabiteth eternity. He opens the door to everyone who will knock.

As I think of how the skillful Physician longs to heal every sin-sick soul, I feel so anxious that those who are drawn to our sanitariums may there find what they need for the cure of their physical and spiritual maladies.

"Come out from among them, and be ye separate, saith the Lord, and touch not the unclean thing; and I will receive you, and will be a Father unto you, and ye shall be my sons and daughters, saith the Lord Almighty." This invitation will be accepted by those who are burdened for souls. They will become members of the royal family, children of the heavenly King.

The law of God is to be obeyed. Obedience is the life of the soul. It brings health and peace and assurance. Seek the Lord in every necessity, and know that you have a friend in Jesus, one who loves you with an everlasting love. He will {234} be as an anchor to the soul, both sure and steadfast. When men and women come just as they are, he cleanses them from their sins, and they become His sons and daughters.

Dear Brother and Sister Burden

May 23, 1905
Takoma Park, Washington, D. C.

I FEEL VERY GRATEFUL TO the Lord that he has strengthened me to speak six times at this meeting. When I left my home in St. Helena, I was suffering from a severe cold, and I thought it rather a risk to run to attempt to attend the meeting. But I decided to start with the party, thinking that I would go as far as Los Angeles, and then, if I could not go any further, I would return to St. Helena. The Lord strengthened me, and I have been able to bear my testimony six times since the meeting began. All seem surprised that my voice is so clear and strong. I have said many things that the Lord has given me to say, and I still have more to say. I attend only those meetings in which I can bear my testimony.

I have been waiting to hear from you again regarding the place near Redlands, about which you wrote not long ago. I hope that this place can be secured, because I think that the Lord has made it possible for us to obtain it. If you have anything further to tell us, please do so. We do not want this place to be a snare to us; for I feel impressed that it will be a great blessing. I hope that you will send me a line when you have come to a decision regarding the place.

Redlands and Riverside must be worked, and they could be worked from the place about which you have written us. If Brother and Sister Haskell can possibly get away from Nashville, I should like them to spend a little time in Southern California.

Dear Brother Burden

May 24, 1905
Takoma Park, Washington, D. C.

W E RECEIVED YOUR LETTER TODAY. I wish to say that I cannot ask the Conference to invest in a sanitarium at Redlands. They have enough responsibilities to carry without taking upon them other responsibilities. If you in Los Angeles will do your best, we will do our best. If you will do nothing, say so, and we will do nothing. If you will work intelligently, as we know you can, then we will do what we can. But if you {235} do nothing, waiting for the Conference, you will lose your chance. If you are going to depend on the Conference purchasing it, I have no hope of your obtaining it.

Can you give us definite terms of payment? Then we shall know what to tell the people. I am anxious to secure the place for a sanitarium, but if you cannot state anything definite as to the terms of payment, we are left without any certain information.

Brother Burden, if you wait for Brother Santee to work out the plans, there will be no hope at all in the matter. I will not write more till I hear something further from you. Telegraph us at once the price of the property, and the best terms of payment you can obtain.

Dear Brother Burden

May 14, 1905
Takoma Park, Washington, D. C.

Y OUR LETTER HAS JUST BEEN read. I had no sooner finished reading it then I said, "I will consult no one; for I have no question at all about the matter." I advised Willie to send you a telegram without spending time to ask the advice of the brethren. Secure the property by all means, so that it can be held, and then obtain all the money you can make sufficient payments to hold the place. This is the very property that we ought to have. Do not delay; for it is just what is needed. As soon as it is secured, a working force can begin operations in it. I think that sufficient help can be secured to carry this matter through. I want you to be sure to lose no time in securing the right to purchase the property. We will do our utmost to help you raise the money. I know that Redlands and Riverside are to be worked, and I pray that the Lord may be gracious, and not allow anyone else to get this property instead of us.

We had a very pleasant trip from San Francisco to Washington. Several times a song-service was held in the car, and this took well. Many of the passengers outside of our party united in the singing.

I am recovering from the cold that I caught about three weeks before leaving home. On Thursday morning I spoke in the large tent, and on Sabbath morning I spoke again. The large tent was crowded, and I am told that my voice could be heard very distinctly even by those on the seats at the very back. I shall send you a copy of my talk when it is written out.

Today, Sunday, Elder Haskell spoke in the forenoon. The afternoon meeting was broken up by a thunderstorm. The rain came through the large tent, and people were {236} obliged to hurry away to the small tents.

A good work is being done on the school and sanitarium land here. Money is coming in for the completion of the one hundred thousand dollar fund. Last Friday morning, at a meeting held for this purpose, about six thousand dollars were handed in by the delegates for the Washington work. A great many Conferences had not at that time reported fully, and at the end of this week, there will be several thousand dollars more to hand in.

We hope that this meeting will be the means of accomplishing much good. If the Lord sees that we are in earnest in seeking

Him, He will be found of us. Oh, it would be sad indeed to get above the simplicity of the work. When we are humble enough to receive wisdom, the Lord will certainly teach us His way. I have such a hungering and thirsting after God: I must have a strong faith, and I must bear a decided testimony, which will not be weakened. Bible truth will prevail, and oh, how my heart longs to see our church members obtaining a deep experience, which will stand the test that is before us.

Let us seek the Lord while He may be found, and call upon Him while He is near. "Let the wicked forsake his way, and the unrighteous man his thoughts; and let him return unto the Lord, and He will have mercy upon him; and to our God; for He will abundantly pardon."

Let us make straight paths for our feet. The Lord will not leave those who love Him and keep His commandments to be spoiled by the enemy. A short work is to be done. Let us read and study the fifty-fifth and fifty-sixth chapters of Isaiah; for they contain wonderful encouragement, and the Lord wants us to bring all the uplifting possible to His people.

"Thus saith the Lord, Keep ye judgment, and do justice; for My salvation is near to come, and My righteousness to be revealed. Blessed is the man that doeth this, and the son of man that layeth hold on it; that keepeth the Sabbath from polluting it and keepeth his hand from doing any evil.

"Neither let the son of the stranger that hath joined himself to the Lord speak saying, The Lord hath utterly separated me from His people; neither let the eunuch say, Behold, I am a dry tree. For thus saith the Lord unto the eunuchs that keep my Sabbaths, and choose the things that please Me, and take hold of My covenant: Even to them will I give in Mine house and within My walls a place and a name better than of sons and of daughters: I will give them an everlasting name, that shall not be cut off.

"Also the sons of the stranger, that join themselves to the Lord, to serve Him, and to love the name of the Lord, {237} to be His servants, everyone that keepeth the Sabbath from polluting it, and taketh hold of My covenant; even them will I bring to My holy mountain, and make them joyful in My house of prayer; their burnt-offerings and their sacrifices shall be accepted upon Mine altar; for Mine house shall be called an house of prayer for all people. The Lord God, which gathereth the out-casts of Israel, saith, Yet will I gather others to Him, beside those that are gathered unto Him."

Here is the word of the Lord. Open up every place possible. We are to labor in faith, taking hold of a power that is pledged to do large things for us. We are to reach out in faith in Los Angeles and in Redlands and Riverside.

DEAR BROTHER BURDEN

June 2, 1905
Takoma Park, Washington, D. C.

I AM MUCH ENCOURAGED BY the letters that I have received from you regarding Loma Linda. From your description of the place, I believe it meets the representation which I have seen of what we should seek for as sanitarium locations. Such a place was presented to me a few miles from an important city. The city has recently been built up.

I have tried to place before our people the representations given me regarding sanitariums in the country, and I have urged upon them the necessity of establishing our sanitariums outside of the cities. I have had repeatedly presented to me the advantage of securing locations some miles out of the cities. Those who follow the counsel of God in providing places where the sick and suffering can receive proper treatment will be guided to the right places for the establishment of their work.

Let our sanitariums be located where there is an abundance of land. I can see the advantage of such a place as Loma Linda. The Lord worked to help us to secure this property. The work of this institution is to be carried forward on pure, elevated lines. It can be conducted in such a way that the truth will be presented as the rock upon which to build.

In order that our institutions shall teach right lessons, there must be connected with them men of such simplicity that they are willing to learn of the great Teacher. "To you it is given," Christ said, to the people who keep My commandments and do those things that I have presented in my work, "to know the mysteries of the kingdom of heaven."

We are to proclaim the truth to the world, for thus the great Medical Missionary has commanded us. "What ye {238} hear in the ear, that preach ye upon the house top; for there is nothing hid that shall not be made known." "The secret of the Lord is with them that fear Him, and keep His commandments." "As many as received Him, to them gave He power to become the sons of God."

The church of Christ is dependent on Him for her very existence. Only through Him can it gain continued life and strength. The members are to live constantly in the most intimate, vital relationship with the Saviour. They are to follow in His steps of self-denial and sacrifice. They are to go forth into the highways and byways of life to win souls to Him, using every possible means to make the truth appear in its true character before the world.

The truth is to be presented in various ways. Some in the higher walks of life will grasp it as it is presented in figures and parables. As men labor to unfold the truth with clearness, that conviction may come to their hearers, the Lord is present as He promised to be. As they go forth on their mission, teaching all things whatsoever Christ has commanded, the promise will be fulfilled, "Lo, I am with you always, even unto the end of the world." Those who are honest in heart will see the importance of the truth for this time, and will take their place in the ranks of those who are keeping and teaching the commandments.

All that can be done to make clear the mystery of godliness is to be done. The earthly has its place in illustrating the heavenly. All nature is a lesson-book, a teacher to everyone who will learn.

In His wonderful sermon on the mount, Christ used the lilies of the field in their natural loveliness to illustrate a great truth. His language is adapted to the opening intellect of child life. The great Teacher brought His hearers in contact with nature, that they might listen to the voice which speaks in all created things; and as their hearts became tender and their minds receptive, He helped them to interpret the spiritual teachings of the scenes upon which their eyes rested. The parables, by means of which He loved to teach lessons of truth, show how open His spirit was to the influences of nature, and how He delighted to gather spiritual teaching from the surroundings of daily life.

The birds of the air, the lilies of the field, the sower and the seed, the shepherd and the sheep,—with these Christ illustrated immortal truth. He drew illustrations from the facts of life, facts of experience familiar to the hearers,—the hid treasure, the pearl, the fishing net, the lost coin, the prodigal son, the houses on the rock and on the sand. In His lessons there was something to interest every mind, to appeal to every heart. Thus the daily task, instead of being a mere round of toil, bereft of higher thoughts, was brightened and uplifted by constant reminders of the spiritual and the unseen. {239}

Our medical workers are to do all in their power to cure disease of the body and also disease of the mind. They are to watch and pray and work, bringing spiritual as well as physical advantages to those for whom they labor. The physician in one of our sanitariums who is a true servant of God has an intensely interesting work to do for every suffering human being with whom he is brought in contact. He is to lose no opportunity to point souls to Christ, the great Healer of body and mind. Every physician should be a skillful worker in Christ's lines. There is to be no lessening of the interest in spiritual things, else the power to fix the mind upon the great Physician will be diverted. While the needs of the body are to be strictly attended to, while all efforts are to be made to break the power of disease, the physician is never to forget that there is a soul to be labored for.

God would draw minds from the conviction of logic to a conviction deeper, higher, purer, and more glorious, a conviction unperverted by human logic. Human logic has often nearly quenched the light which God would have shine forth in clear rays to convince minds that the God of nature is worthy of all praise and all glory, because He is the Creator of all things.

Christ illustrated character-building by a house built on a rock, against which storm and tempest were powerless, and the house built on the sand, which was swept away. We are living in perilous times.

DEAR BROTHER BURDEN

May 31, 1905
Takoma Park, Washington, D. C.

OUR GENERAL MEETINGS closed last night. We have had excellent meetings, but I cannot give you a full report, for I have gone to those meetings only at which I have spoken. I came to the Conference with fear and trembling, but determined to do my best. I have spoken ten times, and have done considerable writing. Night after Night I have been up writing as early as two o'clock, and yet I

am doing well healthwise.

On the whole, we have had beautiful weather. At the first of the meetings there was a heavy thunder storm, but since then the days have been pleasant. Last night there was a little shower, which is a great blessing; for the dust has been settled.

For the rest of the week, committee meetings will continue, and the first of next week we shall start home. On way out we shall stop to see the place that means so much to me. {240}

During the meeting I did not dare to make any call for money; but last Sunday afternoon, when I had finished speaking the thought came to me that perhaps the people standing on the outside of the tent might give something for the colored work, so I made a call. A contribution was taken up, and in a very few minutes word came that one hundred and twenty-eight dollars had been given. The subduing influence of the Spirit of God rested upon the people, and a good impression was made by the meeting. As I walked from the tent to my room, many stopped me, and with tears of rejoicing shook my hand.

The Conference has called forth very weighty testimonies, and I am pleased with the appreciation shown to these testimonies.

We hope to see you soon now, but in regard to the purchase of "Loma Linda", I will say, Go ahead. I hope to be able to help by giving the proceeds from a certain number of copies of "Ministry of Healing". I can do no more, except to borrow. I wish the place purchased. Do not neglect to tell me all I ought to know. I have been looking over your descriptive letter, and I am well satisfied that the place is one we ought to have. It is cheap at forty thousand dollars. We will not leave you, but will stand back of you, and help you to raise the means. In regard to the right man to manage the institution? I am confident that we shall find someone when the right time comes.

As soon as we can be released from here, we shall return to California. I will let you know when we shall leave here, as soon as I can find out.

(Stamped) Ellen G. White

DEAR BROTHER BURDEN

May 28, 1905
Takoma Park, Washington, D. C.

WHEN YOU WROTE TO ME about the advisability of purchasing the property known as "Loma Linda", I did

not consult with anyone, because I thought this would hinder us, and I believed that we could carry the matter forward without putting the burden on the Conference. We do not desire to bring perplexity upon the Conference regarding this matter. Be assured, my brother, that I never advance anything unless I have a decided impression that it should be carried out, and unless I am firmly resolved to assist.

I am glad that means is in sight to make the first payment on the place; for we ought to have it. I do not know just where to look for the rest of the money needed. I have {241} asked Brother Washburn to let me know of anyone who would be willing to lend me some money without interest. He thinks that I could get means on these terms.

We will appropriate the proceeds of the sale of a certain number of copies of "Ministry of Healing" toward the purchase of this property. The book will soon be on the market.

By all means secure the property, if you can; for I believe it to be the very place the Lord desires us to have. We do not desire to burden the Conference. We can as a company raise the required sum, I believe. I hope that we shall see you soon, and then we can talk these matters over. We shall have to stay here for a week after the meetings close, because Willie has some committee work to do.

Since coming to the Conference, I have spoken nine times. Up to today I had not made any call for means. At the close of my talk this afternoon, I called for a contribution for the work among the colored people of the Southern field. One hundred and twenty-eight dollars was raised. I was much pleased. When I left my tent, it looked as if I would not be able to get to my room, there were so many who wanted to speak to me. Edson was present, and he felt very grateful for the donation.

We had a large profitable meeting on Sabbath. The tent was filled, and a number of people stood on the outside. This afternoon I spoke to a large company.

This is a beautiful place, and I am glad that the school is established here. A sanitarium must be erected, and we hope that this can be done soon. Then there is the publishing house to be built, but we hope that after both the school and the sanitarium have been completed, there will be something left for the publishing house.

(Stamped) Ellen G. White

DR. JOHN F. MORSE

July 24, 1905
Loma Linda, Near Redlands, California
(M.-247- 1905)

Dear Brother:

I **WRITE TO INVITE YOU** to connect with our sanitarium work in Southern California.

We now have three sanitariums in this southern part of the State. Loma Linda, the one most recently purchased, is the most desirable place I have ever seen for a sanitarium. We realize that the Lord has been very gracious to us in opening the way {242} for us to secure this plant, which was originally constructed as a sanitarium.

Upon this property there has been made an investment of about a hundred and fifty thousand dollars. Several months ago our brethren spoke to me of the place as a beautiful location with grant buildings, but they supposed that it would be valued so high that we could not possibly secure it.

Until I saw Loma Linda I could not feel that I had seen a place that seemed in every respect to correspond with the representations I had seen of what a sanitarium should be. I had been instructed to say to our brethren that we should have a sanitarium situated near Redlands and Riverside. This institution is about five miles from Redlands and twelve from Riverside. But I had no idea that we would be able to purchase Loma Linda, though we had heard that the owners were very anxious to sell the property.

While I was at Takoma Park attending the General Conference, I received a letter from Brother Burden describing the property at Loma Linda, and informing me that the place was offered for sale for forty thousand dollars. There were others who desired to secure the property, but we were given an option till the brethren could communicate with us. The description given by Brother Burden answered in every respect to that of places that I had been instructed would be offered far below their original cost.

This letter from Brother Burden I received one Friday afternoon. I asked W. C. White to telegraph immediately to Brother Burden that he should by all means secure the property. Some of our brethren connected with the Conference advised otherwise, fearing that the Conference would be more deeply involved in debt. But I followed my telegram with a letter, saying distinctly that the place should be purchased without delay. I considered that the advantages of this location authorized me to speak positively regarding this matter. I said, There is sufficient money in the hands of God's people, and if we seek the Lord, He will make their hearts willing to help in this time of need.

After writing to Brother Burden, the uncertainty so affected me that for several nights I was unable to sleep. I lifted my heart to God in prayer. With great anxiety I waited, till at last word came that a deposit of one thousand dollars had been made and the way was open for us to secure the place.

We now have possession of this valuable property. All the negotiations have been pleasant and agreeable. Brother Burden has been a man in the right place. The former owners have every confidence in him, and seem pleased that we have purchased the place. We thank the Lord for this.

We have just been attending the Los Angeles camp meeting, {243} and before going home I am spending a few days here, and expect to stop for a few days at the Paradise Valley Sanitarium.

Owing to a weakness in my hip, I was unable to go over the building when I was here last spring, but I could see something of the advantages of the place and the beauty of the seventy-six acres. There are many lovely pepper-trees, and other varieties of trees, the names of which I have not learned. Hundreds of happy birds sing in the branches. There is a large orchard set out to orange trees, grapefruit, plums, peaches, nectarines, lemons, pears, etc.

In the cellar I see a large quantity of jellies that have been put up. Shelf after shelf is laden with jars of rich fruit. The work of fruit-canning is now going on, superintended by those who thoroughly understand the business. Some of the fruit will be sent to the sanitarium at San Diego.

The buildings here are completely furnished with nearly every essential necessary to conduct a sanitarium. Every room is furnished with a bed and elegant and substantial furniture. The mattresses and pillows are excellent. The chairs are well selected. Many of them are very expensive. The buildings are lighted with electricity. The main building has four stories. Everything is in first class condition. There are many articles of furniture that we could not have furnished if we had been fitting up the building. We thank the Lord for His providence that has brought us to this beautiful place.

We have also a beautiful property near San Diego. We thank the Lord for such a beautiful location and such excellent buildings at so low a cost. We must put forth every effort to fulfil the purpose of God in this institution. Suitable bathrooms are needed there, and we are asking the people to help us in making the necessary additions.

We are to take advantage of every blessing within our reach. Above all things, let us seek for the excellency of the knowledge of Christ. The apostle Paul, who had received abundant revelations from God, whose judgment had been formed under the special intuition of the Holy Spirit, says: "Yea, doubtless, I count all things but loss for the excellency of the knowledge of Christ Jesus my Lord." That knowledge we must impart to others.

The knowledge of Jesus Christ is obtained through correct views of our Lord. Through the work of our sanitariums the light of truth may shine forth to the world. To these institutions we may invite all classes of people, men and women of every denomination. We must have physicians who will reveal Christ in knowledge and in speech. We want well-qualified physicians, who have a well-grounded hope in Jesus Christ. {244}

It is through the love of Christ that we receive spiritual food, that we may break the bread of life to others. His blessings, which have gladdened our hearts, are to be communicated to those who know not Christ. We must make every provision possible to lead others to become acquainted with the Saviour.

The highest and most noble work we can do in this world is to reflect the glory of God as seen in the face of Jesus Christ. Let Christ appear through those who love the truth. Let Him be seen as the Desire of all ages.

How can we prepare the way of the Lord? We will present our reasonable request that He may open the way before us, then we will walk and work and act our faith. "Faith is the substance of things hoped for, the evidence of things not seen." Christ is all and in all, and we need an increase of faith.

Brother Morse, I feel impressed to ask you to come to California and connect with the sanitarium at Loma Linda. Your talent is needed here. If you but have faith in our Lord and Saviour Jesus Christ, your health will improve physically and spiritually.

(Stamped) Ellen G. White

DEAR BROTHER AND SISTER KRESS

August 29, 1905
Loma Linda, California
(K.-253- 1905)

I HAVE JUST ENJOYED THE pleasure of reading your good letters.

Brother H. W. Kellogg from Battle Creek spent Sabbath and Sunday with us here at Loma Linda. He was astonished that such a beautiful premises and such a complete equipment could be purchased at so low a price as that for which we have secured this property.

We regard this place as one especially provided for us by the Lord. Some of the brethren had spoken to me of Loma Linda as a popular health resort, conducted as a hotel, but it was not considered possible that we would be able to pay so much as it was supposed they would ask. I had supposed we would be obliged to erect buildings for Sanitarium work in the vicinity of the beautiful cities of Redlands and Riverside.

Last spring I asked Brother Burden to look carefully for any opening to secure property suitable for a sanitarium {245} in this vicinity. While I was in Washington, he wrote to me describing the beauty of Loma Linda, and stated that everything connected with the place was offered to us for forty thousand dollars.

When I read the description of the property as written by Brother Burden, I recognized it as answering fully to an ideal sanitarium property such as has been presented to me. I received the letter on Friday afternoon, and I told W. C. White to telegraph Brother Burden immediately that he should secure the place. One of our brethren sent another telegram contrary to this. Some of the men connected with the conference thought that such a large place would be like an elephant on their hands. I was so burdened that for several nights I could not sleep. I feared lest the enemy might, through unbelief, keep this property out of our hands.

In the meanwhile Brother Burden had been obliged to tell the men that we would be unable to purchase the property. But when he received from me a letter of good cheer and hope, and an assurance that this was the place for which I had long been looking to correspond with places such as the Lord had shown me would be offered to us at a small part of their original cost, Brother Burden, in fear and trembling, re-turned to the agent, and told him we would purchase the place. Had he been an hour later, the opportunity might have been lost; for they were sending men to offer the property to other parties.

The main building contains four stories. In its entrance is a most beautiful sun-parlor. There is also a large parlor, carpeted with the very best body Brussels. The furniture in the house is of first class quality,- not fancy but durable and very handsome. We could not have furnished the building as expensively as it has been furnished by others. In this main building the furniture cost twelve thousand dollars and has been in use less than two years.

The long halls are carpeted with fine Brussels carpet, and there are carpets and rugs for the various rooms throughout the building. There is a large roll of rubber carpet that can be used wherever it is thought best. The mattresses on the beds look like new ones. There are two feather pillows, sheets, blankets, quilts, and spreads for every bed. Every room contains chairs, substantial, but very comfortable.

Besides the main building, in which there are about sixty rooms that can be used by patients, there are four four-roomed cottages sitting back on higher ground. Some of these are so arranged that each room is connected with a private veranda, where, in warm weather, a bed can be rolled from the room through the large windows. Besides the four cottages with four rooms each, there is a two story cottage with nine beautiful rooms, splendidly furnished. This of itself is quite a large building.

Between the cottages and the main building is what they {246} called the amusements building. This has been used for a bowling alley and a billiard hall. The billiard table will be sold; and with a few alterations the building may be made into a good meeting house.

There are seventy-six acres of land in this property. Quite a portion of it is set out in orchard. They raise oranges, lemons, grapefruit, peaches, apples, plums, pears, etc. I am having strawberries from the second crop, and they are very nice.

Five horses, three cows, about a hundred hens and a few turkeys were purchased with the place. There were also a number of hogs which have since been sold.

About a hundred and fifty thousand dollars has been expended in making the property what it is at present, and forty thousand dollars seems very reasonable for such a complete equipment as we find here. It would be a heavy tax if we had to pay interest on such an amount, but we believe that our brethren will raise this money, and that we shall soon be free from debt. Every dollar is to be expended with great care. Something must be done to furnish treatment rooms, but this need not incur great expense.

The city of Redlands is five miles from the institution. This city is one of the most beautiful cities in America. When President Roosevelt visited Redlands about two years ago, he expressed the thought that it was as near like heaven as any place he had ever seen. The purchase of Loma Linda will help to give us an influence with the people of this city.

The more we realize of the advantages of this location, the more certain we feel that we are in the line of duty. We shall now endeavor to secure the very best help possible to conduct the work of this institution. Some of the outside stairways need to be painted, and other work must be done before we are ready to open the institution.

For a time we had to work against fearfulness and unbelief in the minds of some of our brethren. There are some who will always be found holding back when any advance move is to be made.

Last June a meeting was called at Los Angeles to consider the question of the purchasing of Loma Linda. I was very glad that Elder Irwin was present. When some expressed themselves as thinking it unwise for the Conference to incur further indebtedness by such a heavy investment, Elder Irwin spoke right to the point, urging them to follow the manifest leadings of God.

I also bore my testimony that the Lord would bless us if we would act in faith. There are some who seem to consider it a virtue to talk unbelief and to hold back when there should be an advance. We are hoping that there may be connected with the work in Southern California men who will act {247} in faith.

Only a few were present at this meeting, but they expressed themselves as favoring the purchase of the property, and they pledged eleven hundred dollars as a gift to start the enterprise.

Last Sunday afternoon quite a number of our brethren from neighboring churches met on the lawn under the trees just back of the main building, and Brother Burden says they had an excellent meeting. One man said he had gone to the camp meeting in Los Angeles as an unbeliever, but had been convicted of the Sabbath truth. He seemed very happy, and made a donation of one hundred dollars to Loma Linda. We shall now endeavor to secure the necessary means, so that we shall not have to carry a heavy burden of interest on borrowed money.

Let us praise the Lord that He is making it possible for us to obtain such advantages, where we can help the sick to take their minds away from themselves, and delight in the beauty of God's handiwork.

DEAR BROTHER AND SISTER KRESS

August 9, 1905
"Elmshaven," Sanitarium, California
(K. 233 1905)

I WISH TO SAY TO YOU that if God opens the way for the brethren in other parts of Australia to purchase property that may be used for sanitarium work, such as the place that Brother Semmens has written about, forbid them not. Utter not one word of remonstrance. There are many cities to be worked, and medical missionary work is not to be confined to a few centers.

For a long time the Battle Creek Sanitarium was the only medical institution conducted by our people. But for many years light has been given that sanitariums should be established near such cities as Melbourne and Adelaide. And when opportunities come to establish the work in still other places, never are we to reach out the hand and say No, you must not create an interest in other places, for fear that our patronage will be decreased. If sanitarium work is the means by which the way is to be opened for the proclamation of the truth, encourage and do not discourage those who are trying to advance this work.

May the Lord increase our faith, and help us to see that He desires us all to become acquainted with His ministry of healing and with the mercy-seat. He desires the light of His grace to shine forth from many places. We are living {248} in the last days. Troublous times are before us. He who understands the necessities of the situation arranges that advantage should be brought to the workers in various places, to enable them more effectually to arouse the attention of the people. He knows the needs and the necessities of the feeblest of His flock, and He sends His own message into the highways and the byways. He loves us with an everlasting love.

There are souls in many places who have not yet heard the message. Henceforth medical missionary work is to be carried forward with an earnestness with which it has never yet been done. This work is the door through which the truth is to find entrance to the large cities, and sanitariums are to be established in many places.

Since we returned from Australia, the Lord has opened the way for the establishment of the sanitarium work in Southern California. The brethren there have found opportunity to buy several properties at a price very much below the original cost. The first of these was an opportunity to purchase the Fernando school buildings.

About seven miles from San Diego our brethren found a building admirably adapted for sanitarium work. . . .

Not long ago a building at Glendale, eight miles from Los Angeles, was purchased and fitted up for sanitarium work. Originally this building was an expensive one, costing the owners about forty thousand dollars. There are seventy-five rooms, many of which are arranged in suites, a small one for a bedroom, and a larger one for a sitting-room. There were two bathrooms on each floor, but they were not such as would be needed in giving treatments, and new treatment rooms have been added.

The rooms in the building are pleasant, and the location of the building is very good. The place is a sightly one.

When Brother Burden first went to see the agent about purchasing this place, twenty thousand dollars was asked for it. Brother Burden then told the agent something of the purpose for which those desirous of purchasing the building wished to use it. He told him about our medical missionary work, and assured him that this work was carried on without any thought of making money except for missionary purposes. The agent was much interested, and was inclined in favor of the idea, and he named a sum considerably lower than the sum first mentioned. But Brother Burden told him that it would be impossible for us to pay that price, and he then said, "You can have it for twelve thousand five hundred dollars, and you may consider the remainder of the price a gift to the institution."

Recently we have purchased what is known as the Loma Linda property. This property is sixty miles from Los Angeles, and is on the main railway line from Los

Angeles to New {249} Orleans. It was owned by a corporation of one hundred and fifty people, seventy of whom were physicians. But the physicians did not agree among themselves, and the place lost money instead of making it; and it was decided to sell. It continued to be a loss financially, and the stockholders became anxious to sell. It was offered for forty thousand dollars, and for this price our brethren have purchased it, paying down five thousand dollars. They will make three other payments of five thousand each, and after that will have two years in which to pay the remainder, at six per cent interest.

The property is a most beautiful one. There are seventy-six acres of land, twenty-three of which are set out to fruit and ornamental trees. There are twelve acres of oranges, and eight acres of plums, apricots, lemons, and grapefruit. The rest of the land is garden, alfalfa, and pasture land.

There is one large building and five cottages, four of which have four rooms each, and one nine rooms. In all there are ninety rooms. The buildings are all furnished throughout, and are ready for use.

There are several good carriages, five horses, four cows, and one hundred and thirty-five chickens.

There is an ample water-supply, the property have two good wells.

I know that it was in the providence of God that we had an opportunity to purchase this property.

I wrote the foregoing last night, and this morning I am roused up to repeat the instruction that the Lord has given me in regard to establishing sanitariums. Again and again this matter has been presented to me, and one case especially has been urged upon my notice. At great cost a sanitarium was erected at Boulder, Colorado. It has been a very difficult matter to make this sanitarium what it should be, and yet meet all expenses. The effort to do this has meant a great deal of hard work and much careful study.

During the past four years one of our doctors established himself in the city of Boulder, just a little distance from our sanitarium, and began to build up a private sanitarium. This was not right, and has been to the injury of our sanitarium, which has always had a struggle to make a success and to accomplish the work which the Lord designed it to do. The action of the one who established this private sanitarium was neither just nor righteous. Were he to continue to do as he has done in the past, constant difficulties would arise. He draws patients away from the sanitarium established in the order of God. More than this, he allows his patients to have meat, while the workers in our sanitariums have always endeavored to show their patients that they would be better off without meat. {250}

The question is, What shall be done? Here are two institutions, one endeavoring to hold up and follow the principles of health reform, and the other allowing its patients to indulge in the use of flesh meat, and because of this, drawing patients away from the first institution. The matter is to be treated in a fair, Christ-like manner. When the one who has established himself so close beside the Lord's institution, is converted in heart and mind, he will see the necessity of carrying out the principles of the word of God, and will harmonize with his neighbors. If he cannot blend with them, he will go to some other place. There are many other places to which he could go.

The question has been asked, Should we sell the Boulder Sanitarium to the one who has set up a practice so close to it? I answer, No, no! The one who has offered to buy it is not keeping up the standard of health reform, and the Lord would not be pleased to have the institution sold to him. The Boulder Sanitarium is to do its appointed work. From it the truth for this time is to shine forth, and the great message of warning be given. . .

DEAR BROTHER AND SISTER BURDEN

June 25, 1905
San Jose, California

IT IS JUST DAYLIGHT, AND I am seated on my couch, beginning a letter to you. Our meeting here began a day or two ago, and I think there will be a good attendance of our people. On Sabbath the brethren and sisters at Mountain View turned out well. On Sabbath morning at half past ten I spoke to a large number in the big tent.

I have an intense desire that this meeting shall be the very kind of meeting that the Lord desires us to have. I hope much for the revival of the Spirit of the Lord.

I have consented to remain here till the close of the camp meeting—one week from Monday. We shall then return to our home at St. Helena.

There are many matters to be consid-

ered, and we all need the guidance of the Holy Spirit. I pray that a right impression may be made on the minds of those present at the meeting.

The school question will receive careful attention, and we hope that matters may be so adjusted that future work in educational lines will be of a more advanced and satisfactory character. The Lord can do much through the teachers and students of our schools, if they will carry the work steadily forward and upward. {251}

I shall be pleased to hear from you at any time. I sincerely hope that the brethren in Southern California will unite in pressing forward the school work and the sanitarium work.

In regard to Sister Burden continuing to hold her place as bookkeeper, I think that if she would take the exercise that she should, the evils I have feared might be avoided. She should not confine herself too closely. She can be a real help in teaching others how to keep books. This is a line of education that is greatly needed, and in no case should it be neglected. But Sister Burden should be left entirely free to take up the work that she chooses. She can help with her experience in many ways. She can give valuable counsel in regard to many matters that will come up for discussion.

I have a great desire that you may both be greatly blessed in your work in the new sanitarium. I hope that Brother Reaser will move understandingly in reference to the sanitariums already in operation, and also in regard to the new sanitarium. I pray that the Lord may provide suitable people to connect with this institution, people who will be a genuine strength to the institution.

Do not be discouraged if in any wise there is some cutting across of your plans, and if you are somewhat hindered. But I hope that we shall never again have to meet the hindrance that we have met in the past because of the way in which things have been conducted on some lines in Southern California. I have seen the holdback principles followed, and I have seen the displeasure of the Lord because of this. If the same spirit is manifested, I shall not consent to keep silent as I have done.

It is the most awful thing a man can do to dethrone God from his heart, refusing to take the Bible as his counselor. The man who does this debases whatever he has connection with. Christ does not abide in his heart. The law of God is to him an empty form. He may be supposed to be a Christian, but he debases whatever he touches.

The gospel of Christ has been dishonored by being handled with sin-stained hands. Professed Christians act and speak in a way that is no honor to God. What men and women need now is thorough conversion. Every part of their intelligence should go out to meet Christ, and every part of their spiritual nature should yearn for more of Him. The Father seeketh such to worship him—those who worship Him in spirit and truth and in the beauty of holiness. Let us separate from the contaminating influences of the world, and hold communication with the Saviour. Let us bring ourselves, in thought, word, and deed, into conformity with the will of Christ. The Redeemer is seeking for those whose highest aim is to serve and glorify God.

The message that the Lord has given me for the church {252} in Los Angeles is, Through faith and diligent service you are to become one with Christ. You are to eat His flesh and drink His blood, making His words a part of the daily life. The great Teacher will accept only the purest integrity, the most distinct representation of His words and His Spirit. Spiritual-mindedness must not be allowed to become a strange thing among us. We are to become more and more nearly conformed to Christ. The joy of the Lord, the praise of God, is to be on our lips and in our hearts. The character is to be transformed from the mist and cloud of uncertainty into the radiance of the light proceeding from heaven. The world is to be eclipsed by the contemplation of heavenly things.

I ask the believers in Los Angeles to seek for a deeper, higher experience in the things of God. The Father seeketh such to worship Him. Arise, and brace your souls for action. Take an extensive survey of the work that is to be done. Read your Bibles with an increasing determination to have a larger experience in the things of God. Stand in the light of the Sun of Righteousness.

What could induce the pure, sinless Son of God to tabernacle with men in a world filled with crime and strife and wickedness? He did this that He might better reach the lost and perishing. He suffered, being tempted. Proportionate to the perfection of His holiness, was the strength of the temptation. Because of the depravity so revolting to His purity, His residence in the world was a perpetual sorrow. On every hand He saw men and women destroying themselves by yielding to perverted appetite and passion.

Christ gave His life for the life of the world. He came to this earth in the likeness of man, to present before human beings an example of the character that all must form in order to be saved. He came to bring them power to overcome all the temptations of the enemy.

O that every soul might be awakened, and led to become a subject of the heavenly kingdom, surrendering all to Christ. The word of God gives us no encouragement that a sinner is pardoned in order that he may continue in sin. He is pardoned on condition that he receives Christ, confessing and repenting of his sin, and becoming renewed. Many who pass under the name of Christian are not converted. Conversion means renovation. The sinner must enter into the renovating process for himself. He must come to Jesus. He must give up the wrong habits in which he has indulged. He must bring his unsubdued, unchristlike tendencies under the control of Christ, else he cannot be made a laborer together with God. Christ works, and the sinner works. The life of Christ becomes the life of the human agent. It is through the renewing power of the divine Spirit that man is fashioned into a perfect man in Christ.

By the character that he is forming, every man is {253} deciding his future destiny. In the books of heaven is made the record. There the character is photographed. There is seen a picture of the unclothed soul.

The promise is given, "As many as received Him, to them gave He power to become the sons of God, even to them that believe on His name." It is the striving souls who receive the assistance of heaven and partake of its elements. It is by test and trial that the followers of Christ are fitted to dwell with Him in the heavenly courts.

(Stamped) Ellen G. White

DEAR BROTHER BUTLER

June 23, 1905
Glendale, California July 24, 1911
(B-183-'05)

SINCE LEAVING WASHINGTON, I have had much writing and speaking to do. I have spoken twice to the Los Angeles church. The Lord gave me a message for the people before leaving San Diego.

On our way to Los Angeles, we stopped off at "Loma Linda" and visited the property that we have purchased for sanitarium work. We were taken through the different buildings. There is one large main building, which was built for sanitarium work, and is well adapted for that purpose. Some changes will have to be made regarding bath and treatment facilities, but otherwise, everything is in readiness for us to begin work at once.

Until this recent visit, I had never before seen such a place with my natural eyes, but four years ago such a place was presented before me as one of those that would come into our possession if we moved wisely. It is a wonderful place in which to begin our work for Redlands and Riverside. We must make decided efforts to secure helpers who will do most faithful medical missionary work. If God will bless the treatment given, and Christ will let His healing power be felt, a wonderful work will be accomplished.

We shall need the very best physicians that can be secured, men and women who are faithful and true, and who will live in constant dependence upon the great Healer, men and women who will humble their hearts before God, and believe his word, men and women who will keep their eyes fixed on their leader and counselor, the Lord Jesus Christ.

This work must be carried on aright. In the past, decided failures have been made in the institutions established for the care of the sick because so much business {254} has been crowded in that the main object for which our sanitariums are established has been lost sight of. Great Loss has thus been sustained. I am to urge upon our people that the proclamation of the principles of truth must be kept prominent, as the main line of work for which our sanitariums were instituted.

The Lord calls for a solemn dedication to him of the sanitariums that shall be established. Our object in the establishment of these institutions is that the truth for this time may through them be proclaimed. In order that this may be done, they must be conducted on right lines. In them business interests are not to be crowded in to take the place of spiritual interests. Every day devotional exercises are to be held. The word of God is in no case to be given a secondary place. Those who come to our sanitariums for treatment must see the word of God, which is the bread of life, exalted above all common, earthly considerations. A strong religious influence is to be exerted. It must be plainly shown that the glory of God and the uplifting of Christ are placed before all else.

The stupidity of soul that has been ev-idenced in our plans must now cease to bear away the victory. "What shall it profit a man, if he gain the whole world, and lose his own soul? Or what will a man give in exchange for his soul?"

Many who should have stood with us in solid rank and file have given themselves up to ambitions which have led to objectionable practices, opposed to honest and righteous dealing. The service of such ones God does not accept. They are drawing into the pattern strange threads, which will spoil the figure, and the Lord cannot endorse their work. Those who become adept in unfair dealing gain their success at altogether too high a price. Their mental powers are used to overreach and defraud, and opposite their names in the books of heaven God writes the words, Unfaithful stewards. God and eternal life become of little account to them when the greed for gain and for the mastery are in the scale. An eternity of blissful experience is exchanged for the flattery of supposed success. Transaction after transaction forbidden by God is entered into. The Voice said, Better, far better the loss of all earthly possessions that the loss of the favor of God and the eternal interests that are at stake.

The time is not far distant when the last venture will be made in giving the enemy the advantage over the soul. And the loss will be for eternity. Success in such ventures is a terrible disaster to those who take part in them. The words were spoken, Better the cross and the disappointment, better the shattered hopes and the world's charge of foolishness, than to gain a name, to sit with princes, and to forfeit heaven.

There is in the world today a power that palsies the {255} spiritual energies, benumbs the sense of right, and robs man of the victory of overcoming. The benumbed soul does not recover. The spiritual paralysis continues until the end. Lies are spoken, lies are acted. Deception is practiced, and dishonesty connived at. This leaves a deadly sting in the soul. The father of lies has taken possession of the citadel of the heart. The false, the deceptive, has turned the whole current of life. Business transactions have become corrupt. And this moral degradation has been chosen instead of a rich current of light from heaven.

The time has come when men who were once chosen of God have become degenerate. The word will soon be spoken, He is joined to his idols; let him alone.

There is much more that I might say, but I will withhold it. God pity those who are deceived by men. I am instructed to say, Lift up your voice like a trumpet, and show my people their transgressions, and the house of Jacob their sins. Now is the time to raise the standard aloft. I am to give the message that all advantage gained by compliance with tainted customs, will leave its slimy trail. Any man, whatever his profession may be, who has committed himself to an objectionable course of action, opposed to that which is pure, lovely, and of good report, will trample upon the word of God. Would that those who have had great light would, in this the day of atonement, humble their souls and confess and forsake their sins, declaring that from henceforth by the grace of God, they will hold fast to their integrity, saying, Get thee behind me, Satan, and taking the word of God as their rule of conduct, their standard of duty.

When men plan and scheme to get the advantage of one another in business dealing, it is because they have cast the word of God behind them. It pains my heart even to trace these words. The word of God does not restrict man's diligence in business transactions that are according to righteousness. But it bears plain witness against underhand dealing. Upon this point it is clear and decided, and no one need err in understanding it. The word of God is a light put into man's hand. God tells him to be guided by its precepts. Thus only can he become an heir of God and a joint heir with Jesus Christ. In obeying the word, man is acquiring immortal treasures, which will never pass away. The peace of God is worth everything to the receiver.

The talents entrusted to us by God are to be used in his service. Thus only can the highest results be obtained from their use. Man will not be deprived of the powers given him, if he uses these powers to the glory of God. I am given a message to bear to the members of our churches. My brethren and sisters, Consecrate all that you have and are to God. The silver and the gold that we possess is but lent us in trust. The sin of covetousness is {256} destroying the value of holy principles. It is leading us to act in opposition to God's will. It is eating out the hearts of men. Let us not cherish it longer.

How disgraceful are the disclosures that are being made regarding men who have occupied high places in the world. Shall the intrigues practiced by these men be practiced by the members of the church of God? Shall we not obey the injunction,

"Honor the Lord with thy substance?" My brethren and sisters, it was the favor of God that enabled you to gather together your substance. All that you have belongs to him, and cheerfully and gladly you are to lay your means and talents upon the altar of service, that they may be used in saving perishing souls.

The Christian in the market place who keeps his soul unspoiled has a credit in the heavenly courts. His means will not be used to carry out the devising of the enemy, but to do good, in the very lines that God has marked out. The Lord will teach us how to employ all our powers to the glory of His name. The gathering of wealth is to be used in the service of the Master. Thus used, it will bring a hundredfold in this life, and in the life to come glorious and eternal riches.

To every church member I would say, Never, never let there be any departing from the strictest integrity. Do not mock God, the Majesty of heaven, by a disregard of his word. Never, never, defraud a fellow-being, and then suppose that your sharpness is something to be proud of. Do not follow maxims of business that are based on false pretensions. There is in this our day a great deal of falsity. The pretender, the deceiver, is increasing in numbers, and truth and integrity are violated. Lies are spoken, lies are acted, and are becoming more and more common among those who do not make the word of God their counselor.

Never was there a time when truth and righteousness should be so highly exalted by those who are in God's service as the present. Let us urge upon our people the necessity of laying hold upon the foundation principles of the truth. Oh, there are so many who fail to enjoy the blessing that comes from a clear conviction of what the people of God must be. There is nothing in self upon which it is safe to rest. In the place of being confused in regard to the foundation of our faith, which has been confirmed by the power of the Holy Spirit, in the place of building flimsy foundations upon the sands of error, let us hold fast to the great principles of truth given us, refusing to be moved. Those who receive theories of Satan's furnishings are building upon the sand. When the storm and tempest come, their building will suddenly collapse, and great will be the fall of it.

Let us thank God, Brother Butler, that there are still some living who have had an experience from the beginning {257} in the proclamation of the great and solemn messages that have come to our world in warning. We know that the Holy Spirit's power has confirmed the word spoken. We can say, as did John, "That which was from the beginning, which we have heard, which we have seen with our eyes, which we have looked upon, and our hands have handled, of the Word of life; . . . that which we have seen and heard declare we unto you, that ye also may have fellowship with us; and truly our fellowship is with the Father, and with his Son Jesus Christ."

From our own personal experience we can speak of the truth that has made us what we are,—Seventh-day Adventists. Truth felt within is most precious, but truth confirmed by the testimony of the word and by the Holy Spirit's power is of the highest value. We can confidently say, The truth that has come to us through the Holy Spirit's working is not a lie. The evidences given for the last half century bear the evidence of the Spirit's power. In the word of God we have found the truth that substantiates our faith. We have watched the influence of the heresies that have come in, and we have seen them come to naught. God has given us sacred, holy truths. Let us hold them fast. I am instructed to say that we are now to present these truths, in plainness and simplicity, to the people of God.

(Stamped) Ellen G. White

ELDER AND MRS. J. E. WHITE

December 1, 1907
Paradise Valley Sanitarium,
National City, California
(W. 392 '07)

Dear Children:

I THANK THE LORD THAT HE has sustained me on this journey. I have done much important writing. On Sabbath a week ago, and again last Sabbath, I spoke in the church at San Diego.

I am hoping and praying that I may understand my duty. It seems to me that I must remain in this section of the country until after Elder Haskell arrives, and then I may not be able to leave for some weeks to come. An important work has been begun in the vicinity of Riverside. The third year class of students at Loma Linda went over to Riverside a few weeks ago, and did their first practical work in canvassing for "Ministry of Healing." There were eight in the class, and their object in visiting the homes of the people was more to become acquainted and to {258} talk of the work at Loma Linda, than it was to sell books for profit. However, in the course of their conversation, they would usually introduce "Ministry of Healing," tell the story of the book, and then offer to sell it as a volume that contained the principles taught in the school at Loma Linda. In this way, about seventy copies of the book were placed in the homes of the people, in a little over one week; and the students made many, many friends for the work at Loma Linda. Wherever they went, they sought to leave a good impression. We believe they did a good work. They were wide awake, and full of courage in the Lord, and seem to have met with success.

The second year class will undertake a similar work soon, while the third year class continue their studies at Loma Linda. Later on, it is hoped that some members of the first year class can go out. Thus each of the several students in the school will assist in working Riverside. I suppose you have seen that place. It is a grand city, and the managers of the Loma Linda school are seeking to gain a foothold there by introducing, first, the "Ministry of Healing." Afterward, they will send out students with "Christ's Object Lessons." They will earnestly endeavor to handle these books wisely.

A similar work is to be carried on in other places besides Riverside. We are all praying that the Lord may abundantly bless these first working forces going out from the school. It means much to our Loma Linda training school and sanitarium, not only with regard to the good impression that they hope to make on the minds of the people, but in a financial way as well. Many new students have come in, and considerable money will be needed to care for them all, and at the same time keep up the other running expenses of the school and sanitarium. At Loma Linda there are now over a hundred under training for medical missionary work.

Oh, how anxious I am to have a small press in operation at Loma Linda, so as to print the discourses that shall be given in the surrounding cities! I have mentioned the matter to Brother Henry W. Kellogg; for he has a special interest in this line of work. We need a small press for printing notices, and for bringing out in printed form, for use in surrounding cities, discourses that will be given from time to time. Now is our time to work. We expect to connect with the W. C. T. U. in some lines of service.

I cannot feel free to return to St. Helena until I see the work fully in running order. The Lord has given light that these cities in the San Bernardino Valley should be worked. The time has come to do this work, and we are to have wise managing forces to carry the work forward intelligently.

There never was a time when we needed more to encourage faith, than at the present time; for these are perplexities on the right hand and on the left.

THE WORK IN SOUTHERN CALIFORNIA

(MS-3-1906) {259}

SOUTHERN CALIFORNIA is a field that should depend more that it has upon its own resources. It should have more facilities, and should not be cramped as it has been in some respects.

Southern California is a missionary field, a large part of which has received but little missionary effort. Henceforth it should receive more attention. The various lines of work that can be carried on should be diligently studied, and the advantages of such cities as Redlands and Riverside, and the need of putting forth decided effort for them, faithfully investigated.

Los Angeles demands constant labor because of its changing population. San Bernardino calls for earnest missionary effort. The work for all these places needs to be done by those who can adapt themselves to the needs of the field. In our work we miss the laborers of Elder Simpson; but we must not leave the work undone because some of the faithful workers fall by the way.

In Loma Linda we have an advantageous center for the carrying on of various missionary enterprises. We can see that it was in the providence of God that this sanitarium was placed in the possession of our people. We should appreciate Loma Linda as a place which the Lord foresaw we should need, and which He gave.

The cities in the San Bernardino Valley were presented before me as places where the truth should go with power. The small printing press that Brother H. W. Kellogg has furnished should prove a blessing to the work in that part of the field, by printing publications that will be needed for the furtherance of the work in the Southern California cities. Our publications must now be greatly multiplied. Papers and leaflets containing the best discourses preached by our ministers are to be published and scattered widely throughout the regions where meetings are being held.

It was the Lord who placed in our possession the sanitariums at Loma Linda, Glendale, and Paradise Valley.

We have been indolent in regard to our duty to Southern California. The many tourists who visit the cities in this conference should be given opportunity to hear the truth for this time. Let us do all in our power to enlighten the people in this large field. It is the privilege of every believer to let the light shine forth. We are drawing near to the close of this earth's history; we have not one hour to devote to needless matters. Our ministers in the Southern California Conference should now devote their best efforts to proclaiming the message of truth in all these large resorts. The Lord will impart His grace to all who {260}

will work in Christ's lines. And hope and faith will strengthen as the workers for God put their trust in Him.

ELDER J. A. BURDEN AND OTHERS BEARING RESPONSIBILITIES AT LOMA LINDA

March 14, 1908
Sanitarium, California
(B.-90-1908)

Dear Brethren:

I FEEL A DEEP INTEREST that careful study shall be given to the needs of our institutions at Loma Linda, and that the right moves may be made. In the carrying forward of the work at this place, men of talent and of decided spirituality are needed.

We may, in the work of educating our nurses, reach a high standard of the knowledge of the true science of healing. That which is of most importance is that the students be taught to truly represent the principles of health reform. Teach the students to pursue this line of study faithfully, combined with other essential lines of education. The grace of Jesus Christ will give wisdom to all who will follow the Lord's plan of true education.

Let the students follow closely the example of the One who purchased the human race with the costly price of His own life. Let them appeal to the Saviour, and depend upon Him as the One who heals all manner of diseases. The Lord would have the workers make special efforts to point the sick and suffering to the great Physician who made the human body. He would have all become obedient children to the faith, that they may come with confidence and ask bodily restoration. Many who come to our sanitariums will be blessed as they learn the truth concerning the word of God, many who would never learn it through any other medium.

It is well that our training schools for Christian workers should be established near to our health institutions, that the students may be educated in the principles of healthful living. Institutions that send forth workers who are able to give a reason for their faith, and who have that faith that works by love and purifies the soul, are of great value.

I have clear instruction that wherever it is possible, schools should be established near to our sanitariums, that each institution may be a help to the other. But I dare not advise that steps be taken at this time to branch out so largely in the educational work at Loma Linda that a large outlay of means will be required to erect new buildings. Our faithful workers at Loma Linda must not be overwhelmed with such great responsibilities that they will {261} be in danger of becoming worn and discouraged.

I am charged to caution you against building extensively for the accommodation of students. It would not be wise to invest at this time so large a capital as would be required to equip a medical college that would properly qualify physicians to stand the test of the medical examinations of the different states.

A movement should not now be inaugurated that would add greatly to the investment upon the Loma Linda property. Already there is a large debt resting upon the institution, and discouragement and perplexity would follow if this indebtedness were to be greatly increased. As the work progresses, new improvements may be added from time to time as they are found necessary. An elevator should soon be installed in the main building. But there is need of strict economy. Let our brethren move cautiously and wisely, and plan no longer than they can handle without being overburdened.

In the work of the school maintain simplicity. No argument is so powerful as is success founded upon simplicity. And you may attain success in the education of students as medical missionaries without

a medical school than can qualify physicians to compete with the physicians of the world.

Let the students be given a practical education. And the less dependent you are upon worldly methods of education, the better it will be for the students. Special instruction should be given in the art of treating the sick without the use of poisonous drugs, and in harmony with the light that God has given. Students should come forth from the school without having sacrificed the principles of health reform.

The education that meets the world's standard is to be less and less valued by those who are seeking for efficiency in carrying the medical missionary work in connection with the work of the third angel's message. They are to be educated from the standpoint of conscience; and as they conscientiously and faithfully follow right methods in their treatment of the sick, these methods will come to be recognized as preferable to the method of nursing to which many have been accustomed, which demands the use of poisonous drugs.

We should not at this time seek to compete with worldly medical schools. Should we do this, our chances of success would be small. We are not now prepared to carry out successfully the work of establishing large medical institutions of learning. Moreover, should we follow the world's methods of medical practice, exacting the large fees that worldly physicians demand for their services, we would work away from Christ's plan for our ministry for the sick.

There should be at our sanitariums intelligent men and {262} women, who can instruct in Christ's methods of ministry. Under the instruction of competent, consecrated teachers, the youth may become partakers of the divine nature, and learn how to escape the corruptions that are in the world through lust. I have been shown that we should have many more women who can deal especially with the diseases of women, many more lady nurses who will treat the sick in a simple, way and without the use of drugs.

There are many simple herbs which, if our nurses would learn the value of, they could use in the place of drugs, and find very effective. . . .

I write these things that you may know that the Lord has not left us without the use of simple remedies which when used will not leave the system in the weakened condition in which the use of drugs so often

leaves us. We need well-trained nurses who can understand how to use the simple remedies that nature provides for restoration to health, and who can teach those who are ignorant of the laws of health, how to use these simple but effective cures.

He who created men and women has an interest in those who suffer. He has directed in the establishment of our sanitariums and in the building up of schools close to our sanitariums, that they may become efficient mediums in training men and women for the work of ministering to suffering humanity. In the treatment of the sick, poisonous drugs need not be used. Alcohol or tobacco in any form must not be recommended, lest some soul be led to imbibe a taste for these evil things. There will be no excuse for the liquor-dealers in that day when every man shall receive according to his works. Those who have destroyed life will by their own life have to pay the penalty. God's law is holy and just and good.

We have seen the poor wrecks of humanity come to our sanitariums to be cured of the liquor habit. We have seen those who have ruined their health by wrong habits of diet, and by the use of flesh-meats. This is why we need to lift up the voice like a trumpet, and "show my people their transgression and the house of Jacob their sins."

The Lord will judge according to their works those who are seeking to establish a law of the nations that will cause men to violate the law of God. In proportion to their guilt will be their punishment. The Lord would have us lift up the Sabbath of the Lord our God. We have a sacred work to do in opening blind eyes in regard to the day that the Lord has set apart and sanctified as the rest day of mankind. He declares, "The seventh day is the Sabbath of the Lord thy God." He has placed His own {263} signature upon that day that He has set apart to be observed as long as time shall last. We should have much to say upon this subject just now.

Let Seventh-day Adventist medical workers remember that the Lord God omnipotent reigneth. Christ was the greatest Physician that ever trod the sin-cursed earth. The Lord would have his people come to Him for their power of healing. He will baptize them with His Holy Spirit, and fit them for a service that will make them a blessing in restoring the spiritual and physical health of those who need healing.

TO THE BRETHREN IN SOUTHERN CALIFORNIA

April 23, 1908
Sanitarium, California
(B.-132-1908)

Dear Brethren:

I AM INSTRUCTED TO SAY to you, Let every soul earnestly seek the Lord. We all need to understand clearly what is our duty, that we may make no false moves. We need to hold fast the experiences which in the past the Lord has given us. I have a great desire to see success attend every movement we shall make.

There is a very precious work to be done in connection with the interests of the sanitarium and school at Loma Linda; and this will be done when we all work to that end. The word of God is to be our lesson book. In the unity that is coming in among our people we can see that God is working in our midst.

"Wherefore be ye not unwise, but understanding what the will of the Lord is." Let us walk and work circumspectly. Let humble prayers go up to God, and let us seek Him with the whole heart. Then the Lord will open the way for us to lay wise plans. My brethren, speak to yourselves in psalms, and hymns, and spiritual songs, "singing and making melody in your hearts to the Lord, giving thanks always for all things unto the Lord."

Ever bear in mind that heaven is interested in every question that agitates your mind in regard to your school and sanitarium. Both are to be strengthened. The Lord is our helper and our God; let us look to Him to open the way for the carrying out of our plans.

We must have a church at Loma Linda, that those in the sanitarium and school may have a suitable place in which to meet for worship; but this should not be an expensive building. We shall build a neat, modest, but roomy chapel, that will show that we believe that we are living in the closing days of this earth's history, in a time when many {264} of the cities because of their sins will be cast down and their lofty buildings destroyed.

In our school at Loma Linda many can be educated to work as missionaries in the cause of health and temperance. The best teachers are to be employed in this educational work,—not men who esteem highly their own capabilities, but men who will walk circumspectly, depending wholly upon the Lord.

Small cottages will have to be built at little cost to accommodate the teachers and students; for these are to gain all the advantages possible from the lectures given at the sanitarium. This work should go forward as fast as means for it be obtained.

If the teachers in medical lines will stand in their lot and place, we shall see a good work done. My soul is drawn out in earnest prayer to God that He will preserve the honest in heart from being led astray by those who are themselves in confusion and darkness.

Teachers are to be prepared for many lines of work. Schools are to be established in places where no efforts have been made. Missionaries are needed to go to other States where little work has been done. Truth, Bible truth, is to be presented in many places. Christ is represented as identifying Himself with all the needy upon earth when He says, "Inasmuch as ye have done it unto one of the least of these, My brethren, ye have done it unto Me."

All should put forth efforts to enlarge their experience. We are in a most critical situation; but Christ identifies Himself with our necessities. Christians are to learn daily of Christ. Spiritual sinew and muscle are now needed to work out right principles in every city and town and village. Varied talents are to be appreciated and cultivated, and with all we need true wisdom. We may not see our need of counseling with God; but the true Christian in every place will inquire what is the will of the Lord concerning his individual work.

All heaven is interested in the work of preparation to be done in our schools. Let the talent that is among us be combined wisely for the accomplishment of the greatest good. "Ye are God's husbandry; ye are God's building." Then link up the powers that God has given for the doing of the special work he designs to have done. If self, is kept humble, the transforming grace of Christ and His wisdom will blend heart to heart. Let us make our gifts and offerings with a single heart. Let us draw upon our talents remembering that for this purpose they were given. To every man God has given His work; and He would have this work done intelligently. The Lord will make it possible for each to do a work that can be accepted by Him. {265}

The Lord expects all, by acts of self-denial, to help in the upbuilding of His work. In the house of worship to be erected, and the additional schoolrooms that will be needed, let all be willing to do their best, willing to deny themselves the unnecessary expenditure for display, that they may have means to give to the cause of God. The work in promulgating the principles of health reform, which the Lord has outlined to us, must be accomplished. When we study the self-denial of Christ, and make His life our example, truth and righteousness will prevail among us. We will esteem as of highest value the ornament of a meek and quiet spirit, which is in the sight of God of great price.

ELDER A. G. DANIELLS

June 20, 1908
Sanitarium, California
(D.-196- 1908)
Tacoma Park Station Washington, D. C.

Dear Brother:

I HAVE BEEN READING LETTERS from you concerning the Bible teacher needed at Union College.

I will say that Elder Owen is needed just where he is, and he is where the Lord would have him be. God has a work of special importance to be done in Southern California, and I know from the light given me that this work must now be perfected.

Loma Linda has been specified to me as a very important place, and one which demands the best Bible teacher we can supply. There are promising youth here who are to be qualified to fill important positions in the work. They should have the best class of instructors, and capable Bible teachers who understand the truths of the word. The truth and righteousness revealed in the word of God is to be the stronghold of our workers.

There has been given to me an outline of the work that must be done at Loma Linda, and I know that we must give to that place our best labors. The Lord wants the wisest talent there, for by means of our very best educational talent we are to train our ministerial laborers. The work is to be carried after the Lord's order, and not according to the supposition of man.

The Lord has given us a wonderful advantage in enabling us to secure Loma Linda for the establishment of the work in progress there. A school is to be built up at Loma Linda that will train Bible workers and missionary nurses for {266} efficient service. The Lord calls for the best talents to be united at this center for the carrying on of the work as He has directed, not the talent that will demand the largest salary, but the talent that will place itself on the side of Christ to work in His lines.

We must have medical instructors who will teach the science of healing without the use of drugs. If physicians refuse to give their services unless they can be paid the highest wage, we shall not bribe them. We are to prepare a company of workers who will follow Christ's methods.

There has been a dearth of means for our educational work because we have neglected to follow fully the Lord's directions. The Lord now asks that energy and zeal be given to the carrying out of His methods. The books "Christ's Object Lessons" and "Ministry of Healing" are the Lord's specified agencies for the financial aid of our institutions. By following the plan that He has laid down, a continual work of education may be carried on. I pray that God may teach us to understand His ways, and help us to learn daily of Christ.

DEAR BROTHER AND SISTER D. H. KRESS

January 14, 1909
(K.-94-'09)

SOON AFTER THE PARADISE VALLEY Sanitarium had been secured, the brethren at Los Angeles, after long search, decided to purchase a hotel property at Glendale, eight miles from the city. This property was offered at a price below its original cost, and within the reach of the conference. As everything seemed favorable, it was secured, and has since been refitted and opened as the Glendale Sanitarium. Some additions have been made to the old building.

When we first saw the Glendale property, so unlike some other properties we had visited in the vicinity of Los Angeles, we believed that this was a place that had been providentially reserved for us, and we have had no reason since for changing our minds.

In less than a year after the establishment of the Glendale Sanitarium, the Loma Linda property was purchased. Thus, within a comparatively short period of time, God wrought marvelously in the establishment of three sanitariums within the territory of the Southern California Conference. {267}

ELIZA MORTON

April 12, 1909
Loma Linda, California
(M.-70-1909)

WE ARE ABOUT TO LEAVE Loma Linda for our journey to College View, Nebraska. I have spoken once while here. Last Sabbath the patients and church members assembled on the beautiful grounds of the sanitarium, and I spoke to them from the 58th chapter of Isaiah.

We hope that in the school established at Loma Linda many will be qualified to go forth and impart the knowledge of truth they have here received. A quick work will the Lord do in our world, for Satan is preparing his forces to seek to overcome the remnant people who love God and keep His commandments. He points to the smallness of their numbers, and flatters his followers that his larger army can outnumber the believers. We know how powerful are the hosts of Satan; but God is more powerful than they. Our risen Saviour is all sufficient for our needs.

ELDER J. A. BURDEN

June 9, 1909
Washington, D. C.
(B.-100-'09)

Loma Linda, California

IN THE NIGHT SEASON I seemed to be conversing with you, and encouraging you to go forward in the name of the Lord, preparing your school to give the education most needed at this time. The education that is to be given by our people in the large cities of Southern California is set before me day and night. The people in these cities are to be made to understand what constitutes "higher education." Higher education means conformity to the plan of salvation.

Obtain facilities for your school work. Let the means that shall come to you be used very economically. Do not spend one dollar unnecessarily.

Endeavor to place yourself where you will not be confused by the representations and forbiddings of human agencies who would misinterpret the true meaning of the higher education. Lift up the Man of Calvary. By the work of teaching and by earnest prayer, endeavor to place the students where they will receive the inspiration of heaven. Jesus Christ is to be presented before them as the Source of all light and knowledge. Let none dishonor Him by choosing to accept the world's interpretation of what the higher education means. Let us leave that to those who do not acknowledge the truths of the word of God as the source of all true knowledge. {268}

Give to the teachers all the advantages possible, to secure a clear understanding of what constitutes the essential education.

Teach the students to look for wisdom to the One who gave His life for the salvation of the world. Now is your time to work. That same Jesus who walked with His disciples on earth, and who taught them from day to day, will teach His servants in this age.

I would call your attention to the eighth chapter of Acts, in which is related Philip's experience with the Ethiopian seeker after truth. The record states:

"And the angel of the Lord spake unto Philip, saying, Arise, and go toward the south unto the way that goeth down from Jerusalem unto Gaza, which is desert. And he arose and went: and, behold a man of Ethiopia, a eunuch of great authority under Candace queen of the Ethiopians, who had the charge of all her treasure, and had come to Jerusalem for to worship, was returning, and sitting in his chariot read Esaias the prophet.

"Then the Spirit said unto Philip, Go near, and join thyself to this chariot. And Philip ran thither to him, and heard him read the prophet Esaias, and said, Understandest thou what thou readest? And he said, How can I, except some man should guide me? And he desired Philip that he would come up and sit with him.

"The place of the Scripture which he read was this, He was led as a sheep to the slaughter; and like a lamb dumb before his shearer, so opened He not His mouth: in His humiliation His judgment was taken away: and who shall declare his generation? for His life is taken from the earth.

"Then Philip opened his mouth, and began at the same scripture, and preached unto him Jesus.

"And as they went on their way, they came unto a certain water: and the eunuch said, See, here is water; what doth hinder me to be baptized? And Philip said, if thou believest with all thine heart, thou mayest. And he answered and said, I believe that Jesus Christ is the Son of God.

"And he commanded the chariot to stand still: and they went down both into the water, both Philip and the eunuch; and he baptized him. And when they were come up out of the water, the Spirit of the Lord caught away Philip that the eunuch saw him no more: and he went on his way rejoicing. But Philip was found at Azotus, and passing through he preached in all the cities, till he came to Caesarea."

The whole of the book of Acts should receive careful {269} study. It is full of precious instruction; it records experiences in evangelistic work, the teachings of which we need in our work today. This is wonderful history; it deals with the highest education, which the students in our schools are to receive.

TALK BY MRS. E. G. WHITE BEFORE THE GENERAL CONFERENCE COMMITTEE

June 11, 1909
(M.-53-1909)

WHEN BROTHER BURDEN WAS leaving for Southern California at the close of this conference, he inquired of me, "What shall we plan to do for Loma Linda?" "Go straight ahead," I replied; "let the truth shine forth in every possible way. Continue to work with all your zeal in the territory surrounding your sanitarium. Help your students to learn how to labor, and keep sending them out into Redlands, and Riverside, and San Bernardino, and the smaller towns and villages round about. Introduce our publications, and do thorough work. Let your light shine as a lamp that burneth. Encourage the students to greater activity in missionary labor while taking their course of study."

Our brethren at Loma Linda are in need of funds with which to carry on their work. But notwithstanding their present necessity, I have encouraged them not to falter, but to go forward in the name of the Lord. And now I appeal to my brethren in Washington not to allow them to suffer. While we are planning to support the educational work in such places as Washington, we must not forget the important work that must be done at Loma Linda, and in other centers of training.

THE RELATION OF LOMA LINDA COLLEGE TO WORLDLY MEDICAL INSTITUTIONS

September 23, 1909
(MS-7-)

Report of interview at the home of Mrs. E. G. White, Sanitarium, California, September 20, 1909.
Present Mrs. E. G. White, W. C. White and J. A. Burden.

E. G. WHITE:

WE WANT NONE OF THAT KIND of "higher education" that will put us in a position where the credit must be given, not to the Lord God of Israel, but to the god of Ekron. The Lord designs that we shall stand as a distinct, sanctified, and holy people, so connected with him that he can work with us. Let our physicians realize that they are to depend wholly upon the true {270} God.

I felt a heavy burden this morning when I read over a letter that I found in my room, in which a plan was outlined for having medical students take some work at Loma Linda, but to get the finishing touches of their education from some worldly institution. God forbid that such a plan should be followed. I must state that the light I have received is that we are to stand as a distinct, commandment-keeping people. The Sabbath is a great distinguishing line, and its observance will separate us from the world. As God's peculiar people we should not feel that we must acknowledge our dependence upon men who are transgressing God's law to give us influence in the world. It is God that gives us influence. He is our exceeding great reward. He will give us advantages that are far beyond all the advantages we might receive from worldlings, by uniting with those who do not recognize the law of God.

J. A. BURDEN: I know that these thoughts are what you have presented to us before. We do not want to cause you to carry a heavy burden. We simply wanted to know if we were moving in right lines. If the Lord gives you light, well and good, we will be glad to receive it; if not, then we will wait.

E. G. WHITE: If we follow on to know the Lord, we shall know that His going forth is prepared as the morning. There are some who may not be able to see that here is a test as to whether we shall put our dependence on man, or depend upon God. Shall we by our course seem to acknowledge that there is a stronger power with unbelievers than there is with God's own people? When we take hold upon God, and trust in Him, He will work in our behalf. But whatever the consequences may be, we are in regard to our faith to stand distinct and separate from the world.

I feel a decided interest in the work at Loma Linda, and I desire that it shall exert a powerful influence for the truth. Your success depends upon the blessing of God, not upon the ideas and views of men who are opposed to the requirements of the law of God. When people see that God blesses us, and gives success to our work as we make Him supreme, then they will be led to give consideration to the truths we teach. Many will be compelled to recognize that our methods are superior to those employed in the schools of the world, as they are commonly conducted.

We need not tie to men in order to secure influence. We need not think that we are dependent upon the knowledge and experience of men who do not recognize the Lord as their Master. Our God is a God of knowledge and understanding, and if we will take our position decidedly on His side to be wholly influenced by His spirit, He will give us wisdom. I would that all our people might see the {271} inconsistency of those who profess to be God's commandment-keeping people, a peculiar people zealous of good works, thinking that they must copy after the world's pattern, in order to make their own successful. Our God is stronger than any human influence. If we will accept Him as our educator, if we will make Him our strength and righteousness, He will work in our behalf.

The following out of these principles may result in a condition of things that is not just as we would desire it to be. We might like to see certain conditions, for the attainment of which we would be dependent on the world, but the result would be an experience that means weakness rather than strength. We should realize a bondage that we do not anticipate.

Jesus Christ is our Saviour today, and He is willing to work in our behalf, if we will not put our dependence upon some other power. If we are sustained by the living God, the superiority of His power will be manifested in His people. This is the testimony that I have borne all the way along, and it is the testimony that I shall continue to bear. We must exalt God who is our wisdom, our sanctification, and our exceeding great reward.

J. A. BURDEN: We love to hear the truth over and over again, that we may be sure it is the truth.

E. G. WHITE: You have the Word which tells you that God's commandment-keeping people are to have His special favor, and that they are to be sanctified through obedience to the truth. Shall we unite ourselves with those that are full of error, who have no respect for God's commandments, and shall our students go forth to obtain the finishing touches of their education from men who, unless they are converted will not be honored with a place in the councils of heaven.

W. C. WHITE: What is to be the final outcome? Will all our medical missionaries be simply nurses? Shall we have no more physicians, or shall we have a school in which we can ourselves give the finishing touches?

E. G. WHITE: Whatever plan you follow, take your position that you will not unite or be bound up with those that do not respect God's commandments.

W. C. WHITE: Does that mean that we are not to have any more physicians, but that our people will work simply as nurses, or does it mean that we shall have a school of our own where we can educate physicians?

E. G. WHITE: We shall have a school of our own. But we are not to be dependent upon the world, we must put our dependence upon a power that is higher than all {272} human power. If we honor God, He will honor us, because we observe all His commandments, which mean eternal life.

J. A. BURDEN: The governments of earth provide that if we conduct a medical school, we must take a charter from the government. That in itself has nothing to do with how the school is conducted. It is required, however, that certain studies shall be taught. There are ten subjects required. Physiology is one of these. It is required that those who labor as physicians shall be proficient in these subjects. In starting our sanitariums for the care of the sick, we must secure a charter from the government; our printing offices must do the same. Would the securing of a charter for a medical school, where our students might obtain a medical education, militate against our depending upon God.?

E. G. WHITE: No, I do not see that it would, if a charter were secured on the right terms. Only be sure that you do not exalt men above God. If you can gain force and influence that will make your work more effective without tying yourselves to worldly men, that would be right. But we are not to exalt the human above the divine.

J. A. BURDEN: That is the vital point, where we have been hanging for three years. The only thing that we have asked for in this matter is to take advantage of the government provision that would give standing room to our students when they are qualified.

E. G. WHITE: I do not see anything wrong in that, as long as you do not in any way lift men above the Lord God of Israel, or throw discredit upon His power. But enter into no agreement with any fraternity that would open a door of temptation to some weak souls to lose their souls on God.

J. A. BURDEN: In planning our course of study, we have tried to follow the light in the Testimonies, and in doing so it has led us away from the requirements of the world. The world will not recognize us as standing with them. We shall have to stand distinct, by ourselves.

E. G. WHITE: You may unite with them in certain points that will not have a misleading influence, but let no sacrifice be made to endanger our principles. We shall always have to stand distinct. God desires us to be separate, and yet it is our privilege to avail ourselves of certain rights. But rather than to confuse our medical work, you had better stand aloof and labor with the advantages that you yourselves can offer.

J. A. BURDEN: Now the proposition in this letter {273} was to deviate from that, so that standing as we do, would enable us to stand with them and to have their advantage. From the instruction that has come, it has seemed to me from the very first, that we were to stand by ourselves in a distinct light, following the light that God has given with reference to physical healing, and that when we do that, God will open the way before us, and give us prestige with the people. But if we deviate and connect with these other schools, we would find ourselves being thrown more and more into the very things that they are doing, and our students would be molded after their similitude instead of after the similitude of truth.

E. G. WHITE: That is what I am trying to guard against all the time. As we read our Bible we see that God is dishonored when His people go to any worldly power, or put their trust in a worldly power. That is where God's people again and again became ensnared, and spoilt their history. You must arrange this matter the best you can, but the principle that is presented to me is that you are not to acknowledge any power as greater than that of our God. Our influence is to be acknowledged of God, because we keep His commandments, and His commandments are not grievous. Here is our standard. Keep God's commandments as the apple of your eye.

W. C. WHITE: Jesus said at one time, "The scribes and the Pharisees sit in Moses' seat: all therefore whatsoever they bid you observe, that observe and do; but do not ye after their works." Now the law says that a man shall not practice medicine un-less he has a diploma from a college, and unless he has passed the examination of the state board, and has a certificate. The law would not recognize the diplomas of our physicians unless they have studied some things that we do not think are really essential. For instance, in their preparation they have to study a number of things that we think they might get along without, but we can teach them. We do not have to teach these subjects in their way; we can teach them in our way. When it comes to the study of drugs, they teach how to give them. We can teach the dangers of using them, and how to get along without them. In some other schools they teach geology on the evolution basis. We can teach geology, and show that the theory of evolution is false.

E. G. WHITE: Well, you must plan these details yourselves. I have told you what I have received, but these details you will have to work out for yourselves.

J. A. Burden: It seems clear to me that any standing we can lawfully have without compromising, is not out of harmony with God's plan.

E. G. WHITE: No, it is not. All I can say is that {274} I have had very distinct light, however, that there is danger of our limiting the power of the Holy One of Israel, in connection with certain plans for connecting our schools with worldly methods. He is the God of the universe, and our influence is dependent upon our carrying out the precepts of His word. We weaken our powers by not placing our dependence upon God, and taking hold of His strength. This is our privilege.

DEAR BROTHER AND SISTER HASKELL

November 3, 1907
Loma Linda, California
(H.-358-'07)

WE THANK YOU FOR YOUR letters, and for the news that they contain. . .

For more than a year the light has been coming to me that here at Loma Linda we should have a school of the highest order, and that the very best talent should be obtained, in order to prepare young men and young women for medical missionary work. This work we are desirous of seeing accomplished. It should not be necessary for students to be placed under the influence of teachers who do not obey the law of God.

I wish that you might have been present at this meeting. I think it would be well for you to be here as soon as possible. The instruction you might give would just now be very timely. You should be here with us to help in molding and fashioning the work. We are all doing the best we can to take advanced steps in the right direction.

There should be a different mold placed upon the work in this Southern California Conference. The president of this field has not had the experience that one should have who occupies such an important position. He seems to be unable to understand the Lord's plans for the carrying forward of the work.

A man lives unto God when he continually recognizes Him as a present Helper. When there is a recognition of the Lord Jesus Christ, there will be a holy fear lest he shall make mistakes. The soul will be drawn out continually in earnest prayer as he realizes his need. As he draws night unto God, God will draw night unto him, the love of God will be kindled in his heart, and he will be able to speak the words of God. The language of the heart will then be, "Whom have I in heaven but Thee, and who on earth do I desire besides Thee?" {275}

We must give evidence of a spiritual relationship to God, in all our ways acknowledging Him. Others will be able to detect Christ as all and in all. When we have the fear of the Lord ever before us, our experience will not be tame and spiritless. Christ formed within will be the hope of glory.

The fear of the Lord is the beginning of wisdom. In Him there is a hope that "maketh not ashamed." The joy of the Lord will break forth from lips that are sanctified. We must now receive rich experiences in the service of God.

Our faith is to be expressed in thanksgiving. "Whoso offereth praise glorifieth God." "In everything give thanks." "Bless the Lord, O my soul, and all that is within me, bless His holy name." Let expressions of praise flow forth from human lips. We are to rejoice in the Lord more than we have done. Let not the heart remain cold and dull and unimpressive.

There are some who think that in matters of practical Christianity, they have a superior intelligence. Whether or not this is so, will be demonstrated by the life actions. Are they self-centered, or are they moved by the Holy Spirit of truth and righteousness? Religion is to become a living, active principle. The one all absorbing motive of the true Christian is to give an expression of the goodness and love of Christ.

We need you here, Brother Haskell, to exert your influence against the presumption of men who feel that their brethren must ask permission of them, before engaging in the Lord's service where and in the manner that He indicates. Such presumption should find no place in the cause of God. We hope that there may be such changes here that the work of the Lord may move on more smoothly. . .

The Lord sends His messages to correct the erring, however highly they may regard themselves. He asks that they submit their judgment to His control. Every soul must be under discipline to God. To occupy an exalted position is not always evidence that the Lord has placed an individual in that position. It is the works, not position, that testify to the value of a man. Hereditary traits of character need to be overcome. A man cannot safely be entrusted with the control of others. unless he himself is under the sanctification of the Holy Spirit.

In the spirit of meekness and lowliness of heart, all methods and plans should be submitted to wise counselors for their prayerful consideration and their endorsement. Otherwise, a restless, speculative energy and ambition may make an evil mark upon the cause of {276} God, and subvert and hinder the very work that the Lord has declared should be done in this Conference.

In order that the great work of sanctification that needs to be carried forward in the churches of Southern California, may be accomplished, the minds and wills of our ministers, and physicians, and teachers should be united, their hearts blending in one spirit to give the trumpet a certain sound. Let every voice proclaim distinctly the third angel's message. In word and act let those who are proclaiming the message, reveal that they are numbered among those "that keep the commandments of God, and the faith of Jesus."

If this had been done faithfully, with the word of the living God as the great lesson book, the third angel's message would have gone with greater power. Had all God's ministers, as faithful stewards of the grace of God, called upon the world to hear the last note of warning, giving the trumpet a certain sound, thousands more might have been converted, and added their voices in proclaiming the message to the world. In distinct notes of solemn warning is to be given the closing message that will prepare a people to receive the seal of the living God.

Satan is working to fill minds with the spirit of ambition and of commercialism. Those whose minds are thus diverted, will lose their opportunity of giving the last message to the world.

If a faithful work had been done during the last few years that have gone into eternity, thousands of souls would now be found with Bibles in their hands, reading the Word of God, and praying for light and guidance. Many of these would be engaged in the work of hunting for souls, and fitting up a people to stand in the great day of God. But some who ought to be missionaries, are filled with the spirit of commercialism, and with an ambition to secure for themselves certain advantages. The truth becomes to them a dead letter, not practiced nor obeyed.

Jehovah is the true God. Let Him be feared and reverenced.

JEHOVAH IS OUR KING

August 15, 1907
(MS.-73)

GOD HAS REVEALED MANY things to me which He has bidden me give to His people by pen and voice. Through this message of the Holy Spirit, God's people are given {277} sacred instruction concerning their duty to God and to their fellow-men.

A strange thing has come into our churches. Men who are placed in positions of responsibility that they might be wise helpers to their fellow workers, have come to suppose that they were set as kings and rulers in the churches, to say to one brother, Do this, to another, Do that, and to another, Be sure to labor in such and such a way. There have been places where the workers have been told that if they did not follow the instruction of these men of responsibility, their pay from the conference would be withheld.

It is right for the workers to counsel together as brethren; but that man who endeavors to lead his fellow workers to seek his counsel and advice regarding the details of their work, and to learn their duty from him, is in a dangerous position, and needs to learn what responsibilities are really comprehended in his office. God has appointed no man to be conscience for his fellow man, and it is not wise to lay so much responsibility upon an officer that he will feel that he is forced to become a dictator.

A Constant Peril

For years there has been a growing tendency for men placed in positions of responsibility to Lord it over God's heritage, thus removing from church members their keen sense of the need of divine instruction and an appreciation of the privilege to counsel with God regarding their duty. This order of things must be changed. There must be a reform. Men who have not a rich measure of that wisdom which cometh from above, should not be called to serve in positions where their influence means so much to church members.

In my earlier experience in the message I was called to meet this evil. During my labors in Europe and Australia, and again at the San Jose camp meeting I had to bear my testimony of warning against it, because souls were being taught to look to man for wisdom, instead of looking to God who is our wisdom, our sanctification, and our righteousness. Recently the same message has again been given me, more definite and decisive, because there has been a deeper offence to the Spirit of God.

An Exalted Privilege

God is the teacher of His people. All who humble their hearts before Him, will be taught of God. "If any man lack wisdom, let him ask of God, that giveth to all men liberally and upbraideth not, and it shall be given him." The Lord wants every church member to pray earnestly for wisdom, that he may know what the Lord {278} would have him do. It is the privilege of every believer to obtain an individual experience, learning to carry his cares and perplexities to God. It is written, "Draw nigh to God, and He will draw nigh to you."

Through His servant Isaiah God is calling His church to appreciate her exalted privilege in having the wisdom of the infinite at her demand: "O Zion, that bringest good tidings, get thee up into the high mountain; O Jerusalem, that bringest good tidings, lift up thy voice with strength; lift it up, be not afraid; say unto the cities of Judah, Behold your God! Behold, the Lord will come with a string hand, and His arm shall rule for Him: behold, His reward is with Him, and His work before Him. He shall feed His flock like a shepherd: He shall gather the lambs with His arm, and carry them in His bosom, and shall gently lead those that are with young." (Isaiah 40:12-17, 28-31)

In the forty-first to the forty-fifth chapters of Isaiah, God very fully reveals His purpose for His people, and these chapters should be prayerfully studied. God does not here instruct His people to turn away from Him and look to finite man for wisdom. (Isaiah 44:21-23; 45:21-25)

I wrote this fully because I have been shown that ministers and people are tempted more and more to trust in finite man for wisdom, and to make flesh their arm. To conference presidents and men in responsible places I bear this message: Break the bands and fetters that have been placed upon God's people. To you the word is spoken, "Break every yoke." Unless you cease the work of making man amenable to man, unless you become humble in heart, and yourselves learn the way of the Lord as little children, the Lord will divorce you from His work. We are to treat one another as brethren, as fellow laborers, as men and women who are, with us, seeking for light and understanding of the way of the Lord, "and who are jealous for His glory.

God declares, "I will be glorified in My people;" but the self-confident management of men has resulted in putting God aside, and accepting the devisings of men. If you allow this to continue, your faith will soon become extinct. God is in every place, beholding the conduct of the people who profess to represent the principles of His word. He asks that a change be made. He wants His people to be molded and fashioned, not after man's ideas, but after the similitude of God. I entreat of you to search the Scriptures as you have never yet searched them, that you may know the way and will of God. O that every soul might be impressed with this message, and put away the wrong! {279}

Paul's Experience

We would do well to study carefully the first and second chapters of First Corinthians. "We preach Christ crucified," the apostle declared, "unto the Jews a stumbling block, and unto the Greeks foolishness; but to them which are called, both Jews and Greeks, Christ the power of God, and the wisdom of God." (1 Corinthians 1:24-28; 2:16

Read also the third chapter of this book, and study and pray over these words. As a people of our faith and practice need to be energized by the Holy Spirit. No ruling power, that would compel men to obey the dictates of the finite mind, should be exercised. "Cease ye from man, whose breath is in his nostrils," the Lord commands. By turning the minds of men to lean on human wisdom, we place a veil between God and man, so that there is not a seeing of Him who is invisible.

In our individual experience we are to be taught of God. When we seek Him with a sincere heart, we will confess to Him our defects of character; and He has promised to receive all who come to Him in humble dependence. The one who yields to the claims of God will have the abiding presence of Christ, and this companionship will be to him a very precious thing. Taking hold of divine wisdom, he will escape the corruptions that are in the world through lust. Day by day he will learn more fully how to carry his infirmities to the One who has promised to be a very present help in every time of need.

This message is spoken to our churches in every place. In the false experience that has been coming in, a decided influence is at work to exalt human agencies, and to lead some to depend on human judgment and to follow the control of human minds. This influence is diverting the mind from God, and God forbids that any such experience should deepen and grow in our ranks as Seventh-day Adventists. Our petitions are to reach higher than erring man, to God. . . God does not confine Himself to one place or person. He looks down from heaven upon the children of men; He sees their perplexities, and is acquainted with the circumstances of every issue of life. He understands His own work upon the human heart, and He needs not that any man should direct the workings of His Spirit.

"This is the confidence that we have in Him, that if we ask anything according to His will, He heareth us. And if we know that He hears us, we know that we have the petitions that we desire of Him." God has appointed the angels that do His will to respond to the prayers of the meek of the earth, and to guide His ministers with counsel and judgment. Heavenly agencies are constantly seeking to impart grace and strength and counsel to God's faithful children, that they may act their part in the work of communicating light to the world. The wonderful sacrifice of Christ has made it possible for every man to do a special work. When the worker receives wisdom {280} from the only true source, he will become a pure channel of light and blessing; for he will receive his capability for service in rich currents of grace and light from the throne of God.

———————

Dear Brother and Sister Burden

August 29, 1907
(B-200)

I HAVE BEEN VERY ANXIOUS to learn something of the meetings you have been holding. W. C. White has written us no particulars. I would be glad if you would bear in mind that I am intensely interested in this meeting, and desire to know about it. Has it meant victory or defeat?

One night this week, I think it was Sunday, I did not sleep any through the entire night; and again on Wednesday I had a wakeful night. I slept for a short time before three o'clock. While I lay awake, I spent the time in prayer that God would give to His people sanctified and converted minds, that individually they might comprehend their duty, and learn to reveal the power of the truth in sound speech that cannot be condemned.

The talent of speech is a precious talent. The riches of the grace of Christ which He is every ready to bestow upon us, we are to impart in true, hopeful words. "Rejoice in the Lord always, and again I say, Rejoice." If we would guard our words, so that nothing but kindness shall escape our lips, we will give evidence that we are preparing to become members of the heavenly family! In words and works we shall show forth the praise of Him who has called us out of darkness into His marvelous light. O what a reformative influence would go forth if we as a people would value at its true worth the talent of speech and its influence upon human minds.

The Sabbath meetings, the morning and evening worship in the home, the services held in the chapel, all should be vitalized by the Spirit of Christ. Each member of the Sanitarium family confess Christ openly and with gladness, expressing the joy and comfort and hope that is written in the soul. Christ is to be set forth as the chiefest among ten thousand, the one altogether lovely. He is to be set forth as the Giver of every good and perfect gift. the one in whom our hopes of eternal life are centered. If we would do this, all narrowness must be set aside, and we must call into exercise the love of Christ. The joy we experience in this love will be a blessing to others.

I am bidden to say to the sanitarium family, let your {281} social meetings, and all your religious exercises be characterized by a deep earnestness and a joy that expresses the love of God in the soul. Such meetings will be profitable to all; for they will bind heart to heart. Let there be earnest seasons of prayer; for prayer will give strength to the religious experience. Confess Christ openly and bravely, and manifest at all times the meekness of Christ.

The Lord would have the family of workers at Loma Linda channels of light. If we will keep the heart and mind opened heavenward, cherishing the comfort of His grace in the heart, the presence of Christ will be revealed. Let earnestness and zeal come into your lives. Make no backward movements. The Lord is our Helper, our Guide, our Shield, our exceeding great Reward. Do not allow levity to come into your experience, but cultivate cheerfulness; for this is an excellent grace. We cannot afford to be unmindful of our words and deportment.

During the past night I seemed to be standing before a large congregation, speaking to the people the words of life. I long to understand more perfectly about this meeting that was presented to me. I seemed to hear the sweet melody of praise to God, and expressions of gratitude were coming from souls that were the recipients of the grace of Christ. The voice of praise and thanksgiving was heard, and countenances were aglow with the light of the love of God. It seemed that angels' voices united with those in the meeting who were offering praise to God.

My father was a very cheerful Christian. No doleful testimony was ever suffered to go forth from his lips. When those about him were giving doleful testimonies, his voice would be heard, "What doth much increase the store? When I thank Him, He gives me more."

We all have very much to be thankful for; let us open our lips in praise and thanksgiving to God. Let us come nearer to the Lord Jesus, and acknowledge our daily obligations to Him. He has made it possible for us to secure for ourselves a very happy life even in this world of sin, and holds out the hope of being continually in His presence in the kingdom He is preparing for His people. Should not these thoughts call forth from us praise and thanksgiving? May the Lord bless you, and bless the sanitarium family, is my prayer.

In Humility and Faith

September 19, 1907

SPECIAL INSTRUCTION has been given me for God's people, for perilous times are upon us. In the world, destruction {282} and violence are increasing. In the church man power is gaining the ascendency; those who have been chosen to occupy positions of trust think it their prerogative to rule.

Men whom the Lord calls to important positions in His work are to cultivate a humble dependence upon Him. They are not to seek to embrace too much authority; for God has not called them to a work of ruling, but to plan and counsel with their fellow laborers. Every worker alike is to hold himself amenable to the requirements and instructions of God.

To our brethren in Southern California I bear this message: The president of your conference has the lesson to learn that he is not to endeavor to rule his fellow laborers who have occupied positions of trust under God in the work; neither is he to consider himself capable of carrying all things after his own ideas. He has thought that it was his right to rule in every branch of the conference work, and this has led him to judge and criticize fellow laborers who were better able than he to do the work. He must first rule himself before he can hope to rule others wisely, or to plan wisely for the advancement of the work. Position will not give to any man an all-round education.

Because of the importance of the work in Southern California, and the perplexities which now surround it, there should be selected no less than five men of wisdom and experience to consult with the presidents of the local and union conferences regarding general plans and policies. The Lord is not well pleased with the disposition some have manifested to rule those of more experience than themselves. By this course of action, some have revealed that they are not qualified to fill the important positions which they occupy. Any human being who spreads himself out to large proportions, and who seeks to have the control of his fellows, proves himself to be a dangerous man to be entrusted with religious responsibilities.

Upon the Union Conference President should rest the greater responsibilities, and I am instructed that he needs other helpers to advise him in his work. He should not cling to the idea that unless money is in hand no move should be made that calls for the investment of means. If in our past experience we had always followed this method, we would often have lost special advantages, such as we gained in the purchase of the Fernando School property, and in the purchase of the sanitarium properties at Paradise Valley, and Loma Linda.

To make no move that calls for the investment of means unless we have the money in hand to complete the contemplated work, should not always be considered the wisest plan. In the up building of His work, the Lord does not always make everything plain before His servants. He sometimes tries the confidence of His people by having them move forward in faith. Often He brings them into strait and {283} trying places, bidding them go forward when their feet seem to be touching the waters of the Red Sea. It is at such times, when the prayers of His servants ascend to Him in earnest faith, that he opens the way before them, and brings them out into a large place.

The Lord wants His people in these days to believe that He will do as great things for them as He did for the children of Israel in their journey from Egypt to Canaan. We are to have an educated faith that will not hesitate to follow His instructions in the most difficult experiences. "Go forward," is the command of God to His people.

Faith and cheerful obedience are needed to bring the Lord's designs to pass. When He points out the necessity of establishing the work in places where it will have influence, the people are to walk and work by faith. By their godly conversation, their humility, their prayers and earnest efforts, they should strive to bring the people to appreciate the good work that the Lord has established among them. It was the Lord's purpose that the Loma Linda Sanitarium should become the property of our people, and He brought it about at a time when the rivers of difficulty were full and overflowing their banks.

The working of private interests for the gaining of personal ends is one thing. In this men may follow their own judgment. But the carrying forward of the Lord's work in the earth is entirely another matter. When He designs that a certain property should be secured for the advancement of His cause and the building up of His work, whether it be for sanitarium or school work, or for any other branch, He will make the doing of that work possible, if those who have experience will show their faith and trust in His purposes, and will move forward promptly to secure the advantages He points out. While we are not to seek to wrest property from any man, yet when advantages are offered, we should be wide awake to see the advantage, that we may make plans for the upbuilding of the work. And when we have done this, we should exert every energy to secure the free will offerings of God's people for the support of these new plans.

Often the Lord sees that His workers are in doubt as to what they should do. At such times, if they will put their confidence in Him, He will reveal to them His will. God's work is now to advance rapidly, and if His people will respond to His call, He will make them the possessors of property willing to donate of their means, and thus make it possible for His work to be accomplished in the earth. "Faith is the substance of things hoped for, the evidence of things not seen." Faith in the word of God will place His people in the possession of property which will enable them to work the large cities that are waiting for the message of truth. {284}

The cold, formal, unbelieving way in which some of the laborers do their work is a deep offense to the Spirit of God. The apostle Paul says, "Do all things without murmurings and disputings: that ye may be blameless and harmless, the sons of God in the midst of a crooked and perverse nation, among whom ye shine as lights in the world; holding forth the word of life, that I may rejoice in the day of Christ, that I have not run in vain, neither labored in vain. Yea, and if I be offered on the sacrifice and service of your faith, I joy and rejoice with you all."

We are to encourage in one another that living faith that Christ has made it possible for every believer to have. The work is to be carried forward as the Lord prepares the way. When he brings His people into straight places, then it is their privilege to assemble together for prayer, remembering that all things come of God. Those who have not yet shared in the trying experiences that attend the work in these last days, will soon have to pass through scenes that will severely test their confidence in God. It is at the time when His people see no way to advance, when the Red Sea is before them, and the pursuing army behind, that God bids them "Go forward." Thus He is working to test their faith. When such experiences come to you, go forward, trusting in Christ. Walk step by step in the path He marks out. Trials will come, but go forward. This will give you an experience that will strengthen your faith in God, and fit you for truest service.

A deeper and wider experience in religious things is to come to God's people. Christ is our example. If through living faith and sanctified obedience to God's word, we reveal the love and grace of Christ, if we show that we have a true conception of God's guiding providence in the work, we shall carry to the world a convincing power. A high position does not give us value in the sight of God. Man is measured by his consecration and faithfulness in working out the will of God. If the remnant people of God will walk before him in humility of faith, He will carry out through them His eternal purpose, enabling them to work harmoniously in giving to the world the truth as it is in Jesus. He will use all, men, women, and children, in making the light shine forth to the world, and calling out a people that will be true to His commandments. Through the faith that His people exercise in Him, God will make known to the world that He is the true God, the God of Israel.

"Let your conversation be as becometh the gospel of Christ," the apostle Paul exhorts, "that whether I come and see you, or else be absent, I may hear of your affairs, that ye stand fast in one spirit; with one mind striving for the faith of the gospel; and in nothing terrified by your adversaries; which is to them an evident token of perdition, but to you of salvation, that of God. For unto you it is given in the behalf of Christ, not only to believe on Him, but also to suffer for His sake." {285}

I have been instructed to present these words to our people in Southern California. They are needed in every place, where a church is established; for a strange experience has been coming into our ranks. It is time now for men to humble their hearts before God, and to learn to work in His ways. Let those who have sought to rule their fellow workers study to know what manner of spirit they are of. They should seek the Lord by fasting and prayer, and in humility of soul. Christ in His earthly life gave an example that all can safely follow. He appreciates His flock and he wants no power set over them that will restrict their freedom in His service. He has never placed man as a ruler over His heritage. True Bible religion will lead to self-control, not to control of one another. As a people we need a larger measure of the Holy Spirit, that we may bear the solemn message that God has given us without exaltation.

Brethren, keep your words of censure for your individual selves. Teach the flock of God to look to Christ, not to erring man. Every soul who becomes a teacher of the truth must bear in his own life the fruit of holiness. Looking to Christ and following Him, He will present to the souls under His charge an example of what a living, learning Christian will be. Let God teach you His way. Inquire of Him daily to know His will. He will give unerring counsel to all who seek Him with a sincere heart. Walk worthy of the vocation wherewith you are called, praising God in your daily conversation as well as in your prayers. Thus, holding forth the word of life, you will constrain other souls to become followers of Christ.

ELDER A. T. ROBINSON

May 22, 1907
Glendale, California
(R.-182- 1907)

Dear Brother Robinson:

AT OUR REQUEST BROTHER BURDEN has consented to visit important gatherings of our people in the Middle West, and to endeavor to secure gifts or loans for some of our Southern California Sanitariums. We desire that wherever he goes, he may be given opportunity to present the word and needs of the Paradise Valley Sanitarium and the Loma Linda Sanitarium. We need help in both these places. Both at Loma Linda and at Paradise Valley it has been necessary to build additions to the main building for bathrooms. This has left us with debts that must be met shortly, and we greatly need financial assistance.

At Loma Linda, a school is being conducted for the training of medical missionary evangelists, and we want this school to be of the highest order. Both the sanitarium {286} and the school can be a help one to the other.

Elder Burden has felt an earnest interest in the advancement of the sanitarium work along right lines. He and Sister Burden have put their whole soul into an effort to make the work at Loma Linda a success. They have put into the institution all the means they could spare to keep the enterprise moving. We have the utmost confidence in the integrity of Brother Burden, and have no reason to doubt that the Lord selected him as the manager of the Loma Linda Sanitarium.

Will you, Brother Robinson, assist Brother Burden in his mission in behalf of these institutions? You may introduce him to some of our loyal brethren who have

means, or you may permit him to speak before gatherings of our people, and raise donations or loans in your conference. We trust that our brethren in Nebraska may be able to assist in relieving the pressure for means that exists at present in these two sanitariums that the Lord has providentially placed in our hands.

ELDER G. I. BUTLER

May 29, 1907
Sanitarium, California
(B.-186-'07)

24th Avenue North,
Nashville, Tennessee

My dear Brother:

I RECEIVED YOUR LETTER, for which I thank you. I am always glad to hear from you.

For nearly six weeks I have been absent from St. Helena, traveling in Southern California . . Sabbath and Sunday, April 20 and 21, I spent at Fernando. Our school this year at Fernando has been greatly blessed. Many of the students have offered themselves for service in the Master's vineyard. On Monday I left for Loma Linda. I remained there a little over a week, and returned again to Loma Linda after a visit to Paradise Valley, San Diego, San Pasqual, and Escondido.

On Sabbath, May 18, the members of several churches gathered at Loma Linda, and we held meetings under the pepper trees on the lawn at the back of the sanitarium. In the forenoon I spoke for one hour, and the Lord helped me wonderfully. Before closing my remarks, I presented to those present the needs of the sanitarium, and expressed the desire that sufficient money be received to complete the payments on the additions that have been made to the main building. Before we {287} purchased the property, the main building had been used mostly as a hotel, and the bathroom facilities were limited. In order to do efficient work in the sanitarium, it was necessary to make additions to the buildings already standing. Dr. White, Brother and Sister Burden, and the sisters of Sister Burden, invested in the sanitarium at Loma Linda all that they could possibly spare, but there still remains an indebtedness that must be cleared off.

After the morning service, a lunch was provided by the sanitarium for the visitors, and served on the lawn. Brother Burden felt that the sanitarium would not be a loser by this entertainment, and

I agreed with him; for I remember the experiences we have had in the past in making similar provision. Such acts of hospitality are sometimes the means of sowing seed in the hearts of those who are inquiring after truth.

In the afternoon Elder Luther Warren gave an excellent discourse. Brother Warren is an able worker, and we hope that he may labor for a time in this needy field. At present he is resting somewhat on account of the condition of his own and his wife's health. After his service, the visitors left for their homes; and all were agreed that they had spent a pleasant day, and had been blessed by the discourses.

After the Sabbath, Brother Nichols came to my room, his face glowing with happiness, and said, "I want to tell you what your words today have accomplished." He then told me that one sister had come to Brother Burden and given him ten dollars and that a gentleman had offered to lend him one thousand dollars for a year without interest. I felt to praise the Lord at this response.

Later, Brother Burden gave me some particulars concerning this man who has loaned the money. He was brought to the sanitarium in such a distressed condition that his case was thought to be hopeless. But he was carefully treated, and the crisis was safely passed. He is one of the most grateful patients they have had. He has become interested in the truth, and by his loan he has shown his appreciation of what has been done for him.

I had promised to speak at Los Angeles on Sunday afternoon, so it was necessary for us to hasten away by the early train from Loma Linda. We had about sixty miles to travel. On our arrival at Los Angeles, we went up to our restaurant and treatment rooms on Hill Street, and while waiting there before the service, I prayed to the Lord for strength for the work before me.

At the church we found that a large crowd had gathered. Every foot of room was occupied, even the aisles being {288} filled, and I was told that some were unable to find entrance to the building. Among those present were a large number not of our faith.

I presented the importance of obedience to the commandments of God, dwelling upon the instruction given in connection with the proclamation of the law from Mt. Sinai. Never before had these Scriptures appealed to me so forcibly. I spoke for a full hour, and the interest was marked throughout. As I felt my voice weakening, I paused to send a prayer to heaven for help. Then the power of the Holy Spirit strengthened me, and I knew that angels of God were by my side. At the last I became somewhat hoarse, but I felt very thankful that the Lord has permitted me to speak for so long and so distinctly.

DEAR BROTHER BURDEN

(B.-276-1907)

I HAVE READ WITH MUCH interest your letter regarding the camp meeting.

I have a message to bear to some who hold positions of responsibility in the Southern California Conference. They have lost from their experience that true fervor which the presence of the Holy Spirit gives, and which would teach them to subdue self and walk humbly in the way of Christ. The responsible worker who will not become a humble follower of Christ will do great harm to the cause of God, by molding and fashioning the experience of the conference to a common, cheap standard. The sacred work that we handle will never, if performed in a spirit of consecration, cheapen the experience of a single soul.

That man is unfit to be the president of a conference or a leader among God's people, who has not broad ideas and views. It is the privilege and duty of those who bear responsibilities in the cause to become learners in Christ's school. The professed follower of Christ must not follow the dictates of his own will; his mind must be trained to think Christ's thoughts, and enlightened to comprehend the will and way of God. Such a believer will be a learner of Christ's methods of work.

A mistake was made in the methods that were adopted to clear the schools in California from debt. The book, "Christ's Object Lessons" was given to relieve the indebtedness of our schools. But this plan has not been presented in our schools as it should have been; the students and teachers have not been educated to take hold of this book and push its sale for the benefit of {289} the educational work. The plan that has been followed of calling on our people to support these schools must not be continued; for this is giving to our teachers and students, and to our people in general a wrong education. They must not be so instructed that they will forget the needs of other fields outside their own.

In the cities of Riverside, Redlands, and San Bernardino a mission field is open to us that we have as yet only touched with the tips of our fingers. A good work has been done there as far as our workers have had encouragement to do it; but there is need of means to carry the work successfully. It was God's purpose that by the sale of "Ministry of Healing" and "Christ's Object Lessons" the necessary means would be raised for the work of our sanitariums and schools, and thus our people be left free to donate of their means for the opening of the work in new fields. If our people had engaged in the sale of these books as God purposed they should, we would now have the means to carry the work in the way the Lord designed.

Wherever the work of selling "Christ's Object Lessons" has been taken hold of in earnest, the book has had a good circulation. And the lessons that have been learned by those who have been engaged in this work have well repaid their efforts. Our people should all be encouraged to take part in this missionary effort. Light has been given me that in every possible way instruction should be given to our people in the best methods of presenting this book to the people. We have been instructed that at our large gatherings, workers should be present who will teach our people how to sow the seeds of truth. This means more than instruction in how to sell the Signs of the Times and other periodicals. It includes such books as "Christ's Object Lessons" and "Ministry of Healing". These are books which contain precious truths, and from which the reader can draw lessons of highest value.

At your recent camp meeting, was anyone appointed to present the interests of this line of work to our people? If this was not done, you lost a precious opportunity of placing large blessings within the reach of the people, and an opportunity of raising means for the relief of our institutions. My brother, let us encourage our people to take up this work without further delay. Let those who have had experience in the sale of health foods interest themselves in the sale of "Christ's Object Lessons" and "Ministry of Healing"; for here is food unto eternal life. Los Angeles has been presented to me as a very fruitful field for the sale of these books. I know that every household in the land would be benefited by their presence in the home.

Those who bear responsibilities in our sanitariums and schools should act wisely in this matter, encouraging {290} all by this means to gather the money required to meet the expenses of the different institutions. We have need of workers in Southern California who have clear spiritual eyesight, men who will weigh matters wisely, and can see afar off. If our workers were more fully consecrated to the cause of God, a much more effective work would be done.

God's Spirit is grieved because His people are so slow to understand that which the Lord requires of them. Our workers should present these books to our people at our large and small gatherings, and call for volunteers who will engage in the sale of them. When this work is entered into with the earnestness which the times in which we live demand, the indebtedness that now rests upon our schools and sanitariums will be wiped out, and the people who are now being called on to give of their means to support these institutions, will be free to donate their offerings to missionary work in other needy places.

Great good will result by bringing these books before the women of the Women's Christian Temperance Union. Invite these workers to your meetings, and give them an opportunity to become acquainted with our people. Place these books in their hands, and tell them the story of their gift to the cause and its object. Explain how by the sale of "Ministry of Healing", patients will be brought to the Sanitarium for healing who could never get there unaided, and how through this means also sanitariums will be established in places where they are needed. If our sanitariums are managed wisely by men and women who have the fear of God before them, the workers in the temperance cause will not be slow to see the advantage of this branch of the work. If you will in earnestness and faith work out the plan that God has laid down, angels of God will attend your steps, and the blessing of heaven will be upon your efforts.

I send you these lines because I see that there is need of a deeper intuition, a wider perception, on the part of our sanitarium and educational workers if they would get all the benefit that God intends shall come to them through these books. I ask you, Brother Burden, to read these words to our people, that they may learn to show the wisdom of a sound mind. The Lord gave me His Holy Spirit to enable me to write the manuscript for this book, the Review and Herald and the Press donated the labor required to prepare it for the public;

and God now calls upon our people, men and women and youth, to make the most of this gift to His cause. Let the students, under wise directors, be set to work to sell the books, and let all understand why they are engaged in this missionary enterprise. The blessing and approval of God will rest upon those who make the effort.

_____

Dr. C. C. Nicola

September 30, 1907
306 Sanitarium, California {291}
Hinsdale, Illinois

Dear Brother and Sister Nicola:

BROTHER BURDEN HAS informed me that you have been considering again going to Loma Linda. I thank the Lord for this, for I know that Loma Linda is the place where you should go. I trust that the snare of the enemy is broken.

A message has been given me for you. I am charged to say to you, Do not go to Battle Creek. You do not understand how the enemy is working to place you in opposition to the truth and the work of God.

A. T. Jones, Dr. Kellogg, and Elder Tenney are all working under the same leadership. They are classing themselves with those of whom the apostle writes, "Some shall depart from the faith, giving heed to seducing spirits and doctrines of devils." In the case of A. T. Jones, I can see the fulfillment of the warnings that were given me regarding him.

I want this message to come to you before you shall make a wrong move. I do not want you to imperil your souls. Heed the message that the Lord sends, and have nothing to do with those at Battle Creek who are opposing the messages of the Spirit of God. Clear light has been given me regarding those who are thus departing from the faith.

I want you to understand that you are both in positive danger. I plead with you to break this influence that would lead you into wrong paths. It proceeds from the one who, if it were possible, would deceive the very elect. Free yourselves from the influence prevailing at Battle Creek, and place yourselves fully on the Lord's side. I do not want you to lose your souls. I beg of you to resist the devil. Make your calling and election sure. Christ gave His precious life for you. Do not let him make this sacrifice in vain.

My brother and sister, this is a life and death question with you. As the Lord's messenger, I urge you to free yourselves

from the snare of Satan, and place yourselves on the platform of eternal truth. I cannot let you take this step without warning you of your danger. If I should do this, I could not be clear before God.

The world is fast becoming as it was before the flood. Wickedness of every description is abroad in the land. Very soon the earth will be ripe for destruction. It is time now for those who believe that Jesus is soon coming to take their stand fully on the Lord's side. I have an {292} earnest desire that you shall stand with God's loyal people.

I believe, Brother and Sister Nicola, that you will heed these words, and decide to connect with the Loma Linda Sanitarium. Will you not write to me as soon as you receive this, and set my mind at rest? May the Lord give you His Holy Spirit to guide and direct you, is my prayer.

_____

Elder J. A. Burden

October 2, 1907
Loma Linda, California
(B.312)

Dear Brother and Sister Burden:

I HAVE JUST WRITTEN A LETTER to Brother and Sister Nicola. I have sent you a copy of this. We should use every opportunity we have to save these souls.

The apostle Paul writes, (Jude 3, 4, 20-23)

We shall have more decided opposition to meet from those who have departed from the faith. Those who were once strong teachers, but who have forsaken the way of the Lord, will be just as strong in their opposition of the truth. There is need now that our people be educated to put their trust in God alone. They must learn that their trust is not to be placed in any human voice or arm of flesh. We need ever to keep in mind the experiences of the children of Israel, and learn the lesson that the record of their failures is intended to teach us. . . .

The Lord wants you to understand your individual responsibility for the salvation of your soul. With the word of God as your guide and instructor, you are to personally work out your own salvation. You are to strive to secure eternal life, when you may dwell forever with the Lord. In studying how you may gain this, seek for that wisdom which God alone can impart. Accept the invitation, "If any man lack wisdom, let him ask of God that giveth to all men liberally, and

upbraideth not; and it shall be given." "My brethren," the apostle James writes, "Count it all joy. . ." James 1:2-8

There is an individual work for all to do before our labors can accomplish anything for others. Blessed is the man who endures temptation, who when he is tried, takes the word of life as his own, brings the promises to the Lord, and claims them as his. This man relies not on any human power, but on the strength of the Lord.

Faith in the word of God will bring to us the {293} fulfillment of His promises. "Whatsoever ye shall ask in My name, that will I do," the Saviour declares. "If ye shall ask anything in My name, I will do it." "And all things whatsoever ye shall ask in faith, believing, ye shall receive." When we learn to place our reliance, not on the words of man, but in God, He will make that word yea and Amen to us in Christ Jesus.

Brother and Sister Burden, study the Word. You are not to go to any man to learn your duty. Take the Bible as your guide; live its teachings. "Ask, and ye shall receive." We all need a deeper spirituality; we should each seek God for ourselves. Let us ever remember that while we seek to follow one pattern Christ Jesus, we are to maintain our individuality. "Do not err, my beloved brethren. Every good gift and every perfect gift is from above, and cometh down from the Father of lights, with whom is no variableness, neither shadow of turning. Of his own will begat he us with the word of truth, that we should be a kind of firstfruits of his creatures. Wherefore, my beloved brethren, let every man be swift to hear, slow to speak, slow to wrath: For the wrath of man worketh not the righteousness of God." James 1:16-20

When the word of God is received and obeyed, your light will shine forth in good works. "But be ye doers of the word, and not hearers only, deceiving your own selves. For if any be a hearer of the word, and not a doer, he is like unto a man beholding his natural face in a glass: For he beholdeth himself, and goeth his way, and straightway forgetteth what manner of man he was. But whoso looketh into the perfect law of liberty, and continueth therein, he being not a forgetful hearer, but a doer of the work, this man shall be blessed in his deed. If any man among you seem to be religious, and bridleth not his tongue, but deceiveth his own heart, this man's religion is vain. Pure religion and undefiled before God and the Father is this, To visit the fatherless and widows in their affliction, and to keep himself unspotted from the world." James 1:22-27

THE WORK HINDERED BY LACK OF FAITH

October 11, 1907
Sanitarium, California
(MS. 117- 1907)

HOW SHALL WE OBTAIN MEANS for our sanitariums, is a question that must be solved. Some of our institutions are prospering; some seem to have come to a standstill; and others are running behind. As I present our perplexities to the Lord, there comes to my mind with considerable force this scripture, "Although the fig-tree shall not blossom, neither fruit be in the vine; and the labor of the olive shall fail, and the flock shall be cut off from the fold; and there shall be no herd in the stall; yet I will rejoice in the Lord, and joy in the God of my salvation."

In the word of God I find these promises, "Behold, the days come, saith the Lord of Hosts, that I will make a new covenant with the house of Israel, and with the house of Judah. Not according to that which I made with their fathers when I took them by the hand to bring them out of the land of Egypt; which my covenant they brake, although I was an husband unto them, saith the Lord. But this shall be the covenant that I will make with the house of Israel: After those days, saith the Lord, I will put My law in their inward parts, and write it in their hearts; and will be their God, and they shall be My people. And they shall teach no more every man his neighbor; for they shall all know Me, from the least of them even unto the greatest, saith the Lord; for I will forgive their iniquity, and I will remember their sin no more." {294} I thank the Lord for these words of comfort and encouragement. I will put my trust in the Lord, and will wait patiently for Him. He will work in our behalf, and make us to rejoice in His mercies. He will surely be the help of His people.

Unbelief is finding an entrance in our churches, in our sanitariums, and in our publishing houses. There are some who have committed the error of turning away from the source of their strength to follow devices and plans of men, plans that are not after the order of the Lord; and because of this, they are weak when they should be strong. This is the reason that God has not wrought more mightily for His people.

Had he done more for us, human beings would have taken to themselves the glory that should be given to God.

God has a purpose in leaving men in their weakness when they turn from Him to follow the dictation of human minds. He wants them to learn where only true light and wisdom dwells. The Lord pities our weakness; he is grieved because of the error that has come in, because of the education that has been given to believers to look to men for wisdom and help. He wants his people to learn lessons of faith and trust in Him, and to stand in the strength of Israel's God.

Our sanitariums should all be in running order, so that they may act their part in influencing that class of people who can be reached in no other way than by the work of the sanitarium. Our physicians are to rebuke in decided terms the sins which are the cause of sickness and disease. We have need of men who, under the inspiration of the Holy Spirit, will rebuke gambling and liquor drinking, which are such prevalent evils in these last days. We need men who will bear their message against the selfishness that is eating out the very vitals of godliness. God calls for men of faith and prayer. "Pray ye therefore the Lord of the harvest that He will send forth laborers into His harvest."

Tremendous responsibilities are ours; and men are called for who will not misinterpret their responsibilities, but will do their appointed work in a spirit of humility and in the fear of God. We should ever be afraid of a spirit that would lead us to place restrictions on the work of others, lest we hinder the advance of the message of truth. Those who have in the past allowed such a spirit to control them have sadly hurt the work. They need to repent and be converted; for the Holy Spirit cannot work with them while they refuse to acknowledge His counsel and control. He cannot use the men who employ the trust He has imposed upon them as an oppressive power to close the lips that He has opened.

This age demands that the servants of God be men of faith and prayer, who realize the responsibilities that rest upon them as bearers of the last message of mercy to a perishing {295} world. "Ye are the light of the world," Christ declared. "Let your light so shine before men, that they may see your good works, and glorify your Father which is in heaven." Many, many souls will be brought to a knowledge of the truth if intelligent labor is put forth in their behalf.

MRS. MABEL WORKMAN

October 30, 1907
Loma Linda, California
(360-1907)

My Dear Granddaughter:

I HAVE JUST READ A LETTER that you wrote to your father, and will now begin a letter to you. . .

Last Sunday night we were on the cars, and I was unable to sleep well. The next night we spent at Loma Linda. I had a good bed, but was wakeful, and had but a short period of rest. At the early morning meeting on Tuesday, I spoke to the people. After breakfast I rode out for an hour.

Tuesday afternoon I met with the stockholders of the Paradise Valley Sanitarium. Their council-meeting was held in the bowling alley. In coming out, we had to pass through the assembly room, where there was a large audience. Brother Burden asked me to stay, as they were speaking of the work of higher education that should be carried on in medical lines, but I thought it best not to do this. After I had climbed the long flight of stairs to my room on the third floor, which was the third time for that day, I found an article that I had written about a year ago, in reference to the establishment of a school of the highest order, in which the students would not be taught to use drugs in the treatment of the sick. With this I went down stairs again, and returned to the meeting.

Elder Burden was reading some extracts from letters that I had written about the school work. When he had finished I read the article I had with me, which was right to the point. It spoke of the school that should be operated here at Loma Linda. Here there are wonderful advantages for a school. The farm, the orchard, the pasture land, the large buildings, the ample grounds, the beauty, all are a great blessings. If all will now take hold intelligently of the work that should be done here, there will be success.

For some weeks before this meeting, I had been feeling very poorly. But the Lord has greatly blessed me here, and for this I am very thankful. The Lord has imparted to me strength as the occasion has demanded.

Thursday morning, Sara came to my room, and told me it was time to go to the early meeting. I had been writing since {296}three o'clock. I attended the meeting, and spoke for about three-quarters of an hour, and then there was a testimony meeting. I could not hear what was said, but I was told that it was an interesting meeting. In all my talks I have tried to present Christ as our wisdom, our sanctification, and our righteousness.

To The Leading Ministers In California

December 6, 1909
Sanitarium, California
(-178-1909)

Dear Brethren:

IN THE NIGHT WATCHES OF November 22, I seemed to be bearing my testimony in a meeting where believers and unbelievers were assembled. I spoke to them in regard to the short work to be done in the earth, and our need of keeping before the world the evidences that the Lord is in our midst. This evidence may be given in words of praise and thanksgiving. "Whosoever offereth praise glorifieth God." The Lord calls for faithful witnesses. With our lips and in our works we should praise Him. As a people we have received special advantages from the Lord, but we do not render to Him sincere thanksgiving. Daily His praise should be spoken by every one of us.

My attention was called to these words, which are profitable for our study:

"I am the Lord and there is none else, there is no God beside me: I girded thee, though thou hast not known Me: that they may know from the rising of the sun, and from the west, that there is none beside Me. I am the Lord, and there is none else. I form the light, and create darkness: I make peace, and create evil: I the Lord to all these things. Drop down, ye heavens from above, and let the skies pour down righteousness: let the earth open and let them bring forth salvation, and let righteousness spring up together; I the Lord have created it." (Isaiah 45:5-8)

"Thus saith the Lord, in an acceptable time have I heard thee and in a way of salvation have I helped thee: and I will preserve thee, and give thee for a covenant of the people, to establish the earth, to cause to inherit the desolate heritages; that thou mayest say to the prisoners, Go forth; to them that are in darkness, Show thyselves. They shall feed in the ways, and their pastures shall be in all high places. They shall not hunger nor thirst; neither shall the heat nor sun smite them; for He that hath mercy on them shall lead them, even by the spring of water shall He guide them. And I

will make all my mountains a way, and my highways shall be exalted. Behold these shall come from far: and lo, these from the north and from the west; and these from the land of Sinim. (Isaiah 49:8-12){297}

"Sing, O ye heaven, and be joyful; and break forth into singing, O mountains: for the Lord hath comforteth His people, and will have mercy on His afflicted. But Zion said, The Lord hath forsaken me, and my Lord hath forgotten me. Can a woman forget her sucking child, that she may not have compassion on the son of her womb? yea, they may forget, yet will I not forget thee. Behold, I have graven thee upon the palms of my hands; thy walls are continually before me." (Isaiah 49:13-16)

"Ho, every one that thirsteth, come ye to the waters, and he that hath no money; come ye, buy and eat; yea, come buy wine and milk without money and without price. Wherefore do ye spend money for that which is not bread? and your labor for that which satisfieth not? hearken diligently unto me, and eat ye that which is good, and let your soul delight itself in fatness. Incline your ear, and come unto Me, hear, and your soul shall live; and I will make an everlasting covenant with you, even the sure mercies of David. Behold, I have given Him for a witness to the people, a leader and a commander to the people. Behold thou shalt call a nation that thou knowest not; and nations that know not thee shall run after thee, because of the Lord thy God, and for the Holy One of Israel; for he hath glorified thee." (Isaiah 55:1-5)

"Seek ye the LORD while he may be found, call ye upon him while he is near: Let the wicked forsake his way, and the unrighteous man his thoughts: and let him return unto the LORD, and he will have mercy upon him; and to our God, for he will abundantly pardon. For my thoughts are not your thoughts, neither are your ways my ways, saith the LORD. For as the heavens are higher than the earth, so are my ways higher than your ways, and my thoughts than your thoughts. For as the rain cometh down, and the snow from heaven, and returneth not thither, but watereth the earth, and maketh it bring forth and bud, that it may give seed to the sower, and bread to the eater: So shall my word be that goeth forth out of my mouth: it shall not return unto me void, but it shall accomplish that which I please, and it shall prosper in the thing whereto I sent it. For ye shall go out with joy, and be led forth with peace:

the mountains and the hills shall break forth before you into singing, and all the trees of the field shall clap their hands. Instead of the thorn shall come up the fir tree, and instead of the brier shall come up the myrtle tree: and it shall be to the LORD for a name, for an everlasting sign that shall not be cut off." (Isaiah 55:6-13)

Let the instruction given in the fifty-eighth chapter of Isaiah be studied in connection with these scriptures. Wonderful would be the results if ministers and church members would be converted, and adopt Christ's manner of witnessing to the power of the Lord.

In many places, and especially in Southern California, plans and methods of labor have been followed that have hindered the Lord's work, so that those upon whom the Lord has laid special burdens could not do the work to which they were appointed. In some cases watchers were sent to restrict the work and to hedge up the way of some who were laboring most earnestly for advancement. Unsanctified plans were laid that worked counter to the plans of God. All this was displeasing to the Lord, and it was work which He repudiated. There were cities that might have been entered and a good work begun, but through lack of faith there developed a counter working influence. With unbelief, jealousies arose, and with sacred missionary enterprises were linked up men who themselves needed to experience the converting power of God, and to learn to walk humbly with Him.

To those who had kept the way hedged up, I wrote out the instruction given me, and trusted the result with the Lord. The burden was heavy, and I feared I should not live to see the results of my efforts to break the yokes which men were placing upon their fellow workers. The Lord presented before me in decided representations that it would take years to root out the evil resulting from placing in the hands of finite men the power to hinder and delay the work of God. Repeated messages of reproof and counsel were necessary, {298} that capable men whom the Lord had specified as the ones to do a special work might be set free to follow the light that God was giving.

There were strong men in Southern California who stood decidedly against the light the Lord was giving His messenger regarding the work to be done. They were following their own counsel and judgment, and were imperiling the cause of God. I was instructed that the only way to counterwork this evil was to have placed in positions of trust men who would be guided by the counsel of the Lord, and who would not be turned aside by those who were deficient in faith.

The Lord has wrought in a remarkable manner to uphold the messages sent to correct the strange work that was being done. The evil has been checked, but it has not yet been fully rooted out, and if there were not a continuation of the messages from the Lord to His people, the will and ways of men would yet prevail to bring in strife and contention, and a deformed work would be the result. I was shown that human power is constantly working to weave itself into the work of God. This brings in disjointed and inharmonious action. The messages of pure and unadulterated truth are in danger of being trampled under feet by self-willed, unconverted men who work to destroy confidence in the warnings that God would speak to the hearts of His people to correct error, and to encourage righteousness.

A great many of the difficulties that have come into our work in California and elsewhere have come in through a misunderstanding on the part of men in official positions concerning their individual responsibility in the matter of controlling and ruling their fellow laborers. Men entrusted with responsibilities have supposed that their official position embraced very much more than was ever thought of by those who placed them in office, and serious difficulties arose as the result.

Simple organization and church order are set forth in the New Testament Scriptures, and the Lord has ordained these for the unity and perfection of the church. The man who holds office in the church should stand as a leader, as an advisor and a counselor and helper in carrying the burdens of the work. He should be a leader in offering thanksgiving to God. But he is not appointed to order and command the Lord's laborers. The Lord is over His heritage. He will lead His people if they will be led of the Lord in the place of assuming a power God has not given them. Let us study the twelfth and thirteenth chapter of First Corinthians, and the fifteenth chapter of Acts.

Let the men carrying responsibilities treat those who labor with them with the same consideration that they would wish to receive, were they the helpers, and others the leaders. "All ye are brethren," the Saviour declares. Position does not give

a man kingly authority. The meekness of Christ is a wonderful lesson given to the fallen world. Learning this {299} meekness from the great Teacher, the worker will become Christlike.

For several years there have been leading men in the Northern California Conference who exercised an authority which they supposed was theirs by virtue of their office, to control the work according to their own disposition and judgment. The work was becoming confused, and the Lord gave me a message regarding the movements that should be made. Because of the strange conditions in the conference, Elder Haskell was to be called to take the presidency.

Elder Haskell and his wife have been engaged in the work for years, and their faith in the truth and in the Testimonies given by the Holy Spirit is strong. They have unitedly served according to the Lord's appointment, and we have sought to sustain them in their work. Conditions in the churches have changed decidedly, but the Lord has shown me that some in responsible positions are not yet converted, and without thorough conversion, they cannot conduct the work in right lines. Some who have been reproved and warned are not established and settled, and fully yielded to the guiding power of the Holy Spirit. Satan is not yet fully cast out of the minds of some, and it would take very little to produce again the conditions that existed ten years ago.

The cause of God in Oakland, San Francisco, and the surrounding places needs men of solid Christian character, who fear God and take counsel of God, or believers will be misled by those who attach themselves to the work, and who desire to guide and control according to human judgment and plans. The Lord desires to work through men of clean purposes and decided experiences, men who will learn from the Testimonies of His Spirit where they have not been in harmony with the Lord's will, and who will be converted. Then decided changes will be made. The perils threatening the work will be seen conversions will be experienced, and our people will be preparing to stand firmly and unitedly with God to build up His kingdom in the earth.

Men who repudiate the teachings of the Spirit of God are not the proper persons to be placed in office as leaders in the church. There is danger that the teachings of men who are not soundly converted may lead

others into bye and forbidden paths. In our efforts to secure consecrated leadership, we may expect to encounter opposition, for the enemy is seeking through unconverted men in positions of trust to mold the work, and he has too much at stake lightly to lose their influence.

Many have refused to see and adopt the light, because they would not humble themselves before God, and be daily converted to Christ. Yet this must be the experience of all who overcome by the blood of the lamb and the word of their testimony. When men humble their hearts, and are daily converted, following the example of the meek and lowly Jesus, then there is hope that they will become wise in their religious experience. . . . {300}

I see a crisis before us, and the Lord calls for His workmen to come into line. Every soul should now stand in a position of deeper, truer consecration to God, than during the years that are past.

God corrects His people when they are in danger of being corrupted by those who obey not the truth. I have been charged to stand faithfully in the position in which the Lord has placed me among His people, that they might be instructed and counseled.

I have been shown that there are men helping to form committees, and men filling important positions in the churches, who are self-righteous, men walking after the counsel of their own hearts. Neither these self-righteous men nor those who have been influenced to hurt the work of God, should now be out in places of large responsibility; for the work of God will be marred by such steps. There are some who will always be deceived. We are living amid the perils of the last days. Let the word of God teach righteousness. Let the chaff be separated from the wheat.

The work of Elder Haskell and others who have labored in Oakland and the nearby places might have been a much greater blessing, had they not been obliged to meet wrong influences in opposition to the counsels that God has given to build up and prepare a people for the final conflict that is before us.

It is not in harmony with the plan of God that men who are working counter to the spirit of the messages that the Lord gives to bless and strengthen His people, should be given places of large influence in our churches. Such men are not a help, but a hindrance. Their work is to unsettle minds, and they sow the seed which will spring up and bear its fruit to make of none effect the counsels that the Lord has so graciously given to His people.

ELDER J. A. BURDEN

November 5, 1909
Sanitarium, California
(B.-140-)

Loma Linda, California

Dear Brother Burden:

SOME QUESTIONS have been asked me regarding our relation to the laws governing medical practitioners. We need to move understandingly, for the enemy would be pleased to hedge up our work so that our physicians would have only a limited influence. Some men do not act in the fear of God, and they may seek to bring us into trouble by placing on our necks yokes that we could not consent to bear. We cannot submit to regulations if the sacrifice of principle is involved; for {301} this would imperil the soul's salvation.

But whenever we can comply with the law of the land without putting ourselves in a false position, we should do so. Wise law have been framed in order to safeguard the people against the imposition of unqualified physicians. These laws we should respect, for we are ourselves by them protected from presumptuous pretenders. Should we manifest opposition to these requirements, it would tend to restrict the influence of our medical missionaries.

We must carefully consider what is involved in these matters. If there are conditions to which we could not subscribe, we should endeavor to have these matters adjusted so that there would not be strong opposition against our physicians. The Saviour bids us be wise as serpents and harmless as doves.

The Lord is our leader and teacher. He charges us not to connect with those who do not acknowledge God. "Verily My Sabbaths ye shall keep, for it is a sign between Me and you throughout your generations." Connect with those who honor God by keeping His commandments. If the recommendation goes forth from our people that our workers are to seek for success by acknowledging as essential the education which the world gives, we are virtually saying that the influence the world gives is superior to that which God gives. God will be dishonored by such a course. God has full knowledge of the faith and trust and confidence that His professed people have in His providence.

Our workers are to become intelligent in regard to Christ's life and manner of working. The Lord will help those who desire to cooperate with Him as physicians, if they will become learners of Him how to work for the suffering. He will exercise His power through them for the healing of the sick.

Intemperance and ungodliness are increasing everywhere. The work of temperance must begin in our own hearts. And the work of the physicians must begin in an understanding of the works and teachings of the great Physician. Christ left the courts of heaven that He might minister to the sick and suffering of earth. We must cooperate with the chief of physicians, walking in all humility of mind before Him. Then the Lord will bless our earnest efforts to relieve suffering humanity. It is not by the use of poisonous drugs that this will be done, but by the use of simple remedies. We should seek to correct false habits and practices, and teach the lessons of self-denial. The indulgence of appetite is the greatest evil with which we have to contend.

The truth brought to light by Christ teaches that humanity through obedience to the truth as it is in Jesus, may realize power to overcome the corruptions that are in the world through lust. Through living faith in the merits of Christ the soul may be converted and transformed into Christlikeness. Angels of God will be by the side of those who in humbleness of mind learn daily the lessons taught by Christ.

ELDER J. A. BURDEN

October 11, 1909
Sanitarium, California
(B.122- 1909) {302}

Dear Brother:

I AM INSTRUCTED TO SAY that in our educational work, there is to be no compromise in order to meet the world's standard. God's commandment-keeping people are not to unite with the world, to carry various lines of work according to worldly plans and worldly wisdom.

Our people are now being tested as to whether they will obtain their wisdom from the greatest Teacher the world ever knew, or seek to the god of Ekron. Let us determine that we shall not be tied by so much as a thread to the educational policies of those who do not discern the voice of God, and who will not hearken to His commandments.

We are to take heed to the warning: "Enter ye in at the strait gate: for wide is the gate, and broad is the way, that leadeth to destruction, and many there be which go in thereat; because strait is the gate, and narrow is the way, which leadeth unto life, and few there be that find it." Those who walk in the narrow way are following in the footprints of Jesus. The light from heaven illuminates their path.

Shall we represent before the world, that our physicians must follow the pattern of the world, before they can be qualified to act as successful physicians? This is the question that is now testing the faith of some of our brethren. Let not any of our brethren displease the Lord, by advocating in their assemblies the idea that we need to obtain from unbelievers a higher education than that specified by the Lord.

The representation of the great Teacher is to be considered an all-sufficient revelation. Those in our ranks who qualify as physicians are to receive only such education as is in harmony with these divine truths. Some have advised that students should, after taking some work at Loma Linda, complete their medical education in worldly colleges. But this is not in harmony with the Lord's plan. God is our wisdom, our sanctification, and our righteousness. Facilities should be provided at Loma Linda, that the necessary instruction in medical lines may be given by instructors who fear the Lord, and who are in harmony with His plans for the treatment of the sick.

I have not a word to say in favor of the world's ideas of higher education in any school that we shall organize for the training of physicians. There is danger in their attaching themselves to worldly institutions, and working under the ministrations of worldly physicians. Satan is {303} giving his orders to those whom he has led to depart from the faith. I would advise that none of our young people attach themselves to worldly medical institutions in the hope of gaining better success, or stronger influence as physicians.

"When Israel was a child then I loved him, and called My son out of Egypt. As they called them, so they went from then: they sacrificed unto Baalim, and burnt incense to graven images. I taught Ephraim also to go, taking them by their arms; but they knew not that I healed them. I drew them with cords of a man, with bands of love: and I was to them as they that take off the yoke on their jaws, and I laid meat unto them."

The Lord gave to His people advantages which they failed to recognize. "My people," he says, "are bent to backsliding from Me: though they called them to the Most High, none at all would exalt Him. How shall I give thee up, Ephraim? how shall I deliver thee, Israel? how shall I make thee as Admah? how shall I set thee as Zeboim? Mine heart is turned within Me, My repentings are kindled together." Read also the promises of blessing to Israel on condition of their repentance, recorded in the fourteenth chapter of Hosea. These scriptures were written in times past, but they have also a present-day application.

The enemy has worked in Southern California, and has tried to thwart the purposes of God. Messages of reproof have been sent to leading men whose work was not done in righteousness. Reformations have been called for. What is now needed is that the leaders in the Lord's work shall be fully converted. It is time that the Lord's voice was heeded, and that men should put away the spirit of self-confidence and self-sufficiency. Should the ideas of some who are wise in their own estimation be carried out, there would result a condition of things that would demand a most thorough reformation.

Let none think that they can pass safely through the perils of these last days, while puffed up with self-sufficiency. Some would unsettle minds by urging the carrying out of false plans. False theories are taught as truth, and I am charged to meet these errors decidedly. We should heed the instruction found in the third and fourth chapters of second Timothy, especially the solemn charge given by Paul to Timothy:

"I charge thee therefore, before God, and the Lord Jesus Christ, who shall judge the quick and the dead at His appearing; preach the word, be instant in season, out of season; reprove, rebuke, exhort, with all long suffering and doctrine. For the time will come when they will not endure sound doctrine; but after their own lusts shall they keep to themselves teachers, having itching ears; and they shall turn away their ears from the truth, and shall be turned unto fables. But watch thou in all things, endure {304} afflictions, do the work of an evangelist, make full proof of the ministry."

"I am now ready to be offered, and the time of my departure is at hand. I have fought a good fight, I have finished my course, I have kept the faith: henceforth there is laid up for me a crown of righteousness, which the Lord, the righteous judge shall give me at that day; and not to me only, but unto all them also that love His appearing."

I am intensely in earnest that our people shall realize that the only true education lies in walking humbly with God. The teachings of the word of God are opposed to the ideas of those who think that our students must receive the mold of an education that is according to human ideas. Some are departing from the faith, as a result of receiving from the world what they regard as a "higher education." The word of God just as it reads contains the very essence of truth. The highest education is the keeping of the law of God.

"Therefore, my brethren dearly beloved and longed for, my joy and crown, so stand fast in the Lord, my dearly beloved, Let your moderation be known unto all men. The Lord is at hand. Be careful for nothing; but in everything by prayer and supplication with thanks giving let your requests be made known unto God. And the peace of God which passeth all understanding, shall keep your hearts and minds through Christ Jesus.

"Finally brethren, whatsoever things are true, whatsoever things are honest, whatsoever things are just, whatsoever things are pure, whatsoever things are lovely, whatsoever things are of good report; if there be any virtue, and if there be any praise, think on these things. Those things which ye have both learned, and received, and heard, and seen in me, do: and the God of peace shall be with you."

A STATEMENT REGARDING THE TRAINING OF PHYSICIANS

(MS.-7- 1910)

(The statement given below, was called forth by a question submitted by Elders I. H. Evans, E. E. Andross, and W. H. Cottrell, reading as follows: "Are we to understand, from what you have written concerning the establishment of a medical school at Loma Linda, that, according from the light you have received from the Lord, we are to establish a thoroughly equipped medical school, and the graduates from which will be able to take State Board examinations and become registered, qualified physicians?")

THE LIGHT GIVEN ME IS, we must provide that which is essential to qualify our youth who desire to be physicians, so that they may intelligently fit themselves to be able to stand the examinations {305} essential to prove their efficiency as physicians. They are to be prepared to stand the essential tests required by the law, and to treat understandingly the cases of those who are diseased, so that the door will be closed for any sensible physician to fear that we are not giving in our school the instruction essential for the proper qualification of a physician. Continually the students who are graduated are to advance in knowledge; for practice makes perfect.

The medical school at Loma Linda is to be of the highest order, because we have a living connection with the wisest of all physicians, from which there is communicated knowledge of a superior order. And whatever subjects are required as essential in the schools conducted by those not of our faith, we are to supply so that our youth need not go to these worldly schools. Thus we shall close the door that the enemy could be pleased to have left open; and our young men and young women, whom the Lord would have us guard religiously, will not then need to connect with worldly medical schools conducted by unbelievers.

ELDER H. W. COTTRELL

January 27, 1910

THOSE WHO HAVE the responsibility of locating and keeping in operation our sanitariums and schools, are ever to bear in mind that these institutions are to be regarded as divinely appointed agencies for the restoration of the entire man, physical, mental, and spiritual. In planning for the establishment of sanitariums in places where God has designated we should do a special work, we are to allow no selfishness, no personal ambition to mar the work. Over and over again I have repeated that the establishment and maintenance of sanitariums is ordained of God for the advancement of His cause in the earth. While Christ was on this earth, He ministered to the needs of suffering humanity. He is our example. We are to labor intelligently; and in planning for the extension of Sanitarium work, we are to seek to secure the very places that God indicates are most suitable for carrying forward this line of our work.

In the providence of God, there come to His people, times of need, favorable opportunities to secure valuable facilities for the rapid advancement of the cause.

At times, the Lord has specified that we should come into possession of properties in certain localities where we needed to gain an entrance for the proclamation of the third angel's message. The idea that we are not to purchase any such properties, unless first the money is in hand, is not in accordance with the mind of God. Again and again, in years past, the Lord has tested our faith by opening the way for us to secure places possessing advantages, at a cost far below their real value, and at a time when we had no money. We have, at such times, met the situation by borrowing money on interest, and advancing in harmony with the {306} command of our divine Leader who made us advance in faith. These experiences have been attended with many perplexing problems, but the Lord has helped us through them all, and His name has been glorified. Had we hesitated, the precious cause would have been retarded rather than advanced, and, in many cases, opportunity would have been given our enemies to triumph over our failure to secure these advantages placed within our reach. In such matters as these, we are to learn to walk by faith, when necessary, as some have walked in the past.

Light has been given that it is best to establish our sanitariums outside the cities. Some of our physicians have spoken in favor of locating our sanitariums in the cities. It is difficult to understand why anyone should plan to establish a large sanitarium in a city. The very atmosphere of the cities is objectionable. We must conduct our sanitarium work in places suitable for the recovery of the sick. The more attractive the surroundings, the better. In the gardens of nature, the sick rapidly find something to please. Their thoughts are uplifted to the Creator. Let us thank God that so many of our sanitariums are established in pleasing country locations, and yet within easy reach of important centers of population where there are many people to whom we are to communicate a knowledge of saving truth.

It is the favorable situation of the property, that makes Loma Linda an ideal place for the recovery of the sick, and for the warning of many who might otherwise never hear the truth for this time. It is God's plan that Loma Linda shall be not only a sanitarium, but a special center for the training of gospel medical missionary evangelists.

ELDER J. A. BURDEN

April 27, 1910
Sanitarium, California
(B.-60-'10)

Dear Brother:

I WISH TO EXPRESS TO YOU some thoughts that should be kept before the sanitarium workers. That which will make them a power for good is the knowledge that the great Medical Missionary has chosen them to this work, that He is their chief instructor, and that it is ever their duty to recognize Him as their Teacher.

The Lord has shown us the evil of depending upon the strength of earthly organizations. He has instructed us that the commission of the medical missionary is received from the very highest authority; He would have us understand that it is a mistake to regard as most essential the education given by physicians who reject the authority of Christ, the greatest Physician who ever lived upon the earth. We are not to accept and follow the {307} views of men who refuse to recognize God as their teacher, but who learn of men, and are guided by man-made laws and restrictions.

During the night of April 26, many things were opened before me. I was shown that now in a special sense we as a people are to be guided by divine instruction. Those fitting themselves for medical missionary work should fear to place themselves under the direction of worldly doctors, to imbibe their sentiments and peculiar prejudices, and to learn to express their ideas and views. They are not to depend for their influence upon worldly teachers. They should be "looking unto Jesus, the author and finisher of our faith."

The Lord has instructed us that in our institutions of education, we should ever be striving for the perfection of character to be found in the life of Christ, and in His instruction to his disciples. Having received our commission from the highest authority, we are to educate, educate, educate, in the simplicity of Christ. Our aim must be to reach the highest standard in every feature of our work. He who healed thousands with a touch and a word is our Physicians. The precious truths contained in His teachings are to be our front guard and our reward.

The standard set for our sanitariums and schools is a high one, and a great responsibility rests upon the physicians and teachers connected with these institutions. Efforts should be made to secure teachers who will instruct after Christ's manner of teaching, regarding this of more value than any human methods. Let them honor the educational standards established by Christ, and following His instruction give their students lessons in faith and in holiness.

Christ was sent of the Father to represent His character and will. Let us follow His example in laboring to reach the people where they are. Teachers who are not particular to harmonize with the teachings of Christ, and who follow the customs and practices of worldly physicians, are out of line with the charge that the Saviour has given us.

It is not necessary that our medical missionaries follow the precise track marked out by medical men of the world. They do not need to administer drugs to the sick. They do not need to follow the drug medication in order to have influence in their work. The message was given me that if they would consecrate themselves to the Lord, if they would seek to obtain under men ordained of God, a thorough knowledge of their work, the Lord would make them skillful. Connected with the divine Teacher, they will understand that their dependence is upon God and not upon the professedly wise men of the world.

Some of our medical missionaries have supposed that a medical training according to the plans of worldly schools is essential to their success. To those who have thought that the only way to success is by being taught by worldly men, and by pursuing a course that is sanctioned by worldly men, I would now say, {308} Put away such ideas. This is a mistake that should be corrected. It is a dangerous thing to catch the spirit of the world; the popularity which such a course invites, will bring into the work a spirit which the word of God cannot sanction. The medical missionary who would become efficient, if he will search his own heart and consecrate himself to Christ, may by diligent study and faithful service, learn how to grasp the mysteries of his sacred calling.

At Loma Linda, at Washington, at Wahroonga, Australia, and in many other sanitariums established for the promulgation of the work of the third angel's message, there are to come to the physicians and to the teachers new ideas, a new understanding of the principles that must govern the medical work. An education is to be given that is altogether in harmony with the teachings of the word of God.

In the first chapter of Ephesians, beginning with verse 2, we read: "Grace be unto you, and peace, from God our Father, and from the Lord Jesus Christ. Blessed be the God and Father of our Lord Jesus Christ, who hath blessed us with all spiritual blessings in heavenly places in Christ: according as he hath chosen us in Him before the foundation of the world, that we should be holy and without blame before Him in love: having predestinated us unto the adoption of children by Jesus Christ to Himself, according to the good pleasure of His will, to the praise of the glory of His grace, wherein he hath made us accepted in the beloved. In whom we have redemption through His blood, the forgiveness of sins, according to the riches of His grace, wherein He hath abounded toward us in all wisdom and prudence; having made known unto us the mystery of His will, according to His good pleasure which He hath purposed in Himself." Study the whole of this chapter, and grasp the assurances that are given again and again for your acceptance.

It is a lack of faith in the power of God that leads our physicians to lean so much upon the arm of the law, and to trust so much to the influence of worldly powers. The truly converted man and woman who will study these words of inspiration spoken by the apostle Paul may learn to claim in all their depths and fullness the divine promises.

I am charged to present these scriptures to our people, that they may understand that those who do not believe the word of God cannot possibly present to those who desire to become acceptable medical missionaries, the way by which they will become most successful. Christ was the greatest physician the world has ever known; His heart was ever touched with human woe. He has a work for those to do who will not place their dependence upon worldly powers.

God's true commandment-keeping people will be instructed by Him. The true medical missionary will be wise in the {309} treatment of the sick, using the remedies that Nature provides. And then he will look to Christ as the true Healer of disease. The principles of health reform brought into the life of the patient, the use of nature's remedies, and the cooperation of divine agencies in behalf of the suffering, will bring success.

Satan will try to place barriers in the way of the true medical missionary. He will seek to bring discouragement upon those who recognize the commandments of God, and are determined to obey them. We must be careful not to carry our views of health reform to extremes, thus making it "health deform." Our food should be plain and free from all objectionable elements, but let us be careful that it is always palatable and good.

A time will come when medical missionaries of other denominations will become jealous and envious of the influence exerted by Seventh-day Adventists who are working in these lines. They will feel that influence is being secured by our workers which they ought to have. We should have in various places, men of extraordinary ability, who have obtained their diplomas in medical schools of the best reputation, who can stand before the world as fully qualified and legally recognized physicians. Let God-fearing men be wisely chosen to go through the training essential in order to obtain such qualifications. They should be prudent men who will remain true to the principles of the message.

These should obtain the qualifications, and the authority to conduct an educational work for our young men and women who desire to be trained for medical missionary work.

Now while the world is favorable toward the teaching of the health reform principles, moves should be made to secure for our own physicians the privileges of imparting medical instruction to our young people who would otherwise be led to attend the worldly medical colleges. The time will come when it will be more difficult than it is now, to arrange for the training of our young people in medical missionary lines.

ELDER J. A. BURDEN

April 30, 1911
Sanitarium, California
(B. 20-1911)

Loma Linda, California

Dear Brother and Sister Burden:

ON WEDNESDAY EVENING we took the train at Los Angeles. We had good accommodations, and nothing in particular transpired to cause any unpleasantness. It was a very long {310} train of cars. We had a good lunch, and were all very comfortable.

My letter must be a short one, as my head is easily wearied. As soon as I begin to use it, I am troubled with disagreeable pains. I have not yet recovered from the severe affliction I suffered at Glendale. After our trip to Fernando my heart and arm were seriously painful. Sara gave me most thorough treatment, and after a long time relief came. I was urged to visit Long Beach, to see how they were situated, in the work there; but I was in such pain that I had to refuse. I dared not venture to go.

In the afternoon of the day that we left for home, Elder Andross took us in an automobile to visit the several churches and the Bible workers' home in Los Angeles. We did not get out of the conveyance, but stopped and spoke to some of those engaged in the work. It was a very pleasant trip, and I was very glad to see so much of the work in Los Angeles. The automobile was an easy-riding machine that did not jolt me, so I was spared any increased suffering.

We reached home in safety, and on Friday I got relief from the pain I had endured for two days and nights. I felt that the Lord had blessed me; and on the next day, Sabbath, I consented to speak in the Sanitarium chapel. I was surprised to meet so large a congregation there, and was thankful for the opportunity of speaking to them.

My mind is settled in regard to the purchase of the land in front of the Loma Linda Sanitarium. We must have that piece of land. I will pledge myself to be depended upon for one thousand dollars. I hope to be favored with an opportunity to hire some money soon; but I shall not worry in regard to this, or I shall not be able to do anything. The effort of speaking on Sabbath and of reading my letters today is all I have been able to do to the present time. But as soon as I can I will make some movement concerning the raising of the one thousand dollars. The piece of land we must have; for it will never do to have buildings crowded in there. Do not fail to carry through the purchase of it. Do your best, and I will do my best. The money from me you may depend upon. We shall be able to send it soon.

J. A. BURDEN

May 18, 1911
Sanitarium, California
(B. 18, 1911)

I WISH TO SAY TO Elder Burden that the money which I pledged to help purchase the eighty-five acres will be sent without fail. Please let me know if a couple of weeks delay will trouble you seriously. I am truly glad that I gave my promise to help to purchase this land, under the influence {311} of the Spirit of God. I felt that the land must be secured; otherwise that we should have reason to regret that we did not obtain it.

DR. D. H. KRESS

June 5, 1911
Sanitarium, California
(K. 32-1911)

IREALIZE THAT A PLACE LIKE Loma Linda needs experienced men and women to conduct the work in its different departments. But the Lord is willing to work with all who will commit their ways to Him, and who will be led by the Holy Spirit. All are to be workers with Christ. He commits to His true followers the power of persuasion, the power of His grace and truth, a deep and constant love for His work in home and foreign fields. He gives them hearts that are in earnest and gathering with Christ. With helpers possessing such gifts as these, the medical missionary work cannot be without fruit.

The power of persuasion is a wonderful gift. It means much to those who would win souls to Christ. Let us keep our souls in the love of God. If Christ is working with His messengers, fruit will be seen as the result of their efforts.

ELDER J. A. BURDEN

June 7, 1911
Sanitarium, California
(B. 34-1911)
Loma Linda, California
Dear Brother and Sister Burden:

IWANT TO SAY TO YOU BOTH that I am thankful I was moved to speak as I did concerning the piece of land in front of the Loma Linda Sanitarium. I was urged by the Spirit of God to make the pledge of one thousand dollars; and I did so hoping that others, who were better able to give than I, would follow my example. I dared not leave the meeting without following the conviction I had; and now I feel that I have done my duty, showing my faith by my works.

I am glad that we were able to send you a part of the first payment a few days ago.

I would like to inquire what progress has been made in the raising of the means for the purchase of the land. My investment was not made in order to lessen the responsibility {312} of others who should help. Do what you can to encourage those who have money that they can use in the cause, to use it wisely and not let it slip away into speculation. Secure pledges from those who have not the money in sight. We need special wisdom to move out at the right time. I thank the Lord that He encouraged me to walk by faith, and I pray that He will help you to show others their privilege in this matter.

True faith is the substance of things hoped for, the evidence of things not seen. Thus far the Lord has led us as we have moved under the guidance of His Spirit. He will continue to work for us if we are careful to follow the counsel He gives.

Medical missionary work is the pioneer work of the gospel, Let us seek to understand the scope of the work to be done in our sanitariums for the saving of the souls and the healing of the bodies of those who come to us for relief. My soul is drawn out to encourage men and women to see in Christ the great Physician. If they will be drawn to Him, He will be their helper. He understands their every need. He stands ready to heal both body and soul. Let physicians and nurses learn to tell of the One who has power and who is willing to do a marvelous work for human beings. Talk of His love, tell of His power to save every sinful soul who will cast himself upon Christ's merits. His power will save to the uttermost all who truly accept Him.

I am glad that your wife is wholeheartedly united with you in the work. Let her stand by you to give help and encouragement.

I have written to you the instruction that has been given me regarding the special work to be done by the lady physicians in our sanitariums. It is the Lord's plan that men shall be trained to treat men, and the women trained to treat women. In the confinement of women, midwives should take the responsibility of the case. In Bible times it was not considered a proper thing for men to act in this capacity; and it is not the will of God that men should do this work today. Very much evil has resulted from the practice of men treating women, and women treating men. It is a practice according to human devising; and not according to God's plan. Long has the evil been left to grow, but now we lift our voice in protest against that which is displeasing to God.

REGARDING THE PURCHASE OF LAND ADJOINING LOMA LINDA

(MS.-13-1911)

LOMA LINDA IS AN important center. We needed this place and all its advantages. We were successful in obtaining it, and we have had success in operating it, notwithstanding the opposition shown by some who should have been acting as {313} helpers in the effort to equip the sanitarium properly. I have a deep interest in Loma Linda. It is a beautiful place. For sanitarium work, we could not have a more favorable situation. And it is well adapted for the other lines of work that we desire to see done there.

Recently the question arose about securing some more of the nearby land that is for sale. One piece, a tract of 86 acres, has already been purchased, and there is another of 47 acres joining the Loma Linda property, which is now for sale. Because this piece of land is so near to our Loma Linda buildings, we do not want to see it sold to outsiders, who will divide it up, and sell it to those who may desire to crowd into this neighborhood. In the night season I was talking to our brethren, telling them that this must not be allowed, and pointing out what unfavorable results would follow. If this piece of land should be purchased by outsiders, and divided up and sold to those who would be no help to our work, the injury to Loma Linda would be serious and lasting. I cannot bear the thought of this. Cannot a group of individuals who are alive to the vital interests of the Lord's work, unite together and make this land our property? Then if we wish to sell a portion of it, let it be sold to our people. There is an orange orchard on the place, and this could be handled to advantage by the sanitarium. The institution is hardly complete without the control of this orchard.

As the number of patients and students increases, more land will be needed. Grape vines could be planted, thus making it possible for the institution to produce its grapes.

Families and institutions should learn to do more in the cultivation and improvement of land. If people only knew the value of the products of the ground, which the earth brings forth in their season, more diligent efforts would be made to cultivate the soil. All should be acquainted with the special value of fruit and vegetables fresh from the orchard and garden.

Will not some of our brethren who thus far have invested but little in Loma Linda, help the Lord's cause by assisting in the purchase of this piece of land? I place this matter before you, feeling sure that you will not allow the land to pass into the hands of unbelievers. We ought not to place ourselves where we shall become unfavorably associated with those who could make it hard for us if they chose to do so, and restrict us to certain limits.

We must have room to keep ourselves distinct as a Sabbath keeping people. The Lord has given directions that we are to make provision which will prevent our being harassed and inconvenienced by having to crowd in with unbelievers. I wish I might make on your minds the impression that has been made on mind regarding this matter.

If a portion of this land must be sold, we can sell it {314} to the friends of the institution.

(Stamp) Ellen G. White

ELDER S. N. HASKELL

September 28, 1911
Sanitarium, California
(H. 78-1911)

I HAVE MADE SOME INVESTMENTS for Loma Linda to enable that institution to secure land adjoining the sanitarium that was for sale. Had this land been sold to unbelievers, and they had crowded in, the institution would have been placed at a disadvantage. I felt that we could not afford to run this risk. The land is now purchased, and to that extent we are safe from elements that might work trouble and confusion to our medical school. I could not rest until I had the assurance that we were safe from this possibility. This purchase may mean the keeping away from the institution a class of people who might have proved burdensome. Now that we have this land a burden is rolled off my heart.

UNION WITH CHRIST

December 11, 1904
Talk given at Riverside [California]

CHRIST HAD BEEN GIVING his disciples the instruction contained in the fourteenth chapter of John. Then he led them from the upper chamber out through the city to the Mount of Olives. On their way they passed a beautiful vine, and the disciples charmed with its loveliness, called the Saviour's attention to it. As they looked upon it, Christ said, "I am the true vine, and my Father is the husbandman. Every branch in me that beareth not fruit, he taketh away; and every branch that beareth fruit, he purgeth it, that it may bring forth more fruit."

God allows trouble to come upon us, that he may test and try us. The pruning will cause pain, but it is God who applies the knife. The divine husbandman prunes away the harmful growth, that the fruit may be richer and more abundant.

"Abide in me, and I in you. As the branch cannot bear fruit of itself, except it abide in the vine, no more can ye, except ye abide in me. I am the vine, ye are the branches. He that abideth in me, and I in him, the same bringeth forth much fruit; for without me ye can do nothing."

"Abide in me, and I in you." How are we to abide in Christ? By a daily, hourly faith. We are not safe in any other position. A man may have his name on the church books, {315} and make a high profession, but this avails nothing unless he has a living connection with Christ, unless his spirit, his words, his deportment, his business transactions with believers and unbelievers, reveal the virtues that come from such a union. A man who is thus united with Christ has a living faith, which takes hold upon divine power; and he is enabled to escape the corruption that is in the world through lust.

"If a man abide not in me, he is cast forth as a branch, and is withered; and men gather them and cast them into the fire and they are burned. If ye abide in me, and my words abide in you, ye shall ask what ye will, and it shall be done unto you."

In thought, word, and deed show that you are abiding in Christ. Let your speech reveal this. Speech is a precious talent. Our words are to be words that God and the holy angels can hear with approval. Our minds are to be storehouses filled with the treasures of the Bible. Let the walls of memory's hall be hung with the treasures of God's word, with his precious promises. Store up these promises, that in time of need you may be able to give them to the weary and heavy laden. You are God's missionary just as soon as you take your stand under his banner. You are to be a laborer together with him.

"Herein is my Father glorified, that ye bear much fruit; so shall ye be my disciples." What is the fruit that ye are to bear?—The fruit of the Spirit,—"Love, joy, peace, longsuffering, gentleness, goodness, faith, meekness, temperance."

"As the Father hath loved me, so have I loved you; continue ye in my love. If ye keep my commandments, ye shall abide in my love, even as I have kept my Father's commandments, and abide in his love." He keeps us in connection with him as he is in connection with the Father. What possibil-

ities, what strength, there are in that promise! Why do we not believe it? If there are hindrances in our way, and if we meet with difficulties, let us not give up in despair, but keep fast hold of the promises.

"These things I have spoken unto you,"—That you may be sad and discouraged, refusing to believe that you can live the Christian life? No. "These things have I spoken unto you, that my joy might remain in you, and that your joy might be full."

Although you may be in trouble, you can go forward with confidence. Knowing that you have an abiding Christ. He tells those who are in trouble and perplexity to bring their burdens to him. He does not tell them to go to their neighbors and talk the matter over. To those who are weary and heavy laden, he says, "Come unto me, and I will give you rest." "Take my yoke upon you, and learn of me; for I am meek and lowly in heart, and ye shall find rest unto {316} your souls. For my yoke is easy, and my burden is light."

Do not wear a yoke of human manufacture; such yokes are heavy and galling. When we learn Christ's meekness and lowliness, and lay our burdens upon him, rest will come to us. He is ever ready to help us. The Lord is more willing to give the Holy Spirit to those that ask him than parents are to give good gifts unto their children. How full, how broad, this statement!

But often we take ourselves in our own hands, thinking that we can arrange matters in a way that will bring us peace and rest. Do we succeed? No. We get into more trouble than before. When things arise to perplex our minds, we fret and worry, and begin to accuse others, and to find fault with them. What ought we to do? Christ tells us. "Verily, verily, I say unto you," He declares, "except ye eat the flesh and drink the blood of the Son of man, ye have no life in you. Whoso eateth my flesh and drinketh my blood, hath eternal life; and I will raise him up at the last day. For My flesh is meat indeed, and My blood is drink indeed. He that eateth My flesh and drinketh My blood, dwelleth in Me and I in him. As the living Father hath sent Me, and I live by the Father, so he that eateth Me, even he shall live by Me." "It is the Spirit that quickeneth; the flesh profiteth nothing; the words that I speak unto you, they are spirit and they are life." These words are clearly explained in John 5:24; "Verily, verily, I say unto you, He that heareth My word, and believeth on Him that sent Me, hath everlasting life, and he shall not come into condemnation; but is passed from death unto life."

Do not talk of the faults of others. Take care of your own garden. See that your own heart is cleansed by the power of God. When trouble comes, instead of getting out of patience instead of fretting and worrying, go to the Lord, and tell Him all about it. Has He not said, "Ask, and it shall be given unto you; seek, and ye shall find; knock, and it shall be opened unto you?" Go right to the Lord, and in humility of mind, tell him about your trouble. Do not go to human friends; for they have all the burdens they can bear. Go to the One who gave his life for you. You have been bought with a price; therefore glorify God in your body, and in your spirit, which are his. Do not walk in self-sufficiency, thinking that you are capable of guiding yourself aright. "Learn of me," Christ says, "For I am meek and lowly in heart."

Kneel before the Lord, and ask him to be a help to you. Tell him your heart is burdened, and ask him to remove the load. Night after night I have told him this, when for hours I have been unable to sleep, because of the thought of what must be done here and elsewhere to lead our people to realize the glorious probabilities and possibilities before those who engage wholeheartedly in the Lord's work, and to get them to take up this load.

"Then answered Jesus and said unto them, Verily, verily, {317} I say unto you, the Son can do nothing of himself, but what he seeth the Father do: for what things soever he doeth, these also doeth the Son likewise. For the Father loveth the Son, and showeth him all things that himself doeth; and he will show him greater works than these, that ye may marvel. For the Father raiseth up the dead, and quickeneth them, even so the Son quickeneth whom he will. For the Father judgeth no man, but hath committed all judgment to the Son; That all men should honor the Son, even as they honor the Father. He that honoreth not the Son honoreth not the Father which hath sent him."

Do not think that by placing your burdens on others, you can find relief. Come right to the Burden-bearer, and tell him about them. Believe that he is able and willing to meet the circumstances of your case. When in contrition you come to the foot of the cross, when you have faith in the merits of a crucified and risen Saviour,

you will receive power through him. As you cast your helpless soul upon him, he gives you peace and joy and strength and courage. Then you are able to tell someone else how precious Christ is to you. You can say, "I sought him, and found him precious to my soul."

"Ye shall find rest." How? By living experience. Because God's yoke is a yoke of patience and gentleness and long-suffering. He, the Prince of the heavenly host, humbled himself. He took upon himself human nature, and stood at the head of humanity that he might teach fallen man how to be a partaker of the divine nature. Those who learn his meekness and lowliness learn also how to love one another as he has loved them. They will reach the place where they refuse to criticize and condemn others. They learn that there is committed to them a work that no one else can do for them, the work of learning of Christ. When we place ourselves in his hands, he shows us the possibilities and probabilities before us, and bids go for help to One infinitely higher than erring human beings.

Christ is our efficiency. How do I know this? I know it by experience. For a while, many years, ago, I was in despair. Then I cast myself on the mercy and love of the Saviour, and his power came upon me. At one time those who were working over me thought me dead. But all at once I raised my voice in prayer. The power of God was upon me all night long, and henceforth I understood that I must look to Christ, and not to any human being for relief. I had been praying and praying for help, and all the time my Saviour was by my side, waiting for me to recognize him as my sufficiency, my strength, my grace. I learned the lesson, and after that, when I kneeled down to pray, I believed that I would receive an answer, whether I felt as if I would or not. Feeling is not to be our guide. Feeling is not faith, but it is as widely separated from faith as the east is from the west.

Why should we have a question as to whether we shall receive the promised blessing? God does not alter the word that has gone forth out of his mouth. When we trust in {318} him, our hearts will be filled with peace and joy. When irritating words are spoken to us, we do not retaliate, but, when opportunity offers, we tell how good the Lord is, and what he is willing to do for those who trust in him.

God wants every one of us to come to him as little children come to their parents.

He wants us to ask him in faith, nothing doubting, for grace to supply our needs. "If any of you lack wisdom, let him ask of God, that giveth to all men liberally, and upbraideth not; and it shall be given him."

We are God's little children, but let us not forget that he expects us to grow up to the full stature of men and women in Christ. Let us talk of God's goodness and tell of his power, putting away gloom and unbelief. Let us talk faith. God wants us to be strong in his strength. He died to save us, and he wants us to reach the high standard that he holds before us.

We are not to stand still in the Christian life. There is an advancement for us to make. We are to lay hold of him who has all power, remembering that every hour, every moment, we need his help. We are to be always ready to speak to others in regard to the grace and the saving power of our Lord Jesus Christ. It is the privilege of everyone to grow in grace, daily reaching higher attainments in the Christian life.

Oh, how I wish that we would honor Christ by realizing what he wants to do for us, and taking him at his word. If we would do this, we should be sunshiny Christians. By beholding Christ, we would be changed into his likeness. But we shall never grow in grace by beholding the faults and mistakes and defects of someone else. Instead, we will become spiritually dwarfed and enfeebled. Let us keep looking to Christ, thinking of what he has done for us and of what he has promised to do. Thus we shall be changed into his likeness. This is true religion. In the future we shall have to contend with difficulties tenfold greater than any we have yet had. Do you ask why I say this? Do you not realize that his time is short? He is working and planning with intensity of effort to place obstacles in the way of God's people, and to hinder their progress. We have the powers of darkness to meet. At this time, more than ever before, willing, unquestioning, obedience is needed, if we come off conquerors.

"This is my commandment, That ye love one another, as I have loved you." My dear friends, for Christ's sake take your stand on higher ground. Every feature of our faith is to be tested in the way that is the most trying. The pillars of our faith are to be tested. Sophistry will be brought in as it was to Adam and Eve. You will be strongly tempted, and unless you have firm faith in the principles of the truth for this time, you will be led astray. Look to Christ as your helper. Take him into your {319} heart as an abiding friend. As you do this, his blessing will rest upon you in large measure. You will be kept by the power of God. The enemy will not be able to lead you to swerve from your allegiance.

My dear friends, I want to ask you in conclusion to do what you can to help in the establishment of Glendale Sanitarium. You may have to make sacrifice in order to respond to this call, but God will richly bless you in so doing. Those who have the work in hand are doing their best, but they are in great need of funds. This institution must be furnished. First give yourselves to the Lord, and then bring your offerings to him. We want to see the Glendale Sanitarium put in working order, so that the sick who come for treatment may hear the truth. Often we meet those who first heard and became interested in the truth while at one of our sanitariums, and who have been keeping the Sabbath ever since.

(Stamped) Ellen G. White

Dear Brethren Palmer and Ballenger

February 20, 1905
Elmshaven, Sanitarium, California
(P.-75- 1905)

WE ARE WELL PLEASED WITH the reports that Brother Ballenger has sent us of the work of the Paradise Valley Sanitarium. What we see being accomplished there is a fulfillment of what I have been instructed we might expect. For this we thank the Lord, and take courage for the future, believing that the Lord will bless and guide.

The patronage you are receiving, even before you are fully prepared to accommodate patients, has exceeded my expectations. The Lord has been good to us, and we must ever bear in mind that this sanitarium is to be made a means of communicating truth to those who know it not.

Treatment rooms should be fitted up soon. Let them be, as we suggested when we were there, outside the main building. Were they inside the sanitarium, the steam from them would make an unhealthful atmosphere, which would pervade the rooms of the patients. Let us take every precaution to make everything connected with the Paradise Valley Sanitarium, healthful and wholesome.

We are made sad as we see in many places so much left undone that should be done. But the Lord will use in the accomplishment of His work means that we do not now see. He will raise up from among the common people, men and women to do His work, even as of old He called fishermen to be his disciples. There will soon be an awakening that will surprise many. Those who do not realize the necessity {320} of what is to be done, will be passed by, and the heavenly messengers will work with those who are called the common people, fitting them to carry the truth to many places. Now is the time for us to awake and do what we can.

I have received a letter from Brother Burrill of Canada, in which he speaks of the Sunday question that is soon to be met there. He says that they especially need Brother Robinson to help them in meeting this issue. He is a native-born Canadian, and can be a great help to them at this time.

Brother Burrill has written to me because he understood that I had encouraged Brother Robinson to come to San Diego. At first I could remember nothing in regard to the matter. But after I received Brother Ballenger's letter stating that Brother Robinson was expected in San Diego soon to act as business manager of the Sanitarium, I remembered that Brother Robinson was one whose name had been mentioned in some of our councils. I think he was presented as one who was not well, and who needed a change of climate. I asked if he were qualified to act as manager. When it was stated that he seemed to have the qualifications necessary for the place, I think I said, "Then by all means let him come." But I did not present this as light that had been given me by the Lord. It was merely my personal judgment, formed from your presentation of the case.

Brother Burrill also stated that Elder W. W. Simpson is a Canadian, and that such men as he are needed in Canada. He seemed to think that it is not right that Elder Simpson should be held in Los Angeles. I know nothing in regard to Elder Simpson's case, except that he has been used by the Lord in His work in Los Angeles, and that he has been greatly blessed. Over one hundred have taken their stand for the truth as a result of his labors. At the close of his last series of tent meetings he thought of changing his field of labor, but he received a petition signed by many of the citizens of Los Angeles, asking him to remain and continue his meetings. The Lord has given Brother Simpson a spirit of adaptability, with wisdom to plan and carry out his work, and He has blessed him in the bringing out of leaflets, notices, and charts that have aroused the interest of the people.

I would say, Let Brother Simpson labor where his message is evidently accomplishing great good. Those who have come to his meetings have given freely of their means to sustain the work that he has carried forward. At this time, when there is such urgent need of workers in Los Angeles, when the brethren are {321} seeking to establish a sanitarium there, I dare not say to Elder Simpson, You must go back to Canada. And besides, such a move might not be best for his health. For the present let him remain in Los Angeles; for the Lord is giving him marked success in bearing the message to the people. Let him give the trumpet a certain sound, arousing those who have never heard the truth. May the Lord encourage him to remain in Los Angeles until the church members are aroused to gird on the armor, and show that they have a burden to give the message. Our ministers are not to hover over the churches. They are to proclaim the truth, as Elder Simpson is doing. Let those who know not the truth be given as opportunity to hear the reasons of our faith.

I believe that Brother Simpson is presenting the truth as God would have many others present it. Some of the brethren in Los Angeles felt that he should do more in the church there. When this was suggested to me, I thought of the answer that Christ gave when the priests and rulers reproached Him for eating with publicans and sinners. "I came not to call the righteous, but sinners to repentance," he declared. Let the work now being accomplished for those who have never before heard the truth, lead our ministers and church members in Los Angeles to arouse. Let them take hold, as they see that God is working. Let them make diligent work in repenting of their coldness and indifference and selfishness. As the church is by repentance cleansed from this neglect, and the members are converted, they will heartily engage in laboring from house to house. By teaching those who are seeking for the light of truth, they themselves will receive a valuable education.

Let no one, by precept or example, seek to draw Elder Simpson from his God-appointed work. Let all take hold with him in an effort to carry the work in clear lines. The members of the Los Angeles church need to heed every message that comes to them bidding them arouse from their stupor. If they will earnestly seek the Lord, he will give them light and life, and the quickening power of the Holy Spirit.

The message that I have to bear to the church in Los Angeles is, Awake, and put on the whole armor of God. There is selfishness in the church that must be rooted out.

[The Next Page is Missing in Manuscript] {322}

. . . . bring the truth before unbelievers.

Let the older members be an example to those who have recently come into the truth. I entreat those who have been long in the truth not to hurt the new converts by living irreligious lives. Lay aside all murmuring, and do thorough work in your own hearts. Break up the fallow ground of your hearts, and seek to know what you can do to advance the work in Los Angeles.

Temptations are being brought in by men who have been long in the truth. The truths that we received in 1841, '42, '43, and '44 are now to be studied and proclaimed. The messages of the first, second, and third angels will in the future be proclaimed with a loud voice. They will be given with earnest determination and in the power of the Spirit.

The members of the Los Angeles church need to have a deep work of grace done in their own hearts. Let everyone build over against his own house. The messages given by Elder Simpson, which convert sinners, should be sufficient to arouse you also. Awake, awake, and give to the unconverted evidence that you believe the truth of heavenly origin. Unless you do awake, the world will not believe that you practice the truth that you profess to hold.

Pray earnestly. Read and study the prayer of Christ, as given in the seventeenth chapter of John, and then seek to live lives that will answer that prayer. Read also the messages given in the third chapter of Revelation. God sent his angel from heaven to give these messages. The message to the Laodicean church belongs to the church in Los Angeles, and to our churches generally. Will they arouse, and do the work that God has given them to do?

Dear Brother Ballenger

February 26, 1905
Elmshaven, Sanitarium, California

I RECEIVED YOUR LETTER ON Friday, and we feel deep sympathy with you in your emergency. I wish that Sister Hall could spend some time with you, but she is under engagement to leave us in two or three weeks to stay with her relatives for a while.

I have been trying to think of someone who could go to your assistance. But we do not know exactly what you want. Sister Hall has been telling me of a friend of hers, a Miss Webber, who worked with her for a time in {323} the Battle Creek Sanitarium. Miss Webber has had a long experience in sanitarium work, and has diplomas from two schools at least. She is thorough in all that she does, and is as firm as a rock to duty and principle. I think she would answer your purpose. She would come to California if we asked her to.

But even though we should decide to send for Miss Webber, I suppose it would be necessary to get someone to fill the place till she could get here. If necessary I could spare my matron, Mrs. Nelson, who is an excellent cook and caretaker, and who has taken part of the nurses' course in Battle Creek.

I have asked Mrs. Ings to consider the matter, and see if there is any one at the Sanitarium here who could fill the bill. I could barely mention the matter to her, as it was Sabbath, and I had only a few minutes in which to talk with her before going to the Chapel to speak. I asked her to report to me after the Sabbath, and I shall doubtless hear from her soon.

Please let me know whether you have any one in mind who could fill the vacancy. Of course, you will stand by, and your wife might be able to help until we can make other arrangements. Perhaps Sister Howard could come in for a while, until a suitable matron could be found.

I can think of no one more competent than Miss Webber. I know her to be a faithful woman, one who will show a care for things indoors and out of doors. Sister Hall has just received a letter from her, saying that she will be coming to California in about two months.

Brother Ballenger, I am very desirous that the buildings and land that we designed to purchase shall not be allowed to pass into other hands. I think we ought to obtain this property, even if four thousand dollars are asked for it. If we had only purchased it before the rain came, what a good thing it would have been. We must ask the Lord so to arrange matters that we can obtain this property. We shall need every foot of the land.

I hope, Brother Ballenger, that when you see a suitable place in Redlands, which could be used as a sanitarium, offered for sale at a reasonable price, you will let us know about it. We shall need a sanitarium in Redlands. Unless we start an enterprise of this kind, others will. I understand that the property-owners are afraid that consumptives will come in, and thus the reputation of the place be spoiled. But, of course, we should make it clear that we were not going to establish a consumptives' home.

I merely mention this matter so that you and Brother {324} Burden may keep it in view. We shall not take any steps to establish a sanitarium in Redlands until we can be assured that we are doing the right thing. Brother Burden and you can visit the place from time to time, and see what openings there are. And in all that you do, be as wise as serpents and as harmless as doves.

Our sanitarium work is one of the most successful means of reaching such people as live in Redlands, and bringing the truth before them. We must educate, educate, educate, pleasantly and intelligently. We must preach the truth, pray the truth, and live the truth, bringing it, with its gracious, health-giving influences within the reach of those who know it not. As the sick are brought into touch with the Life-giver, their faculties of mind and body will be renewed. But in order for this to be, they must practice self-denial, and be temperate in all things. Thus only can they be saved from physical and spiritual death, and restored to health.

When the human machinery moves in harmony with the life-giving arrangements of God, as brought to light through the gospel, disease is overcome and health springs forth speedily. When human beings work in union with the life-giver, who offered up His life for them, happy thoughts fill the mind. Body and mind and soul are sanctified. Human beings learn of the great Teacher, and all upon which they look ennobles and enriches the thoughts. The affections are drawn out in gladness and thankfulness to the Creator. The life of the man who is renewed in the image of Christ is as a light shining in darkness.

Adam listened to the specious sophistry of Satan, and received it as truth. He had originally the wonderful gift of a sinless nature. But he listened to the falsehoods of the one who fell from his first estate. Satan exercised his hypnotism upon him, and Adam, listening to him, sinned, and thus opened the door through which the enemy could ever after gain access to human beings. Adam and Eve lost the spiritual life that would have been theirs by continual endowment.

Christ came to this world bearing a message freighted with redemption. To all who receive him as a personal Saviour he gives power to become the sons of God. "The Word was made flesh, and dwelt among us. . . full of grace and truth. . .And of his fullness have all we received, and grace for grace."

All who become the sons of God are possessed of his nature. They are the objects of his love and special affection. They dwell in Christ as Christ dwells in God. Knowing the power of his grace, they are commissioned and qualified to bear the message of salvation to a sinful world, to make known his grace and truth. As they consecrate themselves wholly to God, the grace {325} they impart will be continually renewed in increased measure. Converted to the truth, imbued with the Holy Spirit, they are under the transforming influence of divine grace. The life of self-indulgence they once lived has been changed to a life of service. They become sons of God, spiritual children, adopted into the Lord's family.

(Stamped) Ellen G. White

THE LOMA LINDA TRAINING SCHOOL

June 21, 1906
(Extract from "Review and Herald")

ONE OF THE CHIEF advantages of situation at Loma Linda is the pleasing variety of charming scenery on every side.

But more important than magnificent scenery and beautiful buildings and spacious grounds, is the close proximity of this institution to a densely populated district, and the opportunity thus afforded of communicating to many, many people a knowledge of the third angel's message. We are to have clear spiritual discernment, else we shall fail to understanding the opening providences of God that are preparing the way for us to enlighten the world. The great crisis is just before us. Now is the time for us to sound the warning message, by the agencies that God has given us for this purpose. Let us remember that one most important agency is our medical missionary work. Never are we to lose sight of the great object for which our

sanitariums are established, the advancement of God's closing work in the earth.

Loma Linda is to be not only a sanitarium, but an educational center. With the possession of this place comes the weighty responsibility of making the work of the institution educational in character. A school is to be established here for the training of gospel medical missionary evangelists.

Much is involved in this work, and it is very essential that a right beginning be made. The Lord has a special work to be done in this part of the field. He instructed me to call upon Elder and Mrs. S. N. Haskell to help us in getting properly started a work similar to that which they had carried on in Nashville and at Avondale. They came, and are now laboring with all the powers of their being to do a solid work. They conduct classes regularly in the institution, and have established a Bible training-school at San Bernardino, from which center is {326} extending an influence throughout this district. Prof. W. E. Howell and his wife have consented to unite with the forces at Loma Linda in an effort to develop the school that must be carried on there. As they go forward in faith, the Lord will go before the, preparing the way.

TO THE WORKERS IN THE GLENDALE SANITARIUM

March 14, 1905
Elmshaven, Sanitarium, California
(B. 97 1905)

WE ARE GLAD THAT notwithstanding some delay, the property at Glendale has been secured for a sanitarium. Years ago the Lord gave me instruction that there should be a sanitarium near the city of Los Angeles. Instruction was also given that we should find properties for sale on which there would be buildings suitable for sanitarium purposes, and that we might secure such properties at a very low cost. The location of the Glendale Sanitarium meets the representation given me of places God has reserved for us. The electric cars running close by the institution make access to it very convenient.

Let all connected with this sanitarium keep in mind the purpose for which this property has been secured. The institution is to act a special part in bringing souls to Christ, leading them to love God and keep His commandments. Unless the workers have a living connection with God, unless there is seen in the institution a spirit of kindness and compassion, establishment

of the sanitarium will have been in vain. Spiritual as well as physical healing is to be brought to those who come for healing.

Brother and Sister Burden, I am glad that you have a part in the work of the Glendale Sanitarium. May the Lord increase your wisdom and courage and faith. I am glad that Dr. Simpson and her husband can unite with you. You and Dr. Abbott and the other workers may do a precious work in letting the light of present truth shine forth in clear rays. Remember that you are doing a work for time and for eternity. You should have an ever-increasing faith in the promises of God's word. It is your privilege to seek wisdom and help from God. Come to the Saviour in humility, confessing your sins, and asking for strength and grace.

The Holy Spirit enlightens the mind of the one who depends on the merits of a crucified and risen Saviour, and indites a prayer of confession and repentance that is acceptable to the Lord. "We know not what we should pray for as we ought; but the Spirit itself maketh intercession for us, with groanings that cannot {327} be uttered," "He that searcheth the heart knoweth what is the mind of the Spirit, because he maketh intercession for the saints according to the will of God."

Let no man boast that he does not confess the sins that the Lord has pointed out to him. If he makes no confession, he receives not forgiveness and pardon from God. He must go forth in sorrow, to work in his own strength. The enemy finds him in this position, a subject to be deceived.

There are many, many of this class. May the Lord open their eyes, that they may see the danger of their self-sufficiency. A superficial work is always a snare to every professed Christian. Satan finds easy access to the heart of the one who is careless and slack in his experience, and beguiles him with seducing theories that will destroy his faith in God. "He that cometh to God must believe that He is, (as He has declared Himself in His personality) and that He is a rewarder of those who diligently seek Him."

In every sanitarium there must be kept before all in the institution the principles of true service. From the institution is to go forth light and knowledge. All connected with it are to act their part intelligently, as representatives of the truth for this time. It is that they may be trained to do true missionary work, that young people are brought to our sanitariums.

If you will co-operate with God, He will go before you, and the glory of the Lord will be your reward. Heavenly angels will break forth into singing as souls receive the great gift of God through Jesus Christ. You may assure the sick and afflicted that Christ is the great Healer. They may believe on Him, and trust in His word; for it will never fail.

"Thus saith the Lord, Keep ye judgment, and do justice; for My salvation is near to come, and My righteousness to be revealed. Blessed is the man that doeth this, and the son of man that layeth hold on it; that keepeth the Sabbath from polluting it, and keepeth his hand from doing any evil."

What a representation is here given! "My salvation is near to come,"—that great salvation wrought out for each soul through Jesus Christ, the salvation for which the prophets have inquired and searched diligently. Our Lord is soon to come to us in mercy and compassion and love. We must go forth to receive Him as a welcome guest.

The Lord Jesus calls upon everyone to become interestedly engaged in the work of becoming a channel of light through which the grace of Christ may flow. Jesus has said, "Ye are the light of the world. . . Let your light so shine before men that they may see your good {328} works, and glorify your Father which is in heaven." In the great salvation wrought through Jesus Christ, the unbelieving world is to be helped through the work of believers. In the work you do in the sanitarium, many may become convinced that you are indeed the children of God.

"Seek ye the Lord while He may be found, call ye upon Him while He is near: let the wicked forsake his way, and the unrighteous man his thoughts: and let him return unto the Lord, and He will have mercy upon him; and to our God, for He will abundantly pardon."

"For My thoughts are not your thoughts, neither are your ways My ways, saith the Lord, For as the heavens are higher than the earth, so are my ways higher than your ways, and My thoughts than your thoughts. For as the rain cometh down, and the snow from heaven, and returneth not thither, but watereth the earth, and maketh it bring forth and bud, that it may give seed to the sower, and bread to the eater; so shall My word be that goeth forth out of My mouth: it shall not return unto Me void, but it shall accomplish that which I please, and it shall prosper in the thing whereto I sent it."

All the promises of God's word are made on gospel terms. If we on our part will fulfill the conditions, if we will seek the Lord, while He may be found, we may claim the promise:

"For ye shall go out with joy, and be led forth with peace: the mountains and the hills shall break forth before you into singing, and all the trees of the field shall clap their hands. Instead of the thorn shall come up fir tree, and instead of the brier shall come up the myrtle tree: and it shall be to the Lord for a name, for an everlasting sign, that shall not be cut off."

Let this message be sounded to all people, Seek the Lord while He may be found. Seek Him against whom you have been in rebellion. Let us make every effort to check the seducing sentiments that would come into our ranks. Let every soul be wide-awake to close every avenue of the soul to the sophistry of Satan, as revealed in heaven and in Eden. Let us be armed with that vigilance that shall resist his enchantments.

ELDER DANIELLS AND PRESCOTT AND DR. HARE

February 15, 1904
Elmshaven, Sanitarium, California

My Dear Brethren:

THE INSTRUCTION THAT HAS been given me in regard to {329} the buildings to be erected in Washington is that it is not the Lord's will for an imposing display to be made. The buildings are to show, to believers and to those not of our faith, that not one dollar has been invested in needless display. Every part of the buildings is to bear witness that we realize that there is before us a great, unworked missionary field, and that the truth is to be established in many places.

If the buildings erected correspond to the truth that we are proclaiming, a telling influence will be exerted on minds. Actions speak louder than words. Say frankly, God has charged us not to invest a large amount of means in one place, and He has charged us also not to invest means in gratifying the desire for display. The principles that we are to follow in our work are exemplified in the life of Christ. He was the Majesty of heaven, and yet He worked at a carpenter's bench.

A few words more in regard to buildings. In reference to the question of building with wood, or brick, or stone, the instruction given me in the past is that brick buildings are not the most healthful, and that wooden buildings, while properly put up, are preferable to brick or stone buildings. And while we are under the keeping power of God, a wooden building is as safe from fire as a stone building.

In planning for the erection of the buildings that you propose to put up, do not follow the counsel of those who would invest means for the sake of display. Do not launch out into expensive investments. In laying plans for the sanitarium building, remember that this is to be a building for the sick and suffering. To those who plead for buildings of brick or stone, say, "We believe that the Lord is soon to come, and we cannot consent to launch out into the erection of expensive buildings." For years the erection of such buildings has borne the rebuke of God, but His warnings were not heeded, and at last He permitted His judgments to fall upon the Sanitarium and the publishing house in Battle Creek.

The buildings that you erect must be solid and well-constructed. No haphazard work is to be done. The buildings are to be thoroughly presentable, but no extravagance is to be seen. We are not to make it possible for worldlings to say that we do not believe what we preach—that the end of all things is at hand.

The buildings should be put up at as little cost as possible. No money is to be spent on them merely for show. We are living in a time of fearful depravity. The whole world has thrown off the restraints of religion. Worldlings and church members are making void the law of God. We are to bend every energy to the proclamation of the message of warning. {330}

There are many other places where memorials for God are to be established, many other places in which sanitarium work is to be started. In many countries gospel medical missionary work is to be done. God's agencies are to act their appointed part. In all that is done, in all the institutions that are established, the example of economy that Christ has set in His life is to be followed.

On no account is the course followed in the erection of the Boulder Sanitariums to be followed in the erection of the Washington Sanitarium. If this course were followed places in which sanitariums should be established, would be left destitute.

My brethren, in your work at the capital of the nation, let the principles of unselfishness revealed in Christ's life be carried out. Remember that in many other places, as well as in Washington, gospel medical missionary work is needed, to open doors for the entrance of the truth.

Ellen G. White

EXTRACTS FROM LETTER TO G. W. AMADON

September 19, 1906
Regarding Battle Creek

I WISH TO SAY TO YOU and to the leading men in the church: and to the trustees of the Tabernacle, that light has been given to me very distinctly that Elder A. T. Jones has taken a position that divorces him from the privileges of the use of the Tabernacle. He does not know what spirit is leading him. Efforts are being made in an underhand way to get possession of the Tabernacle.

Brethren, be on guard. Keep burnished for action the weapons of your warfare, which is the Word of God. Pray, believe, and walk humbly with God, and let all your prayers be without ceasing that God shall be glorified. Make a most earnest effort to call to Battle Creek the very best ministerial talent, men of experience in the early days of the message, men who will give the trumpet a certain sound. Hold the fort. Do not let it be taken by those who have placed themselves decidedly in a position of opposition to the truth which God has given us for these last days.

Our call is, Come out from among them and be ye separate; and the Tabernacle should be set apart decidedly to those who are true and loyal.

Those who have denied their faith, and who would now tear down that which is past years they have labored to build up, should understand that they have no lot nor {331} part in the faith that has firmly held the people of God in unity. You do not know how earnestly they will work to get possession of the Tabernacle. But this must not be permitted. In no case should a decidedly opposing element be permitted in the Tabernacle.

EXTRACTS FROM LETTER TO DR. AND MRS. KRESS

July 27, 1906
Regarding Battle Creek

I FEEL INTENSELY SORROWFUL when I see some of our brethren in Battle Creek taking a course that is leading them away from the truth: for I have had

a presentation of the first apostasy in the heavenly courts. The warnings of the Holy Spirit have been disregarded, and there has been persistent work of deception. A. T. Jones has permitted himself to be used as the voice of Dr. J. H. Kellogg.

It is our privilege to believe in a personal Father, who has made a gift of His only Begotten Son, that a fallen world might repent, and accept of a personal Saviour, and be permitted to eat of the leaves of the tree of life. Thank God, we may uplift the Saviour before the people, as had been done at these meetings. The work will advance more and more, as we humble our hearts, and bring our wills in submission to God. Some will place themselves under Satan's rule, but we will not fail nor become discouraged.

Brother Kress, I am thankful that you have not been deceived by the representations of Dr. Kellogg. At the Berrien Springs meeting, the Lord showed me what He was willing to do for Dr. Kellogg. The most blessed invitation was given to Him. But the doctor wrenched himself away from the outstretched hand of Christ. It seemed that in the agony of my soul I should die.

I have seen how Dr. Kellogg has united with the arch deceiver in using hypnotic influence upon souls to deceive them. Those who sustain him in his course are guilty with him of resisting the Spirit of God. Such blindness of understanding seems strange in one who has known the truth for this time.

A. T. Jones has a theory of the truth, as expressed in his books. He does not repudiate these, but he virtually goes back upon their teachings, by the course of action he is following.

Dr. Kellogg places himself before the world in the position of one who is greatly abused. He writes many letters, as he has to you, making such a representation as would call forth sympathy. But he is still at work with all subtlety. I have felt compelled to warn our people: for they do not understand his cunning. {332}

I have seen that the leaders in the medical work in Battle Creek will try to secure possession of the Tabernacle. Their scheming is so subtle, that I greatly fear that this may be accomplished.

If Dr. Kellogg can destroy the faith of any of our people in the testimonies, he will do it. He sometimes takes the nurses and others, sometimes alone in the night season, and talks with them for hours framing a tissue of falsehood, to make

them believe himself a much abused man. Some of these poor souls have heard the truth, and they wish to get out of Battle Creek. They realize that their safety consists in leaving the place where they are so deceived. The doctor will take advantage in every way to make an impression upon human minds in destroying all confidence in the testimonies. If we are not constantly on guard, he will destroy by his sophistries, if possible, the very elect. And those associates who have upheld him will have to answer before God for their individual course of action.

The messages of encouragement given to Dr. Kellogg have been many. They have been tender and true, but there have always been conditions involved. We might say much more than we do, but we do not wish to expose before the world the things we might say. But we should so far as possible overcome the impression that we sustain and honor one who follows such a course as has the doctor and his associates. Our only object in publishing any of those things has been to save some of our own people from being destroyed.

EXTRACTS FROM LETTER TO ELDER G. I. BUTLER

October 30, 1906

R ECENTLY I HAVE WRITTEN letters to different ones who are in danger of being misled by the deceptive influence that prevails at B. C. The disaffected ones will make every effort possible to secure the Tabernacle, and to gain other advantages by which to disseminate their wrong theories and carry forward their apostasies. But the Lord lives and reigns. I am writing out the cautions He gives me. I will not give up. I must relieve my soul of its burden. It may be that I shall have to visit Battle Creek.

I have been pleading with the Lord to help His people on every point: for He alone can control the elements of wickedness in B. C. He will shortly bring something to pass. What a privilege it is to be able to bring our perplexities to the Lord in prayer. He has invited us to do this, and why should we not avail ourselves of this privilege. "Ask, and it shall be given you: seek and ye shall find: knock and it shall be opened unto you." We need much more faith and much more earnest prayer. We need to humble our hearts before God, and put all selfishness out of the way. We must have that strength, that wisdom

{333} that cometh from our Lord and Saviour Jesus Christ. With the hand of faith we must grasp the hand of infinite power, and hold on believing with the whole heart the promises God has made. Our will and way are to be submerged in the Lord's will and way. Self must surrender not to discouragement, though difficulties be piled mountain high, but to God.

AN ADDRESS IN REGARD TO THE SUNDAY MOVEMENT

December 24, 1889
(R. & H. Extra)

Dear Brethren and Sisters:

I HAVE BEEN MUCH BURDENED in regard to movements that are now in progress for the enforcement of Sunday observance. It has been shown to me that Satan has been working earnestly to carry out his designs to restrict religious liberty. Plans of serious import to the people of God are advancing in an underhand manner among the clergymen of various denominations, and the object of this covert maneuvering is to win popular favor for the enforcement of Sunday sacredness. If the people can be led to favor a Sunday law, then the clergy intend to exert their united influence to obtain a religious amendment to the Constitution, and compel the nation to keep Sunday.

There are many who, if they understood the spirit and the result of religious legislation, would not do anything to forward in the least the movement for Sunday enforcement. But while Satan has been making a success of his plans, the people of God have failed at their post. God had an earnest work for them to do; for the honor of his law and the religious liberty of the people are at stake. God would have us see and realize the weakness and depravity of men, and put our entire trust in him; "For we wrestle not against flesh and blood, but against principalities, against powers, against the rulers of the darkness of this world, against spiritual wickedness in high places. Wherefore take unto you the whole armor of God, that ye may be able to withstand in the evil day, and having done all, to stand."

There are many who are at ease, who are, as it were, asleep. They say, "If prophecy has foretold the enforcement of Sunday observance, the law will surely be enacted," and having come to this conclusion, they sit down in calm expectation of the event, comforting themselves with the thought that God will protect his people in the day of trouble. But God will not save us if we make no effort to do the work he has committed to our charge. We must be found faithfully guarding the outposts, watching as vigilant soldiers, lest Satan shall gain an advantage {334} which it is our duty to prevent. We should diligently study the word of God; and pray in faith that God will restrain the powers of darkness; for as yet the message has gone to comparatively few, and the world is to be lightened with its glory. The present truth—the commandments of God and the faith of Jesus—has not yet been sounded as it must be. There are many almost within the shadow of our own doors for whose salvation no personal effort has ever been made. We are not prepared for the time when our work must close. We must take a firm stand that we will not reverence the first day of the week as the Sabbath, for it is not the day that was blessed and sanctified by Jehovah, and in reverencing Sunday we should place ourselves on the side of the great deceiver. The controversy for the Sabbath will open the subject to the people, and an opportunity will be given that the claims of the genuine Sabbath may be presented. Blindness, disloyalty to God, so prevails that his law is made void, but the psalmist says of such a condition, "It is time for thee Lord to work; for they have made void thy law."

It is time for God's people to work as never before, because of the increase of wickedness. The God-fearing, commandment-keeping people should be diligent, not only in prayer, but in action: and this will bring the truth before those who have never heard it. The world is over-borne with falsehood and iniquity and those whom God has made the depositaries of his law, and of the pure religion of Jesus, must be determined to let their light shine. If they do nothing to disabuse the minds of the people, and through ignorance of the truth our legislatures should abjure the principles of Protestantism, and give countenance and support to the Roman fallacy, the spurious sabbath, God will hold his people who have had great light, responsible for their lack of diligence and faithfulness. But if the subject of religious legislation is judiciously and intelligently laid before the people, and they see that through Sunday enforcement the Roman apostasy would be re-enacted by the Christian world, and that the tyranny of past ages would be repeated, then whatever comes, we shall have done our duty.

The man of sin thinks to change times and laws. He is exalting himself above God, in trying to compel the conscience. But God's people should work with persevering energy to let their light shine upon the people in regard to the law, and thus to withstand the enemies of God and his truth. When the law of God has been made void, and apostasy become a national sin, the Lord will work in behalf of his people. Their extremity will be his opportunity. He will manifest his power in behalf of his church.

My brethren, you must have Jesus enthroned within, and self must die. We must be baptized with the Holy Spirit, and then we shall not sit down, saying unconcernedly, {335} "What is to be will be; prophecy must be fulfilled." O awake, I pray you, awake! for you bear the most sacred responsibilities. As faithful watchmen, you should see the sword coming, and give the warning, that men and women may not pursue a course through ignorance that they would avoid if they knew the truth. The Lord has enlightened us in regard to what is coming upon the earth, that we may enlighten others, and we shall not be held guiltless if we are content to sit at ease, with folded hands, and quibble over matters of minor importance. The minds of many have been engrossed with contentions, and they have rejected the light given through the Testimonies, because it did not agree with their own opinions.

God does not force any man into his service. Every soul must decide for himself whether or not he will fall on the Rock and be broken. Heaven has been amazed to see the spiritual stupidity that has prevailed. You need individually to open your proud hearts to the Spirit of God. You need to have your intellectual ability sanctified to the service of God. The transforming of power of God must be upon you, that your minds may be renewed by the Holy Spirit, that you may have the mind that was in Christ.

If the watchmen sleep under an opiate of Satan's and do not recognize the voice of the true Shepherd, and do not take up the warning, I tell you in the fear of God, they will be charged with the blood of souls. The watchmen must be wide awake, men who will not slumber at their post of duty, day nor night. They must give the trumpet a certain sound, that the people may shun the evil, and choose the good. Stupidity and careless indifference cannot be excused. On every side of us there are breakers and hidden rocks which will dash our bark in pieces, and leave us helpless wrecks, unless we make God our refuge and help. Every soul should now be distrustful of self. Our own ways, our own plans and ideas, may not be such as God can approve. We must keep the way of the Lord to do his will, making him our counselor, and then in faith work away from self.

Light must come to the people through agents whom God shall choose, who will give the note of warning, that none may be in ignorance of the purposes of God or the devices of Satan. At the heart of the work, Satan will use his hellish arts to the utmost. He will seek in every possible way to interpose himself between the people and God, and shut away the light that God would have come to his children. It is his design to keep them in ignorance of what shall come upon the earth. All should be prepared to hear the signal trumpet of the watchmen, and be ready to pass the word along the walls of Zion, that the people may prepare themselves for the conflict. The people must not be left to stumble their way along in darkness, not knowing what is before them, and unprepared for the great issues that are coming. There is a work to be done for this time in fitting a people to stand in the day of trouble, {336} and all must act their part in this work. They must be clothed with the righteousness of Christ, and be so fortified by the truth, that the delusions of Satan shall not be accepted by them as genuine manifestations of the power of God.

Years have been lost, but will you now awake? Will those in responsible positions take in the situation, or will they by their indifference and inactivity, say to the people, "Peace and safety"? May God help everyone to come up to the help of the Lord now. The watchmen have been asleep, but may God grant that they may not sleep the sleep of death. Let all who are standing upon the walls of Zion give the trumpet a certain sound. It is a solemn time for God's people, but if they stand close by the bleeding side of Jesus, he will be their defense. He will open ways that the message of light may come to great men, to authors, and law makers. They will have opportunities of which you do not dream, and some of them will boldly advocate the claims of God's downtrodden law.

Instead of increased power as we enter the perils of the last days, weakness,

dissension, and strife for supremacy, are apparent. But if we had a connection with the God of heaven, we should be mighty in him, and yet we would walk with all lowliness of mind, having self hid in Jesus. But now both spiritual and natural feebleness and death are depriving us of workers. God alone, by his Holy Spirit, can arouse us from the slumber of death. There is now need of earnest working men and women who will seek for the salvation of souls; for Satan as a powerful general has taken the field, and in this last remnant of time he is working through all conceivable methods to close the door against light that God would have come to his people. He is sweeping the whole world into his ranks, and the few who are faithful to God's requirements are the only ones who can ever withstand him, and even these he is trying to overcome. Much upon these things has been shown to me, but I can only present a few ideas to you. Go to God for yourselves, pray for divine enlightenment, that you may know that you do know what is truth, that when the wonderful miracle working power of Satan shall be displayed, and the enemy shall come as an angel of light, you may distinguish between the genuine work of God and the imitative work of the powers of darkness. Ministers may do a great work for God if Jesus abides in the heart by faith. "Without me," says Christ, "ye can do nothing." I would that I had the power to present before you your sacred responsibility.

It is now too late in the day for men to please and glorify themselves. Ministers of God, it is too late to be contending for the supremacy. The solemn time has come when ministers should be weeping between the porch and the altar, crying, "Spare thy people, O Lord, and give not thine heritage to reproach." It is a day when instead of lifting up their souls in self-sufficiency, ministers {337} and people should be confessing their sins before God and one another. The law of God is made void, and even among those who advocate its binding claims, are some who break its sacred precepts. The Bible will be opened from house to house, and men and women will find access to these homes, and minds will be opened to receive the word of God; and when the crisis comes, many will be prepared to make right decisions even in the face of the formidable difficulties that will be brought about through the deceptive miracles of Satan. Although these will confess the truth and become workers with

Christ at the eleventh hour, they will receive equal wages with those who have wrought through the whole day. There will be an army of steadfast believers who will stand as firm as a rock through the last test. But where in that army are those who have been standard bearers? Where are those whose voices have sounded in proclaiming the truth to the sinning? Some of them are not there. We look for them but in the time of shaking they have been unable to stand, and have passed over to the enemy's ranks.

Brethren and sisters, the Lord wants to impart to us increased light. He desires that we shall have distinct revealings of his glory; that ministers and people shall become strong in his strength. When the angel was about to unfold to Daniel the intensely interesting prophecies to be recorded for us who are to witness their fulfillment, the angel said, "Be strong, yea, be strong." We are to receive the very same glory that was revealed to Daniel, because it is for God's people in these last days, that they may give the trumpet a certain sound. God help us to work unitedly and as we never have worked before, is my prayer. There is need now of faithful Calebs, whose voices will be heard in clear, ringing notes, saying of the immortal inheritance, "Let us go up at once and possess it, for we are well able." We need now the courage of God's faithful servant of old; not one wavering, uncertain note should come from the watchers' trumpets. They must be true to the sacred, solemn work that has been entrusted to them, and lead the flock of God in right pathways.

(Signed) Mrs. E. G. White

CAMP MEETING APPEAL

December 23, 1890
Review and Herald

"THE LORD HAS SEEN OUR backslidings, and he has a controversy with his people." Their pride, selfishness, their opening of the mind to doubt and unbelief, are manifest in his sight and grieve his heart of love. Many gather darkness about their souls as a garment, and virtually say, We want not a knowledge of thy way, O {338} God; we choose our own way. These are the things which separate the soul from God. There is in the soul of man an obstacle which he holds there with stubborn persistency, and which interposes between his soul and God. It is unbelief. God gives sufficient evidence, but man with his unsanctified will refuses to receive evidence unless it comes in his own way, to favor his own ideas. With a spirit of bravado he cries, "Proof, proof, is what we want," and turns away from the evidence that God gives. He talks doubt, unbelief, sowing the seeds of evil, which will spring up and yield their harvest. He is separating his soul farther and farther from God.

"Why is it that men do not believe upon sufficient evidence—because they do not want to be convinced. They have no disposition to give up their own will for God's will. They are willing to acknowledge that they have cherished sinful unbelief in resisting the light of God has given them. They have been hunting for doubts, for pegs upon which to hang their unbelief. They have been willing to accept testimony which is weak and insufficient, testimony which God has not given them in his word, but which pleases them because it agrees with their ideas and is in harmony with their disposition and will. These souls are in great peril. If they will bow their proud wills and put it on God's side of the question, if they will, with humble, contrite hearts, seek for light, believing that there is light for them, then they will see the light because the eye is single to discern the light which comes from God. They will acknowledge the evidence of divine authority. Spiritual truths will shine forth from the divine page. But the heart must be open for the reception of light, for Satan is ever ready to obscure the precious truth which would make them wise unto salvation. If any do not receive it, it will forever remain a mystery of mysteries to them.

"We should earnestly seek to know and appreciate the truth, that we may present it to others as it is in Jesus. We need to have a correct estimate of the value of our own souls; them we would not be as reckless in regard to our course of action as at present. We would seek most earnestly to know God's way; and we would work in an opposite direction from selfishness, and our constant prayer would be that we might have the mind of Christ, that we might be molded and fashioned after his likeness. It is in looking to Jesus and beholding his loveliness, having our eyes steadfastly fixed upon him, that we become changed into his image. He will give grace to all who keep his way and do his will and walk in truth. But those who love their own way, who worship their ideas of opinion and do not love God and obey his word, will continue to walk in darkness. Oh, how terrible is unbelief! As well let light be poured upon the blind as to present truth to these souls; the one cannot see; the other will not see.

"I beseech you whose names are registered on the church books as worthy members, to be indeed worthy through the {339} virtue of Christ. Mercy and truth and the love of God are promised to the contrite soul. The displeasure and judgments of God are against those who persist in walking in their own ways, loving self, loving the praise of men. They will certainly be swept into the Satanic delusions of these last days because they receive not the love of the truth. Because the Lord has in former days blessed and honored them, they flatter that they are chosen and true, and do not need warning, instruction, and reproof. The True Witness says, "As many as I love, I rebuke and chasten; be zealous therefore and repent! The professed people of God have the charge against them. Nevertheless I have somewhat against thee, because thou hast left thy first love. Remember therefore from whence thou hast fallen, and repent, and do the first works; or else I will come quickly, and will remove thy candlestick out of its place, unless thou repent.

"The love of Jesus that once burned in the heart has become dim and almost extinguished. Spiritual strength has become enfeebled. The displeasure of the Lord is against his people. In their present condition it is impossible for them to represent the character of Christ. And when the True Witness has sent them counsel, reproof, and warning because he loves them, they have refused to receive the message; they have refused to come to the light, lest their deeds should be reproved. Jesus said, "I lay down my life for the sheep. . .Therefore doth my Father love me." By taking your sins upon myself, I am opening a channel through which his Grace can flow to all who will accept it. In giving myself for the sins of the world, I have prepared a way for the unrepressed tide of his love to flow to men.

"All heaven is filled with amazement that when this love, so broad, so deep, so rich, so full, is presented to men who have known the grace of our Lord Jesus Christ, they are so indifferent, so cold and unmoved. What does it mean that such amazing grace does not soften our hard hearts? Oh, it is because of the power of unbelief—because "thou hast left thy first love." This is why the Word of God has so little influence. It is as a fire, but it cannot penetrate nor warm the ice bound heart that cherishes unbelief.

"The infinite treasures of truth have been accumulating from age to age. No representation could adequately impress us with the extent, the richness of those vast resources. They are waiting the demand of those who appreciate them. These gems of truth are to be gathered up by God's remnant people, to be given by them to the world; but self-confidence and obduracy of soul refuse the blessed treasure. God so loved the world that he gave his only begotten Son, that whosoever believeth on him should not perish, but have everlasting life." Such love cannot be measured, neither can it be expressed. John calls upon the world to "Behold what manner of love the Father hath bestowed upon us that we should be called the sons of God." It is a love that passeth knowledge. In the fullness of the sacrifice nothing was withheld. Jesus gave himself. God designs that his {340} people should love one another as Christ love us. They are to educate and train the soul for his love. They are to reflect this love in their own character, to reflect it to the world. Each should look upon this as his work. In his prayer to the Father, Jesus said, "As thou hast sent me into the world, even so have I sent them into the world." Christ's fullness is to be presented to the world by those who have become partakers of his grace. They are to do that for Christ which Christ did for the Father, represent his character.

"There is a lack of moral and spiritual power throughout our Conferences. Many churches do not have light in themselves The members do not give evidence that they are members of the True Vine by bearing much fruit to the glory of God, but appear to be withering away. Their Redeemer has withdrawn his light, the inspiration of his Holy Spirit, from their assemblies; for they have ceased to represent the self-denial, the sympathy and compassionate love of the world's Redeemer; they have not love for the souls for whom Christ died. They have ceased to be true and faithful. It is a sad picture—the lack of consecration and devotion to God. There has been a separation of the soul from God; many have cut off the communication between him and the soul by refusing his messengers and his message.

"In our largest churches the greatest evils exist because these have had the greatest light. They have not a true knowledge of God and of Jesus Christ whom he has sent. The leaven of unbelief is working, and unless these evils which bring the displeasure of God are corrected in its members, the whole church stands accountable for them. The deep movings of the Spirit of God are not with them. Many come to the assembly as worshippers like a door upon its hinges. They understand not the true application of the Scriptures nor the power of God. They have eyes but they see not; ears have they but they hear not; they continue in their evil ways yet regard themselves as the privileged obedient people, who are doers of the word. A carnal security and ease in Zion prevail. Peace, peace, is sounded in her borders when God has not spoken peace. They have forfeited the terms of peace; there is reason for an alarm to be sounded in all my holy mountain. The sinners in Zion should be afraid; in a time when they do not expect it, sudden destruction will surely come upon all who are at ease.

"The Holy Spirit strives to make apparent the claims of God, but men pay heed only for a moment and turn their minds to other things. Satan catches away the seeds of truth; the gracious influence of the spirit of God is effectually resisted. Thus many are grieving away the Holy Spirit for the last time and they know it not.

Will the church see where she has fallen? A coldness, a hardness of heart, a want of sympathy for the brethren exists in the church. An absence of love for the erring is manifested. There is a withdrawing from the very ones {341} who need pity and help. A severity, an overbearing spirit, such as existed among the Pharisees, exists in our churches, and especially in those entrusted with sacred responsibilities. They are lifted up in self-esteem and self-assurance. The widow and the fatherless have not their sympathy or their love. This is entirely unlike the spirit of Christ. The Lord looks with displeasure upon the coarse, harsh spirit that has been manifested by some—a spirit so devoid of sympathy, of tender appreciation of those whom he loves. Brethren, you who close the heart against Christ's suffering ones, remember that as you deal with them, God will deal with you. When you call, he will not say, "Here am I;" when you cry, he will not answer. Satan is watching, preparing his delusions to ensnare those who are filled with self-importance while they are spiritually destitute.

"The road to Paradise is not one of self-exaltation but of repentance, confession, humiliation, of faith and obedience. The message to the Laodicean church is appropriate to the church at this time: "And unto the angel of the church of the Laodiceans write: These things saith the Amen, the Faithful and True Witness, the beginning of the creation of God: I know thy works that thou are neither cold nor hot; I would thou wert cold or hot. So then because thou are lukewarm, and neither cold nor hot, I will spew thee out of my mouth. Because thou sayest, I am rich, and increased with goods, and have need of nothing; and knowest not that thou are wretched, and miserable, and poor, and blind, and naked; I counsel thee to buy of me gold tried in the fire, that thou mayest be rich; and white raiment that thou mayest be clothed, and that the shame of thy nakedness do not appear; and anoint thine eyes with eye salve that thou mayest see. As many as I love, I rebuke and chasten; be zealous therefore, and repent." There are many who are priding themselves upon their spiritual riches, their knowledge of the truth, and are living in guilty self-deception. When the members of the church humble themselves before God by zealous, not half-hearted, lifeless action, the Lord will receive them. But he declares, "I will come unto thee quickly and remove thy candlestick out of its place except thou repent." How long shall this warning be resisted? How long shall it be slighted?

"The True Witness declares: "I know thy works," "Repent, and do the first works." This is the true test, the evidence that the Spirit of God is working in the heart to imbue with his love. "I will come unto thee quickly, and will remove thy candlestick out of his place, except thou repent." The church is like the unproductive tree, which, receiving the dew, and rain, and the sunshine, should have produced an abundance of fruit, but on which the divine Searcher finds nothing but leaves. Solemn thought for our churches, solemn {342} indeed for every individual. Marvelous is the patience and forbearance of God, but "except thou repent," it shall be exhausted; the churches, our institutions, will go from weakness to weakness, from cold formality to deadness while they are saying, "I am rich and increased in goods, and have need of nothing." The True Witness says, "And knowest not that thou art wretched, and miserable, and poor, and blind, and naked. Will they ever see clearly their true condition?

"There is to be in the churches a wonderful manifestation of the power of God, but it will not move upon those who have not humbled themselves before the Lord and opened the door of the heart by confession and repentance. In the manifestation of that power which lightens the earth with the glory of God, they will see only something which in their blindness they think dangerous, something which will arouse their fears, and they will brace themselves to resist it. Because the Lord does not work according to their ideas and expectations they will oppose the work. "Why," they say, "should not we know the spirit of God when we have been in the work for so many years?" Because they did not respond to the messages, the warnings, and entreaties of the Lord, but persistently said, "I am rich and increased in goods, and have need of nothing." Talent, long experience, will not make men channels of light, unless they place themselves under the bright beams of the Sun of Righteousness, and are called and chosen and prepared by the endowment of the Holy Spirit. When men who handle sacred things will humble themselves under the mighty hand of God, the Lord will lift them up. He will make them men of discernment, men rich in the grace of his Spirit.

"The end is near. We have not a moment to lose. Light is to shine forth from God's people in clear, distinct rays, bringing Jesus before the churches and before the world. God will give additional light, and old truths will be recovered and replaced in the framework of truth; and wherever the laborers go they will triumph. As Christ's ambassadors, they are to search the Scriptures to seek for the truths that have been hidden beneath the rubbish of error, and every ray of light received is to be communicated to others. One interest will prevail, one subject will swallow up all others, Christ our Righteousness. This is life eternal, "That they might know thee, the only true God, and Jesus Christ whom thou hast sent." "Thus saith the Lord, Let not the wise man glory in his wisdom, neither let the mighty man glory in his might, let not the rich man glory in his riches; but let him that glorieth, glory in this, that he understandeth and knoweth me, that I am the Lord which exerciseth loving kindness, judgment, and righteousness in the earth; for in these things I delight, saith the Lord." {343}

"As the Saviour came to glorify the Father by the demonstration of his love, so the Spirit came to glorify Christ by revealing to the world the riches of his love and grace. If the Holy Spirit dwells in us, our work will testify to the fact. We will lift up Jesus. Not one can afford to be silent now. The Burden of the work is to present Christ to the world. All who venture to have their own way, who do not join the angels who are sent from heaven with a message to fill the whole earth with its glory, will be passed by. The work will go forward to victory without them, and they will have no part in its triumph."

FROM E. G. WHITE

May 9, 1892
Preston, Melbourne, Victoria

THERE HAS BEEN AN abundance of slipshod work done. The only conclusion that the world can come to is that those who profess to believe that the end of all things is at hand, do not really believe the tremendous truth that Christ is at the door. Do they believe the mission of Christ was to save the lost and perishing; that Christ is the only remedy for sin; that the world's Redeemer came to the world all seared and marred with the curse to lift up fallen man, to reveal to the perishing the love of the Father, and bring them to look and live, and thereby bring many sons and daughters to glory. . . .

The most grievous sin of idolatry exists in the church. Anything that interposes between the Christian and the whole hearted service to God, takes the form of an idol, and the most grievous sin of idolatry is idolatry itself. The testimonies of God's word are plain and clear in regard to the snares of the devil. But these are not only church members on the devil's ground, but those who are opening the Scriptures to others, practice evil, and defile soul and body. They are guilty before God because they are unholy. Were the church living by faith and had they the oil of grace in their vessels with their lamps, the guilty repose would end. Those who believe the sacred, elevating truths for this time, they cannot sleep over them. . .

Is this exclusively addressed to the few individuals who have been ordained to the ministry? No; but to every Christian young or old, rich or poor. If Christ has forgiven them of their sins, if the truth has made them free, have they not a work to do for the Master? If they are Christians, they will present the truth to others. They will not consider that all they have

to do is to serve themselves, live to please and glorify themselves.

Sins of a grave character are in our borders, and unless there is an awakening such as we have not seen for some time which will convict and convert professed Sabbath keepers, they will die in their sins; and the punishment of Sodom and Gomorrah will be light in comparison with those who have had great light and {344} precious opportunities, but have been worldly minded, corrupt in thoughts and practices, and have not purified their souls by obeying the truth.

Now we see need of workers in the opening fields before us, but where are the men who can be trusted, men who have been year by year growing into a better knowledge of God and his ways, and the movings of his providence? I want to sound in the ears of these sleepy, half paralyzed souls the words spoken to Nicodemus, "Except a man be born again he cannot see the kingdom of God." There is need to ask God with all the heart, to elevate the standard. The commonness, the cheapness of conversation reveal the measure of spirituality of the members of the church. Now, those who have lived years in this same experience know not God nor Jesus Christ whom he hath sent; and should such go forth as representatives of Jesus Christ? These men will never give the right mold to other minds. They have not grown up to the full stature of men and women in Jesus Christ. They simply live the name of Christian, but are not fitted for the work of God, and never will be until they are born again, and learn their A.B.C.'s in the religion of Jesus Christ. There is hope in one direction. Take the young men and women and place them where they will come as little as possible in contact with our churches, that the low grade of piety which is current in this day shall not leaven their ideas of what it means to be a Christian. The worshippers of God are in need of transforming grace to subordinate the world to religion. In the place of making the temporal interest first, exhausting soul, body, and spirit to secure temporal advantages, Jesus points us to the heavenly treasure, and tells us not to lay up our treasure in earth which will perish, but to lay up for ourselves treasure in heaven which will not perish, for where our treasure is there will our heart be also. Jesus would have all that profess to believe in him deal in the currency of heaven, handling those things upon which God has

stamped his image and superscription. These he presents before us of infinite value. We see the need of a deep and thorough work in our churches; but the Lord alone can by his Holy Spirit make the hearts that are as steel, soft and sympathetic, and true to the service of Christ. We are far behind because the churches have folded their hands in a peace and safety attitude, and are at ease in Zion, doing almost nothing when the living zeal should be in their hearts as never before. Satan is stirring the powers from beneath to make one last desperate effort to convert the world to his own principles. He has his plans laid with Satanic subtlety, and destruction cometh suddenly while these that have the light, the warnings that such a crisis is before us are almost unmoved. . .

Those who quibble over the authenticity of the Scriptures, and question the authenticity of Revelation will not be influenced. Their hearts are not sound. {345} They are not at enmity with Satan. The heart is the treasure house of sin. Not being expelled, it is hidden until an hour of opportunity, and then is revealed and springs into action. The first work is with the heart. Truth, the love of Jesus must supply the vacuum, Saith Christ, Make the tree good and the fruit will be good. . . .

We must as a people rise up from our formality. We must enter the straight gate. Satan has placed his active agents all along the passage to dispute the way of every soul. Christ has encouraged his followers not to be intimidated, but to press, urge your way through. Strive to enter in at the straight gate, "For many I say unto you, shall seek to enter in, but shall not be able." Darling cherished idols will have to be given up, the sins that have been indulged in, even if it comes as close as the plucking out of the right eye, or cutting off the right arm. Arouse! Force your way through the very armies of hell that oppose your passage.

Oh, we must be terribly in earnest to impress every soul that there is a hell to shun and a heaven to be won. Every energy of the soul must be aroused to force their passage, and seize the kingdom of heaven by force. Satan is active, and we must be active. Satan is untiring and persevering, and we must be. This is no time now to make excuses and blame others for our backslidings; no time now to flatter the soul: if circumstances had only been more favorable, how much easier for us to work the work of God. We must tell even those who profess the truth that they must cease to offend God by their sinful excuses. Jesus has provided for every emergency. If they will walk where he leads the way, he will make rough places plain. He, with his presence, will create an atmosphere for the soul. He closes the door and brings the soul into seclusion with God, and the needy soul is to forget everyone and everything but God. Satan will walk with him; but speak aloud to God, and he will drive back the hellish shadow of Satan. With humble, subdued, thankful hearts, they will come forth saying, Thy gentleness hath made me great. The sincere seeker comes forth from the audience with God, rich in the assurance of his love to go forth to distill a heavenly fragrance wherever he goes. He can talk of the righteousness of Christ; he can talk the love of God with sincerity. He has tested, and he knows the Lord is good. This work is to be done in all our churches. Christ his love, his forgiveness, his purity is to be the theme upon which we dwell. The charms of Jesus are to be kept ever before our minds, charged with the elevated character of the true model that every soul should copy. Let us turn our hearts from everything that would dishearten and discourage. Satan will seek to distort everything to {346} our vision, and make a mountain of a mole hill. Our eyes must be steadily fixed on Jesus. The Lord Jesus is our leader. We must follow where he leads the way. We are not to commence to plan for the second step. We are not to say, Lord, after I have taken this step, what shall I do, for I shall meet with difficulties? But by faith we must take that one step, come what will, and trust in Jesus.

The reason why our ministers are so inefficient is, that they go to their labors and come from their labors, if they have any success, full of themselves. The disciples of Christ did this when they came and said, "Even the devils are subject unto us." Jesus could discern their danger, and he said, "Come ye yourselves apart into a desert place, and rest awhile—come out of the din of the battle, away from the conflict, and hold communion with God." Thus it is with many workers, they are too strong, too full of self. The Lord cannot lead them or teach them, or use them to his glory, for they are wise in their own conceit, and vainly imagine that the Lord cannot do without them. Self must be buried. We must educate the people to seek the Lord. We must speak plain words to the ministers who are walking in the sparks of their

own kindling. The praise and flattery of men make ministers hungry for more, until they think as did Elder Daniels, the praise and flattery of men of more value than the approval of God.

We must, if saved, imbibe the spirit and power of Christ, self must be hidden in Christ, and Christ alone appear. Our work is to elevate, not by praising anyone, but by upholding Jesus, bringing the mind to Jesus. Lift him up, the Man of Calvary, before the people, and he can do all things for the humble, trusting, believing soul.

SELECTIONS FROM SEVERAL SOURCES
Prior to July, 1915

BUT OF HOW MANY WILL CHRIST say in the judgment, "Good and faithful servant." I think of how the angels must feel seeing the end approaching and those who claim to have a knowledge of God and Jesus Christ whom he hath sent, huddle together, colonize, and attend the meetings, and feel dissatisfied if there is not much preaching to benefit their souls, and strengthen the church while they are doing literally nothing. If they are branches really and truly of the true vine, nourished by the sap which flows from the vine to the branches, they are indeed partakers of the divine nature. They have moral power from Christ to overcome Satan, to hate sin; and these cannot be silent. Souls are perishing for the light and knowledge of the truth which they have. It is their duty to put that knowledge to use to save souls. {347}

What self-denial have our churches as a whole manifested? They may have given donations as a whole in money, but have withheld themselves. The heavenly agencies are waiting to cooperate with human agencies in a grand work of reflecting light to the world. Wherever there is even one soul converted on earth, there is a response of joy circulated through-heaven. Whenever one soul is snatched from Satan's hand and given as a trophy to Jesus Christ, there is joy in the presence of God, Jesus Christ and Holy angels, because the lost is found. I send my appeal to the churches to "Arise, shine, for the light is come, and the glory of the Lord is risen upon thee." "Ye have not," said Christ, "chosen me, but I have chosen you and ordained you, that you should go and bring forth fruit, and that your fruit should remain: that whosoever ye shall ask the Father in my name, he may give it to you."

Have you tasted of the powers of the world to come? Have you been eating the flesh and drinking the blood of the Son of God? Then if ministerial hands have not been laid upon you in the world, Christ has laid his hands upon you, and said, "Ye are my witnesses" go trade on the talents I have given you. . . .

Let us ask why there are so few martyrs now? What is the reason that Christians and the world confederate together in confidence. Has the world become converted, or has the church lost her holy and peculiar character and assimilated to the world? They do not come out and separate from the world, and do not maintain her high and holy character. Many of the professed followers of Christ feel no more burden for souls than does the world. The lusts of the eye, and the pride of life, the love of display, the love of ease has separated the professed Christians from God, and the missionary spirit in reality exists in but few. What can be done to open the eyes of these sinners in Zion, and make hypocrites tremble?

I have been alarmed for some years because I have seen the line of demarcation between the church and the world almost obliterated. The design of God in the formation of the church, was that the very action of the separation from the world, is itself sufficient to attract attention.

It is a solemn statement that I make to the church that not one in twenty whose names are registered upon the church books are prepared to close their earthly history, and would be as verily without God and without hope in the world as the common sinner. They are professedly serving God, but they are very earnestly serving mammon. This half and half work is a constant denying of Christ rather than a confessing of Christ. So many have brought their own unsubdued spirit, unrefined, their spiritual taste is perverted by their own immoral, debasing {348} corruptions, symbolizing the world in spirit, in heart, in purpose, confirming themselves in lustful practices, and are full of deception through and through in their professed Christian life; living as sinners claiming to be Christians. Those who claim to be Christians and will confess Christ, should come out from among them and touch not the unclean thing and be separate. There is a Satanic policy that is practiced by those who are spirit-blind, that they can mingle safely with the worldly element, confederate with them, be in co-operation with them, but it will not require a great length of time to discern that they are no longer with Christ, or place the least value upon living one with their brethren. They have left the cool snows coming from Lebanon for the putrid stream of the valley. The words of God, "Come out from the world, and be ye separate, and touch not the unclean thing" has to a great extent lost its effect upon many. The words of the great deceiver are, you will greatly augment your influence if you confederate with the world. Your influence in receiving their knowledge will greatly increase your popularity, and will by connection with them be much larger. Let all who are not completely deluded pray as never before that they may be kept from the bewitching snares of Satan to delude unwary souls in these last days. The work of every Christian has ever been to sprinkle the door posts with blood, gather their children into their houses with them, that the destroying angel might see the mark of God pointing to the only begotten Son of the Father.

"He is the rock, his work is perfect; for all his ways are judgment; a God of truth, and without iniquity, just and right is he. They have corrupted themselves, their spot is not the spot of their children; they are a perverse and crooked generation." Is he not thy Father that hath brought thee? Hath he not made thee and established thee?"

I lay down my pen and lift up my soul in prayer, that the Lord would breathe upon his backsliding people, which are as dry bones, and they shall live. The end is near, stealing upon us stealthily, so imperceptibly, no noiselessly, like the muffled tread of the thief in the night to surprise the sleepers off guard and unready. May the Lord grant to bring his Holy Spirit to bear upon the hearts of all who are now at ease, that they may no longer sleep as others but watch and be sober.

Who will consent even now, after wasting much of your lifetime, to give your will as clay into the hands of the potter, and you cooperate with God in becoming in his hands molded a vessel unto honor.—L. T. {349}

"As Christ was riding into Jerusalem, on the crest of Olivet, He broke forth in uncontrollable grief, exclaiming in broken utterances, as he looked upon Jerusalem, "If thou hadst known, even thou, at least in this thy day, the things which belong unto thy peace! but now they are hid from thine eyes. " He wept not for himself, but for the despisers of his mercy, long suffering

and forbearance. The course taken by the hardhearted and impenitent inhabitants of the doomed city, is similar to the attitude of churches and individuals toward Christ at the present time. They neglect his requirements and despise his forbearance. There is a form of godliness, there is ceremonial worship, there are complimentary prayers; but the real power is wanting. The heart is not softened by grace but is cold and unimpressionable. Many like the Jews are blinded by unbelief, and know not the time of their visitation. So far as the truth is concerned, they have had every advantage; God has been appealing to them for years, in warnings, in reproofs, corrections, and instructions in righteousness but special directions have been given only to be disregarded and placed on a level with common things." T. 32, p. 14

"The only hope for our churches of today is to repent and do their first work. The name of Jesus does not kindle the heart with love. A mechanical, formal orthodoxy has taken the place of deep, fervent charity and tenderness to one another. Will any give heed to the solemn admonition, "Turn ye, turn ye; for why will ye die?" Fall upon the rock and be broken; then let the Lord Jesus prepare you, mold and fashion you, as a vessel unto honor. Well may the people fear and tremble under these words: "Except thou repent, I will come unto thee quickly, and will remove thy candlestick out of his place." What then? "If therefore the light that is in thee be darkness, how great is that darkness!"

One matter burdens my soul; the great lack of the love of God, which has been lost through continued resistance of light and truth, and the influence of those who have been engaged in active labor, who in the face of evidence piled upon evidence, have exerted an influence to counteract the message God has sent. I point them to the Jewish nation and ask, Must we leave our brethren to pass over the same path of blind resistance, till the very end of probation? If ever a people needed true and faithful watchmen, who will not hold their peace, who will cry day and night, sounding the warning God has given, it is the Seventh-day Adventists. Those who have had great light, blessed opportunities, who like Capernaum have been exalted to heaven in point of privileges, shall they, by nonimprovement, be left to darkness corresponding to the greatness of the light given?" T. to Ministers No. 2 pp. 25-28, September 1892.

We have been plainly told that the standard of the {350} ministry must be raised, and also that if we do not come where we will meet the mind of God; we will be severed from the work. These are very solemn words to me, and I desire that they shall have their full effect upon my own heart. Nothing can be more certain than that if we do not take heed to the counsel from the Lord, we shall be left to go into a still greater darkness. O. A. Olsen 1892

Leaving Pitcairn, Tahiti was reached August 25. The boat remained just long enough to take on needed supplies. . . Those connected with the enterprise feel that the cruise has been a successful one in every respect. No accident or harm has come to the ship, and wherever she has touched prejudice has been disarmed. The workers were very careful not to press upon the people the peculiar views held by Seventh-day Adventists, but to preach Christ Jesus and Him crucified. Clipping from article published in Oakland Times, January 18, 1893, furnished by our people.

FORWARDNESS AND CONSOLIDATION

May 31, 1896
Sunnyside, Cooranbong, N. S. W.
Elder O. A. Olsen
Battle Creek, Michigan, U. S. A.

My dear Brother:

SCENES THAT WERE A SHAME to Christians, have been presented to me, as taking place in the council meetings held after the Minneapolis meeting. The loud voice of dispute, the hot spirit, the harsh words, resembled a political meeting more than a place where Christians were met for prayer and counsel. These meetings should have been dismissed as an insult to heaven. The Lord was not revered as an honored guest by those assembled in council, and how could they expect divine light to shine upon them; how could they feel that the presence of Jesus was molding and fashioning their plans? The place of meeting was not held as sacred, but was looked upon as a common business place. Then how could those assembled receive an inspiration which would lead them to enthrone truth in their hearts, to speak words in the tender, loving spirit of the Master?

In your council meetings and committee meetings, decisions are made, plans devised and matured, which, when put into practice, leave an impression on the work at large; and no vestige of a spirit of harshness should appear. Loud, impatient words should never be heard. Remember that in all your council meetings, there is a {351} heavenly Watcher. Do not allow one word of vanity to be spoken; for you are legislating for God, and he says to you, "Be still, and know that I am God."

If your committee meetings and council meetings are not under the direct supervision of the Spirit of God, your conclusions will be earth-born, and worthy of no more consideration than are any man's expressions. Christ says, "Without me ye can do nothing." If he is not honored in your assemblies as chief counselor, your planning comes from no higher source than the human mind.

Brother Olsen, you speak of my return to America. For three years I stood in Battle Creek as a witness for the truth. Those who then refused to receive the testimony given me by God for them, and rejected the evidences attending these testimonies, would not be benefited should I return.

I shall write to you; but should I return to Battle Creek, and bear my testimony to those who love not the truth, the ever ready words would rise from unbelieving hearts, "Somebody has told her." Even now unbelief is expressed by the words, "Who has written these things to Sister White?" But I know of no one who knows them as they are, and no one could write that which he does not suppose has an existence. Someone has told me, He who does not falsify, misjudge, or exaggerate any case. While at Minneapolis he bade me follow him from room to room that I might hear what was spoken in the bed chamber. The enemy had things very much his own way. I heard no word of prayer, but I heard my name mentioned in a slurring, criticizing way.

I shall never, I think, be called to stand under the direction of the Holy Spirit as I stood at Minneapolis. The presence of Jesus was with me. All assembled in that meeting had an opportunity to place themselves on the side of truth by receiving the Holy Spirit, which was sent by God in such a rich current of love and mercy. But in the rooms occupied by some of our people, we heard ridicule, criticism, jeering, laughter. The manifestations of the Holy Spirit were attributed to fanaticism. Who searched the Holy Scriptures as did the noble Bereans, to see if the things they heard were so? Who prayed for divine guidance? The scenes which took place at this meeting made the God of heaven

ashamed to call those who took part in them, his brethren. All this the heavenly Watcher noticed, and it is written in the book of God's remembrance.

The Lord will blot out the transgression of those who, since that time, have repented with a sincere repentance, but every time the same spirit wakens in the soul, the deeds done on that occasion are endorsed, and the doers of them are made responsible to God, and must answer {352} for them at his judgment throne. The same spirit that actuated the rejecters of Christ, rankles in their hearts and had they lived in the days of Christ, they would have acted toward him in a manner similar to that of the godless and unbelieving Jews.

God's servants have no tame testimony to bear at this time, whether men will hear or whether they will forbear. He who rejects the light and evidence God has been literally bestowing upon us, rejects Christ; and for him there is no other Saviour.

The Work at Battle Creek

The spirit of the Lord has outlined the condition of things at the Review and Herald Office. Speaking through Isaiah God says, "I will not contend forever, neither will I be always wroth, and he went on frowardly in the way of his heart."

This is precisely what has been done in the office of publication at Battle Creek. Covetousness has been woven into nearly all the business transactions of the institution, and has been practiced by individuals. This influence has spread like the leprosy, until it has tainted and corrupted the whole. As the publishing house has become corrupted, the General Conference Association has stepped in, and proposed to take the diseased child off its hands, and care for it. But it is a snare for the General Conference Association to take the publishing work on its shoulders. This puts no special sanctity upon the work, but upon the General Conference Association a burden which will weigh it down, cripple it, and weaken its efficiency unless men who have firm principle, mingled with love, shall conduct the business lines.

In this step there has been a change of responsibility, but the wrong principles remain unchanged. The same work that has been in the past will be carried forward under the guise of the General Conference Association. The sacred character of this association is fast disappearing. What will then be respected as pure, holy, and undefiled? Will there be any voice that God's people can regard as a voice they can re-

spect? There certainly is nothing now that bears the divine credentials. Sacred things are mixed and mingled with earthly business that has no connection with God.

To a large degree the General Conference Association has lost its sacred character, because some connected with it have not changed their sentiments in any particular since the Conference held at Minneapolis. Some in responsible positions go on "Frowardly" in the way of their own hearts. Some who came from South Africa and from other places to receive an education which would qualify them for the work, have imbibed this spirit, {353} carried it with them to their homes, and their work has not borne the right kind of fruit. The opinions of men which were received by them, still cleave to them like the leprosy; and it is a very solemn question whether the souls who became imbued with the spiritual leprosy in Battle Creek, will ever be able to distinguish the principles of heaven from the methods and plans of men. The influences and impressions received in Battle Creek have done much to retard the work in South Africa.

As things now exist in Battle Creek, the work of God cannot be carried forward on a correct basis. How long will these things be? When will the perceptions of men be made clear and sharp by the ministration of the Holy Spirit? Some there do not detect the injurious effects of the plans which for years have been working in an underhanded manner. Some of the managers at the present time are walking in the light they have received, and are doing the best they can, but their fellow workers are making things so oppressive for them that they can do but little. The enslaving of the souls of men by their fellow men are deepening the darkness which already envelopes them. Who can now feel sure that they are safe in respect the voice of the General Conference Association? If the people in our churches understood the management of the men who walk in the light of the sparks of their own kindling, would they respect their decisions? I answer, No, not for a moment. I have been shown that the people at large do not know that the heart of the work is being diseased and corrupted at Battle Creek. Many of the people are in a lethargic, listless, apathetic condition, and assent to plans which they do not understand. Where is the voice, from whence will it come, to whom the people may listen, knowing that it comes from the true Shepherd? I am called upon by the Spirit of God to present these things before you, and they are correct to the life, according to the practice of the past few years. . . .

Consolidation of the Publishing Work

The Lord has presented before me matters that cause me to tremble for the institutions at Battle Creek. He has laid these things before me, and I shall not be consistent if I do not seek to repress the spirit in Battle Creek, which reaches out for more power, when for years there have not been men who were qualified to preside, with Christian faithfulness, over the charge they already have.

The scheme for consolidation is detrimental to the cause of present truth. Battle Creek has all the power {354} she should have. Some in that place have advanced selfish plans, and if any branch of the work promised a measure of success, they have not exercised the spirit which lets well enough alone, but have made an effort to attach these interests to the great whole. They have striven to embrace altogether too much, and yet they are eager to get more. When they can show that they have made these plans under the guidance of the Holy Spirit, then confidence in them may be restored.

Twenty years ago, I was surprised at the cautions and warnings given me in reference to the publishing house on the Pacific Coast, that it was ever to remain independent of all other institutions; that it was to be controlled by no other institution, but it was to do the Lord's work under his guidance and protection. The Lord says, "All ye are brethren;" and the Pacific Press is not to be envied and looked upon with jealousy and suspicion by the stronger publishing house at Battle Creek. It must maintain its own individuality, and be strictly guarded from any corruption. It must not be merged into any other institution. The hand of power and control at Battle Creek must not reach across the continent and manage it.

At a later date, just prior to my husband's death, the minds of some were agitated in regard to placing these institutions under one presiding power. Again the Holy Spirit brought to my mind what had been stated to me by the Lord. I told my husband to say in answer to this proposition, that the Lord had not planned any such action. He who knows the end from the beginning, understands the matter better than erring man.

At a still later date the situation of the publishing house at Oakland was again presented to me. I was shown that a work was to be done by this institution which would be to the glory of God if the workers would keep his honor ever in view; but that an error was being committed by taking in a class of work which had a tendency to corrupt the institution. I was also shown that it must stand in its own independence, working out God's plan under the control of none other but God.

The Lord presented before me that branches of this work would be planted in other places, and carried on under the supervision of the Pacific Press, but that if this proved a success, jealousy, evil surmisings, and covetousness would arise. Efforts would be made to change the order of things, and embrace the work among other interests at Battle Creek. Men are very zealous to change the order of things, but the Lord forbids such a consolidation. Every branch should be allowed to live, and do its own work.

Mistakes will occur in every institution, but if the managers will learn the lessons that all must learn to {355} move guardedly, these errors will not be repeated, and God will preside over the work. Every worker in our institutions needs to make the Word of God his rule of action. Then the blessing of God will rest on him. He cannot with safety dispense with the truth of God as his guide and monitor. If man can take one breath without being dependent upon God, then he may lay aside God's pure, holy, word, as guide book. The truth must take control of the conscience and the understanding in all the work that is done. It is to direct in all temporal and spiritual actions.

It is well pleasing to God that we have praise and prayer, and religious services, but Bible religion must be brought into all we do, and give sanctity to each daily duty. The Lord's will must become men's will in everything. The Holy One of Israel has given rules of guidance to all, and these rules of guidance are to be strictly followed, for they form the standard of character. No one can swerve from the first principles of righteousness without sinning. But our religion is misinterpreted and despised by unbelievers because so many who profess to hold the truth, do not practice its principles in dealing with their fellow men.

To my brethren at Battle Creek, I would say, You are not in any condition to consolidate. This means nothing less than placing upon the institutions at Battle Creek the management of all the work, far and near.

God's work cannot be carried forward successfully by men who, by their resistance to light, have placed themselves where nothing will influence them to repent or change their course of action. There are men connected with the work at Battle Creek whose hearts are not sanctified and controlled by God.

If those connected with the work of God will not hear his voice and do his will, they should be separated entirely from the work. God does not need the influence of such men. I speak plainly, for it is time that things were called by their right name. Those who love and fear God with all their hearts are the only men that God can trust. But those who have separated their souls from God, should themselves be separated from the work of God, which is so solemn and so important.

E.G. White

CRITICIZING, CONDEMNING AND ALL EVIL SPEAKING TO BE PUT AWAY

December 26, 1896 {356}

IT IS THE DUTY OF GOD'S servants to work constantly with an eye single to his honor and glory. No man's person is to be respected or looked upon with admiration if his heart and soul is not enlisted in the work of God, unless he seeks to carry forward that work with self-sacrificing efforts. There are those who think more highly of themselves than they ought to think. They speak evil of their brethren because after a thing is done, they can look back and tell how differently they would have done it. But their forethought would not have been any better than that of their brethren had they been in their place. God sees that faults and imperfections have characterized the lives of the very ones who speak evil of their brethren.

Keep yourselves off the judgment seat. All judgment is committed unto the Son of God. Your words and your works will not be judged according to the light in which you view them, but according to God's unerring standard. By uniting and talking with those who have grievances, by emptying your heart of all the hard feelings and wounds and bruises you have sustained, you have made great blunders. God will hold you accountable for every seed of that kind which you have sown in human hearts. Satan will water that seed, and inspire you with all the bitterness and evil speaking and wrath and malice that he can.

O how can anyone suppose that he can be in harmony with Christ and indulge in this cruel and wicked work? All who do so are departing from the word of God, disregarding that word, and failing to act out the lessons of Jesus Christ. Talking with solemn earnestness the Counselor has said: "There are many who, when their own ideas and will is crossed, reveal a bitterness of spirit. They cherish the same feelings as an unconverted man. They watch for an opportunity to complain, and thus set a wrong example for others. In that day, declares the word of God, "shall the deaf hear the words of the book, and the eyes of the blind shall see out of obscurity, and out of darkness. The meek shall also increase their joy in the Lord, and the poor among men shall rejoice in the Holy One of Israel. For the terrible one is brought to nought, and the scorner is consumed, and all that watch for iniquity are cut off; that make a man an offender for a word, and lay a snare for him that reproveth in the gate, and turn aside the just for a thing of nought."

Here is one man professing to be a Bible Christian. But if everything does not harmonize with his ideas, he looks upon himself as abused. He feels justified in making a great fire out of a spark. Another brother in connection with the work of God thinks that he has {357} been treated unjustly. What if he has? Does not the Lord know all about that? It would not be surprising if the human agent did not know himself; for the heart is deceitful above all things, and desperately wicked; who can know it?

A condition of things has been coming into existence that is not after the order of Christ. Those who look for evil, who are ready to charge those who do not meet all their expectations by accommodating them and carrying out their ideas with evil, who feel at liberty to judge their brethren and misconstrue their motives, are not Christians. Those who encourage and sustain persons who are not walking in the ways of the Lord, are aiding Satan by doing his work. They are not feeding on Christ, the bread from heaven. They have ever lived for self. Self has been their center. As long as they can be first, all goes well.

I wish all my brethren who shall read the words I am placing on paper to carefully consider that which I present before them. No man liveth for himself. Whatever course of action the human agent may pursue, others are influenced. God alone knows the extent of this individual responsibility. Apparent influence may be deceiving; real influence requires all that there is of a man. Whatever the position of surroundings of old or young, they carry with them an influence. Their responsibility is great. No one can be lax, self-indulgent, self-serving, and be counted worthy of eternal life.

Never let your tongue and voice be employed in discovering and dilating upon the defects of your brethren; for the record of heaven identifies Christ's interests with those he has purchased with his own blood. "Inasmuch as ye have done it unto one of the least of these my brethren," he says "ye have done it unto me." We are to learn to be loyal to one another, to be true as steel in the defense of our brethren. Look to your own defects. You had better discover one of your own faults than ten of your brother's. Remember that Christ has prayed for these, his brethren, that they all might be one as he is one with the father. Seek to the uttermost of your capabilities to be in harmony with your brethren to the extent of Christ's measurement, as he is one with the Father. Then your evil thinking and evil speaking will cease. You will not become bitter and hard against them because they do not make enough of your merits and show special partiality to you. Those who are missionaries for the Master will have the spirit of truth and righteousness.

"Love as brethren; be pitiful; be courteous." True moral worth does not seek to have a place for itself by evil thinking and evil speaking, by demeriting others. All envy, all jealousy, all evil speaking, with all {358} unbelief, must be put away from God's children.

Satan works zealously to cause men to offend on this point. Those whose tongues are so free to utter words of criticism, the adroit questioner, who draws out expressions and opinions which have been put into the minds by sowing seeds of alienation, are his missionaries. They may repeat the expressions they draw from others as originating with the ones they so slyly led on to forbidden ground. These persons seem always to see something to criticize and condemn. They treasure up everything of a disagreeable nature, and then leaven others. Their tongues are ready to exaggerate everything evil. What a great matter a little fire kindleth. They scatter their fire brands, putting doubts and mistrust into other minds, falsifying because they view everything in a false light. Thus neighbors and churches are leavened.

Jesus said to his disciples, "Take heed and beware of the leaven of the Pharisees and Sadducees." His voice comes sounding down the lines of our time, "Beware of that misrepresenting tongue, which is not content unless leagued with the disaffected, with those who are tempted to think that they have been misused.' Self, self, self is their theme. They have become envious and jealous, and Satan has helped them, putting his magnifying glass before their eyes, until a mote looks to them like a mountain, and they thing themselves the most abused persons in the world. With a beam on their own eye, they are very much interested in pulling the mote out of their brother's eye.

It is Satanic to be an accuser of the brethren, to delight to tell of the imperfections and wrongs of others. Those who suppose themselves to be God's missionaries and yet work upon the minds of those who are weak and inexperienced in the faith, may see the time, if they are converted, when they will wish to counteract their past work. But it is not an easy matter to do this. Eternity alone will reveal on whose side everyone has been working, and the good or ill they have wrought.

Shall the attributes of the enemy be revealed in the life practice of professed Christians? Shall men who put on the armor and stand as faithful sentinels for God, refusing to favor any man, and seeking to do the work God has given them to do with humble faith and sincerity, be despised by men who know not that they have given themselves to do the work of Satan? O how much better it would be if those who thus judge others would themselves feed on the flesh and blood of the Son of God, studying and practicing the word of God.

Men who have large opinions of themselves are often in error, but they will not confess this. Envy and {359} jealousy are diseases which disorder all the faculties of the being. They originated with Satan in Paradise. After he had started on the track of apostasy, he could see many things that were objectionable. After he fell he envied Adam and Eve in their innocency. He tempted them to sin, and to become like himself, disloyal to God. Those who accept of his attributes will demerit others, misrepresent and falsify in order to build up themselves. These persons are generally incurable, and as nothing that defileth can enter heaven, they will not be there.

They would criticize the angels. They would covet another's crown. They would not know what to do, or what subjects to converse upon unless they could be finding some errors, some imperfections, in others. O that such ones would be changed by following Christ. O that they would become meek and lowly of heart by learning in the school of Christ. Then they would go forth, not as missionaries for Satan, to cause disunion and alienation, but as missionaries for Christ, to be peacemakers to work with Christ in restoring, not to bruise and mangle character. Let the Holy Spirit of God come in and expel this unholy passion, which cannot in the slightest degree survive in Heaven. Let it die. Let it be crucified. Open the heart to the attributes of Christ, who was pure, holy, undefiled, without guilt.

"Keep thy heart with all diligence; for out of it are the issue of life." The word of God tells us that the heart is to be kept as a temple holy unto God. The unconverted heart is represented as a habitation for the evil one, who brings in a whole brood of unholy thoughts, and stirs up the natural passions. But the Spirit of God must cleanse the soul from its defilement. Every room must be purified. The conscience must be quickened by the Holy Spirit. Truth must take hold of the thoughts and actions. Holy vigilance must keep guard to spy out the approach of the enemy. Woe unto that man who falls asleep and lets the enemy take possession of his house.

Genuine conversion is needed, not once in years, but daily. This conversion brings a man into new relation with God. Old things, his natural temper, natural passions, and hereditary traits of character pass away, and the man is renewed, converted, sanctified. But this work needs to be continued, or else the heart will become estranged from God; for just as long as Satan lives, he will make an effort to carry out his will. The human agent will constantly encounter a strong undercurrent. His heart needs to be barricaded by faithful watchfulness and unceasing prayer, else the embankment will give way, and like a mill stream, the undercurrent of natural and cultivated tendencies will sweep away the safeguard. Then the old objectionable traits of character will assert their sway. No renewed heart can keep in a condition of {360} sweetness and grace without the application of the salt of the word. Divine grace must be applied daily, else no man will stay converted.

It is the sufferings of our Redeemer in his life and death that makes it possible for fallen man to become refined and elevating. As the divine substitute and surety, he elevates the fallen race in character, and brings their minds into healthful sympathy with the divine mind. Those who are partakers of the divine nature see that true-heartedness means continual humiliation, self-denial, and self-sacrifice. Those who have spiritual eyesight will discern that God does not honor those who are honored by the world, but those who are true to principle.

THE USE OF FLESH FOODS
[Prior to July 1915]

I HAVE BEEN CALLING TO mind the light God has given me on health reform. Have you carefully and prayerfully sought to understand the will of God in this matter?

The use of meats is entirely out of harmony with health reform principles. If we would allow reason to take the place of impulse and love of sensual indulgence, we should not taste the flesh of dead animals. What is more repulsive to the sense of smell than a shop where flesh meats are kept for sale? The smell of the raw flesh is offensive to all whose senses have not been depraved by culture of the unnatural appetites. What more unpleasant sight to a reflective mind than the beasts slain to be devoured? If the light God has given in regard to health reform is disregarded, he will not work a miracle to keep in health those who pursue a course to make themselves sick.

You may think, you cannot work without meat. I thought so once, but I know that in his original plan, God did not provide for the flesh of dead animals to compose the diet of man. It is a grossly perverted taste that will accept such food. Then the fact that meat is largely diseased should lead us to make strenuous efforts to discontinue the use entirely.

My position now is to let meat altogether alone. It will be hard for some to do this—as hard as for the rum-drinker to forsake his dram—but they will be better for the change.

You know how you would answer a tobacco devotee if he urged, as a plea for the use of tobacco, the arguments {361} some advance as a reason why they should continue the use of the flesh of dead animals as food. The weakness some experience with-

out the use of meat is one of the strongest arguments that can be presented why they should discontinue its use. Those who eat meat feel stimulated after eating this food, and they suppose they are made stronger. After one discontinues the use of meat, he may for a time feel a weakness, but when his system is cleansed from the effect of this diet, he no longer feels the weakness, and will cease to wish for that which he had pleaded for as essential to his strength.

I have a large family which often numbers sixteen. In it there are men who work at the plow and who fell trees. These men have vigorous exercise, but not a particle of flesh of animals is placed upon our table.

I have felt urged by the Spirit of God to set before several the fact that their suffering ill health was caused by a disregard of the light given them upon health reform. I have shown them that their meat diet, which was supposed to be essential, was not necessary, and that, as they were composed of what they ate, brain, bone and muscle were in an unwholesome condition because they lived on the flesh of dead animals; that their blood was being corrupted by this improper diet; that the flesh which they ate was diseased, and their entire system was becoming gross and corrupted.

There is an alarming lethargy shown on the subject of unconscious sensualism. It is customary to eat the flesh of dead animals. This stimulates the lower passions of the human organism. In the preparation of food, the golden rays of light are to be kept shining, teaching those who sit at the table how to live. Physicians are not employed to prescribe a flesh diet for patients, for it is this kind of diet that has made them sick. Seek the Lord. When you find him, you will be meek and lowly of heart. Individually, you will not subsist upon the flesh of dead animals, neither will you put one morsel in the mouth of your children. Physicians will not prescribe flesh, tea or coffee for their patients, but will give talks showing the necessity of a simple diet. They will cut away injurious things from their bill of fare. To have the physicians of our institutions educating by precept and example those under their care to use a meat diet, after years of instruction from the Lord, disqualifies them to be superintendents of our health institutes. The Lord does not give light on health reform that it may be disregarded by those who are in positions of influence and authority. The Lord means just what he says, and he is to be honored in what he says. Light is to be given upon these subjects. It is the diet question that needs close investigation and prescriptions should be made in accordance with health principles. {362}

The Lord intends to bring his people back to live upon simple fruits, vegetables, and grains. He led the children of Israel into the wilderness, where they could not get a fresh diet, and he gave them the bread of heaven. Men did eat angels' food, but they craved the fleshpots of Egypt, and mourned and cried for flesh, notwithstanding that the Lord had promised them if they would submit to his will, he would carry them into the land of Canaan and establish them there, a pure, holy, happy people, and there should not be a feeble one in all their tribes, for he would take away all sickness from among them. But, although they had a plain thus saith the Lord, they mourned and wept and murmured and complained until the Lord was wroth with them, and because they were so determined to have the flesh of dead animals, he gave them the very diet he had withheld from them. The Lord would at first have given them flesh if it had been essential for their health; but he created and redeemed them, and led them a long journey in the wilderness to educate and discipline and train them into correct habits. The Lord understood what the influence of flesh eating is upon the human system. He would have a people that would, in their physical appearance, bear the divine credentials notwithstanding their long journey.

When I hear those who profess to believe the truth for this time pleading for the use of flesh meats, I am forcibly reminded of the complainings of the children of Israel because they were not favored with a meat diet. The diet of animals generally used for food is vegetables and grains. Must the vegetables be animalized before we can eat them? Must they be incorporated into the system of an animal before we can digest them? Must we obtain our vegetable diet by eating the flesh of dead creatures? God provided fruit in its natural state for our first parents. He gave Adam charge of the garden to dress it and to care for it, saying, "To you it shall be for meat." The plan was not for one animal to destroy another animal for food. After the fall, the eating of flesh was suffered in order to shorten the period of the existence of the long-lived race. It was allowed because of the hardness of the hearts of men. One of the great errors that many insist upon is,

that muscular strength is dependent upon animal food. But the simple grains, fruits of the trees, and vegetables have all the nutritive properties necessary to make good blood. This a flesh diet cannot do.

When a limb is broken, physicians recommend their patients not to eat meat, as there will be danger of inflammation setting in. Condiment and spices used in the preparation of food for the table aid in digestion in the same way that tea, coffee and liquor are supposed to help the laboring man perform his tasks. After the {363} immediate effects are gone, they drop as correspondingly below par as they were elevated above par by these stimulating substances. The system is weakened, the blood is contaminated, and inflammation is the sure result.

After all the light that has been given on the diet question, for the people of God to lament because they cannot exercise freedom in meat eating is very similar to the complainings, lamentations and weeping of the children of Israel in the ears of the Lord.

Our sanitariums should never be conducted after the fashion of the hotel. A meat diet changes the disposition and strengthens animalism. We are composed of what we eat, and eating much flesh will diminish intellectual activity. Students would accomplish much more in their studies if they never tasted meat. When the animal part of the human agent is strengthened by meat eating, the intellectual powers diminish proportionately. A religious life can more successfully be gained and maintained if meat is discarded, for this diet stimulates into intense activities lustful propensities, and enfeebles the moral and spiritual nature. "The flesh warreth against the spirit, and the spirit against the flesh."

We greatly need to encourage and cultivate pure, chaste thoughts and to strengthen the moral powers rather than the lower and carnal powers. God help us to break from our self-indulgent appetites! The idea of eating dead flesh is abhorrent to me; the thought of one living animal eating the flesh of another animal is shocking. There is no call for it.

Cancers, tumors, and all inflammatory diseases are largely caused by meat eating. From the light God has given me, the prevalence of cancers and tumors is largely due to gross living on dead flesh. I sincerely and prayerfully hope that our physicians and our people will not forever be blind on this subject, for blindness

is mingled with a want of moral courage to deny appetite, to lift the cross, which means, to take up the very duties which cut across the natural passions.

The juices and fluids of what we eat pass into the circulation of the blood, and, as we are composed of what we eat, by feeding on flesh we become animalized; thus a feverish condition is created, because the animals are diseased, and by partaking of their flesh we plant the seeds of disease in our own tissue and blood. Then when exposed to the changes in a malarious or poisonous atmosphere, these are more sensibly felt; also when we are exposed to prevailing epidemics and contagious diseases the system is not in condition to resist disease.

I have the subject presented to me in different aspects. The mortality caused by meat eating is not discerned; if it were, we would hear no more {364} arguments and excuses in favor of the indulgence of the appetite for dead flesh. We have plenty of good things to satisfy hunger without bringing corpses upon our tables to compose our bill of fare.

I might go to any length upon this subject, but I forbear. I do hope that our physicians will not, by precept and example, counterwork that which the Lord has given me to enlighten minds and bring in thorough reforms. I am working earnestly along these lines, and shall never cease working against the practice of meat-eating. I have had opened before me the stumbling block which this diet question has been in the spiritual advancement of some, and what a stumbling block they in turn have placed in the paths of others, and all because their own sensibilities were blunted through the selfish gratification of the appetite. For Christ's sake, look deeper, study deeper, and act in accordance with the light God has been pleased to give on this subject.

DEAR BROTHER

March 1, 1886
Basle, Switzerland

YOUR LETTERS HAVE BEEN received. Your last in reference to the College came this morning. I was not aware that our College was in debt twenty thousand dollars. This must make it a necessity to call for donations.

The evils of centering so many responsibilities in Battle Creek have not been small. The dangers are great. There are unconsecrated elements that only wait for circumstances to put all their influence on the side of wrong. I can never feel exactly safe in regard to B. C. or Battle Creek College. I cannot at this time state all my reasons. That which led me to write as I did was the great need of business managers—godly, devoted men to take hold of the work and push it in a God fearing manner.

Whatever may have been the object in placing the tuition of students at so low figures, the fact that the College has been running behind so heavily is sufficient reason for changing the price, that this shall not be the showing in the future. The low price is not in its favor, even if at higher rates the College is not so largely patronized. Those who really want the advantages to be obtained at B. C. will make extra exertions to receive these advantages, and a large class who would be induced to come because of the low tuition would be of no benefit to other students or to the church. The larger the number, the more tact, skill, and vigilance {365} are required to keep them in order, and from becoming demoralized.

Some provision should be made to have a fund raised to loan to the worthy poor students who desire to give themselves to the missionary work; and in some cases they should receive donations. Then these youth should have it plainly set before them that they must work their way as far as possible and partly defray their expense.

The churches in different localities should feel that a solemn responsibility rests upon them to train youth and educate talent to engage in missionary efforts. When they see any in the church who give promise of making useful workers, but who are not able to educate themselves, they should lift that responsibility and send them to the College to be instructed, and developed, with the object in view of becoming workers in the cause of God. There is material that needs to be worked up, and that would be of good service in the Lord's vineyard; but they are too poor to obtain the advantages of the College. The churches should feel it a privilege to take the responsibility of defraying their expenses.

The tuition should be placed higher, and if there are some who need help, let them be helped as above stated. When the College was first started there was a fund placed in the Review and Herald office for the benefit of those who wished to obtain an education but had not the means. This was used by several students until they could get a good start, and earn enough to replace what they had drawn, so that others could be benefited by it. That which costs little will be appreciated little, but that which costs something near its real value will be estimated accordingly.

If there were fewer students, and they were of a hopeful character, it would be a blessing to Battle Creek. If there are men as teachers in the College and associated with it, who are well balanced, and have a strong moral influence, who know how to deal with minds, and possess the true missionary spirit; then if the College was crowded so as to necessitate the building of another equally as large, that would be the best missionary field in the world. It is this ability that is greatly needed in the College.

If these superior qualities were found in the men connected with the office at Battle Creek, the outlook would be more encouraging. Great and important interests are in danger of being misshaped, and of coming forth defective from their hands. If some felt their ignorance more, and would depend less on self, be less self-sufficient, they might learn of the Great Teacher meekness and lowliness of heart.

In regard to the College I would say, Raise the price of tuition and have a better class of students. But {366} provision should be made to do the very best for those who come, to secure for them every healthful, intellectual, and moral advantage. I see the need of still another boarding house, and there may be need of another building for the students. I cannot see how you can do better than you have in calling for means while this debt is against the College. It ought not to be there, and if there had been the right kind of planning it would not exist; that is, if those especially employed in the College were all enterprising men of broader ideas. They would constantly be exercising ingenuity and tact, and devising means whereby the College should not become burdened with debt.

If we only had devoted, spiritually-minded workers connected with our important institutions, who relied upon God more than upon themselves, we might certainly look for far greater prosperity than we have had hitherto. But where there is a decided want of humble trust, and of an entire dependence upon God, we are sure of nothing. Our great need today is men who are baptized with the Holy Spirit of God. Men who walk with God as did Enoch; men who are not so narrow in their outlook that they will bind about the work in place of enlarging it; men who will not say, "Business is business, religion is religion." We need men who can take in the situation; men who are far seeing; men who can reason from cause to effect.

I will here give some extracts from a letter written November 8, 1880:

"The interest of every part of the cause is as dear to me as my life. Every branch of the work is important. I was shown that there is great danger not of making the tract and missionary work so absorbing that it will become intricate through a multiplicity of plans: that it will become perplexing and absorb every other interest. It was also brought before me that there was too much machinery in the tract and missionary, and in the Sabbath school work. There was a form and arrangement, but little of Christ-like simplicity felt or practiced by the workers. We want less machinery and mechanical arrangement, and more heart work, more real piety and true holiness; especially in the missionary work everywhere. There needs to be piety, purity, and wise generalship, and then far greater and much better work would be done with less expenditure of means.

There is a broad field to be covered, and a getting above the simplicity of the work. Now is the time to work, and to work in the wise counsel of God. If you connect unconsecrated persons with mission fields and with the Sabbath schools, our work will take on a formal mold and be without Christ. The workers must study carefully, prayerfully, in every part of the field, how to work with the simplicity of Christ, and in an economical manner; to plan and devise the most successful manner of reaching hearts. {367}

We are in danger of spreading over more territory, and starting more enterprises than we can possibly attend to properly. There is danger of overdoing some branches of the work, and leaving some important parts of it to be neglected. To undertake a large amount of work and do nothing perfectly, would be a bad plan. We are to move forward, but must not get so far above the simplicity of the work that it will be impossible to look after the enterprises entered into without sacrificing our best helpers to keep things in order. Life and health must be regarded.

While we should ever be ready to follow the opening providence of God, we should lay no larger plans, nor occupy more ground than there is help and means to bind off the work well, keep up and increase the interest already started. While there are broader plans and fields constantly opening for the laborers, our ideas and views must broaden in regard to the workers who are to labor to bring souls to the truth. Our young ministers must be encouraged to take hold of the work with energy, and labor in educating, as well as encouragement must be given to these men. They must be trained and disciplined to carry forward the work in simplicity. I am astonished to see how little some of our young ministers are appreciated, and how little encouragement they receive. Yet some of them cling to the work and do anything and everything with unselfish interest; but some will yet be lost to the cause because they are not receiving proper encouragement.

There must be more of Christ's ways and less of self. Sharp criticisms should be repressed. Sympathy, compassion, and love should be cultivated in every worker. Unless Jesus comes in and takes possession of the heart; unless self is subdued, and Jesus exalted, we shall not prosper as a people. I testify that which I have seen. I beseech of you brethren, to labor wholly in God. Do not have too many plans, but strive to have the work carried on healthfully, circumspectly, and with such thoroughness that it will not ravel out.

There is another subject which I wish to mention to you. It is the matter of royalties on books. W. C. W. has received letters since he returned from America, from A. R. Henry of a very decided character on this point. W. C. W. has stated the positions taken by your board in B. C. I am very sorry that they are not far seeing in judgment. They evidence that they are narrow in their views and comprehension. They will arouse much unpleasantness of feeling in the bookmakers, and will not accomplish that which they have undertaken. This movement will create a want of harmony. God will not sanction any such means as they have in view, because they are not just. Here is the danger of depending on unsanctified men to make decisions.

Selfish policy is not heaven-born, but earthly. The leading maxim is, "The end justifies the means." And {368} in pursuing the course entered upon, it stops at nothing, but seeks its own success. This may be traced in every department of business; it is the prevailing element in every class of society; in the grand councils of nations, and in every meeting where the Spirit of Christ is not the ruling principle. Prudence and caution, tact and skill, need to be cultivated by everyone who is connected with our institutions. But the laws of justice and righteousness must not be left to one side, nor the all-prevailing principle to be to make their own branch of the work a success regardless of other branches. The interests of others should be investigated to see that no one's right is invaded.

The policy plan is a snare. While the council may pride themselves in the thought that they are doing a very nice thing, they show a shortsighted wisdom which will cripple their own efforts for success. The structure must be built upon a right foundation in order to stand. When the Board of the Publishing Association takes it upon themselves to urge that all the profits from books shall go to the Publishing Association, they are seeking to control matters which do not come under their jurisdiction. They are taking upon themselves a work which they cannot carry out.

These brain-workers have as much interest in the cause of God as those who compose the Board, which is willing to be conscience for them. Some of these have had a connection with the work almost from its infancy. God has not placed upon this Board the work of being conscience for others. They should not seek so persistently to force men to their terms. The policy plan is not to be classed with discretion; although it is too often mistaken for this. It is a species of selfishness in whatever cause it is exercised, and stops at nothing which promises success: but discretion uses judgment, and is never narrow in its workings, and has broad ideas, and the eye of the mind is capable of taking in more than one object, and views questions from all sides. While policy has a short range of vision, seeing every object near at hand, but failing to discover those at a distance. It is ever watching to obtain advantages which do not belong to it; and would build itself up by pulling out the foundation from another's building.

Let it not be necessary for God to send rebuke to men in responsible positions, who should be guardians of the people, especially of the interests of those who have long served in the cause of God; whose pen and voice have been active in bringing up the work to its present proportions. I wish I could lay these matters before these men in their true light. Ever since the Publishing Association was formed, light has been given in cases of perplexity. The Lord has often spoken, laying down principles and rules which must be carried out by all the workers. The grave responsibilities resting upon those in positions of trust have been continually kept before us, and we have sought the Lord from three to five times a day to give us heavenly wisdom that we might sacredly guard the interests of the cause, and of his chosen people. I have been repeatedly shown that we must do this. It was shown me that {369} those who preside over these institutions should ever bear in mind that there is a Chief Director, even the God of Heaven. There should be strict honesty in the business transactions in every department of the work. While there should be firmness in preserving order, there should also be compassion, mercy and forbearance incorporated into the character. Justice has a twin sister—love—and they should stand side by side.

It has been repeatedly presented before me that God is observing every transaction in that office. "Thou God seest me," should be ever in mind; courtesy and Christian politeness should be exercised by everyone who bears responsibilities in the office. They should have a sense of the encroachment upon others' rights which is so common in the world's practice, but which is an offense to God. The board of directors should ever act as under the divine eye, with a continual sense that they are finite men, and are liable to make mistakes in judgment, decisions, and plans, unless they are closely connected with God, and seeking to have every deficiency removed from their characters. As they are only weak and erring men themselves they should feel kindness and pity for others who may err. The divine standard must be met. You should take the Lord with you into every one of your councils. If you sense that God is in your assemblies every transaction will be conscientiously carefully and prayerfully considered. Every unprincipled act will be repressed, and uprightness will characterize the dealings in small as well as in large matters. There should be cultivation of universal kindness with the workers. First seek counsel of God, for this is necessary for you to properly counsel together.

There should be a watchcare lest the busy activities of life, the accumulating business, should so engross the workers that it would lead them to neglect prayer when the strength it would give them is most needed. Here comes in all the evils, because they deprive their souls of the strength and wisdom of heaven which is waiting their demand upon it. We need that illumination which God alone can give, and we are unfitted to transact business unless we have this wisdom. There are a few words of prayer uttered at the commencement of the meetings, but the heart is not brought into sympathy and harmony with God by earnest, importunate prayer, offered by broken hearts and contrite spirits, in living faith. If they divorce themselves from the God of wisdom and power, they cannot preserve that high integrity in dealing with their fellow men which God requires. Without divine wisdom, the objectionable traits of their characters will be woven into the decisions they make. And if these men are not in communication with God, Satan will just as surely be one in their councils, and take advantage of their unconsecrated state in their decisions. There will be acts of injustice because God is not presiding in their councils. The spirit of Christ must be an abiding, controlling power over the hearts and mind. In the world the god of traffic is the god of fraud. It must not be so with those who are dealing with God's cause. The worldly principle and standard is not to be the standard of those who are connected with {370} sacred things.

Some years ago the matter of publication of books came up, and plans were laid which I cannot now fully call to mind. A decision was made something like this: that no one individual was to be benefited by the publication of his own book. A proposition was then made to us which my husband, without ability to fully consider, assented to, that the Publishing Association should have the benefit of his books. I was considering the matter, and thought like this: I wish the Testimonies to go to as many as possible: they are a message from God to this people, and I wish no personal benefit from this work. Thus we stated the matter. But shortly after I was shown that this was not wisdom, to relinquish our right to control our own writings: for we would know better how to use the profits of these books, than would those who had far less experience; publications were to be multiplied, and the profits we would receive would enable us to lead out in the advancing work, to build up the interests of the cause, and to carry others with us in the work. There was a principle to be maintained to guard the interests of the true workers. We were not the only ones who

would be affected by this decision. Justice must be maintained: the cause of God would be continually widening, it would embrace the whole world as its field: the wants of the cause would not be determined by one man's mind and one man's obscure vision: there would be important work done in God's moral vineyard, and no man should feel that that part of the work over which he presides is to swallow all other interests.

I have been shown that brain workers have a God-given capital. The improvement of their brain belongs to God, and not man. If the worker gives the time to his employer for which he receives his pay, the employer has no further claim upon him. But if by close and diligent economy of moments he prepares matter for publication, it is his to do with as he, in the fear of God, thinks he can serve the cause of God the best. If he gives up all except a small royalty, he should not be urged to do more: he has already done a good work for those who handle the books; but if the publishers want it all, and cannot see that they are exceeding their rights in the demand, it would be the worst thing that could be done for the author to accede to their grasping, avaricious spirit, even though the plea be that it is for God's cause. The authors are responsible for the manner in which they use means received. There will be many calls for it. It was shown me that there would be many interests to build up, and that my husband and myself would be called upon to invest in meeting houses that would have to be erected which would never be built unless someone should feel and know the needs of the cause, and lead out in investments themselves.

I was also shown that there would be mission fields to be entered, and this would require means. Those to whom God has entrusted talents are to trade upon these talents according to their ability, for they are to act their part in carrying forward these interests. And that we would not be working for the best and most successful interests of the cause of God to have our income barely enough to sustain life, {371} as our experience would enable us to set many ways and opportunities of helping the cause which others would not discern. God, in his wise providence, gives the ability to write, and he designs that means should come into our hands to be used wisely, as his stewards, unrestricted by compromise. It is not our duty to shift our stewardship upon

any man or set of men, but to invest our means in his cause when and where the Spirit of God shall indicate. God himself has given us the ability to write, and calls upon us to use this entrusted talent for the advancement of his cause.

It was presented to me that there were poor men whose only means of obtaining a livelihood was their brain work. There are men who have not grown up with our institutions, and been benefited by the instruction which God has given from time to time, business men who will not incorporate in their business management the religion and spirit of Christ. They would separate religion, in a large degree from their business; therefore, even the Publishing Association should not be an all-controlling power. Individual talent and individual right must be respected. Should rules be established and arrangements entered into to invest the benefits of personal talent in the Publishing Association, other important interests would be crippled. Men would at times have a controlling power in connection with the Publishing Association who would not have compassion, and guard the interests of those in poverty and distress. There would be one iron rule, after the policy of the world rather than after the spirit of Christ, to bear upon all. The principles established would mean more to others than to us, therefore, we must be guarded in every decision.

Years ago it was shown me that my husband and myself should not be dependent upon others, because there would be men connected with our institutions who have been educated and trained as business men of the world, and they would work, acting out their spirit to make us feel our dependence if they had the chance; for all men are not, in character, as God would have them, tender, compassionate, and Christlike. He would have us guard the means entrusted to us, and use it in different branches of his work; stimulating others by our example to invest in the different enterprises, We should not invest largely in any one institution, for our message is a worldwide one, and there are necessities continually arising that demand means. To every man he has given his work, and talents of means and influence, and those who have the cause of God at heart will understand the voice of God telling them what to do. They will have a burden to push the work where it needs pushing, but others will only see the needs of their own respective branches, and other branches will be left to suffer for want of far seeing judgment.

It has several times been pointed out to me that there has been a close, ungenerous spirit exercised toward Brother _____, from the very first of his labors in Battle Creek. It makes me sad to state that the reason is that he came {372} to them in poverty, and a stranger. Because of this poverty he has been placed in unpleasant positions and made to feel his poverty. Because men connected with our institutions have thought they could bring him to their terms, he has had a very unpleasant time. There are unpleasant chapters in his experience which would not have been recorded if his brethren had been kind and dealt with him after the manner of Christ. The record in heaven is of such a character as some will not be proud to meet in the day of final settlement of all accounts. The Lord's cause should always be free from the slightest act of littleness, injustice, or oppression.

There were some men and women who invested means in the Publishing Association as a donation. Afterwards, through misfortune they were brought to actual distress and want. When my husband was stricken down by disease they came to the ones who occupied his place, and begged that some of the means which they had invested in good faith should be returned to them. The matter was treated on the policy plan, that business is business, religion is religion. The managers reasoned that nothing donated to the cause should be returned to the donors under any circumstances, and they took no measures to relieve the situation of those in distress. When my husband returned to his position in the office, these persons laid the matter before him. In the case of means donated by widows, my husband had objected when it was freely offered, and had entered upon the books the statement that the money should be repaid when donors needed it. Notwithstanding this, their cases were passed by with indifference. Such management may be dictated by worldly policy, but it is not in accordance with the character of Christ. We can best serve the cause of God by ever considering in tenderness the needs of suffering humanity.

In the cause of God, Christ's Spirit and manner of working are to be carried out in every particular. Mercy and justice will be the ruling principles where Christ abides. In order to be qualified for their positions of trust, men who are connected with the work of God, must be Christ like in all their dealings with each other. These principles we have labored to have maintained from the very first in our Publishing Association. We have had to fight the battle over and over with men connected with the Publishing Association. This is God's institution, and we prize it too highly to allow one blot or stain to rest upon this instrumentality, if we can do or say anything to prevent it.

The policy which worldly business men adopt is not to be chosen or carried out by men connected without institutions. I think it was in 1881 that the precious light was given me upon the scenes of the judgment. The books registering the deeds of men revealed the {373} dealings of those professing godliness in our institutions, showing that it was after the world's standard, and not in strict accordance with God's great standard of righteousness. That which bears a close relation to the question of dealing with others, especially with those connected with the work of God, was opened to me quite fully. The Spirit of Christ did not enter into and control the brethren's business arrangements. Their dealings were too much after the sharp policy plan, and not according to God's rule of right and justice. Some were suspicious and jealous, imagining that others were trying to gain advantages at their expense. Their attitude toward each other was not such as should exist between Christians.

I saw that there should be no close, sharp dealing between these brethren who were representatives of two important institutions of a different character, but branches of the same work. They should ever maintain a noble, generous, Christlike spirit; the spirit of grasping avarice should have no place in their dealings with each other. God's cause cannot be advanced by any acts which are contrary to the Spirit and character of Christ. Men should show an unselfish interest, seeking to advance one another's interest; for the cause of God can afford to be fair. Even a single instance of sharp dealing is an offense to God; and that which is sown will be reaped again. A selfish manner of dealing will provoke the same spirit in others. So with the manifestation of a Christian gentleman in spirit and word and deed; liberality, courtesy awaken the same spirit in others.

There is a spirit of worldly policy coming into the council and board meetings; a critical spirit in which personal feelings mold in a greater of less degree, decisions that are being made. A hard, unsympathetic spirit is ruling out the spirit of kindness, compassion, and love. Those who compose our councils need to sit daily at the feet of Christ, learning in his school to be meek and lowly of heart. They are not prepared to deal justly, to love mercy, and to exhibit that true courtesy which characterized the life of Christ, unless they see the necessity of yoking up with Christ and bearing the burdens of his cause. The love of Christ must be incorporated into the work of the several departments in the office, not only to do justice to the work, but to the workers also.

Your council and board meetings in 1886 need this instruction just as much, and even more, than in 1881. Let men receive a mold of character in the school of Christ; learning meekness and lowliness of heart from Jesus, and they will be less self-sufficient, less self-confident, and will not have too high an opinion of their own ability, but will be regarded by those in the office as Christian brethren, walking humbly with God, {374} trying to serve in whatever capacity they can do the most good without trying to exalt themselves. This lesson has not been learned by some. Therefore, they have a new character to form, a new experience to gain, which shall fit them to come close to the hearts of their brethren, and to deal with those who have a part to act in the work. They will have to guard themselves closely, or they will be dictatorial and officious, ready to give orders, to speak of, and to take the oversight of, things of which they are ignorant, and will thus disgust the workers in the office. If they take hold in a humble way, trying to learn as much as they can, maintain the position of learner rather than a director, they will make themselves friends in the office. Everyone that serves in the board meetings, needs to seek most earnestly the wisdom from above. The influence of the Spirit of Christ upon their hearts will then place a right mold upon the work. The transforming grace of Christ will be manifest in every board meeting, quelling tumultuous actions, and charming away the unhallowed effects of business, and checking the sharp critical, worldly policy which makes men overbearing and ready to accuse. There will have to be most earnest reformation in the characters of those who are now connected with our important institutions. Some of these men possess valuable talents, but they must fashion their lives after the divine character of Christ. Everyone must remember that they have not yet "attained"—the work of character building is not yet finished. If they will improve every ray of light God has given, and walk in this light, they will learn lessons from Christ. By comparing their lives with Christ's character, they will be able to discern where they have failed to meet the requirements of God's holy law; and will seek to make themselves perfect in their sphere even as God is perfect in his sphere. If men of today had realized the importance of their positions, they would have been far in advance, far better qualified to fill positions of trust than they are.

In these hours of probation we are to seek for perfection of character. We must learn daily of Christ. We are connected with the cause of Christ, not because we are perfect and unerring, but notwithstanding these defects, and God expects those connected with his work to be constantly studying how to copy the pattern.

Jesus connected John, Peter, and Judas with him in his work, making them colaborers with him, and at the same time they were to be constantly learning lessons of Christ gathering from the divine Teacher instructions that would correct their wrong ideas and incorrect views of what constituted a Christian character. John and Peter were not perfect, but they improved every opportunity to learn. Peter did not learn to be jealous and distrustful of himself, until he was overcome by the devil {375} and denied the Lord. Judas had the same opportunities to learn as did the other disciples, but he was a hearer only, and not a doer. The result was manifested in the betrayal of His Lord. God has connected men with his instrumentalities, and he wants them to be learners; they must not feel self-sufficient, or self-important, but must ever realize that they are treading on holy ground. Angels of God are ready to minister unto them, and they must receive light and heavenly influences daily, or they are no more fit for the work than are unbelievers. Transformation will be wrought in those who will repress unfavorable traits of character, and develop Christlike dispositions; this alone will bring them up to the highest standard of Christian character. Judas failed to be benefited because he did not see the importance of having his character molded after the example of Christ.

The Lord guards every man's interest. He was always the poor man's friend, and would have his interests sacredly guarded.

There is a most wonderful dearth of the love of Christ in the hearts of nearly all of those who are handling sacred things. I would echo from one part of the earth to the other, that the love of Christ should be cultivated; it should well up in the soul of the Christian like streams in the desert, refreshing the heart, bringing gladness, peace, and joy into their own as well as into other lives. No man liveth unto himself. If there is the least of depression practiced toward the poor, or unjust dealing with them either in large or small things, God will hold the actor accountable. The very first work, my brethren, is to secure the blessing of God in your own hearts. This is where the work begins. Then take the blessing into your homes; let the atmosphere of cheerfulness and kindness prevail; put away your criticisms, overcome your exacting spirit. The atmosphere that surrounds you in your homes will also envelop you in the office. Wherever the love of Jesus reigns, there is pity, tenderness, and thoughtful care for others. The most precious work that my brethren can engage in is that of forming a Christlike character that they may enter into the mansions which Christ has gone to prepare for them. I cannot be a party to any unjust dealing with any of God's children.

Do not seek to make with Elder Smith, Professor Bell, or any other brain-worker terms that are not perfectly just and fair. Do not urge nor compel them to accept terms dictated by those who do not know what it is to make books. They have a conscience and are accountable to God for the use and improvement of their entrusted talents; and they want the privilege of investing the means which they acquire by hard labor, when and where the Spirit of God shall indicate. My brethren must remember that the cause of God includes more than the publishing house, and other institutions established {376} at Battle Creek. No one understands better than Brother Smith the difficulties through which the Publishing Association was brought into existence, for he has been connected with it from its earliest years when it was oppressed by poverty, and self-denial had to be carried into our practical life. The table was hardly supplied with sufficient food to sustain our lives; there was economy in dressing and in wages paid. This was positively necessary in order that the paper might live. Those who passed through these experiences would be ready, under similar circumstances, to undergo the same privations

again. It does not show very good grace for those who have had no part in raising the work up to its present prosperous condition, to press and urge, and even try to force the early workers to submit to terms which they can see no justice in. Brother Smith loves the cause of God. He loves the truth, and will invest his means to advance it wherever he sees that it is necessary. But leave this burden upon those with whom God has entrusted talents and means; they are responsible to him, and the Publishing Association or its chief workers, are not to assume their stewardship.

If the Board should succeed in bringing the workers to their terms, would the writers feel that they had been dealt with justly, would it not rather open a door of temptation to them, and break up sympathy and harmonious action between the brethren? If they should carry out this plan to grasp all the profits for the Publishing Association, it would be worse than they can imagine. A train of evils would grow out of such an arrangement that would be disastrous to the Association. And it would encourage a spirit of intolerance, a narrow conceited spirit, which God cannot approve but which Satan enjoys, and longs to have take possession of those who are connected with God's sacred work. The Bible precepts must be carried out in everyday life. They will be a lamp to your feet and a light to your path. The greatest of all deceptions is for a man to think that he can find a better guide through difficulties than is found in the word of God. It is the worst kind of policy to leave the Lord out of your councils and put your confidence in the wisdom of men. In your positions of trust you are, in a special sense, to be the light of the world, and in order that you may be clean channels of light you should feel an intense desire to place yourselves in connection with the God of light, of wisdom and knowledge. Important interests that relate to the prosperity and advancement of present truth are to be considered; and how can you be competent to arrive at right decisions, to give wise counsels, and to make proper plans unless you are connected with the source of all wisdom and righteousness? Your councils have been regarded in altogether too cheap a light, and common talk, and comments upon others' doings have found a place in these important meetings. You should bear in mind that the all-seeing {377} eye of Jehovah is a witness in all your councils; he measures every one of your decisions, and compares them with his holy law, the great moral standard of righteousness. Those holding the positions of counselors should be unselfish men, men of faith, men of prayer, men that will not dare to rely upon their own human wisdom, but will seek earnestly for light and intelligence as to what is the best manner of conducting their business. Joshua, the commander of Israel, searched the books diligently in which Moses had faithfully chronicled the directions given by God; his requirements, reproofs, and restrictions, lest he should move unadvisedly. Joshua was afraid to trust his own impulses, or his own wisdom. He regarded everything that came from Christ, who was enshrouded with a pillar of cloud by day and a pillar of fire by night, as of sufficient importance to be sacredly cherished. He meditated day and night upon the words which had been spoken to Moses, the servant of God. Joshua desired to know and to do, God's will, and he was commanded by God to study and meditate upon all the directions which had been given: "For then, shalt thou make thy way prosperous, and thou shalt have success." The secret of Joshua's victories was that, even amid his accumulated cares and responsibilities, he dared not trust to his own finite wisdom, but made God his counselor and guide.

The Pharisee, scribes, and elders, in Christ's days manifested an avaricious spirit which brought them under the control of Satan, and was the main cause of their hatred toward Christ; for his teaching and example rebuked everything of this character. If such a spirit should be cherished in our institutions under any pretense, God cannot abide there. There should not be a grasping spirit manifested toward brethren, for it is not born of heaven, but from beneath. Any injustice done to God's children is registered in the books of heaven as done unto Christ. That success which is attained through taking advantage of another by sharp dealing, will prove to be a loss in the end; but that which appears to be loss through the practice of principles that represent the life of Christ, is divine success.

Those connected with the work of God have not yet the crown of immortal glory upon their brows, but are still engaged in earthly battles. They are still on probation, being tried and tested by God's great standard of righteousness and it is their business to prove themselves true men, lovers of righteousness and haters of ev-

ery evil practice, which makes our world today like the world before the flood. They must be men willing to venture something in order to carry out the precious principles laid down by the word of God. They should make determined efforts to be representative men after God's pattern, rejoicing in success only when it arises from obedience to duty and truth. They need to strive {378} to show their wisdom by the confession of weakness and inefficiency; for this throws them on the strength and all sufficiency of Christ. They that be whole need not a physician, but they that are sick. The most deplorable lack any can suffer is that of an earnest determination to do right at whatever cost to self. The lack of humility, the loss of faith and sterling integrity, should cause intense sorrow. If the soul is filled with earthly things; if the heart has not maintained close communion with God; there is no room for heavenly intelligence to work, and there is an earthliness in every project that is devised. The communication with heaven must be kept open; clear the channel in some way. He that is to plan and devise in the interests of God's cause must see that his connection with heaven is not cut off, before he should dare to come into the room for counsel, otherwise Satan will accompany him and manipulate his thoughts and plans to suit his satanic majesty. The atmosphere of heaven must surround you if you would have your plans and works in harmony with heaven. O, how important it is that the representative men keep themselves in the love of God, so that they may be quick to discern, and respond to the signals from heaven.

March 2. My head became so weary I could not complete this in time to mail it last night. I wish to say to my brethren that Michigan has been shown to me as being bound about with too extreme caution, a determination to save means for the Conference; but while economy and caution are essential in our work, unless the mind is broad enough to take in its real needs, these elements will be a block before the wheel of its progress.

There is talent in Michigan, but it needs to be discerned and educated and disciplined. There are some who have experience, who should put forth every effort, in the dying churches as well as in new places, to select suitable young men, and men of mature age, to assist in the work. Thus they will obtain useful knowledge by interesting themselves in personal efforts,

and scores of helpers may be fitted up for usefulness as Bible workers canvassers, and family visitors. But his kind of work is being neglected because there is such great fear of using the Conference money, and men reluctant to bear essential responsibilities to educate men to do the work.

Our brethren should always go out two and two, taking as many as they can really to engage in personal visiting, seeking to interest families. But those who would work in these lines are not encouraged; when mistakes are made, they are not corrected in tender compassion, but are disheartened. Michigan is one of the best mission fields in the world, but it needs men with far-seeing judgment to push the work. {379}

God would have those in responsible positions show tact, skill, and wise generalship in detecting, seizing upon, and putting talent to use. He will not work miracles to advance the truth, without human agents cooperating. He has material in men and women, and he wants the generals in his army to have intelligence to bring it out and act their part to put it to use, not be constantly studying how to bind about the work, so that it shall not branch out and create a demand for more means. Set men to work under those who have some knowledge of the work, and who can educate them. Thrust the workers out into the harvest field. All that they want is encouragement.

Elder _____'s mind must grow with the work, or he must be replaced by someone who will take a more extensive view of what needs to be done to warn the world. Do something, do it now. Let the pull-back principle go, and the go-forward principle come in. The angel with the third message flies swiftly.

(Signed) E. G. White

I have spoken to you the truth because I dare not withhold it. My words are not designed to discourage, but to open before you the fact that although you may have good business qualities and tact, yet something higher than this is necessary in the work in which you are engaged. You may become men as valuable as gold, and this is why I have written as I have. Your character must reflect the character of Christ.

(Signed) Ellen G. White

DEAR BROTHER BUTLER

October 1, 1885
Christiania, Norway

I WAS MORE SORRY THAN I can express, to learn that under your instruction Brother Farnsworth and Burrill sought to restrict the work at the New York camp meeting. You could not have advised them to do a worse thing, and you should not have put a work into their hands that they were not fitted to do in a wise manner. Be careful how you repress advancing work in any locality. There is little enough being done in any place, and it certainly is not proper to seek to curtail operations in missionary lines.

After looking matters over carefully and prayerfully, I wrote as I did in my notes of travel. I wanted to leave the matter in such a shape as not to discourage the laborers in New York in their efforts to do something, {380} although I desired to give them caution, so that they would not make any extreme moves in their plans. The workers were doing well, and ought to have been encouraged and advised to go on with their work. There are men in New York who should have helped them by making needed donations to invest in the cause. They will have to give to the work before they will grow in grace and the knowledge of the truth.

You and your workers should have looked at this matter from different points of view than you did. You should have investigated the work thoroughly, and asked yourselves if five thousand dollars was too large a debt to incur in the important work in which these workers were engaged. Your influence should have been exerted in such a way as to cause the people to see the importance of the work, and to realize that it was their duty to rise to the emergency. You should have done as I have tried to in my notes of travel. But if our brethren feel at liberty to stop the work when they cannot see where money is coming from to sustain it, then the work will not only be contracted in Michigan and New York, but in every other State in the Union. If our workers are going forward in any place, do not put up the bars, and say, "Thus far shalt thou go and no farther." I feel sad that you have closed up the school at Rome, N. Y. I see that the brethren sent to look after this enterprise have not taken measures to advance the work by soliciting donations from men who could give. There are rich men in the Conference who have made complaints about the debt that has been incurred, who ought to have sustained these workers. While reproach and discouragement have been cast upon the workers, the impression has been left upon those who have means that they have a perfect right to question every enterprise that calls for money.

God does not require you to take such a course that the workers in New York or anywhere else shall not feel at liberty to make advance movements unless they can consult you, and ask what your judgment of the matter is before they advance. I cannot sanction the idea that you must have a personal oversight of all the details of the work. If I did the result would be that no worker would dare to exercise his own judgment in anything. The workers would have to rely upon one man's brain and one man's judgment, and the result would be that men would be left in inefficiency because of their inactivity. There are altogether too many of this class now, and they amount to next to nothing. I write this because I feel deeply on this point. We are not doing one half that we ought to do.

It is true that the South Lancaster school must be sustained, but this need not hinder us from sustaining other schools. We should have primary schools in different localities to prepare the youth for our {381} higher schools. It may seem to you that it is wise to close up the school in Rome, N. Y., but I fail to see the wisdom of it. To close up this school will seem to reflect discredit upon all that the people have done, and will discourage them from making further advancement. I cannot see that you have gained anything in making the move that you have, nor can I feel that it is in accordance with God's order. It will work nothing but injury, not only to those that have complained about the debt, but also to the workers. Men who have property, and could have helped this enterprise, will breathe more freely. These moneyed men will be encouraged not to do more for the cause than they have done, but to do less. They will feel at liberty to complain concerning anything that calls for an outlay of means.

O that the Lord might guide you. You should never in a single instance allow hearsay to move you to action, and yet you have sometimes done this. Never take action to narrow and circumscribe the work unless you know that you are moved to do so by the Spirit of the Lord. Our people are doing work for foreign missions, but there are home missions that need their help just as much as these foreign missions. We should make efforts to show our people the wants of the cause of God, and to open before them the need of using means that God has entrusted to them to advance the work of the Master both at home and abroad. Unless those who can help in New York are roused to a sense of their duty, they will not recognize the work of God when the loud cry of the third angel shall be heard. When light goes forth to lighten the earth, instead of coming up to the help of the Lord, they will want to bind about his work to meet their narrow ideas. Let me tell you that the Lord will work in this last work in a manner very much out of the common order of things, and in a way that will be contrary to any human planning. There will be those among us who will always want to control the work of God, to dictate even what movements shall be made when the work goes forward under the direction of the angel who joins the third angel in the message to be given to the world. God will use ways and means by which it will be seen that he is taking the reins in his own hands. The workers will be surprised by the simple means that he will use to bring about and perfect his work of righteousness. Those who are accounted good workers will need to draw nigh to God, they will need the divine touch. They will need to drink more deeply and continuously at the fountain of living water, in order that they may discern God's work at every point. Workers may make mistakes, but you should give them an opportunity to learn caution by leaving the work in their hands.

(Signed) Ellen G. White

DEAR BRETHREN BUTLER AND HASKELL

October 28, 1885
Orebo, Sweden {382}

MY PRAYER IS THAT THE Lord may be with you in great power during the coming Conference. Some may be absent that you might wish were present; but Jesus is your helper. I sincerely hope and pray that those who bear responsibilities in Michigan, New England, Ohio, Indiana, and other States, shall take broader views of the work than they have done. I hope Michigan will take a step in advance. I feel to regret the fact that there is such a dearth of breadth of mind and of far seeing ability. Workers should be educated and trained for the fields of labor. We need missionaries everywhere. We need men and women who will give themselves without reserve to the work of God, bringing many sons and daughters to God.

I have been shown that there is one

practice which those in responsible places should avoid; for it is detrimental to the work of God. Men in position should not lord it over God's heritage, and command everything around them. Too many have marked out a prescribed line which they wish others to follow in the work. Workers have tried to do this with blind faith, without exercising their own judgment upon the matter which they had in hand. If those who were placed as directors were not present, they have followed their implicit directions just the same. But in the name of Christ, I would entreat you to stop this work. Give men a chance to exercise their individual judgment. Men who follow the leading of another, and are willing that another should think for them, are unfit to be entrusted with responsibility. Our leading men are remiss in this matter. God has not given to special ones all the brain power there is in the world. Men in responsible positions should credit others with some sense, with some ability of judgment and foresight, and look upon them as capable of doing the work committed to their hands. Our leading brethren have made a great mistake in marking out all the directions that the workers should follow, and this has resulted in deficiency, in a lack of the care taking spirit in the worker, because they have relied upon others to do all their planning, and have themselves taken no responsibility. Should the men who have taken this responsibility upon themselves step out of our ranks, or die, what a state of things would be found in our institutions. Leading men should place responsibilities upon others and allow them to plan and devise and execute, so that they may obtain an experience. Give them a word of counsel when necessary, but do not take away the work because you think the brethren are making mistakes. May God pity the cause when one man's mind and one man's plan is followed without question. God would not be honored should such a state of things exist. All our workers must have room to exercise their own judgment and discretion. God has given men talents which he means that they should use. He has {383} given them minds, and he means that they should become thinkers, and do their own thinking and planning, rather than depend upon others to think for them.

I think I have laid out this matter many times before you, but I see no change in your actions. We want every responsible man to drop responsibilities upon others.

Set others at work that will require them to plan, and to use judgment. Do not educate them to rely upon your judgment. Young men must be trained up to be thinkers. My brethren, do not for a moment think that your way is perfection, and that those who are connected with you must be your shadows, must echo your words, repeat your ideas, and execute your plans. There are men today might be men of breadth of thought, might be wise men, men to be depended upon, who are not such, because they have been educated to follow another man's plan. They have allowed others to tell them precisely what they should do, and they have become dwarfed in intellect. Their minds are narrow, and they cannot comprehend the needs of the work. They are simply machines to be moved by another man's thought. Now do not think that these men who do follow out your ideas are the only ones that can be trusted. You have sometimes thought that because they do your will to the letter, that they were the only ones in whom you could place dependence. If anyone exercised his own judgment, and differed with you, you have disconnected from him as one that could not be trusted. Take your hands off the work, and do not hold it fast in your grasp. You are not the only man whom God will use. Give the Lord room to use the talents he has entrusted to men, in order that the cause may grow. Give the Lord a chance to use men's minds. We are losing much by our narrow ideas and plans. Do not stand in the way of the advancement of the work, but let the Lord work by whom he will. Educate, encourage young men to think and act, to devise and plan, in order that we may have a multitude of counselors.

How my heart aches to see presidents of conferences taking the burden of selecting those whom they think they can mold to work with them in the field. They take those who will not differ from them, but will act like mere machines. No president has any right to do this. Leave others to plan, and if they fail in some things, do not take it as an evidence that they are unfitted to be thinkers. Our most responsible men had to learn by a long discipline how to use their judgment. In many things they have shown that their work ought to have been better. The fact that men make mistakes is no reason that we should think them unfit to be caretakers. Those who think that their ways are perfect, even now make many grave blunders, but others are none the wiser for it. They present their success,

but their mistakes do not appear. Then be kind and considerate to every man who conscientiously enters the field as a worker for the Master. Our most responsible men have made some unwise plans, and have carried them out because they thought {384} their plans were perfect. They have heeded the mingling of other elements of mind and character. They should have associated with other men who could view matters from an entirely different point of view. Thus they would have helped them in their plans.

This same character of spirit is found here in Europe. For years Elder Andrews held the work back from advancing, because he feared to entrust it to others lest they would not carry out his precise plans. He would never allow anything to come into existence that did not originate with him. Elder Loughborough also held everything in his grasp while he was in California and England, and as a result the work is years behind in England. Elder Wilcox and Sister Thayer have the same spirit of having everything go in the exact way in which they shall dictate, and no one is being trained in such a way as to know how to get hold of the work for himself. What folly it is to trust a great mission in the hands of one man, so that he shall mold and fashion it in accordance with his mind, and after his own diseased imagination. Men who have been narrow, who have served tables, who are not far seeing, are disqualified for putting their mold upon the work. Those who desire to control the work think that none can do it perfectly but themselves, and the cause bears the marks of their defects.

(Signed) Ellen G. White

FROM PRUSSIA
1886

IN ANOTHER LETTER I HAVE spoken in reference to your accumulating so many responsibilities in Battle Creek, when there is so little managing talent that is consecrated to the work of God to take care of these interests. I have spoken in disapproval of the enlargement of the Sanitarium, on the ground that so large a share of its responsibilities are resting upon one man. Doctor Kellogg has to be both physician and manager. Now, my brother, these things are not as God would have them. He is not pleased that so much means should be invested in one locality. Other men should be educated to share in the responsibility that Doctor Kellogg is burdened with, in order that if he fails, another will be prepared to carry the institution forward. We feel to thank God that Dr. Kellogg has the good health that he has, but he may not always have it, and the fact that he has it now, is no reason why our people should sleep till the last moment. They should manage this matter wisely. Great interests are at stake, and unless Dr. Kellogg has less responsibilities, he will not be enabled to stand the pressure for a great while.

There is great need that someone should also stand at the side of Brother C. J. Jones, in order to share the {385} responsibility that he carries, so that if he should fail another could go forward with the work without a disagreeable break. If he were relieved of some of his burdens, he would last the longer. He should not have so great cares, and so heavy burdens to carry, and should not be obliged to work when he should rest. The children of this world are wiser in their generation than the children of light. Jesus said this, and we see that the world works on a different plan in these matters. Weighty responsibilities connected with the business of the world, are not placed wholly upon one man. In large business enterprises, responsible men choose others to share their burdens, and lift their responsibilities, so that in case one should fail, there is someone ready to step into his place. Someone should feel a burden over these matters, and a decided change should take place in the manner of our work.

(Signed) Ellen G. White

FROM BROOKLYN, NEW YORK

November 25, 1890

"John to the seven churches which are in Asia; Grace be unto you, and peace, from him which is, and which was, and which is to come; and from the seven Spirits which are before his throne; and from Jesus Christ, who is the faithful witness, and the first begotten of the dead, and the prince of the kings of the earth. Unto him that loved us, and washed us from our sins in his own blood, and hath made us kings and priests unto God and his Father; to him be glory and dominion forever and forever. Amen. Behold he cometh with clouds; and every eye shall see him, and they also which pierced him: and all kindreds of the earth shall wail because of him. Even so, Amen. I am Alpha and Omega, the beginning and the ending, saith the Lord, which is and which was, and which is to come, the Almighty." After this is given a message revealing future events; for John is commanded to write "the things which thou hast seen, and the things which are, and the things which shall be hereafter."

MATTERS OF DEEP importance were opened before John which were to be given to the world to be read, understood, and appreciated, in the ages to come. Again and again the true witness says, "He that hath ears to hear, let him hear what the Spirit saith unto the churches." But it is evident from what is written that some who have ears to hear, will not hear, will not receive the message, and will not become wise in the scriptures. The Lord Jesus, the Alpha and Omega, gave a message to John in regard to the work of the churches; for he understood how great would be the danger of neglecting their God given work, and thus make a failure of diffusing light to others. The invitation {386} of the gospel was to extend from Christ to the church, and from the church to the world. "And the Spirit and the Bride say, Come. And let him that heareth say Come. And let him that is a thirst say Come, and whosoever will, let him take of the water of life freely." The work of diffusing the gospel is neglected by those who are specified as hearing. But when the professed people of God hear the message to some purpose, when they take on the burden of the work and say to others, "Come," then they will become laborers together with God.

During the night I have been in communion with God. I have been brought by my guide into councils in Battle Creek, and I have a message to bear to you whether you will hear or not, whether you will receive it or reject it. The people must know that they are not moving in the order of God. They have left Christ out of their councils. Leading men are giving a mold to the work that will result in a loss of many souls; for they are moving away from the safe path. Many come here from foreign countries, thinking that Battle Creek, from whence come the publications of truth, will be next to heaven. How disappointed they feel, when they hear in this place, the message of God spoken of lightly, when they hear the messengers of God, by some in responsible places, made a subject of ridicule, and why is this? It is because the message of the messengers does not coincide in every particular with the ideas of these whom the Lord names of his scorners, although it is a message sent from heaven.

Where the truth is rejected, it opens up a way where false waymarks will be set up, and perils will rise on all sides. Through neglect of seeking the earnest counsel of God, men will be connected with the office, who will form themselves into a ring, to echo the sentiments of him whom they consider most influential, and who pleases their human ideas. My guide spoke slowly and solemnly, "Associate yourselves, O ye people, and ye shall be broken in pieces; and give ear all ye far countries; gird yourselves, and ye shall be broken in pieces. Take counsel together, and it shall come to naught; speak the word, and it shall not stand; for God is with us."

Men may be selected by the Conference to connect with the office of publication, but unless these men look to God, and with a transformation of character, unless they seek counsel of God in large and small matters, concerning things connected with the sacred work of God, unless they are emptied of vanity and self, they will be turned from the safe path, and will turn others from the path cast up for the ransomed of the Lord. Unless these associated together are converted men, and they walk in, see, and realize the sacredness of the work of God, for these last time, they will surely imperil the work of God, and discouragement will come upon the people. It is not enough that they assent to the truth; the question is, "Are they sanctified through the truth? Has the truth been brought into the inner sanctuary of the soul?" {387} The past, present, and future, was plainly revealed to me.

When Brother Chadwick was connected with the office at first, he needed a decided change in his character; he needed the gentleness of Christ. His connection has not been to his advantage, or to the benefit of those with whom he was connected; but the atmosphere he has breathed, the words, the precepts, and the example of strong minds and firm wills, sat in the wrong way, brought to the front objectionable traits in his character. He has become sick at heart and desperate in impulse when opposed, and he is man with another spirit. Saul became another man, because the Spirit of the Lord rested upon him, and he had another heart given him. But in the case of Brother Chadwick, the change is of a different character, and from a different source. I have no words to speak individually, to the men from whom this influence has come; my words must be spoken to them as a whole. It is not to be left to them to repeat my words as they have done, interpret them as they please, and thus transmit them to others. I wish to present the matter to them from my own lips as God has presented it to me. How long shall blindness be upon men who have evidence piled on evidence that the Testimonies are indicted by the Spirit of God to his people? How long shall men in positions of trust fail to discern how and where God is working? Eyes have they but they see not, ears have they but they hear not, understanding have they, but they understand not the things of God. Reproofs should not harden you, for "Behold, happy is the man whom God correcteth: therefore despise not the chastening of the Almighty; for he maketh sure, and he bindeth up; he woundeth, and his hands maketh whole."

Many of the old, experienced hands have fallen in death. Those who led out in the work of God, and who could tell how it came into existence, have passed away from the scene of action. In every branch of the work, men have been departing from the principles laid down by the Lord Jehovah to control the working of the cause. Inexperienced hands and unsanctified minds have been placing their mold upon the work, and self has been woven into it in every branch.

Before the destruction of the old world, there were talented men, men who possessed skill and knowledge; but they became lifted up in their own imaginations; just as men are doing today, and because they left God out of their plans and councils, they became wise to do that which God had never told them to do, wise to do evil. Their wisdom would have worked destruction to those who should be born who should come in contact with them, and the Lord took the matter in hand, and cut them off from the earth. After sending them warnings for a hundred and twenty years, God's mercy and forbearance was exhausted, and then the day of probation was ended. The probation given them in mercy, they devoted to ridiculing Noah, {388} whom God had sent with a message. They caricatured and criticized him, just as some who thought themselves wise have done; they have laughed at the messengers just as they did in Noah's day for his peculiar earnestness, and for his intense feelings in regard to the judgments that were sure to come. Noah warned them that God would fulfill his word; but they reasoned among themselves, they talked of science, and of the laws controlling nature, and they laughed Noah to scorn, calling him a crazy fanatic. Men who believe themselves to be wise in our day, will do good to their own souls, and to the souls for whom Christ died, if they recognize that there is a wisdom, an unsanctified wisdom, that comes from beneath, which has been in the world ever since the fall.

I have been shown that there is a great want of personal piety among the workers in the office, nearly every one of them, and that their unsanctified wisdom is a result of a lack of connection with God. They take very little time to seek God's counsel with humble contrition of soul, with earnest searching of heart; self-sufficient they walk in the sparks of their own kindling. The spiritual atmosphere which surrounds their soul, does not make manifest that they have constant reliance upon God. The most sacred truths are fast losing their preciousness and sanctity to them, because they do not have a full connection with God, and receive the things that be of God. Unless the converting power of God shall be felt upon the hearts and characters of men in positions of trust, they will not, cannot, be one with Christ, keeping the way of the Lord, but like the Pharisees in the days of Christ, they will teach the doctrines and commandments of men, and the Lord will have no more use for them. They cannot be laborers together with God, while they keep the spirit that has actuated them in the past. They have felt but little respect for those who have stood under the direction of God in seeking counsel from him who is mighty in wisdom, in founding and building up his great work in the earth. The consecration, the vital piety, the humility which God requires, does not exist among them. Self is exalted, and Jesus is not glorified. Jesus, the blessed and only potentate between God and man, is not working with them. Satan's insinuations are credited, and plain commands of God in regard to mercy and tender compassion are ignored. Those who are handling sacred truths in the publishing work or in any branch of the cause of God, are invited of God to put forth their highest mental and moral energies, to study continually, in their business line, not the will of men, but the will of God.

The office is fast losing its peculiar character of the Lord directed in its establishment, and it is never to take a worldly mold. Those who are welded together to sustain each other, determined to carry out certain plans without the counsel of the church or the people, any succeed for a time, but not long; for God will not permit it. {389} There is too much self, too much confidence in what men can do, too little confidence and dependence upon God, the divine ruler. Men handling sacred things, are not to speak lightly, but with trembling of the work of God. God's grace must be manifested in all the work, of whatever kind it may be. The proud heart must be humbled every day before God, lest he shall humble it. Success of the right kind will attend your efforts in proportion to your consecration, self-denial, and self-sacrifice.

I was instructed that the Lord's will was not fulfilled when the leaders in the office were willing to take such large wages; but how quickly was the bribe taken, how quickly selfishness was manifested. This is greatly at variance with the principles upon which the publishing house was established; and it is not in harmony with the spirit and work of God. There have been serious mistakes made in exalting business above the service and worship of God. Here is where thousands have made shipwreck of faith, and made the greatest possible mistake. The Lord says we are to be "Not slothful in business; fervent in spirit; serving the Lord." The Lord has left a wide door open for those who would go into his work, but energy must be mingled with another element, with living zeal in the service of God. We must be not only diligent in business, but "fervent in spirit, serving the Lord." Devotion and piety and godliness must be interwoven with every transaction. Without this in your business, you will commit robbery toward God, while professing to serve him. We see family and home religion neglected, altars broken down, first love abandoned, and the religion of Christ expelled from the soul, to give place to engaging in speculation and business enterprises, and these things are constantly multiplying. Men are leaving God and Heaven out of their calculations, and time spent in searching the heart is considered wasted. The Bible is neglected, and a multitude of cares overbalance the precious truth of God in the heart, and spiritual eyesight is put out. How much men need the heavenly anointing!

(Signed) Ellen G. White

DEAR BRETHREN IN RESPONSIBLE POSITIONS IN THE REVIEW AND HERALD OFFICE

January 13, 1894
Brighton, Victoria, Australia
(Copy for Elder O. A. Olsen)

I AM MUCH PLEASED THAT YOU have restored Henry Kellogg to his old position, who I trust is born again, not of the flesh but of the Spirit of God. I greatly feared that his long separation from the work would disqualify him to stand in the position he is now occupying; but if the Lord has indeed accepted him, and I know he is {390} always ready to accept any soul who will return from his wanderings and accept of Jesus Christ, he will be qualified to do the work to which God has called him. The arms of Jesus are open to accept him, and he is willing to bless and to teach him. He will realize the force of the word that Christ spoke to Joshua, the high priest, "And the angel of the Lord protested unto Joshua, saying Thus saith the Lord of Hosts; for if thou wilt keep my charge, (the Lord has in his messages shown what this charge is) then thou shalt also judge my house, and shalt also keep my courts, and I will give thee places to walk among these that stand by.

I long to see the righteousness of Christ upon everyone who has any official standing in the office, For a long time warnings, invitations, entreaties, reproofs have been given of God in order that decided reforms should be made in those who were not revealing the life of Christ in their characters. God has sent messages in order that there might have been a transformation of the natural temperament. So that men, leaning on Christ, might be laborers together with God. Men should heed the instruction, "Learn of me; for I am meek and lowly in heart: and ye shall find rest unto your souls." Many moves have been made, many decisions have been carried out in your counsels, that have not been after Christ's likeness. Why? Because self has not been under the control of the Spirit of Christ. You have too often revealed in your counsels a hard, harsh, iron like spirit, to those who differ with you, that has been as unlike the meekness and gentleness of Christ, as Satan is unlike Christ. The Spirit of Christ has been grieved, and his great heart of love has been wounded, because souls have been torn and bruised that might have been healed and bound up, and

saved, that might today have been doing acceptable service in the Lord's army.

What great need there is of cultivating tenderness and gentleness. None should be ashamed to manifest a tender, compassionate spirit for those who err; for those who think they make no mistakes, are far from being without fault before God. No one needs to think that the manifestation of compassion is something for which they need be ashamed, Thorough and decided reformation must be made that this hard, iron like spirit which has been so often and easily brought to the front and made manifest in words and measures that savor more of the attributes of Satan than of the Spirit of Christ, should be overcome. I have a message for the workers in both high and low position in the office to each one of them in their several departments. It is that unless the transforming grace of Christ conforms you to his character, you will never be numbered with the family of God in heaven. Now is the testing time. Angels of God are watching the development of character. {391} Angels of God are weighing moral worth and nothing can make a man truly great in God's estimation except being truly good, being a partaker of the divine nature, escaping the corruption of the world through lust. The world's Redeemer demands that those who are called by his name, who claim to stand under his banner shall represent his character; Christianity is intensely practical. When Christianity is brought into the circumstances of actual life, it is a safeguard to the soul in all daily cares, perplexities, and annoyances, and then it is that the sympathy, tenderness, and gentleness of Christ is manifested in the deportment, and revealed in the character of those in whose heart God abides; and then it is that the kingdom of God comes in through his representatives into the world.

The whole man is then molded after the divine likeness, and he manifests the character of Christ in the home, in the office, and in the congregation where saints assemble to worship God. Christianity then becomes a working power, and has a transforming effect upon the agents in a working world; for then men cooperate with divine agencies in their daily occupations whatever they may be, or wherever they may be. At the present time there is not a thorough, correcting, transforming power circulating through the publishing institution, such as God requires. A deeper and more thorough work is needed in the hearts of those who hold

positions, from the lowest to the highest. "And whatsoever ye do in work or deed, do all in the name of the Lord Jesus, giving thanks to God and the Father by him." Again comes the requirement, "Whether ye eat or drink, or whatsoever ye do, do all to the glory of God."

The truth of God revealed in his word is to be a living, abiding principle. It is not to be looked upon as an influence among many others. It will exercise a power over the life and conduct until the whole being is assimilated to the image of the perfect pattern, and the human agent is complete in Jesus Christ. "As ye have therefore received Christ Jesus the Lord, so walk ye in him, rooted and built up," not in self, not after man's ideas, but "in him established in the faith as ye have been taught, abounding therein with thanksgiving. Beware lest any man spoil you through philosophy and vain deceit, after the traditions of men, after the rudiments of the world, and not after Christ." Your greatest danger will be that you will not see the need of contemplating the character of Christ with a set purpose to imitate his life, and conform your character to his character. You are to show a marked difference between your character and that of the world. "For in him dwelleth all the fullness of the Godhead bodily, and ye are complete in him, which is the head of all principality and power." "Epaphras who is one of you, a servant of Christ, saluteth you always laboring for you in prayers, that ye may stand perfect and complete in all the will of God." {392}

The grand truths of the Bible are for us individually, to rule, to guide, to control our life; for this is the only way in which Christ can be properly represented to our world in grace and loveliness in the characters of all who profess to be his disciples. Nothing less than heart service will be acceptable with God. God requires the sanctification of the entire man, body, soul, and spirit. The Holy Spirit implants a new nature, and molds through the grace of Christ the human character, until the image of Christ is perfected; this is true holiness. Will the workers in the office give heed to the light which God has sent you in the lines which I trace this morning?

You are handling sacred things, and the spirit and word and influence you carry are making impressions upon the minds of others. The atmosphere which surrounds the soul, if it is evil, will be like a spiritual malaria, which will be poisoning to those around. But it is profitable for the soul to have an atmosphere that will be as a savor of life unto life to others. When the soul is weighted with the truth which works by love and purifies the soul, a heavenly atmosphere will pervade the soul. "He that walketh with wise men, shall be wise; but a companion of fools shall be destroyed." Everyone who claims to believe the truth should manifest uprightness of character, devotion to God, steadfastness of purpose, and represent the character of Christ in a well-ordered life and godly conversation, you should render service to God with an eye single to his glory. You should cultivate true respect for every soul with whom you come in contact, because the soul is of great value with God. Saints and sinners are to be treated with courtesy, with kindness, with love, that Christ has manifested for all souls. He died that we might live.

Satan uses human agents to bring the soul under the power of temptation, but the angels of God are searching for human agents through whom they may cooperate to save the tempted ones. Angels are looking for those who will work in Christ's lines, who will be moved by the realization that they belong to Christ. They are looking for those who will feel that those who fall under temptation, whether high or low, are the ones who need their special labors, and that Christ looks on those who are passed by, neglected, wounded and bruised by the enemy, and ready to die, and is grieved at the hardness of men, who refuse to exercise the faith that works by love, which will purify the soul. Angels of God will work with, and through, and by those who will cooperate with the heavenly agencies for the saving of a soul from death, and the hiding of a multitude of sins. That will lead them to consider themselves, lest they also be tempted. It is the sick that need a physician, not those who are whole. When you expend labor on those who do not need it, and take no notice of the very ones that your words and actions could bless, you are forming a character that is not after the likeness of Christ. Christ says, "I come not to call the righteous but sinner to repentance." Let none dream that these obligations do {393} not belong to this time; for they do rest upon all. "Moreover it is required of stewards that a man be found faithful." Those who are making it manifest that they are not faithful in doing the very work that God has enjoined upon them, are working in an exactly opposite direction to Christ. "First cast out the beam out of thine own eye, and then thou

shalt see clearly to cast out the moat of thy brother's eye." Be careful yourselves not to become tempters in evil things.

When a soul is in peril, one who knows little of sympathy and has little of the meekness and lowliness of Christ, by unadvised words, may bruise where he should bind up, and fail to draw to Christ. They are likely to fail to give the words of tenderness and love that they should, to stand back in cold dignity, which is most hateful in the sight of God, and drive souls into the very snare that Satan has laid for their feet. Those who do this will have the blood of souls on their garments, because they obeyed the orders of Satan and disregarded the words of Christ.

When a crisis comes in the life of any soul, and another attempts to give advice, that advice and counsel will have only the weight of influence for good that the example and spirit of the adviser has accumulated for him. It is the consistent life, the revelation of a sincere, Christlike interest for the soul in peril, that will make counsel effectual to persuade and win into safe paths. Those who are quick to advise others, who speak words that cut and bruise the already wounded soul, are doing Satan's work, and are laborers with the prince of darkness. But the True Witness says: "I know thy works," every work shall be brought into Judgment with every secret thing whether it be good or whether it be evil." They will have to give an account for their neglect of those whom they might have blessed, strengthened, upheld, and healed.

"And unto the angel of the church in Sardis write: These things saith he that hath the seven spirits of God, and the seven stars. I know thy works that thou hast a name that thou livest, and are dead. Be watchful and strengthen the things that remain that are ready to die: for I have not found thy works perfect before God. Remember therefore how thou hast received and heard, and hold fast and repent. If therefore thou shalt not watch, I will come unto thee as a thief, and thou shalt not know what hour I shall come unto thee." How many times the human agent fails and, when the urgency arises, is all unprepared to do service for Christ. Had he watched, he would have proved himself a friend indeed, and an ambassador of Jesus. But the Spirit of Christ is not in him, it is another Spirit.

Let the tempted and tried souls remember that when chastisement comes upon them, it is the Lord who would save them

from death. Let the souls to whom reproof comes, remember that "As many as I love, I rebuke and chasten." The human agent imbued with the Spirit of Christ will watch for souls as they that must give an account. {394} The claims of Christ are upon us, and we must understand our duty, and do it in the fear of God, with an eye single to his glory, and not prove unfaithful. Let no thought of self or of natural feelings be cherished to keep the lips silent. Speak, and be not afraid, with the heart full of tenderness and love for souls, care, exhort, and entreat. Never cease to labor for a soul while there is one ray of hope. Your words may cut to the soul. Oh, then be cautious and clothe them with the love and tenderness of Jesus. Soften every accent with love and sympathy, remembering that you are not to be ignorant of the plague of your own heart, and that if Christ should mark your every word and action, there would be an array of figures written in his book, showing that you yourself are greatly out of harmony with his holy will. As you deal with others, as you judge others, so the Lord will judge and deal with you. Let the agent who claims to be a child of God, practice the lessons of Christ. If he is compelled to wound, let him feel the duty of healing as compulsory upon him. The truth is ever to be spoken in love, with the Spirit of God abiding in the soul.

God calls upon you to conquer your own spirit, to correct your own mistakes, to confess your sins before God that pardon may be written off against your own names. With earnest prayer seek wisdom of God, and be careful how you judge and pass sentence upon your brother. God has not placed you on the judgment seat. Great and grand truths for this time are to be brought into practical life. Christ says, "I will sanctify myself, that as head and representative of the human family, the soul may believe on me, and may be sanctified." A religion that does not touch the heart, cannot transform the character, and sanctify the life. Religious vigilance can never be laid to rest. We must stand as faithful sentinels over the mind and soul, lest Satan steal away the heavenly gifts. Dare not to cast the first stone at your neighbor, lest Christ shall say to you, as you parade the sins of others, presenting them in an aggravated light, "Let him that is without sin cast the first stone." Would you not then be covered with confusion of face, as you consider the daily record of sins in your practical life, and remember what is written in the books of heaven? It is these things that are bringing the wrath of God on the children of disobedience. The discrepancy of profession and practice is doing a baleful work, and misrepresenting the character of Christ. Oh that all would realize what great harm is done to souls by little acts, and by sinful inconsistencies! Oh that all might see this and be converted!

The Lord is soon to come and the perils of the last days are upon us. Probation will soon close. Will you fall upon the rock and be broken? Self must die . Your heart can be made tender only by the grace of Jesus Christ. Redeem the time, and no longer pull down with one hand what you are striving to build up with the other, The influence of your words is too often destroyed by the {395} inconsistency of your example. The power of your principles is neutralized by your practice. The unsubdued passions of the human heart, the hard judgment that if meted out to others in your manner and words, does not reveal the meekness of Christ, and in the records of heaven you are judged as you have judged others, and your hard heart has become more unfit for heaven. Take away the stumbling blocks for the sake of your own soul and for the sake of the souls of others for whom Christ died. Open the door of the heart to the love and gentleness of Christ. Let it pervade the soul, and brighten the lives of others, and you will know what the blessing of God is.

(Signed) Ellen G. White

QUALIFICATIONS ESSENTIAL FOR THE WORK OF GOD

April 23, 1896

IN HIS WORD THE LORD enumerates the gifts and graces that are indispensable for all who connect with his work. He does not teach us to ignore learning or despise education, for when controlled by the love and fear of God, intellectual culture is a blessing; yet this is not presented as the most important qualification for the service of God. Jesus passed by the wise men of his time, the men of education and position, because they were so proud and self sufficient in their boasted superiority, that they could not sympathize with suffering humanity, and become colaborers with the Man of Nazareth. In their bigotry they scorned to be taught by Christ. The Lord Jesus would have men connected with his work who appreciate that work as sacred; then they can cooperate with God. They

will be unobstructed channels through which his grace can flow. The attributes of the character of Christ can be imparted to those only who distrust themselves. The highest scientific education cannot in itself develop a Christlike character. The fruits of true wisdom come from Christ alone.

Every worker should test his own qualifications by the word of God. Have the men who are handling sacred things a clear understanding, a right perception of things of eternal interest? Will they consent to yield to the working of the Holy Spirit, or do they permit themselves to be controlled by their own hereditary and cultivated tendencies? It becomes all to examine themselves, whether they be in the faith.

Those who occupy positions of trust in the work of God should ever bear in mind that these positions involve great responsibility. The right performance of the solemn work for this time, and the salvation of the souls connected with us in any way, depend in a great degree upon our own spiritual condition. All should cultivate a vivid sense of their responsibility; for their own present, {396} wellbeing, and their eternal destiny will be decided by the spirit they cherish. If self is woven into the work, it is as the offering of strange fire in the place of the sacred. Such workers incur the displeasure of the Word. Brethren, remove your hands from the work, unless you can distinguish the sacred fire from the common.

Those who have stood as representative men are not all Christian gentlemen. There is prevalent a spirit that seeks the mastery over others. Men regard themselves as authority, they express their opinions, and pass resolutions about matters of which they have no experimental knowledge. Some who are connected with the publishing house at _____, pass through the office, speaking with different ones, giving directions which they suppose it proper for them to give, when they do not understand what they are talking about.

Great injustice and even dishonesty have been committed in the board meetings, in bringing matters before those who have not an experience that will enable them to be competent judges. Manuscripts have been placed in the hands of men for criticisms, when the eyes of their understanding were so blinded that they could not discern the spiritual import of the subject with which they were dealing. More than this, they had no real knowledge of bookmaking. They had had neither study

nor practice in the line of literary productions. Men have sat in judgment upon books and manuscripts unwisely placed in their hands, when they should have declined to serve in any such capacity. It would have been only honest for them to say, "I have had no experience in this line of work, and should certainly do injustice to myself and to others, in giving my opinion. Excuse me, brethren; instead of instructing others, I need that someone should teach me." But this was far from their thoughts. They expressed themselves freely in regard to subjects of which they knew nothing. Conclusions have been accepted as the opinions of wise men, when they were simply the opinions of novices.

The time has come when, in the name and strength of God, the church must act for the good of souls and for the honor of God. A lack of firm faith and of discernment in sacred things should be regarded as sufficient to bar any man from connection with the work of God. So also the indulgence of a quick temper, a harsh, overbearing spirit, reveals that its possessor should not be placed where he will be called to decide weighty questions that affect God's heritage. A passionate man should have no part to act in dealing with human minds. He cannot be trusted to shape matters which have a relation to those whom Christ has purchased at an infinite price. If he undertakes to manage man, he will hurt and bruise their souls; for he has not the fine touch, the delicate sensibility which the grace of Christ imparts. His own heart needs to be softened, subdued by the Spirit of God; the heart of stone has not become a heart of flesh.

Those who are thus misrepresenting Christ, are placing a wrong mold upon the work; for they encourage all who are {397} connected with them to do as they do. For their souls' sake, for the sake of those who are in danger from their influence, they should resign their position; for the record will appear in heaven that the wrongdoer has the blood of many souls upon his garments. He has caused some to become exasperated, so that they have given up the faith; others have been imbued with his own Satanic attributes, and the evil done, it is impossible to estimate. Those only who make it manifest that their hearts are being sanctified through the truth, should be retained in positions of trust in the Lord's work.

Let all consider that whatever their employment, they are to represent Christ, with steadfast purpose, let every man seek to have the mind of Christ. Especially should those who have accepted the position of directors or counselors feel that they are required to be in every respect Christian gentlemen. While in dealing with others we are always to be faithful, we should not be rude. The souls with whom we have to do are the Lord's purchased possession, and we are to permit no hasty, overbearing expression to escape the lips. Brethren, treat men as men, not as servants, to be ordered about at your pleasure. He who indulges a harsh, overbearing spirit, might better become a tender of sheep, as did Moses, and thus learn what it means to be a true shepherd. Moses gained in Egypt an experience as a mighty statesman, and as a leader of the armies, but he did not there learn the lessons essential for true greatness. He needed an experience in more humble duties, that he might become a caretaker, tender toward every living thing. In keeping the flocks of Jethro, his sympathies were called out to the sheep and lambs, and he learned to guard these creatures of God with the gentlest care. Although their voice could never complain of mistreatment, yet their attitude might show much. God cares for all the creatures he has made. In working for God in this lowly station, Moses learned to be a tender shepherd for Israel.

The Lord would have us learn a lesson also from the experience of Daniel. There are many who might become mighty men, if, like this faithful Hebrew, they would depend upon God for grace to be overcomers, and for strength and efficiency in their labors. Daniel manifested the most perfect courtesy, both toward his elders and toward the youth. He stood as a witness for God, and sought to take such a course that he might not be ashamed for heaven to hear his word or to behold his works. When Daniel was required to partake of the luxuries of the king's table, he did not fly into a passion, neither did he express a determination to eat and drink as he pleased. Without speaking one word of defiance, he took the matter to God. He and his companions sought wisdom from the Lord, and when they came forth from earnest prayer, their decision was made. With true courage and Christian courtesy, Daniel presented the case to the officer who had them in charge, {398} asking that they might be granted a simple diet. These youth felt that their religious principles were at stake, and they relied upon

God whom they loved and served. Their request was granted, for they had obtained favor with God and with men.

Men in every position of trust need to take their place in the school of Christ, and heed the injunction of the Great Teacher; "Learn of me; for I am meek and lowly in heart, and ye shall find rest unto your souls. For my yoke is easy, and my burden is light." We have no excuse for manifesting one wrong trait of character. "Not by might nor by power, but by my Spirit, saith the Lord of Hosts." In your dealing with others, whatever you see or hear that needs to be corrected, first seek the Lord for wisdom and grace, that in trying to be faithful, you may not be rude. Ask him to give you the gentleness of Christ; then you will be true to your duty, true to your position of trust, and true to God, a faithful steward, overcoming natural and acquired tendencies to evil.

None but a whole hearted Christian can be a perfect gentleman, but if Christ is abiding in the soul, his Spirit will be revealed in the manner, the words, and the actions. Gentleness and love cherished in the heart, will appear in self-denial, in true courtesy. Such workers will be the light of the world.

(Signed) Ellen G. White

RIGHT RELATIONS IN THE WORK OF GOD

[Prior to July 1915]

MEN, FALLIBLE MEN, are not to think it is their prerogative to control, to mark out, or to prescribe the labors of their fellow men. When God works upon the human instrumentality, let men be very careful how they intermeddle; for it is its process, the work of God is divine. The work of God has often been hindered by men considering that they had power to say, "Go here" or "Go there" "Do this" or "Do that," without consulting the individual himself, or respecting his convictions as a laborer together with God. God has promised his presence to every believer; and let those who are in positions of authority, presidents of conferences and board councils, and everyone who has to do with the human mind, respect the individuality of mind and conscience. These workers are in copartnership with Jesus Christ, and you may interpose yourself so as to interfere with God's plans; for the human agent is under his special authority and dictation.

When men composing boards and councils, are themselves walking at a distance from God, of what value is their discernment and wisdom to decide in reference to the work {399} of God's delegated servants? The human mind is open to jealousies, evil surmisings, and selfish considerations, and God's plans are often turned aside by the caprice and by the plans of unconsecrated men. If the door is not closed to the enemy, he will enter and will figure largely in human inventions. The Lord requires the men who have a directing influence in his work, to be wholly consecrated to him. He wants them to have hearts of flesh, and not of steel.

Men who do not control their own impulses are not chosen by the Lord to deal with human minds. For this work, there is need of much prayer, much humiliation before God, much deep sensibility of the value of the human soul, for whom Christ has paid so great a price. It was to seek for the pearl of great price that he left the enjoyments of heaven. And when the pearl is found, all heaven rejoices. When this is the case, why do not men tremble when they see the pearl in danger of being lost? Why are they not working conscientiously to secure that pearl for Jesus Christ? God sees that men in official positions are lifted up by self-confidence and self-importance. He sees that they are speaking and acting wrongly toward those who need wise instruction, and who need to come in contact with men who have hearts of flesh and not of steel.

Christ is our example, and everyone placed in a position of trust, needs the subduing influence of the Spirit of God upon the heart day by day. Christ wept with those that wept. In all their afflictions he was afflicted, and was touched with the feeling of their infirmities. He is a tender and faithful High Priest. He considers the cases of the tried and tempted ones as verily his own, and he ministers unto them. These weak ones of the flock are to be carefully nourished with the manna Christ has supplied. They are to be educated not to look to men and trust in men, whatever may be their calling.

God would have all such confederacies broken to stone and remodeled upon Christlike principles. The foundation stone must be mercy. Human minds are not to be trampled, and bound and driven by human hands. The Lord Jesus must hold the reins in his own hands that were pierced to bring peace and comfort and hope to every soul who will believe on him. He gives to the purchase of his blood the guardianship of his grace; they shall move in his light, clad in the robes of his righteousness. To every man is given his work; and while souls are brought into church capacity, work is assigned them of God. They are to move as winds that are under the controlling influence of God.

Men are educated to look to men, and to depend on men. One man, by virtue of his position, exercises authority over others as if they were to be led by lines, this way and that, as dumb animals. God has not directed in this way. God is our chief, God is our instructor, and to him we must look. We must ask the Holy Spirit's guidance, {400} and expect to be led and controlled by it. The church organization is to be respected, but it is not to be made in any way a galling yoke. Men are not to assume the prerogative of God, and think to rule and coerce and oppress the souls of God's purchased possessions. All heaven is indignant at what men, with complacency, will do to their fellow men, claiming at the same time to be representatives of Jesus Christ. They too often represent the spirit and character of Satan.

Christ has found his pearl of great price in lost, perishing souls. He sold all that he had to come into possession, even engaged to do the work, and run the risk of losing his own life in the conflict. How then should man regard his fellow man? Christ has demonstrated the way. He says, "A new commandment I give unto you, that ye love one another; as I have loved you, that ye also love one another."

When these words are heeded and obeyed in the spirit and in the letter, we will be doers of the word, and not hearers only. When these words are practiced by those who claim to have wisdom to guide the sheep of the Lord's pasture, there will be far less selfishness, far less boasting, far less putting forth the finger and speaking vanity. Jesus is to superintend all events in the present and future of his church. John was instructed to write the things which he had seen "and the things which are, and the things which shall be hereafter; the mystery of the seven stars which thou sawest in my right hand, and the seven golden candlesticks. The seven stars are the angels of the seven churches; and the seven candlesticks which thou sawest are the seven churches."

Oh, that men would revere the great Head of the Church, and would manufac-ture less human methods, bringing down spirituality to the very dust with human inventions. God has been left out, and the church is not prepared to advance to the conflict under the banner of Jesus Christ. It is not doing the work for suffering souls, which Christ owns as if done to himself. But the church, defective as it is, and enfeebled with so much chaff, is the only object on earth upon which He bestows His highest regard. In His estimation, the church in heaven and the church on earth are identical. He has promised to come personally into the midst of his church. He says to everyone holding a position of trust, "Learn of me; for I am meek and lowly in heart, and ye shall find rest unto your souls. For my yoke is easy, and my burden is light."

Men in official position must realize that their position gives them no license to be unkind or uncourteous, no license to be oppressive, and to let their tongues, which should be sanctified, speak words which will open a door of temptation, and help the great adversary in his work of discouraging souls. God has given us a work to do in saving souls from the companionship of Satan.

(Signed) Ellen G. White

GENERAL INTERESTS OF THE CAUSE

[Prior to July 1915] {401}

Dear Brother:

AT HALF PAST TWO IN THE morning, while the house is locked in slumber, I commence penning these lines to you. I think of the large church at Battle Creek, and of the important interests centered there, which makes it a missionary field in the highest sense. People are coming from all parts of the world to the Sanitarium, and many youth from the different States are attending the College. That field requires the very best methods of labor, that the strongest religious influence may be constantly exerted upon all. God would have men cultivate their abilities, that they may have broader ideas in planning and executing his work. When this is done, the saving power of the grace of Christ will be manifested by those who believe present truth.

As the work grows, if the workers will rely firmly upon the wisdom and power of God, their minds will expand to keep pace with his opening providence. Those who possess piety and ability should be encour-aged to obtain the necessary education, that they may assist in the great work of spreading the light of truth. Progress will then be seen in the great closing message for these last days.

God has different sets of work men for the different branches of his cause. When those whom he has called to do a certain work, have carried that work along as far as they can with the ability he has given them, the Lord in his providence will call and qualify other men to come in and work with them, still making advance moves, that together they may carry it still farther, and lift the standard higher. He will never allow his work to diminish in strength for efficiency, if those to whom he has given their work will act their part with unswerving fidelity. There must be no (belittling) the men whom God has accepted as his workmen.

This great and solemn work is not to be carried to its completion by a few men who have been selected as opportunity has offered, to bear responsibility. There are some minds which do not grow with the work, but allow the work to grow far beyond them, and they find themselves tired and worn before they comprehend the circumstances. Then when those whom God is qualifying to assist in the work, take hold of it in a little different way from that in which these responsible men have tried to do it, they should be very careful not to hinder these helpers, or to circumscribe the work. Since they did not see the work in all its bearings, and did not have the burden which God has specially laid upon others, why should they say just how that work should be done? Those who do not discern and adapt themselves to the increasing demands of the work, should not stand blocking the wheels, and thus hindering the advancement of others. {402}

The case of David is to the point. He made large provisions for building a temple for the Lord; but the Lord told him that he was not the one to do that work; it must devolve on Solomon, because of his large experience; but the younger man must do the work.

The weary, worn minds of all the older brethren do not take in the greatness of the work in all its bearings, and are not inclined to keep pace with the opening providences of God. Therefore, the responsibilities of the work should not rest wholly with them, as they would not bring into it all the elements essential for its advancement, and thus the work would be retarded.

The work in Battle Creek, and in the State of Michigan is far, far behind. For several years there has been on the part of the Conference Committee and the laborers, a want of wise planning and discreet management in regard to it. While the President of the General Conference was willing to do much work he did not see the necessity of training the powers of mind and qualifying himself to plan to discern the talents of young men and set them to work, associating with himself those who could help him. It is well to see and understand the situation, and the needs of foreign missions, so as not to neglect them, we should also be able to comprehend the needs of the work at our very doors. Home missions should not be neglected. There has been an oversight in doing this.

There is a sad neglect at Battle Creek in not using the many advantages right at hand, to keep the heart of the work in a healthy condition. Vigorous heart beats from the center should be felt in all parts of the body of believers. But if the heart is sickly and weak in its action, its inefficiency affects all branches of the work. A sound, healthy, working power at the center of the work, is positively essential, in order that the truth may be carried to the world. It must be diffused through families and communities. This will require wise generalship in devising plans, and educating others to assist in the work. Persons of talent must be sought out, and encouraged to labor in various places, according to the capabilities God has given them. Let every instrumentality of God that is brought within the reach of those older in experience, be encouraged by them to find a place in the work, and these to be educated with the advancing work.

Much ability has been lost to the cause of God; because many in responsible positions were so narrow in their ideas, that they did not discern the increasing responsibilities. They did not have extended vision to see that the work was becoming altogether too large to be carried forward by the workers then engaged in it. The work had outgrown them. Much, very much is now left undone which should have been done because men have held things in their own finite hands, instead of proportioning the work to a larger number of workers and trusting that God would help them. They have {403} tried to take all branches of the work upon themselves, fearing others would not prove as efficient. Their wills have therefore controlled in everything,

and through some unwise decisions, made because of their inability to grasp all the wants of the cause in its various parts, and as the result, great losses have been sustained. The work has been bound about, not from design, but from not discerning the necessity of a different order of things to meet the demands for the time. This is largely due to the feeling of Elder Butler that position gave unlimited authority. Greater responsibilities were pressed upon him and accepted, than one person could carry; and the consequence was a demoralized condition of affairs, notwithstanding he may have done the very best he himself could do under the circumstances. But the infinite God saw there was different kind of qualifications needed to place a different mold on the work. On the part of his brethren there was a fear that others desired Brother's place, which has caused suspicions, and has resulted in keeping in the background those men whom God would have used, could they have had sufficient encouragement, and an opportunity to work. God has not wrought as he would, because of surmisings and suspicions, and because there was not discernment and planning to let every man do the work that God is fitting him to perform, in an understanding, intelligent manner. The lesson must be learned, that when God appoints means for a certain work, we are not to neglect these means, put them aside, and then pray and expect that he will work miracles to supply our neglect. To every man God has appointed his work, according to his capacities and capabilities. Wise planning is needed to place each one in his proper sphere in the work, in order that he may obtain an experience which will fit him to bear increased responsibility.

In God's dealings, in temporal as well as spiritual things, blessings come to man through the use of means. If the husbandman neglects to till his ground, God works no miracle to make up for his neglect; and when the harvest time comes, he has no crops to gather. As in the natural world, so in the spiritual; God always honors the use of the means he has ordained to do his work. It is by practice that men must be qualified for any emergency that may arise. Men need to become better acquainted with themselves and be discerning in regard to their own weak points of character, and then make every effort to strengthen these points, for God makes this their duty.

No one should lean wholly upon an-

other's mind; but as God's free agent, each should ask wisdom of him. When the learner depends in a large degree upon another man's thoughts and goes no farther than to accept his plans, he sees only through that man's eyes, and is so far only an echo of the other. God will, by his own Spirit, work directly through the mind he has put in man, if the man will only give him a chance to work, and will recognize {404} his dealings with him. God designs that men shall use their minds and consciences for themselves. He never designed that one man should become the shadow of another, and utter only another's sentiments. But this error has been coming in among us, that a very few are to be mind, conscience, and judgment for all God's workers. The foundation of Christianity is "Christ, our Righteousness." Men are individually responsible to God and must act as God acts upon them, not as another human mind acts upon their mind; for if this method of indirect influence is kept up, souls cannot be impressed and directed by the great I Am. They will, on the other hand, have their experience blended with another, and will be kept under a moral restraint, which allows no freedom of action or of choice.

God deals with his creatures as with responsible beings. He has issued no command that the leaders of the Battle Creek church shall remain anchored, until by some mighty miracle-working power the church is sent forward and upward to the harbor God has appointed. If we would be wise, and use diligently, prayerfully, and thankfully the means whereby light and blessings are to come to his people, then no voice nor power upon earth would have authority over us to say, "This shall not be."

The Lord has presented before me that men in responsible positions are standing directly in the way of the workings of God upon his people, because they think that the work must be done and the blessings must come in a certain way they have marked out, and they will not recognize that which comes in any other way. "We are laborers together with God." Copy the ways of the Lord Jesus. He was a perfect character.

May the Lord place this matter before you as it is. God works, not as men plan, nor as men wish, but "in a mysterious way, his wonders to perform." Why treat God's ways as worthless, because they do not coincide with our private ideas? God has appointed channels of light, but these are not necessarily through the minds of any particular man or set of men. When all shall take their appointed places in God's work, and not allow others to mold them at will, then one great advance will have been made toward letting the light shine upon the world.

The efforts made here to close every avenue to light and truth which is supposed to disagree with the opinions of some leading men, are very unreasonable. Are these men infallible? Has God appointed them supreme judges of how light shall come to his people? I answer, No.

During the Conference at Battle Creek, when the question of the law in Galatians was being examined, {405} I was taken to a number of houses, and heard the unchristian remarks and criticisms made by delegates. Then these words were spoken: "They must have the truth as it is in Jesus, else it will not be a saving truth to them." "Without me," says Christ, "ye can do nothing." When finite men shall cease to put themselves in the way, to hinder, then God will work in our midst as never before.

It was shown me that broader plans should be laid but at the same time the work in each branch of the cause should be harmoniously united with that in every other branch, all making a perfect whole; but now, selfish ideas and principles are interwoven with the plans of the workers, which makes the work defective. One man, who has the oversight of a certain line of work, magnifies his responsibilities until that one branch, in his mind, is above every other branch, when in reality all are equally important. When this narrow, selfish idea is received, all his energies are set to imbue the people with the same idea. This is human nature, but not after Christ's order. Just in proportion as this policy is followed, Christ is pushed aside, and self appears prominent. When the Saviour is allowed his part in the work, none will become entirely absorbed in any one branch of it, but all will have broad ideas, and will attribute to all parts of the work their due importance.

The Jews, in Christ's day, in the exercise of their own spirit of self exaltation, brought in rigid rules and exactions, and so took away all chance for God to work upon minds, until mercy and the love of God were entirely lost sight of in their work. It was this which caused rulers to lay upon the people the heavy burdens of which they justly complained, which our Saviour condemned. Do not follow in their track. Leave God a chance to do something for those who love him, and do not impose upon them rules and regulations, which, if followed, will leave them as destitute of the grace of God as were the hills of Gilboa, without dew or rain. Your very many resolutions need to be reduced to one third their number, and great care should be taken as to what resolutions are framed. Ours is missionary ground, having many advantages; and if wisely improved, a much larger number of workers would be fitted to go out into the field, as pastors and evangelists; but shortness of vision, and the narrowness of mind in some, have circumscribed the work. There is need of having vigorous efforts put forth in the churches in every conference. A living message, showing the living features of our times should be presented to them, not in a tame, lifeless style, but in the {406} demonstration of the Spirit, and in the power of God. Responsibilities must be laid upon individual members of the church. A missionary spirit should be awakened, and wise workers appointed as they are needed, who will be active pastors, making personal efforts to bring the church up to that condition where spiritual death will not be seen in all her borders.

There was much said to me in reference to other departments of the work, which I will not at this time write. When I came to know where I was, I was sitting up in bed, weary, and my heart very, very sad. I arose and prayed, and tried to write. The knowledge, Brother _____, communicated to me at that time and since then in regard to your positions and feelings, has distressed me beyond measure. The positions and ideas also which are entertained by Elder _____ are of that character to lead you both to occupy incorrect positions, where it would be impossible for me to stand with you; and if you maintain these positions, I shall be compelled, not only to differ with you in some things, but to withstand your ideas and your influence. I was never more conscious of this than during the experience I have had here at this meeting. I have not the least hesitancy in saying that a spirit has been brought into this meeting, not of seeking to obtain light, but to stand barricading the way, lest a ray should come into the hearts and minds of the people, through some other channel than that which you had decided to be the proper one.

PERSONAL APPEAL

May 30, 1895 {407}

GOD CALLS UPON YOU WHO are connected with his instrumentalities, to do his work according to his plans, not your own. He calls for an entire consecration of yourselves to him. If you heed the requirement, it will be a blessing to you in this life and the inheritance of life eternal. There is now a precious period, though short, allotted to you for repentance and improvement.

Brethren A. R. Henry and Harmon Lindsay, God is in earnest with you. Your duty is plain and imperative. Your minds need cultivation, that you may discern heavenly things, and choose them above the common and the earthly. Let not the present opportunity pass unimproved. Unless the warnings that God in his mercy is sending to you, are heeded, before a long time shall elapse you will make shipwreck of faith. You have sown the seeds of unbelief all along the line. And you have so long refused the evidence of the operation of the Holy Spirit that it is questionable whether you will ever again recognize the light from heaven. It may even appear as darkness to you, until the time shall come when every knee shall bow, and every tongue shall confess to God. Instead of regarding it as your imperative duty to cultivate personal piety, with a zeal proportionate to the preciousness of the holy faith you profess and the responsibility of your position, you have suffered yourselves to drift along, your impulses controlled by unholy imaginations and prejudices, until your course is an offense to God. What wonder that you lead the minds of others into the same channels? What wonder that some, following you, turn away from the rock foundation of eternal truth, to build, as you are building, upon the sand? It is a grievous robbery of God to become so blinded as you are today because you have refused heaven's light, slighted the appeals that God has sent you, and have done your best to prove them inconsistent, and have declared them untrue. Your assertions have not made them untrue, but by your resistance against God your hearts have become hard and stubborn.

Again I appeal to you: Will you now be zealous and repent? You have shown your zeal in strong words and oppressive measures towards your brethren. Now I beseech you to give evidence of earnest repentance before it shall be forever too late.

Those who, notwithstanding the light given, have yoked up with you as men imbued with the Spirit of God, and actuated by a self-denying interest in his cause, make yourselves responsible for the influence you have exerted and will exert contrary to the truth. Guilt will rest upon those who have placed increasing responsibilities upon you, when you have no living connection with God. {408}

A condition of things has been brought about that, unless God in mercy shall interpose, will work disaster to his cause. Inexperienced minds are being troubled at the outlook. For reasons that you can give, God is not moving upon the hearts of his people to supply the treasury. When you shall receive the Holy Spirit's unction by returning unto the Lord with full purpose of heart, you will see yourselves in a new light altogether. You who are finite, erring, and unsanctified, have supposed that God's children were put under your jurisdiction, for you to plan for them, and bring them to your terms. The policy you have labored so hard to establish in your connection with the work is an offense to God. He has never justified any arrangement, through organization, discipline, or laws, whereby men who have evidenced that they are not susceptible to the Holy Spirit's moving, shall use their power to sustain others in a like disregard of the Spirit's work. But such has been the arrangement that has prevailed. You have made it hard for those whom you do not especially like, while others who are self-serving have been favored and exalted. Partiality and hypocrisy have excluded the Spirit of God from many hearts, and left them as destitute of his grace as the hills of Gilboa were destitute of dew or rain. Let it no longer be regarded as your privilege to control God's heritage.

The Lord himself will turn and overturn, and set things in order. He has the responsibility of his own work, and he has not entrusted the management of his people to unsanctified human minds.

It is hard for men to learn their real weakness and ignorance and inefficiency. It is hard for the ambitious heart to receive God's ideas and plans with unquestioning faith and obedience. Some have very high ideas of the importance of their own individuality, and by their headstrong course are saying, We want not God's way, but our own way.

The time is near when God by his providence will make manifest what principles have been cherished by the men connected with the management of his work. Unless these men are converted, they will be separated from the work. But the appeals and warnings given have had no more effect upon their hearts than the messages of Christ had upon the Pharisees, and I greatly fear in their behalf, lest they shall continue to walk in the same path, manifesting the same exacting and intolerant spirit, as did the ruling Pharisees. I fear that the same judgments will fall upon them because they have rejected the Lord's reproof, and have set the stumbling block of their iniquity before their eyes.

My brethren, in the name of the Lord I counsel you to seek him by repentance and confession. Let your sins of omission and commission go beforehand to judgment, that pardon may be written against your names, that you may {409} be accounted worthy to stand before him when he shall appear.

(Signed) Ellen G. White

TO MEN IN RESPONSIBLE POSITIONS IN BATTLE CREEK

September, 1895
Granville, N. S. W.

Dear Brethren:

YOU HAVE NO RIGHT TO ABSORB in Battle Creek the means that is sent in by our people, and leave mission fields impoverished. The funds that accumulate in Battle Creek have not been created by those who handle the means. It is the faith of the people in the cause and work of God that has brought tithes and offerings to the treasury.

The efforts made to induce our people to move away from Battle Creek have not succeeded. And why? Because the enlargements constantly going forward have been encouraging people to move in. There was represented to me a mammoth vineyard, requiring much labor to tend and care for it. Men were working in one part of the vineyard, while other parts were left unworked, to grow thorns and briers. One of dignified bearing said, Why are you setting out so many plants in this part of the field? Take some of the plants to other portions of God's vineyard. More ground may be brought under cultivation. Thus the work will be greatly extended, and new elements will be brought in. When the people are congregated together as they are in Battle Creek, it requires more labor to keep the church in a right condition than would be required to minister to the same number if they were scattered as they should be in different parts of the field.

Consolidation means that all institutions are to be merged into the Battle Creek institutions. For years something of this kind has been proposed by one and another. But according to the light I have had, the plan is wrong, decidedly wrong. Let every institution stand in its own individuality, doing its respective work in its own locality. There are not in Battle Creek men of sufficient clearness of discernment, sanctified by the grace of Christ, to carry the responsibilities which they now assume. If there is any action taken to merge everything into one institution under the dictation of those now presiding, it will be one of the worst pieces of business that were ever transacted in Battle Creek in connection with the cause of God. {410}

The Pacific Press should stand in its own moral independence, carrying on its work beyond the Rocky Mountains, in a little world of its own. Its managers are responsible to God to do their work as in full view of the universe of heaven.

Men are coming to trust in men, and to make flesh their arm; and when that arm is not linked in the arm of Christ, they will find that they are leaning upon a broken reed. The publishing houses were established in America in the counsel of God, under his direction and supervision, and they should stand in their own individuality, as sister institutions. Never should they be so related to each other that one shall have power to control the running of the other. If one institution shall adopt a policy which the other does not sanction, the other institution is not to be corrupted, but is to stand in its God given responsibility, true to the principles that were expressed in its establishment, and carrying forward the work in harmony with those principles.

Our people do not know what they are about. In some of their movements they act like blind men. The managers at Battle Creek are taking altogether too much on their hands; but they do not understand the result of this confederacy. Every institution should work in harmony with the other institutions, but farther than this they should not go toward confederacy or merging into one. Already there are men, who, supposing themselves wise, are trying to shape matters according to their ideas. Things may for a time appear to prosper in their hands, but the result will be that which they do not now anticipate.

For years a spirit of oppression has been coming into Battle Creek. The human agents are lifting up themselves unto selfishness and domination. Not a work can be published but they try to gain control of it, and if authors do not concede to their propositions, those who publish the work will exert an influence with canvassers and other agents that will hinder its sale, and this wholly irrespective of the value of the book. And when every institution is merged into the one that is greatest—that is, measured by her power of control—that one will indeed be a ruling power, and if the principles of action in the most powerful institution are corrupted, as is now the case, and as has been in the history of the past, every other institution must follow the same path, also a determined influence will be brought to bear against it. The difficulty is not in the institution, but in the members.

This disposition to press men into hard places if you cannot bring them to your ideas, is not according to God's order. Those who do this when it suits them, are bringing souls into unbelief and temptation, and driving them on Satan's battle-field. They forget that God will deal with them as they deal with their fellow men. God's cause is not to be molded by one man, {411} or half a dozen men. All his responsible stewards are to bear a share in the devising, as well as in the execution of the plans. Men must not forget that the God of heaven is a God of justice; with him is no partiality, no hypocrisy. He will not serve with men's selfishness, nor sanction their plans to rob one soul of his rights because they can press him inconsiderately, and make statements and plans that compel surrender or leave him helpless.

Shall everything pass under the control of men whom we know have not a living connection with God? He who says, "I know thy works," hears all their suggestions, listens to all their plans. The institutions of God's creating, which he established upon principles of justice and equity, they are seeking to make a means of oppression, forcing the Lord's workers to accept terms which they themselves were the situation reversed, would not accept.

God's instrumentalities are not chosen of men, or under their jurisdiction. They are to prepare a people to stand in the day of the Lord. God is a party to every transaction, and He is sinned against and misrepresented. The Lord's powerful instrumentalities are made as a cutting sword to weaken and destroy, because those who are managing these instrumentalities possess attributes that lead them to do this. When men swerve from truth and righteousness, violate justice in deal, making contracts that bind others according to their will, and violate contracts, let them remember that for all this, God will bring them into judgment. By no sharp dealing or underhand advantage is the Lord to be glorified or his truth served. Money acquired in this way to supply the treasury will benefit no one; for God will not serve with the sins of oppression and selfishness.

It should be written on the conscience as with a pen of iron upon a rock that no man can achieve true success while violating the eternal principles of right. There must be a cleansing of the institutions similar to Christ's cleansing of the temple of old. "It is written," saith the Lord, "my house shall be called a house of prayer, but ye have made it a den of thieves." There are in our institutions today transactions similar to those that took place in the temple court in Christ's time; and all heaven is looking on.

God is dishonored by those who are in responsible places of stewardship, yet do not realize the necessity of being, both in spirit and words, an example to those connected with them, who have learned to do as they require. Everyone must have the grace of God for his own soul, he must confide in the pardoning mercy of God through the merits of Christ. Then he will not manifest a harsh zeal to bruise and wound, but a sanctified zeal {412} to answer the prayer of Christ, which he offered before his crucifixion, zeal not for human uplifting, but for the glory of God.

The change of the natural, inherited, and cultivated tendencies of the human heart, is that change of which Jesus spoke when he said to Nicodemus, "Except a man be born again, he cannot see (discern) the Kingdom of God." Nicodemus did not understand Christ's words. He inquired, "How can these things be?" The answer comes home to every man in responsible positions, "Art thou a master of Israel, and knowest not these things? Verily, verily, I say unto thee, We speak that we do know, and testify that we have seen: And ye receive not our witness. If I have told you earthly things, and ye believe not, how shall ye believe if I tell you of heavenly things? And no man hath ascended up to heaven but he that came down from heaven, even the Son of Man which is in heaven."

The change of heart represented by the new birth can be brought about only through the effectual working of the Holy Spirit. Self-love and pride resist the Spirit of God. Every natural inclination of the soul withstands and opposes the change from self-importance and pride to the meekness and lowliness of Christ. It is only through receiving divine light, only through the cooperation of heavenly intelligences, that we can discern the spiritual character of the kingdom of God. Only thus can we have a lively sense of the duties due to all with whom we are connected in labor, or with whom we are brought in contact. We are under contract to God. The express requirements of the Old Testament are in perfect agreement with the teaching of the New Testament.

The Lord Jesus spoke from the pillar of cloud, "And now, Israel, what doth the Lord require of thee, but to fear the Lord thy God, to walk in all his ways, and to love him, and to serve the Lord thy God with all thy heart and with all thy soul, to keep the commandments of the Lord and his statutes, which I command thee this day for thy good? For the Lord your God is a God of gods, and Lord of lords, a great God a mighty, and a terrible, which regardeth not persons, nor taketh regards: he doth execute the judgment of the fatherless and widow, and loveth the stranger, and giveth him food and raiment." Compare this with the words of Christ in the New Testament: "A certain lawyer stood up, and tempted him, saying, Master, what shall I do to inherit eternal life? He said unto him, What is written in the law, how readest thou? And he answering said, Thou shalt love the Lord thy God with all thy heart, and with all thy soul, and with all thy strength, and with all thy mind; and thy neighbor as thyself. And he said unto him, Thou hast answered right: this do, and thou shalt live." "A father of the fatherless and a judge of the widow is God in his holy habitation." "The Lord preserveth the strangers: he relieveth the fatherless and the {413} widow: but the way of the wicked he turneth upside down." "If thy brother be waxen poor, and falleth into decay with thee; then thou shalt relieve him; yea, though he be a stranger, or a sojourner; that he may live with thee; Thou shalt not give him thy money upon usury, nor lend him thy victuals for increase. I am the Lord your God, which brought you forth out of the land of Egypt, to give you the land of Canaan, and to be your God. Thou shalt not rule over him with vigor, but shall fear thy God." See also Deuteronomy 15:7-11; 24:14, 15, 19-21; Leviticus 19:32-37. "Owe no man anything, but to love one another." The oppression of the poor, which is nothing less than actual robbery, is not punishable by human course, except in very extreme cases; but it is marked by the God of heaven as the abhorred practice which he would in no case tolerate.

The apostle James says to the rich, "Behold, the hire of the laborers who have reaped down your fields, which is of you kept back by fraud, crieth: and the cries of them which have reaped are entered into the ears of the Lord of sabbaoth." God condemns injustice wherever manifested, whoever the person, whatever the business. Wherever schemes are devised to withhold money from those to whom it is due, or to deprive any man of his rights, there God's disapprobation rests. It is for the interest of every soul connected with the work of God to receive his warnings and reproofs, and die to that stubborn will which has opposed the will of God.

The publishing houses were brought into existence in a spirit of sacrifice, and no persons should have been permitted to hold a responsible position in the work, who desired to work according to the world's policy. The consecration and purity of the worker will be evidenced by the principles manifested in his attitude toward every child of God. The publishing house was established for the purpose of doing business upon the principles of justice and equity, judging every case without partiality and without hypocrisy. In our institution the Spirit of Christ was to be a witness to the world of the character of God, a living epistle, known and read of all men. These institutions were to reveal nothing like oppression; the managers were to be those who showed decidedly that they were under the control of God. Selfishness and the love of money was not to set aside those principles of sacrifice which characterized the establishment of these instrumentalities.

No one should be allowed to engage in the sacred work who could be bought or sold for money. No one is to take advantage of any man's ignorance or necessity, in order to charge exorbitant prices for work done or for goods sold. The managers are not obeying the commandments of God when by any selfish devising they secure the benefit of the time or talents of the workmen. Such a course is robbery of

your neighbor. God has given every one of his {414} workers certain qualifications for which he is responsible, not to any man or set of men, but to God. He is so to use them that they will be a blessing to himself by having it in his power to be a blessing to others. The practices that have prevailed in the Review and Herald office, and which are now leavening the managers of the Conferences, are not correct. I cannot specify all the departures from righteousness; they are too many to be enumerated, and I am not told to do this.

Some will urge that in dealing with sharpers, those who have no conscience, one must conform in a large degree to the customs that prevail; that should he adopt a course of strict integrity, he will be compelled to give up his business, or fail to secure a livelihood. Where is your faith in God? He owns you as his sons and daughters on condition that you come out from the world and be separate and touch not the unclean thing. There will be violent temptations to diverge from the straight path; there will be innumerable arguments in favor of conforming to custom, and adopting practices that are really dishonest.

When one worker enters into a confederacy with another, as has been done, seeking to supply that other's lack of aptitude or knowledge, he is doing that one an injury, and assisting in a deception. That worker receives pay for qualifications which he has not, and his failures in duties which he is supposed to perform, are many. Yet the largest wages are received, and the treasury is robbed. God has been greatly displeased by these things.

These may be regarded by men as little things, but was it a little thing for Adam and Eve to eat of the fruit which God had forbidden them to eat? The smallness of the act did not avert the consequences. It was disobedience to God's commandments, and the floodgates of woe were opened upon our world. We cannot be Christians and connive at any dishonest practice or breach of trust. The Christian will not be found spending extravagantly means that he has not earned. God requires every man to be punctual, just, and without guilt in his lips or in his heart. Be righteous in all dealings with your fellow men if you would have not only the name but the character of a Christian. Those who depart from Bible principles, and vindicate their defects as righteous, have never received the true knowledge of Christ or the experience of being in truth doers of the

word. There is nothing in the word of God that glosses over or excuses one phase of selfishness, one approach to overreaching or dishonesty.

God pledges his most holy word that he will bless you if you will walk in his way, and do justice and judgment. "Thou shalt not have in thy bag divers weights, a great and a small: thou shalt not have in thine house divers {415} measures, a great and a small: but thou shall have a perfect and just weight, a perfect and just measure shalt thou have: that thy days may be lengthened in the land which the Lord thy God giveth thee. For all that do such things, and all that do unrighteousness, are an abomination unto the Lord thy God. Remember what Amalek did unto thee by the way when we were come forth out of Egypt; how he met thee by the way, and smote the hindermost of thee, even all that were feeble behind thee, when thou wast faint and weary: and he feared not God." Notwithstanding that the children of Israel had often grieved the Lord by departing from his counsel, he still had a tender care for them. The Lord Jesus Christ saw their enemies taking advantage of their circumstances, to do them an injury; for that work was to bring suffering against the weary, who were journeying under God's leading. Hear the judgments which God pronounced: "Therefore it shall be, when the Lord thy God hath given rest from all thine enemies round about, in the land which the Lord thy God giveth thee for an inheritance to possess it, that thou shalt blot out the remembrance of Amalek from under heaven; thou shalt not forget it."

I pen these words of God that those who profess to be his children may not receive the curse pronounced upon Amalek because they have followed the practices of Amalek. If the heathen received this denunciation from their course for overcoming the faint and weary, what will the Lord express toward those who have had light, great opportunities, and privileges, but have not manifested the Spirit of Christ toward their own brethren? The Lord sees all the dealings of brother with brother, which weaken faith, and which destroy their own confidence in themselves as men dealing with justice and equity. In the most positive language he expresses his displeasure at the iniquity practiced in trade. He says, "Shall I count them pure with the wicked balances, and with the bag of deceitful weights?" The very wrong here mentioned may not have been committed in our institutions, but acts which these things represent have been, and are still being done. Page after page might be written in regard to these things. Whole conferences are becoming leavened with the same perverted principles. "For the rich men thereof are full of violence, and the inhabitants thereof have spoken lies, and their tongue is deceitful in their mouth." The Lord will work to purify his church. I tell you in truth, the Lord is about to turn and overturn in the institutions called by his name. Just how soon this refining process will begin, I cannot say, but it will not be long deferred. He whose fan is in his hand will cleanse his temple of its moral defilement. He will thoroughly purge his floor. God has a controversy with all who practice the least injustice; for in so doing they reject the authority of God, and imperil their interest in the atonement, the redemption which Christ has undertaken for every son and daughter of Adam. Will it pay to take a course abhorrent to God? Will it pay {416} to put upon your censors strange fire to offer before God, and say it makes no difference?

It has not been after God's order to center so much in Battle Creek. The state of things now exists that was presented before me as a warning. I am sick at heart at the representation. The Lord gave warnings to prevent this demoralizing condition of things, but they have not been heeded. "Ye are the salt of the earth; but if the salt have lost his savor, wherewith shall it be salted? It is thenceforth good for nothing, but to be cast out, and to be trodden under foot of men."

I appeal to my brethren to wake up. Unless a change takes place speedily, I must give the facts to the people; for this state of things must change; unconverted men must no longer be managers and directors in so important and sacred work. With David we are forced to say, "It is time for thee, Lord, to work; for they have made void thy law."

(Signed) Mrs. E. G. White

ELDER O. A. OLSEN

November 26, 1894
Norfolk Villa, Prospect St., Granville, N. S. W.

Dear Brother:

OF LATE I HAVE NOT addressed so many communications to you as heretofore, fearing to lay upon you responsibilities that would be a tax. When we left Michigan, I placed in your hands Testi-monies in regard to matters in the office. They were important and explicit, and I enjoined upon you to have a most faithful work done in reading the Testimonies to those concerned, in order to correct the existing evils. But you did not follow the directions, and the same things went on accumulating in their objectionable features until the matter was again presented to me in an aggravated character, with these words for those in responsible positions: "Neither will I serve with your sins, nor be with you anymore, unless you put away the wrongs from among you."

I learned from letters received from you that you did not read the Testimonies to those concerned and decidedly point out their errors. Here you failed to do your duty as President of the General Conference. You were presented to me in council meetings, listening to the statements and decisions of strong minded and hard hearted men who were not under the controlling influence of the Spirit of God. You knew that these decisions were not according to God's order, yet you did not protest against them, and thus suffered them to pass as having received your sanction. Thus things have been going according to the will and impulse of men who are opposed to God's will, and are {417} bringing in an order of things that God cannot accept or sanction.

You thought that you would deal with these matters in your discourse, by dwelling upon general principles, and hoped that this would prove the best method of correcting the wrongs. But you should have spoken in the board and council meetings. The wrong principles advanced should not have been permitted to take form in wrong practice, because you held your peace or gave such a feeble protest that those who were pursuing the wrong course thought you were with them. The sanction which you gave by your silence strengthened their hands in an evil work.

You yourself have not been able to discern clearly the right and justice, the tenderness and mercy and strict integrity, which should have been maintained in all your decisions. These matters have several times been presented before me, and I dare not withhold them. You might better have done far less preaching, and reserved your energies to take your stand personally against the wrong in spirit, in mind, in judgment, that has struggled for the mastery, and in a large degree obtained it, leading to a wrong course of action. Had you thus taken your stand, your dis-cernment would have been a sharper, and you would have been able to give your decision against the slightest act of injustice toward God's heritage. Those who are working contrary to the will of God, and misrepresenting his character, would have been given to understand distinctly that you could not permit these things to go on; you could not let them pass in heaven as your action. It was your duty to speak decidedly, but you kept silent.

I send this to you because I do not wish you to feel that I am in harmony with your course in these things. I beseech you to serve God with your mind, might, and strength, and make straight paths for your feet, lest the lame be turned out of the way. I have deep, earnest interest and love for you, and I am so anxious that you shall not in any case give your endorsement to wrong doing.

I have recently sent very earnest, decided Testimonies to men in responsible positions, which they should not have occupied up to this time without evidence of a thorough transformation of character. Whatever their business tact, these men who have so long been evidently resisting light and evidence, fighting against God, should have been separated from the work, both for their own soul's sake and for the sake of the cause. For while they are kept in positions of trust, their voice and influence sway many things in the wrong direction. When matters of the greatest importance have come up for decision, their judgment on the questions has depended on the state of mind they chanced to be in. The mind and heart are not under the influence of the Spirit of God. They are men of strong temperament, decided preferences, and much force of character, and their will and influence have decided matters under the control of another spirit than the Spirit of God. {418}

If these men had a sense of what they have been doing, of what they must meet in that great day, when all shall see as they are seen, and know as they are known, they would feel an anguish of heart, an agony of soul, that would be somewhat proportionate to the harm they have done the cause of God. At times temptations come into such minds with overpowering force, for Satan never sleeps, and never takes a vacation. He is always watching his chance to crowd into your important meetings, to reveal his own attributes through the workers, and make of no effect the spirit of testimony that has been appealing to them in reproof and warnings for many years.

The only hope for these men of iron will and hearts of stone is to fall on the Rock and be broken. Contact with Christ brings currents of divine power into the soul, so that the old cherished, natural tendencies, habits, and practices, are changed by the Spirit of God. What they need is a genuine conversion . When they have this experience, these weak, tempted souls will look unto Jesus, and say, "I can do all things through Christ which strengthen me." They need to appreciate every ray of light that comes from the throne of God into their pathway. They need to catch the Spirit and principle of the holy law of God, and conform their life to the character of Christ. A new power takes possession of the new heart. Man can never work out this change for himself. It is a supernatural work, bringing supernatural element into weak and wicked human nature. This power will cast out the devils that possessed the mind and will, and whose power has been revealed even in the words and works of those who claim to be the children of God.

The truth of God has been resisted and trampled down by men who hated its pure and heavenly principles. Men have walked in the fire of the sparks of their own kindling. God wants every man who is connected with his sacred work to be a man with whom he can communicate, a man of humble, teachable spirit, and a contrite heart. Workers who possess this character will not creep and grovel in earthliness, they will not be in bondage to men not to Satanic agencies. They will quit themselves like men, and be strong. They will turn their faces to the Sun of Righteousness, rising above all baser things into an atmosphere pure from all spiritual and moral defilement.

He who has become a partaker of the divine nature knows that his citizenship is above. He catches the inspiration from the Spirit of Christ. His soul is hid with Christ in God. Such a man Satan can no longer employ as his instrumentality to insinuate himself into the very sanctuary of God, to defile the temple of God. He gains victories at every step. He is filled with ennobling thoughts. He regards every human being as precious, because Christ has died for every soul.

"They that wait upon the Lord shall renew their strength; {419} they shall mount up with wings and eagles." The man who waits upon the Lord is strong in His

strength, strong enough to hold firm under great pressure. Yet he is easy to be entreated on the side of mercy and compassion, which is the side of Christ. The soul that is submissive to God is ready to do the will of God; he diligently and humbly seeks to know that will. He accepts discipline, and is afraid to walk according to his own finite judgment. He communes with God, and his conversation is in heaven.

O, how much evil has been committed by placing a high estimate on human talent, when the possessor was unconsecrated unsanctified. All human talent is valueless before God until the superscription of Jesus is placed upon it. Then in and through Christ the possessor becomes an efficient agent for good because he has a living connection with God. When truth gets full possession of a man's conscience, it sanctifies the soul. All his sensibilities are aroused, his sympathies are not fitful. The light from the Sun of Righteousness shines into his heart, and he becomes a earnest, living representative of truth. It is not the most eloquent men or the so called great men in business matters that are essential but men who may be looked upon as having little talent, yet who are true, simple, humble great hearted men; these may attain to wide usefulness blessing humanity everywhere. Jesus says, "Ye are the salt of the earth. Would that every man in the office of publication would practice the lesson taught by this symbol, and represent the saving salt. God is not deceived; he knows every grain of pure salt.

Enoch walked with God, and he was not, for God took him. The Lord would have us walk with him. If he directs the work, it will move in his way, and will bear his impress.

I write you this because I dare not do otherwise. I do not want you to bear all the responsibility, therefore I will send this to others who should understand the situation and help you. We are praying for you, that God will give you his supporting grace.

With sincere desire that you may be wholly and ever on the Lord's side, I will wait and watch and pray.

(Signed) Mrs. Ellen G. White

ELDER O. A. OLSEN

September 10, 1895
Norfolk Villa, Granville

Dear Brother:

FOR YEARS I HAVE CARRIED a consuming burden for the cause of God in

Battle Creek. I am now deeply troubled over the {420} shape which matters are taking there, and the influence which is being exerted on the work everywhere. I ask you, my brother, how can you entrust A. R. Henry and Harmon Lindsay with so much responsibility in the work, and send them hither and thither to all parts of the field? They are not by precept or example giving the third angel's message. The atmosphere which surrounds their souls, and which is revealed in spirit and influence, shows that they have lost the Spirit of God out of their hearts and their experience. They are made responsible for many, many things, while they do not feel their accountability to God.

Brother Nelson who is in the office, cannot be regarded as in exactly the same position as these men; but he needs a different mold of character. He has not that kind, Christian courtesy that will have a saving, fragrant influence upon the minds of those who associate with him or do business with him. Though he may hold to right principles, his manner of representing these principles is such as to make a disagreeable impression upon the minds of those associated with him. His words, his manner of expression, creates thoughts and feelings that are very objectionable. A good man is to manifest his principles, but he can do this in a way that will not make such a disagreeable impression upon those with whom he does business. God requires Brother Nelson to learn his lessons more perfectly in the school of Christ. His principles should be kept more vividly before his own mind, that they may bring forth in him the peaceable fruits of righteousness. His unfortunate manner of expression, and his spirit of criticism, destroy his influence, that, if sanctified, might be of real value.

The Lord wants Brother Nelson to clothe himself with the garments of righteousness, and to bring into his practical life the sweetness and fragrance of the character of Christ. This brother possesses qualifications of mind and character that, if sanctified daily for the Master's use, would enable him to become a vessel of honor. But he needs the molding and fashioning of Jesus. "The love of money is the root of all evil: which while some coveted after, they have erred from the faith, and pierced themselves through with many sorrows. But thou, O man of God, flee these things: and follow after righteousness, godliness, faith, love, patience, meekness. Fight the good fight of faith, lay hold on eternal life, whereunto thou art also called, and hast professed a good profession before many witnesses."

I would say to Brother Nelson, Let your heart be joined to the heart of Infinite love; let your life be knit by hidden links to the life of Jesus. Let your life be hid with Christ in God; then because Christ liveth, you will live also. God wants you to let him manage you that you may be a lovable Christian. The Lord would have the natural and hereditary traits of character come under the pruning knife. Look steadfastly unto Jesus, that you may catch his spirit, and cherish the qualities of Christlike character. Then it will be recognized by all who have {421} any connection with you, that you have learned of Christ his meekness, his affection, his tenderness, his sympathy. Never rest satisfied until you possess a loving and lovable spirit. Your words may come from the good treasure of the heart, to strengthen, help, bless, and win all around you. True conscientiousness will make the religious life attractive. But your religion has altogether too much acidity to be palatable. You sour your influence by a stubborn, set determination; your critical censoriousness sets the teeth on edge. God help you, my brother, for you need melting.

Others catch your spirit. The seeds we sow will bear a harvest, in goodness, patience, kindness, and love, or exactly the opposite. It is not your purpose to do wrong acts, but you do not see the necessity of doing pleasant acts, so that from you men would receive a better impression of the Christian character. More of the spirit of the beloved disciple John would make you more fragrant and lovable, and a far better example of what constitutes a true Christian life.

Many, many need melting over. Be sound in principle, true to God, but do not manifest one stern, ungenial phase of character. God does not want you to incur contempt by manifesting a disposition like a ball of putty, but he does want you to be a principle as sound as a rock, yet with a healthful mellowness. Like the Master, be full of grace and truth. Jesus was incorruptible, undefiled, yet in his life were mingled gentleness, meekness, benignity, sympathy and love. The poorest were not afraid to approach him, they did not fear a rebuff. What Christ was, every Christian should strive to be. In holiness and winsomeness of character he is our model.

"Learn of me," says Christ; for I am meek and lowly in heart, and ye shall find rest unto your souls." We should all learn of Christ what it means to be a Christian. Let us learn of him how to combine firmness, justice, purity, and integrity with unselfish courtesy and kindly sympathy. Thus the character becomes lovable and attractive. The beauty of holiness will disarm scoffers.

The workers at the Review and Herald office will not enter into the kingdom of heaven, unless their character reflects the character of Christ. The heart must receive the divine current, and let it flow out in rich streaks of mercy and grace to other hearts. All who would win souls to Christ must be winsome. A word to the wise is sufficient.

(Signed) Mrs. E. G. White

AUTHORITY OF THE GENERAL CONFERENCE

Selections 1877-1901 {422}

THE HIGHEST AUTHORITY under God among Seventh-day Adventists is found in the will of the body of that people, as expressed in the decisions of the General Conference, when acting within its proper jurisdiction.—Action Of General Conference, 1877 Year Book, 1914 page 255.

I have been shown that no man's judgment should be surrendered to the judgment of any one man. But when the judgment of the General Conference, which is the highest authority that God has upon the earth, is exercised, private independence and private judgment must not be maintained, but surrendered.—Testimonies For The Church, Vol. III page 492 (1875)

God has ordained that the representatives of his church from all parts of the earth, when assembled in a General Conference, shall have authority. The error that some are in danger of committing is in giving to the mind and judgment of one man, or of a small group of men, the full measure of authority and influence that God has vested in his church, in the judgment and voice of the General Conference assembled to plan for the prosperity and advancement of his work.

At times, when a small group of men entrusted with the general management of the work have, in the name of the General Conference, sought to carry out unwise plans and to restrict God's work, I have said I could no longer regard the voice of the General Conference, represented by these few men, as the voice of God.—Testimonies For The Church, Vol. IX page 260

That these men (leaders) should stand in a sacred place, to be as the voice of God to the people, as we once believed the General Conference to be, that is past.—General Conference Bulletin 1901 page 25

Let those in America who suppose the voice of the General Conference to be the voice of God, become one with God before they utter their opinions.—Testimony To Elder Haskell, November 16, 1899.

Do not understand me as approving of the recent action of the General Conference Association, of which you write, but in regard to that matter it is right that I should speak to them. They have many difficulties to meet, and if they err in their action, the Lord knows it all, and can overrule all for the good of those who trust in him.—Testimony To Elder Littlejohn, August 3, 1894

Who can now feel sure that they are safe in respecting the voice of the General Conference Association? If the people in our churches understood the management of the men who walk in the light of the sparks of their own kindling, would they respect their decisions? I answer, No, not for a moment. I have been shown that the people at {423} large do not know that the heart of the work is being diseased and corrupted at Battle Creek. Many of the people are in a lethargic, listless, apathetic condition, and assent to plans which they do not understand—Special Instruction Relating To The Review And Herald Office And The Work In Battle Creek, pp. 19, 20 (1896)

After the truth has been proclaimed as a witness to all nations, at a time when every conceivable power of evil is set in operation, when minds are confused by the many voices crying, "Lo, here is Christ; Lo, he is there; This is truth, I have the message from God, he has sent me with great light." and there is a removing of the landmarks and an attempt to tear down the pillars of our faith—then a more decided effort is made to exalt the false sabbath, and to cast contempt upon God himself by supplanting the day he has blessed and sanctified.—To Brethren In Responsible Positions, 1892.

There seems to be a burning desire to get up something fictitious and bring it in as new light. Thus men try to weave into the web as important truths a tissue of lies. This fanciful mixture of food that is being prepared for the flock will cause spiritual consumption, decline and death. When those who profess to believe present truth come to their senses, when they accept the Word of the living God just as it reads, and do not try to wrest the Scriptures, then they will build their house upon the eternal Rock, even Christ Jesus.

There are those who say, not only in their hearts, but in all their works, "My Lord delayeth his coming." They show the effect of error upon them by smiting their fellow servants and eating and drinking with the drunken. As in the days of Noah, those who have had great light will show their inconsistency. Because Christ's coming has been long foretold, they conclude that there is a mistake in regard to this doctrine. But the Lord says, "If the vision tarry, wait for it: for it will surely come. It will not tarry past the time that the message is borne to all nations, tongues and people."—Testimony To Elder A. G. Daniells, October 14, 1900.

In ours, as in Christ's day, there may be a misreading or misinterpreting of the Scriptures. If the Jews had studied the Scriptures with earnest, prayerful hearts, their searching would have been rewarded with a true knowledge of the time, and not only the time, but also the manner of Christ's appearing. They would not have ascribed the glorious second appearing of Christ to his first advent. They had the testimony of Daniel; they had the testimony of Isaiah and the other prophets; they had the teaching of Moses; and here was Christ in their very midst, and still they were searching the Scriptures for evidence in regard to his coming. And they were doing unto Christ the very things that had been prophesied they would do. They were so blinded they knew not what they were doing. {424}

And many are doing the same things today, in 1897, because they have not had experience in the testing messages comprehended in the first, second and third angels' messages. There are those who are searching the Scriptures for proof that these messages are still in the future. They gather together the truthfulness of the messages, but they fail to give them their proper place in prophetic history. Therefore such are in danger of misleading the people in regard to locating the messages. They do not see and understand the time of the end, or when to locate the messages. The day of God is coming with stealthy tread; but the supposed wise and great men are prating about "Higher Education." They know not the signs of Christ's coming, or of the end of the world—Testimony dated December 20, 1896

————————

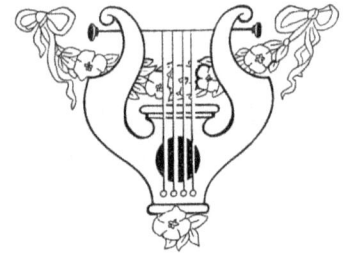

THE KRESS COLLECTION
OF ELLEN G. WHITE LETTERS

LESSONS FROM THE PAST

August 27, 1903-7

A S NOAH'S DESCENDANTS increased in number, apostasy soon led to division. Those who desired to forget their Creator, and to cast off the restraint of His law, decided to separate from the worshipers of God. Accordingly they journeyed to the plain of Shinar, on the banks of the river Euphrates. Here they decided to build a city, and in it a tower reaching unto heaven—so high that no flood could rise to the top, so massive that nothing could sweep it away. Thus they hoped to make themselves independent of God.

But among the men of Babel there were living some God-fearing men who had been deceived by the pretensions of the ungodly, and drawn into their wicked schemes. These men would not join this confederacy to thwart the purposes of God. They refused to be deceived by the wonderful representations and the grand outlook. For the sake of these faithful ones, the Lord delayed His judgments, and gave the people time to reveal their true character. They heeded not the counsel of the Lord, but carried out their own purposes. The great majority were fully united in their heaven-daring undertaking. Had they been permitted to go on unchecked, they would have demoralized the world by their wonderful plans.

This confederacy was born of rebellion against God. The dwellers on the plains of Shinar established their kingdom for self-exaltation, and not for the glory of God. Had they succeeded, a mighty power would have borne away, banishing righteousness, and inaugurating a new religion. The mixture of certain religious ideas with a mass of erroneous theories would have resulted in closing the door of peace, happiness, and security. These suppositions, erroneous theories, carried out and perfected, would have banished a knowledge of the law of Jehovah from the minds of men, who would not think it necessary to obey the divine statutes. These statutes, which are holy, just, and good, would have been ignored. Determined men, inspired by the first great rebel, would have urged on by him, and would have permitted nothing to interfere with their plans, or to stop them in their evil course. In the place of the divine precepts they would have substituted laws framed in accordance with the desires of their selfish hearts in order that they might carry out their purposes.

But God never leaves the world without witnesses for Him. Those who loved and feared Him at the time of the first great apostasy after the flood, humbled themselves, and cried unto him. "Oh God," they pleaded, "interpose thyself between thy cause and the plans and methods of men "and the Lord came down to see the city and the tower (the great idol-building), which the children of men builded." He defeated the purpose of the tower builders, and over-threw the memorial of their rebellion. God bears long with the perversity of men, giving them ample opportunity for repentance; but He marks all their devices to resist the authority of His just and holy law. As an evidence of His displeasure over the building of the tower, he confounded the language of the builders, so that none could understand the words of his fellow-worker.

The Lord has not ordered some of the arrangements that have been made in Battle Creek. He has declared that other places have been robbed of the light {2} and advantages that have been centered and multiplied in Battle Creek. Through a circular letter sent out to the leading men and the church elders of our conferences, a call has been made for the names of young men and young women of capability, in order that they may be corresponded with and invited to come to Battle Creek to receive a training for missionary work.

Through the light given in the Testimonies, the Lord has indicated that He does not desire students to be educated in Battle Creek. He instructed us to remove the College from this place. This was done, but the institutions that remained failed of doing what they should have done in sharing with other places the advantage still centered in Battle Creek. The Lord signified His displeasure over this matter by destroying two of the principal institutions remaining there.

Notwithstanding the plain evidences of the Lord's providence in these destructive fires, men in council meetings have not hesitated to stand before their brethren and make light of the statement that these buildings were burned because men had been swaying things in directions the Lord could not approve.

Principles have been perverted. Men have been departing from right principles, for the promulgation of which these institutions were established. They have failed in doing the very work that God ordained should be done to prepare a people to "build the old waste places" and to stand in the breach, as is represented in the fifty-eighth chapter of Isaiah. In this scripture the work we are to do is clearly defined as being medical missionary work. This work is to be done in all places. God has a vineyard; and He desires that this vineyard shall be worked unselfishly. No parts are to be neglected. The most neglected portion needs the most wide awake missionaries to do the work portrayed in the fifty-seventh chapter of Isaiah.

"Thou are wearied in the greatness of thy way; yet saidst thou not. There is no hope; thou hast found the life of thine hand; therefore thou wast not grieved. And of whom hast thou been afraid or feared, that thou hast lied, and hast not remembered me, nor laid it to thy heart? Have not I held my peace even of old, and thou fearest me not? I will declare thy righteousness, and thy works; for they shall not profit thee."

"When thou criest, let they companies deliver thee; but the wind shall carry them all away; vanity shall take them, and shall inherit my holy mountain: and shall say, Cast ye up, cast ye up, prepare the way, take up the stumbling block out of the way of my people for thus saith the high and lofty one that inhabiteth eternity, whose name is Holy; I dwell in the high and holy place, with him also that is of a contrite and humble spirit, to revive the spirit of the humble, and to revive the heart of the contrite ones. For I will not contend forever neither will I be always wroth; for the spirit should fail before me, and the souls which I have made. For the iniquity of his covetousness was I wroth, and smote him, I hid me, and was wroth, and he went on frowardly in the way of his heart. I have seen his ways, and will heal him; I will lead him also, and restore comforts unto him and to his mourners. I create the fruit of the lips; peace to him that is far off and to him that is near, saith the Lord; and I will heal him. But the wicked are like the troubled sea, when it cannot rest, whose waters cast up mire and dirt." {3}

For their spirit should fail before me, saith the Lord, if I were to deal with my people in accordance with their perversity they could not endure my displeasure and my wrath. I have seen the perverse ways of every sinner. He who repents and does the works of righteousness I will convert and heal, and restore unto him my favor.

I am instructed to say that in his judgments the Lord will remember mercy. For His own name's sake He will not permit the froward and independent to carry out their unsanctified plans. He will visit them for their perversity of action. "There is no peace, saith my God to the wicked."

Concerning those who have been deceived and led astray by unconsecrated men, the Lord says: "Their course of action has not been in accordance with my will; yet for the righteousness of my own cause, for the truth's sake, for the sake of those who have preserved their fear and love of God, I, who create the fruit of the lips, will put my message in the lips of those who will not be perverted. Although some may be deceived and blinded in their ideas of men and the purposes of men, I will heal everyone who honors my name. All the penitent of Israel shall see my salvation. I, the Lord do rule, and I will fill with praise and thanksgiving the hearts of all who are nigh and afar off even all the penitent of Israel who have kept my way."

When iniquity abounds among the nations; when presentations are as marked as they have been during the past few years in America; when the Lord's money is freely circulated by those who do not take the Word of God as their guide, when multitudes are honored, and great festivities are held, when all are interested in making everything possible of men, and are seeking their own pleasure (and we see all these things taking place now), then we may know that the condition of things is similar to the condition that existed in the days of Noah, when the Lord caused the inhabitants of the earth to drink the waters of the flood.

Lot's Experience

The state of the world now is similar to that which existed in the days of Lot, when Sodom's corruption called for the angels visit to that wicked city, to see whether the cries coming up before heaven were of such a character that the inhabitants of beautiful Sodom—a city that had been so highly favored of God—had so corrupted their ways before the Lord that there was no hope of redemption. God's wrath was revealed so signally because the corruption of the Sodomites was extended so deep. The heavenly visitants could see for themselves that the Sodomites had passed the limits of divine forbearance.

The angels took Lot and his wife and daughters by the hand, to hasten their flight from the city, lest the storm of divine judgment should break upon the place they hesitated so much to leave. They were solemnly commanded to hasten; for the fiery storm would be delayed but little longer. But one of the fugitives presumptuously ventured to cast a regretful look backward to the doomed city, and she became a monument of God's judgment,—showing how He regards unbelief and presumptuous rebellion.

This visitation of God's wrath upon Lot's wife hurried the remaining three on their way from the city. But Lot, not desiring to flee to the mountains, had pleaded with the Lord to spare a smaller city a few miles from Sodom where he could flee. What unbelief he manifested. His faith was very weak. But God in His mercy spared [Zoar], in answer to Lot's petitions. {4}

The result of their going into [Zoar] is plainly recorded in the Scriptures. All the cities surrounding Sodom were corrupted with the sins of the Sodomites.

When iniquity abounds in a nation, there is always to be heard some voice giving warning and instruction, as the voice of Lot was heard in Sodom. Yet Lot could have preserved his family from many evils had he not made his home in this wicked, polluted city. All that Lot and his family did in Sodom could have been done by them, even if they had lived in a place some distance from the city. Enoch walked with God, and yet he did not live in the midst of any city, polluted with every kind of violence and wickedness, as did Lot in Sodom.

I have not time now to present all that I hope the Lord will strengthen me to present to his people in regard to this matter.

Seductive Influence

At this time, Jude's testimony is of great force to all who desire to be under the influence of the Holy Spirit:

"Jude, the servant of Jesus Christ, the brother of James, to them that are sanctified by God the Father, and preserved in Jesus Christ and called; mercy unto you and peace, and love be multiplied. Beloved, when I gave all diligence to write unto you of the common salvation, it is needful for me to write unto you, and exhort you that ye should earnestly contend for the faith which was once delivered unto the saints. For there are certain men crept in unawares, who were before of old ordained to this condemnation, ungodly men, turning the grace of our God into lasciviousness, and denying the only Lord God, and our Lord Jesus Christ. I will therefore put you in remembrance though ye once knew this, how that the Lord, having saved the people out of the land of Egypt afterwards destroyed them that believed not. And the angels which kept not their first estate, but left their own habitation, he hath reserved in everlasting chains under darkness unto the judgment of the great day. Even as Sodom and Gomorrah and the cities about them in like manner, giving themselves over to fornication, and going after strange flesh, are set forth for an example, suffering the vengeance of eternal fire."

"Likewise also these filthy dreamers defile the flesh, despise dominion, and speak evil of dignities. Yet Michael the archangel when contending with the devil he disputed about the body of Moses, durst not bring against him a railing accusation, but said, The Lord rebuke thee. But these speak evil of those things which they know not: but what they know naturally, as brute beasts, in those things they corrupt themselves."

"Woe unto them! for they have gone in the way of Cain, and ran greedily after the error of Balaam for reward, and perished in the gainsaying of Core. These are spots in your feasts of charity, when they feast with you, feeding themselves without fear; clouds they are without water, carried about of winds; trees whose fruit withereth, without fruit, twice dead, plucked up by the roots, raging waves of the sea, foaming out their own shame; wandering stars, to whom is reserved the blackness of darkness forever."

"And Enoch also, the seventh from Adam, prophesied of these saying, Behold, the Lord cometh with ten thousands of his saints, to execute judgment {5} upon all, and to convince all that are ungodly among them of all their ungodly deeds which they have ungodly committed, and of all their hard speeches which ungodly sinners have spoken against him. These are murmurers, complainers, walking after their own lusts; and their mouth speaking great swelling words, having man's persons in admiration because of advantage. But beloved, remember ye the words which were spoken before the apostles of our Lord Jesus Christ: how that they told you there would be mockers in the last time, who should walk after their ungodly lusts. These be they who separate themselves, sensual, having not the Spirit."

"But ye, beloved, building up yourselves on your most holy faith, praying in the Holy Ghost, keep yourselves in the love of God, looking for the mercy of our Lord Jesus Christ unto eternal life. And of some have compassion, making a difference, and others save with fear, pulling them out of the fire; hating even the garment spotted by the flesh. Now unto Him that is able to keep you from falling, and to present you faultless before the presence of His glory with exceeding joy, to the only wise God our Saviour, be glory and majesty, dominion and power, both now and ever. Amen."

Jude bears this message to guard believers against the seductive influence of false teachers, men who have a form of godliness but who are not safe leaders. In these last days, false teachers will arise and become actively zealous. All kinds of theories will be presented to divert the minds of men and women from the very truth that defines the position we can occupy with safety in this time when Satan is working with power upon religionists, leading them to make a pretense of being righteous, but to fail of placing themselves under the guidance of the Holy Spirit.

False theories will be mingled with every phase of experience, and advocated with satanic earnestness in order to captivate the mind of every soul who is not rooted and grounded in a full knowledge of the sacred principles of the Word. In the very midst of us will arise false teachers, giving heed to seducing spirits whose doctrines are of satanic origin. These teachers will draw away disciples after themselves. Creeping in unawares, they will use flattering words, and make skillful misrepresentations with seductive tact.

A Message to Church Members

The only hope of our churches is to keep wide awake. Those who are well grounded in the truth of the Word, those who test everything by a "Thus saith the Lord" are safe. The Holy Spirit will guide those who prize the wisdom of God above

the deceptive sophistries of satanic agencies. Let there be much praying, not in human lines but under the inspiration of love of the truth as it is in Jesus Christ. The families who believe the truth are to speak words of wisdom and intelligence,—words that will come to them as the result of searching the scriptures. Now is our time of test and trial. Now is the time when the members of every believing family must close their lips against speaking words of accusation concerning their brethren. Let them speak words that impart courage, and strengthen the faith which works by love and purifies the soul. {6}

Christian fathers and mothers are now called upon to fulfill their duties in the home. They must try to save their children unto eternal life. Let them not advise their children to connect with the Sanitarium at Battle Creek, or with the schools that shall be set in operation at Battle Creek. There is tenfold more danger now in our youth going there, than there has been in any period in the past.

"There were false prophets also among the people," says the apostle Peter concerning the church anciently, "even as there shall be false teachers among you, who privily shall bring in damnable heresies, even denying the Lord that bought them, and bring upon themselves swift destruction. And many shall follow their pernicious ways; by reason of whom the way of truth shall be evil spoken of. And through covetousness shall they with feigned words make merchandise of you; whose judgment now of a long time lingereth not, and their damnation slumbereth not. For if God spared not the angels that sinned, but cast them down to hell, and delivered them into chains of darkness, to be reserved unto judgment; and spared not the old world, but saved Noah the eighth person, a preacher of righteousness, bringing in the flood upon the world of the ungodly; and turning the cities of Sodom and Gomorrah into ashes condemned them with an overthrow, making them ensamples unto those that after should live ungodly; and delivered just Lot, vexed with the filthy conversation of the wicked; (for that righteous man dwelling among them, in seeing and hearing, vexed his righteous soul from day to day with their unlawful deeds): the Lord knoweth how to deliver the godly out of temptation, and to remove the unjust unto the day of judgment to be punished."

The Lord is guarding His people

against a repetition of the errors and mistakes of the past. There have always abounded false teachers, who, advocating erroneous doctrines and unholy practices, and working upon false principles in a most specious, covert, deceptive manner, having endeavored to deceive, if possible, the very elect. They bind themselves up in their own fallacies. If they do not succeed, because their way becomes hedged by warnings from God, they will change somewhat the features of their work, and the representations they have made, and bring out their plans again under a false showing. They refuse to confess, repent, and believe. Confession may be made, but no real reformation takes place, and erroneous theories bring ruin upon unsuspecting souls, because these souls believe and rely upon the men advocating these theories.

Word of Caution

I am instructed to charge parents to take heed, to keep their children guarded and away from Battle Creek. And let all take heed how they hear. Many things are reported in regard to Sister White. Some say one thing, and some say another. There are those who say that Sister White does not object to our having a college in Battle Creek. Until Sister White herself makes this statement, do not believe it. To those who know the messages from the Lord, I would say Hold fast: for soon all will be fulfilled. Hold fast to the Bible. "Search the Scriptures," Christ said, "for in them ye think ye have eternal life: and they are they which testify of me."

Many will become so pleased with erroneous sentiments that they will engage in the promulgation of these sentiments and of specious, deceptive {7} theories. And more than this, they will liberally pay anyone who will assist in promulgating these sentiments.

Let our churches beware of any effort made to draw our youth from their home churches to unite with an institution in order to wait upon worldlings. I call upon those in charge of our churches to beware. You are shepherds, set to watch over the sheep and lambs of Christ's flock. Our youth better far receive their education in a limited sphere than to go to Battle Creek. But because our youth should not go to Battle Creek, they are not to be bound about, so that they cannot develop. They should daily be given the highest motives to advance. They should attend our schools, and the teacher should work with them, and pray with them. They should leave these schools true medical missionaries firmly bound up with the gospel ministry.

Our churches who have a deep interest in the children and youth and in the work of training workers to carry forward the work essential for this time, need not blunder; for God will open ways before all who are perfecting Christian characters. He will have places already for them in which to begin to do true missionary work. It was to prepare workers for this work, that our schools and sanitariums were established.

Let us make no mistakes. The word declared, "Many shall come in my name saying, I am Christ." There shall arise false prophets and false christs and shall show great signs and wonders: insomuch that if it were possible, they shall deceive the very elect." Shall we receive these into our confidence, No No. We are to receive only those who give the surest evidence that they are doing the work appointed them by God.

The Work Before Us

I say to our people, Let not those on whom we must depend to do gospel missionary work in places where the truth should be represented, be drawn away by any pretense from their work. The cause of God needs the very best workers. God's workers are ever to cherish a clear idea of what constitutes pure and undefiled religion. In the cities where the truth is to be established there will be needed workers of Bible faith and practice. The work of God is to be carried forward in the South, and the youths whose talents makes them most desired in Battle Creek are to be ready to step into the places prepared for them in institutions where they can obtain a training for work without being thrown into companionship of worldly people, who know not God, and whose wrong sentiments will leaven the mind of those with whom they are brought in contact. We cannot afford to allow the minds of our youth to be thus leavened; for it is on these youth that we must depend to carry forward the work in the future.

The work at Washington will demand the best and most earnest missionaries. This place, the headquarters of the nation, is a most important field, and there must be those there who are able to state wisely the reasons of their faith. There will be needed young men and young women of capability, who can take up the work as pioneers, and carry it forward in the strength of the Lord.

God's people are to keep their lamps trimmed and burning amid the moral darkness and the unbelief of the world. Canvasser—evangelists are needed to circulate the publications containing the messages of warning for this time. {8}

I call upon the Presidents of our Conferences to exert their God-given influence to open the fields that have never yet been worked. These fields stand as a reproach to our people. Organize your work intelligently, and then proceed to action. Let your simplicity of speech and your simplicity and neatness of dress, speak of your work as missionaries. Educational advantages will be provided and the Lord will go before those who will take up the work in the spirit of self-sacrifice.

Study the life and teachings of Christ. Men may bid for your services, offering large inducements. Remember that Christ paid for you the price of His own life, and that you are not your own. You are to glorify God in your body and in your spirit, which are His.

Humility and benevolence are traits of character that God acknowledges. The Word of God inculcates humility, and encourages benevolence. Humility places man on vantage ground, through the grace of Christ. Christ came to this world to reveal these precious graces as an illustration of the graces that those must reveal who are received as members of the royal family, children of the heavenly king.

To all Christ says, "Come unto me, all ye that labour and are heavy laden, and I will give you rest. Take my yoke upon you, and learn of me; for I am meek and lowly in heart; and ye shall find rest (in the daily experience) unto your souls." Rest will come to all who follow the example given them in the life of Christ. The one whose life practice shows that he has savingly embraced the gospel of Christ will gain access to many souls. This is true of both men and women, and especially of the youth.

"Of the times and seasons brethren, we have no need that I write unto you. For yourselves know perfectly that the day of the Lord so cometh as a thief in the night. For when they shall say peace and safety; then sudden destruction cometh upon them, as travail upon a woman with child, and they shall not escape. But ye, brethren, are not in darkness, that that day should overtake you as a thief. Ye are all the children of light, and the children of the day; we are not of the night, nor of darkness.

Therefore let us not sleep as do others; but let us watch and be sober."

Professed Christians who are being transformed into the likeness of Christ, and who love him with all the heart, will earnestly labor to establish the truth in many places. This is the very work the great Medical Missionary has given us to do. Steadfast faith and perseverance in practical godliness will open the way before every true Christian. And when souls are converted through the instrumentality of such workers, they will give all the glory to God, and will rejoice with exceeding great joy.

Ellen G. White

DEAR BROTHER GRIGGS

August 26, 1903
"Elmshaven" Sanitarium, California

I HAVE RECEIVED YOUR LETTER of August 18. Yesterday I sent you a telegram, in which I told you to publish in the Review and Herald the articles you have written regarding the reopening of the Battle Creek College. I felt {9} that I could not but consent to the publication of this article. The light given me by the Lord— that our youth should not collect in Battle Creek to obtain their education has in no particular been changed. The fact that the Sanitarium has been rebuilt in Battle Creek does not change the light. All that in the past made Battle Creek a place unsuitable for our youth exists today, so far as influence is concerned.

Word has come to me that letters have been sent out to our churches in the different States, offering our youth special inducements to connect with the Battle Creek Sanitarium. The leading men in our conferences are requested to send their most promising young men and young women to the Battle Creek Sanitarium to be educated and trained as nurses. This is an effort to counter-work the counsel of the Lord. Those who present these inducements are working contrary to the will of the Lord.

Had the Sanitarium been re-established in accordance with the Lord's design, it would not now be in Battle Creek. The Lord permitted the Sanitarium to be destroyed by fire, to take away the objection raised to moving out of Battle Creek. It was His design, not that one large building should be erected, but that plans should be made in several places. These smaller sanitariums were to be established where they could have the benefit and advantage of land for agriculture purposes. It is God's plan that agriculture shall be carried on in connection with our sanitariums and schools. Our youth need the education to be gained from this line of work. It is well and more than well—it is essential—that efforts be made to carry out the Lord's plan in this respect.

When the call came to move out of Battle Creek, the plea was made, "We are here, and all settled. It would be an impossibility to move without enormous expense."

The Lord permitted fire to consume the Sanitarium building and thus removed the greatest objection to fulfilling His purpose. Then a large building, different in design, but capable of accommodating as many patients, was erected on the same site as the old building. Since the opening of this institution a very large number of people have come to it. Some of these are patients, but some are merely tourists. But the large number at the Sanitarium is no evidence that it is the will of God that such a condition of things should be. Our Sanitariums were not designed to be boarding places for the rich people of the world.

The care of the large number of guests at the Sanitarium requires a large number of youth, and those in charge of our churches are asked to send in to our Sanitarium the names of the most promising young men and young women in the church, that these youth may be communicated with by the managers of the Sanitarium, and invited to come to the Sanitarium to take the nurses' course.

I would say, Be careful what moves are made. It is not God's design that our youth should be called into Battle Creek. Calling them to this place, and associating them with worldly people of all grades, high and low, is like Lot taking his family into Sodom. {10}

The Lord said, It is for the interest of our youth to be educated in some other place than Battle Creek. He declared it to be His will for the Battle Creek College to be removed to some place in the country.

At this time there was a heavy burden on our schools. I prayed that some way might be opened whereby these debts would be lifted. But Christ heard my prayers and the prayers of many others, and a way was opened. I was instructed to give the manuscript of the book, "Christ's Object Lessons" to our schools. Our publishing houses were to share in the gift by giving the work of printing and binding the book and our people were to sell it, and give their time.

The Lord has blessed the effort put forth to relieve our schools from debt, and I am told that three hundred thousand dollars have been raised toward lifting the debt. While engaged in selling Christ Object Lessons, students and church members have obtained an excellent experience. As they have taken up this work disinterestedly great blessing has come to them. Many have gained a knowledge of how to handle our large books. The Lord himself has co-operated in this work.

It was about the time the light was given regarding "Christ's Object Lessons" that the Lord instructed me that the College in Battle Creek should be removed from that place, and established in some other place. There were too many interests in Battle Creek. Smaller schools were to be established in different places away from the cities.

The establishment of the school at Berrien Springs had the commendation of God. Those in charge of the school at that place have much to encourage them.

Shall we now let the enemy manage for us? Because the Sanitarium is where it should not be, shall the Word of the Lord be no account? Shall we allow the most intelligent of our youth in the churches throughout our conferences be called to Battle Creek, to become servants to worldlings, to be spoiled and robbed of their simplicity, by being brought in contact with men and women who have not the fear of God in their hearts? Such men and women will come in large numbers to Battle Creek Sanitarium, and a large number of helpers will be needed. Shall those in charge of our conferences allow our youth, who, in the schools away from Battle Creek could be fitted up for the Lord's work, to be drawn to Battle Creek, when for many years the Lord has been calling upon His people to move away from Battle Creek.

Human minds may not see the necessity for the call to families to leave Battle Creek, and settle in places where they can do medical missionary evangelistic work. But the Lord has spoken. Shall we question His word.

Our youth are to be prepared to take charge of church school in which the children in our churches will be taught the first principles of education. This is a very nice work, demanding the highest ability and the most careful study. Our young men and young women should be preparing to advance this line of work. Then shall we allow our most promising youth to be called into a work that is not fulfilling the specifications of God? {11}

The Family Firm

The truth, in all its important bearings needs to have a much deeper hold on parents than it has heretofore had. Parents are to work for their own children, helping them while they are still in the home to gain a fitness to work as missionaries for Christ when they leave the home. They are to be taught to be faithful in labor. They are to learn to relieve the weary mother, sharing her burdens. The older children may greatly assist her by helping to care for the little ones. And the younger ones may learn to perform many of the simple duties of the home.

The young men and women should regard a training in the home duties as a most important part of their education. The family firm is a sacred social industry, in which each member is to act a part, each helping the other. The work of the household is to move smoothly, like the different parts of well-regulated machinery. The mother should be relieved of many burdens that the sons and daughters can take upon themselves.

How important that fathers and mothers should give their children, from their very babyhood, the right instruction. They are to teach them to obey the command, "Honor thy father and thy mother, that thy days may be long in the land which the Lord thy God giveth thee." And the children as they grow in years, are to appreciate the care that their parents have given them, and should find their greatest pleasure in helping father and mother.

Fathers and mothers should do all in their power to carry forward the work of the home in right lines. The law of God with its holy principles and solemn injunctions, is ever to bear rule. The principles of the Bible are to be taught and practiced. The parents are to teach their children lessons from the Bible, making them so simple that they can readily be understood.

The more closely the members of a family are united on their work, in the home, the more uplifting and helpful will be the influence that father and mother and sons and daughters will exert outside the home.

It is a serious matter to send children away from home, thus depriving them of the care of their parents. It is of the greatest importance that church schools shall be established to which the children can be sent, and still be under the watch-care of their mothers, and still have opportunity to learn the lessons of helpfulness that it is God's design that they shall learn in the home.

In our larger schools provision should be made for the education of younger children. This line of work is to be managed wisely, in connection with the work of the more advanced students. The older students should be encouraged to take part in teaching the lower classes.

These things are not trifles unworthy of our consideration. I wish to state especially that very much more can be done to save and educate the children of those who at present cannot get away from the cities. Church schools are to be established in these cities and in connection with these schools provision is to be made for the teaching of higher studies, where {12} these are called for. These schools can be managed in such a way, part joining part, and they will be a complete whole. The Lord has His methods, His plans and His wisdom.

God's Design in Establishing Sanitariums

It is God's design to manifest through His people the principles of His kingdom. That in life and character they may reveal these principles. He desires to separate them from the customs, habits and practices of the world. He seeks to bring them near to Him that He may make known to them His will.

This was His purpose in the deliverance of Israel from Egypt. At the burning bush, Moses received from God the message for the king of Egypt, "Let my people go, that they may serve me." Exodus 7:16. With a mighty hand and an outstretched arm God brought out the Hebrew host from the land of bondage. Wonderful was the deliverance He wrought for them, punishing their enemies who refused to listen to His word, with total destruction. God desired to take His people apart from the world, and prepare them to receive His word. From Egypt He led them to Mount Sinai, where He revealed to them His glory. Here was nothing to attract their senses or divert their minds from God: as the vast multitude looked at the lofty mountains towering above them, they could realize their own nothingness in the sight of God. Beside these rocks, immovable except by the power of divine will, God communicated with men. And that His word might ever be clear and distinct in their minds,

He proclaimed amid thunder and lightning and with terrible majesty the law which He had given in Eden, and which was the transcript of His character. And the words were written on tables of stone by the finger of God. Thus the will of the infinite God was revealed to a people who were called to make known to every nation, kindred, and tongue the principles of His government in heaven and in earth.

To the same work He has called His people in this generation. To them He has revealed His will, and of them He requires obedience. In the last days of this earth's history the voice that spoke from Sinai is still saying to men, "Thou shalt have no other gods before me." Exodus 20:3. Man has set his will against the will of God, but He cannot silence this word of command. The human mind can never fully comprehend its obligation to the higher power, but it cannot evade the obligation. Profound theories and speculations may abound, may try to set science in opposition to revelation, and thus do away with the law of God: but stronger and still stronger will the Holy Spirit bring before them the command, "Thou shalt worship the Lord thy God, and Him only shalt thou serve." Matthew 4:10.

How is the world treating the law of God? Everywhere men are working against the divine precepts. Even the churches are taking sides with the great apostate. Men in their blindness boast of wonderful progress and enlightenment, but the heavenly see the earth filled with corruption and violence. Because of sin the atmosphere of our world has become as the atmosphere of a pesthouse.

A great work is to be accomplished in saying before men the saving truths of the gospel. This is the means ordained by God to stem the tide of moral {13} corruption. This is His means of restoring His moral image in man. It is His remedy for universal disorganization. It is the power that draws men together in unity.

To present these truths is the work of the third angel's message. The Lord designs that the presentation of this message shall be the highest, greatest work carried on in our world at this time. That this work may be carried forward on correct lines, He has directed the establishment of schools, sanitariums, publishing houses, and other institutions. In these institutions the attributes of God are to be unfolded, and the glory and excellence of the truth is to be made to appear more vivid.

The Lord years ago gave me special light in regard to the establishment of a health institution where the sick could be treated on altogether different lines from those followed in any other institution in our world. It was to be founded and conducted on Bible principles as the Lord's instrumentality. Those who had any connection with this institution were to be educated in health restoring principles.

The human family is suffering because of the transgression of the laws of God. Satan is constantly urging men to accept his principles, and thus he is seeking to counterwork the work of God. He is constantly presenting the chosen people of God as a deluded people. He is an accuser of the brethren, and his accusing power he is constantly using against those who work righteousness. The Lord desires through his people to answer Satan's charges by showing the result of obedience to right principles.

He desires our health institutions to stand as witnesses for the truth. They are to give character to the work which must be carried forward in those last days in restoring man through a reformation of the habits, appetites, and passions. Seventh-day Adventists are to be represented to the world by the advance principles of health reform which God has given us.

Still greater truths are unfolding for this people as we draw near the close of time, and God designs that we shall everywhere establish institutions where those who are in darkness in regard to the needs of the human organism may be educated, that they in turn may lead others into the light of health reform. The blind leaders of the blind must learn the truth in regard to healthful living as taught in the Scriptures.

"For God so loved the world that He gave His only begotten Son, that whosoever believeth in Him should not perish, but have everlasting life." John 3:16. Our health institutions must be conducted on life saving principles. Those who are suffering because of transgression of physical laws are to be taught that transgression of the laws of nature is the transgression of the law of God. "If thou wilt enter into life," Christ says, "keep the commandments." Matthew 19:17. Live out my law "as the apple of thine eye." Proverbs 7:2.

And in our medical institutions the people are to be brought in contact with the special truths for this time. God says, "There shall be institutions established under the supervision of men who have been healed through a belief in God's word, and who have overcome their defects of character." In the world all kinds of provisions have been made for the relief of suffering humanity, but the truth in its simplicity is to be brought to the suffering ones through the agency of men and women who are loyal to the {14} commandments of God. Sanitariums are to be established all through the world, and managed by a people who are in harmony with God's laws, a people who will co-operate with God in advocating the truth that determines the case of every soul for whom Christ died.

The truth is to be lived out by everyone who has any connection with the work of God in our Sanitariums. Physicians, nurses, and helpers are to work in harmony, to heal not merely the maladies of the body, but the disorders of the soul. When this is done, a power from God will go with the workers. Physicians, managers, and nurses will be living channels of light. The Lord will work with the people who will honor Him.

All the light of the past, which shines unto the present, and reaches forth into the future, as revealed in the word of God, is for every soul who comes to our health institutions. The Lord designs that the Sanitariums established among Seventh-day Adventists shall be symbols of what can be done for the world. Types of the saving power of the truths of the gospel, they are to be agencies in the fulfillment of God's great purposes for the human race.

To God's people and his institutions in this generation as well as to ancient Israel belong the words written by Moses through the Spirit of inspiration:

"Thou art an holy people unto the Lord thy God: the Lord thy God hath chosen thee to be a special people unto him above all people that are upon the face of the earth." Deuteronomy 7:6

"Behold, I have taught you statutes and judgments, even as the Lord my God commanded me. Keep therefore and do them: for this is your wisdom and understanding in the sight of the nations, who shall hear all these statutes, and say, Surely this great nation is a wise and understanding people. For what nation is there so great, who hath God so nigh unto them, as the Lord our God is in all things that we call upon him for? And what nation is there so great, that hath statutes and judgments so righteous as all this law, which I set before you this day? Deuteronomy 4:5-8.

Even these words fail of reaching the greatness and the glory of God's purpose to be accomplished through his people. Not to this world only, but to the universe, are we to make manifest the principles of His kingdom. The apostle Paul, writing by the Holy Spirit, says, "Unto me, who am less than the least of all saints, is this grace given, that I should preach among the Gentiles the unsearchable riches of Christ: and to make all men see what is the fellowship of the mystery, which from the beginning of the world hath been hid in God, who created all things by Jesus Christ, to the intent that now unto the principalities and powers in heavenly places might be known by the church the manifold wisdom of God." Ephesians 3:8-10.

Brethren, "we are made a spectacle unto the world, and to angels, and to men." "What manner of persons ought ye to be in all holy conversation and godliness, looking for and hasting the coming of the day of God?" 1 Corinthians 4:9. 2 Peter 3:11, 12. {15}

The Medical Missionary Work and the Gospel Ministry

As the medical missionary work becomes more extended, there will be a temptation to make it independent of our conferences. But it has been presented to me that this plan is not right. The different lines of our work are but parts of one great whole. They have one center.

In Colossians we read, "The body is of Christ. Let no man beguile you of your reward in a voluntary humility and worshipping of angels, intruding into those things which he hath not seen, vainly puffed up by his fleshly mind, and not holding the Head, from which all the body by joints and bands having nourishment ministered, and knit together, increaseth with the increase of God." Colossians 2:17-19. Our work in all its lines is to demonstrate the influence of the cross. The work of God in the plan of salvation is not to be done in any disjointed way. It is not to operate at random. The plan that provided the influence of the cross provided also the method of its diffusion. This method is simple in its principles and comprehensive in its plain, distinct lines. Part is connected with part in perfect order and relation.

God has brought his people together in church capacity in order that they may reveal to the world the wisdom of Him who formed this organization. God knew what plans to outline for the efficiency and success of his people. Adherence to these plans will enable them to testify of the divine authorship of God's great plan for the restoration of the world.

Those who take part in God's work are to be led and guided by God. Every human ambition is to be submerged in Jesus Christ, who is head over all the institutions that God has established. He knows how to set in operation and keep in operation his own agencies. He knows that the cross must occupy the central place, because it is the means of man's atonement, and because of the influence it exerts on every part of the divine government. The Lord Jesus, who has been through all the history of our world understands the methods that should be invested with power over human minds. He knows the importance of every agency, and understands how the varied agencies should be related to one another.

"None of us liveth to himself." Romans 14:7. This is the law of God in heaven and on earth. God is the great center. From Him all life proceeds. To Him all service, homage, and allegiance belong.

For all created beings there is the same great principle of life, dependence upon and co-operation with God. The relationship existing in the pure family of God in heaven was to exist in the family of God on earth. Under God, Adam was to stand at the head of the earthly family to maintain the principles of the heavenly family. This would have brought peace and happiness. But the law that none liveth to himself Satan was determined to oppose. He desired to live for self. He sought to make himself a center of influence. It was this that brought rebellion in heaven, and it was man's acceptance of this principle that brought sin to earth. When Adam sinned, man broke away from the heaven-ordained censor. A demon became central power in the world. Where God's throne should have been, Satan had placed his throne. The world laid its homage, as a willing offering, at the feet of the enemy. {16}

Who could bring in the principles ordained by God in his rule and government to counterwork the plans of Satan, to bring the world back to its loyalty? God said, I will send my Son, "For God so loved the world that He gave His only begotten Son, that whosoever believeth in Him should not perish but have everlasting life." John 3:16.

This is the remedy for sin. Christ says, Where Satan has set his throne, there shall stand my cross. Satan shall be cast out, and I will be lifted up to draw all men unto me. I will become the center of the redeemed world. The Lord God shall be exalted. Those who are now controlled by human ambition, human passions, shall become workers for me. Evil influences have conspired to counterwork all good. They have confederated to make all men think it righteous to oppose the law of Jehovah. But my army shall meet in conflict with the Satanic forces. My Spirit shall combine with every heavenly agency to oppose them. I will engage every sanctified human agency in the universe. None of my agencies are to be absent. I have a work for all who love me. I have employment for every soul who will work under my direction. The activity of Satan's army, the danger that surrounds the human soul, call for the energies of every worker. But no compulsion shall be exercised. Man's depravity is to be met by the love, the patience, the long-suffering of God. My work shall be to save those who are under Satan's rule.

Through Christ, God works to bring man back to his first relation to his Creator, and to correct the disorganizing influences brought in by Satan. Christ alone stood unpolluted in a world of selfishness, where men would destroy a friend or a brother in order to accomplish a scheme put into their minds by Satan. Christ came to our world, clothing His divinity with humanity, that humanity might touch humanity, and divinity grasp divinity. Amid the din of selfishness he could say to men, Return to your Center, God. He Himself made it possible for man to do this by carrying out in this world the principles of heaven. In humanity He lived the law of God. To men in every nation, every country, every clime, He will impart heaven's choicest gifts if they will accept God as their Creator and Christ as their Redeemer.

Christ alone can do this. His gospel, in the hearts and hands of His followers, is the power which is to accomplish this great work. "O the depth of the riches both of the wisdom and knowledge of God." Romans 11:33. Christ made it possible for the work of redemption to be accomplished, by Himself becoming subject to Satan's misrepresentations. Thus was Satan to show himself to be the cause of disloyalty in God's universe. Thus was to be forever settled the great controversy between Christ and Satan.

Satan strengthens the destructive tendencies of man's nature. He brings in envy, jealousy, selfishness, covetousness, emulation, and strife for the highest place. Evil agencies set their part in operation through the devising of Satan. Thus the enemies' plans, with their destructive tendencies, have been brought into the church. Christ comes with His own redeeming influences, proposing through the agency of His Spirit to impart His efficiency to men, and to employ them as his instrumentalities, laborers together with him in seeking to draw the world back to its loyalty.

Men are bound in fellowship, in dependence, to one another. By the golden links of the chain of love they are to be found fast to the throne of God. This can be done only by Christ's imparting to finite man the {17} attributes which man would ever have possessed had he remained loyal and true to God.

Those who, through an intelligent understanding of the Scriptures, view the cross aright, those who truly believe in Jesus, have a sure foundation for their faith. They have that faith which works by love and purifies the soul from all its hereditary and cultivated imperfections.

God has united believers in church capacity in order that one may strengthen another in good and righteous endeavor. The church on earth would indeed be a symbol of the church in heaven if the members were of one mind and one faith. It is those who are not worked by the Holy Spirit that mar God's plan. Another spirit takes possession of them, and they help to strengthen the forces of darkness. Those who are sanctified by the precious blood of Christ will not become the means of counterworking the great plan which God has devised. They will not do anything to perpetuate division in the church. They will not bring human depravity into things small or great.

It is true that there are tares among the wheat; in the body of sabbath-keepers evils are to be seen, but because of this shall we disparage the church? Shall not the managers of every institution, the leaders of every church, take up the work of purification in such a way that the transformation in the church shall make it a bright light in a dark place?

What may not even one believer do in the exercise of pure, heavenly principles, if he refuses to be constrained, if he will stand as firm as a rock to a "Thus saith the Lord"? Angels of God will come to his help, preparing the way before him.

Paul writes to the Romans, "I beseech you therefore, brethren, by the mercies of God, that ye present your bodies a living sacrifice, holy acceptable unto God, which is your reasonable service. And be not conformed to this world: but be ye transformed by the renewing of your mind, that ye may prove what is that good, and perfect, will of God. Romans 12:1, 2. This entire chapter is a lesson which I entreat all who claim to be members of the body of Christ to study.

Again Paul writes, "If the first fruit be holy, the lump is also holy: and if the root be holy, so are the branches. And if some of the branches be broken off, and thou, being a wild olive tree, wert graffed in among them, and with them partakest of the root and fatness of the olive tree; boast not against the branches. But if thou boast, thou bearest not the root, but the root thee. Thou wilt say then, The branches were broken off, that I might be graffed in. Well, because of unbelief they were broken off, and thou standest by faith. Be not high-minded, but fear: For if God spared not the natural branches, take heed lest He also spare not thee. Behold therefore the goodness and severity of God: on them which fell, severity; but toward thee, goodness, if thou continue in his goodness: otherwise thou also shalt be cut off." Romans 11:16-22. Very plainly these words show that there is to be no disparaging of the agencies which God has placed in the church.

Sanctified ministry calls for self-denial. The cross must be uplifted, and its place in the gospel work shown. Human influence is to draw its efficacy from the One who is able to save and to keep saved all who recognize {18} their dependence upon him. By the union of church members with Christ and with one another, the transforming power of the gospel is to be diffused throughout the world.

In the work of the gospel the Lord uses different instrumentalities, and nothing is to be allowed to separate these instrumentalities. Never should a Sanitarium be established as an enterprise independent of the church. Through their labors, souls are to be saved, that the name of Christ may be magnified.

Medical missionary work is in no case to be divorced from the gospel ministry. The Lord has specified that the two shall be as closely connected as the arm is connected with the body. Without this union, neither part of the work is complete. The medical missionary work is the gospel illustration.

But God did not design that the medical missionary work should eclipse the work of the third angel's message. The arm is not to become the body. The third angel's message is the gospel message for these last days, and in no case is it to be overshadowed by other interests and made to appear an unessential consideration. When in our institutions everything is placed above the third angel's message, the gospel is not there the great leading power.

The cross is the center of all religious institutions. These institutions are to be under the control of the Spirit of God; in no institution is any one man to be the sole head. The divine mind has men for every place.

Through the power of the Holy Spirit, every work of God's appointment is to be elevated and ennobled, and made to witness for the Lord. Man must place himself under the control of the eternal mind, whose dictates he is to obey in every particular.

Let us seek to understand our privilege of walking and working with God. The gospel, though it contains God's expressed will, is of no value to men, high or low, rich or poor, unless they place themselves in subjection to God. He who bears to his fellowmen the remedy for sin, must first be worked himself by the Spirit of God. He must not ply the oars unless he is under divine direction. He cannot work effectually, he cannot carry out the will of God in harmony with the divine mind, unless he finds out, not from human sources, but from Infinite wisdom, that God is pleased with his plans.

God's benevolent design embraces every branch of the work. The law of reciprocal dependence and influence is to be recognized and obeyed. "None of us liveth to himself." The enemy has used the chain of dependence to draw men together. They have united to destroy God's image in man, to counterwork the gospel by perverting its principles. They are represented in God's word as being bound in bundles to be burned. Satan is uniting his forces for perdition. The unity of God's chosen people has been terribly shaken. God presents a remedy. This remedy is not one influence among many influences, and on the same level with them: it is an influence above all influences upon the face of the earth, corrective, uplifting, and ennobling. Those who work for the gospel should be elevated and sanctified: for they are dealing with God's great principles. Yoked up with Christ, they are laborers together with God. Thus the Lord desires to bind his followers together, that they may be a power

for good, each acting his part, yet all cherishing the sacred principle of dependence on the great Head.

TAKOMA PARK, WASHINGTON, D. C.

May 24, 1905{19}

I DESIRE THAT ALL SHOULD understand matters in the right light. The messages given at the Conference of 1901, and since that time, that our sanitariums should not be linked up with the Medical Missionary Association at Battle Creek, were plain enough to be understood by all our medical workers. Had our physicians, whom God has greatly honored by giving them light and encouragement, listened to the counsels and warnings then given them, they would have saved themselves and our people generally from many perplexities and temptations. The Lord designed that these men should be his physicians, light bearers to the world; but they have misappropriated the words of warning, and the enemy has been permitted to work a strange work among those who should have stood as standard-bearers of the truth.

The book, "Living Temple," contains specious, deceptive sentiments regarding the personality of God and of Christ. The Lord opened before me the true meaning of these sentiments, showing me that unless they were steadfastly repudiated, they would deceive the very elect. Precious truth and beautiful sentiments were woven in with false, misleading theories. Thus truth was used to substantiate the most dangerous errors. The precious representations of God are so misconstrued as to appear to uphold falsehoods originated by the great apostate. Sentiments that belong to the revealings of God are mingled with specious, deceptive theories of Satanic agencies.

In the controversy over these theories it has been asserted that I believed and taught the same things that I have been instructed to condemn in the book, "Living Temple." This I deny. In the name of Jesus Christ of Nazareth, I say that this is not so.

Truths are being used to serve the purpose of upholding theories that I have repeatedly condemned. There are those who persist in taking the precious representations given me by God, and weaving them in with sentiments that God never designed should be presented to his people. I protest against this use of my writings, and I am forced to speak to this conference, saying,

Be not deceived; God is not mocked. He who misplaces and misapplies the precious things of God is sinning against Heaven.

I had hoped that these matters would be straightened out at this conference. I hope that after the many decided warnings that have been sent to our medical workers at Battle Creek, they would take a stand for the right, and remove the stumbling blocks out of the way. But another opportunity has passed by unimproved; and I cannot and will not keep silent. The truth of God is imperiled. The students who have gone to Battle Creek to obtain an education in medical missionary lines are in danger of receiving specious errors. In the name of the Lord I say to our people: Let your children receive instruction in medical missionary lines from those who are true and loyal to the faith which has been delivered to the people of God under the ministration of the Holy Spirit. Amidst the perils of these last days, this truth is to shine forth as a lamp that burneth.

When Dr. Kellogg receives the messages of warning given during the last twenty-years; when he is sincerely converted; when he acts as a consistent, level-headed Christian worker; when his energies are devoted to carrying {20} forward, medical missionary work in right lines; when he bears a testimony that has in it no signs of double meaning or of a misconstruction of the light God has given, then we may have confidence that he is following the light. But until then, we have no right to regard him as a safe leader in the interpretation of the Scripture. He will confuse minds, and will co-mingle specious scientific errors with the instruction that he gives. It is not right to allow this seductive influence to be breathed by men and women who are training to be Christian missionaries; for thus they will be deceived, and led away from the truths that Christ gave to John to give to the churches.

It has been presented to me that in view of Dr. Kellogg's course of action at the Berrien Springs meeting, we are not to treat him as a man led of the Lord, who should be invited to attend our general meetings as a teacher and leader.

Ellen G. White

SUNNYSIDE, COORANBONG, N.S.W.

November 20, 1898

T HE LIGHT GIVEN ME in your case, Brother_____ is that you have made a mistake. You have tried to put all that there is of you into the work. You have not observed regular hours for eating or for rest. For a long time, Brother_____, you have abused your physical powers; you have labored above your strength. This is not to be the example minister, but if you do as you have done in the past, you will be able to work only as a broken-down piece of machinery.

Call a halt, I beg of you; for it does not please the Lord to have you in this state of health. Present yourself to God, I beseech of you. Ask Him to forgive your transgressions, and to help you to bring into your future life all the cheerfulness that you possibly can.

You are to apply the laws of life and health to your own case. In violating the laws of health, even in doing the service of God, you misrepresent your maker. He is not unmindful of your work of diligence, of your fervor, but you must remember that you are not a sound man. Your digestive organs are in a very bad state. You ought to be where you can have the most nutritious food. Vegetables should not come into your diet. Some can subsist upon vegetable food, but you cannot. When your food produces gases and an offensive breath, you should know that things are not as they should be. You need a better circulation. Your imagination is very active. The Lord would have the human machinery better cared for. You do not bring yourself to time. You cannot keep up this strain as you have done; for you are lessening your physical, mental and moral powers. You must have a period of rest.

The Lord values his children. He would have them happy, not suffering. The system must have nourishment. Your food need not be measured; you have an observing mind, study the foods you can best assimilate. But that which is of the greatest importance is regularity and simplicity in your diet. Do not have a starvation diet, but do not take a variety at one meal. Get the very best things, if they cost you more, and eat not more than two or three articles at a meal. Two is better. Then there will not be so much quarrelling going on in your stomach. Some have tried to keep a precise measurement of the food {21} they eat. This keeps the mind upon themselves, and is fully as bad as eating too much. You must try to govern your eating. It will be a difficult matter for you to follow this plan when you go to other places as you have to do. But eat a plain food. Do not drop out

the third meal but eat light food. This will call the blood from the brain. Many who eat the third meal would be better without it, but there are cases where three light meals are better than two full meals.

You have not given nature a chance to do her work. You have abused yourself. Now bring yourself to time just as soon as you can. Leave the work for a few weeks, and place yourself under treatment. Do not keep up your work. Brother Olsen who died in Colorado, might have lived to labor many years had he realized that it was his duty to take care of the temple of God. The Lord would have used him as His co-laborer.

There are many now under the shadow of death who are prepared to do a work for the Master but who have not felt that a sacred obligation rested upon them to observe the laws of God. There are many who have limited themselves to a diet that cannot sustain them in health. In the efforts to discard a meat diet, there has not sufficient care been taken to provide nourishing food to take the place of meat. It is really contrary to health reform to cut off the great variety of dishes, and then go to the opposite extreme, taking no pains to understand that the living machinery must be fed in order to work, and reducing the quantity and quality of the food to a low degree. Instead of health reform, this is a health deform. After some have made the change in their diet, they have not considered that they must have tact and energy to prepare their food in the most healthful manner. Brother_____ your stomach is in such a condition that you must give yourself into skillful hands; you must have proper food prepared for you, without having to give particular thought to it yourself. It is your duty to guard the citadel of the soul, and the brain power by taking weeks of rest and not trying to labor until a change takes place in you for the better. Your system must have nourishment. Your whole system will become deranged if you have to take charge of your own diet. This continual mental anxiety is a tax you must not bear. If any physician prescribes meat for you, say No; the flesh of dead animals does not compose my diet. Flesh meat is not necessary for the health and strength of mind or body. If the Lord had not furnished all that is essential in the vegetable world, there would be an excuse for meat eating, but animals are now so diseased that it is now really dangerous; it is unclean to eat meat. Flesh meat formed no

part of the food provided for man in the beginning. It was after the transgression and fall, when death was to be man's portion, that God permitted that long lived race to eat the flesh of clean animals.

Ellen G. White

DEAR BROTHER AND SISTER KELLAR

February 5, 1902
St. Helena, California

I AM SOMEWHAT TROUBLED IN regard to you, my dear friends. I am so anxious for you to take hold of the work in Australia in the right way. I am very desirous that you shall avoid the mistakes some have made. At the beginning, your work may not be pleasant. But if you will take hold unitedly {22} to do your best, to improve your capabilities and talents, you will come very close to the Saviour. You are in a new country, on missionary ground, and you need to be very careful to do all the Saviour requires. You need to be ever under the supervision of Him who has purchased you with His own life.

My sister, I wish to say a few words to you. You can be a great blessing to your husband. But you need a work done for you before you can be a blessing to those with whom you are brought in contact. You know little in regard to heart-consecration. Will you not make an unreserved surrender of all you have and are to the Lord? Do not spoil your record by cheapness of word or action.

I feel a deep interest in both of you. I desire to see you working as the Lord's helping hand to bring others to the knowledge of the truth. You can be either a savor of life unto life, or of death unto death.

To all his followers the Lord gives talents; and he calls upon all to work while the day lasts. For everything received from God we must render a strict account. By faithful, diligent use we are to increase our talents. God will expect a return proportionate to the amount we have received. If we have been-given five talents, he will call for the increase of five. It is by the faithful use of our talents that means are to be brought to the Lord's treasury, to supply the necessities of his ever-enlarging work.

Many, instead of taking up the work God has given them, are looking for some service that will distinguish them as workers of marked talent. Do not aspire to do some great thing. Take up the work waiting to be done near you. Every word prompted by the Spirit of God, every duty faithfully performed, is a seed sown unto eternal life.

A few pence well-handled are of more use than pounds that lie unused. The one who uses one talent faithfully for the Master is of far more value in his sight than the one who has many talents, but who refuses to use them aright, who looks down on the one who does humble service. The faithful performance of small duties fits us for larger responsibilities. Of those who take up their appointed work, no matter how small it may seem, who perform faithfully the humble duties nearest them, Christ says, "He that is faithful in that which is least is faithful also in much."

We have no time to complain or to disparage others. God calls upon us to carry our work forward in right lines, for Christ's sake exerting a correct influence in the daily life. He calls upon us to lead others to His throne. He teaches us to pray, "Thy kingdom come, they will be done on earth as it is.."

THE WORK OF CHRISTIAN PHYSICIANS

June 3, 1907
Sanitarium, California

AMONG CHRISTIAN PHYSICIANS there should ever be a striving for the maintenance of the highest order of true refinement and delicacy, a preservation of those barriers of reserve that should exist between men and women.

We are living in a time when the world is represented as in Noah's time, and as in the days of Sodom. I am constantly being shown the great dangers {23} to which youth, and men and women who have just reached manhood and womanhood, and also men and women of mature years, are exposed, and I dare not hold my peace. There is need of greater refinement, both in thought and association. There is need of Christians being more elevated and delicate in words and deportment.

The work of a physician is of that character that if there is a coarseness in his nature, it will be revealed. Therefore the physician should guard carefully his speech, and avoid all commonness in conversation. Every patient he treats is reading the traits of his character, and the tone of his morals by his action and conversation.

The light given me of the Lord regarding this matter is that, as far as possible, lady physicians should have the care of lady patients, and gentlemen physicians the care of gentlemen patients. Every physician should respect the delicacy of the patients. Any unnecessary exposure of ladies before male physicians is wrong. Its influence is detrimental.

Delicate treatments should not be given by male physicians to women in our institutions. Never should a lady patient be alone with a gentleman physician, either for special examination or for treatment. Let physicians be faithful in preserving delicacy and modesty under all circumstances.

In our medical institutions there ought always to be women of mature age and of good experience who have been trained to give treatments to the lady patients. Women should be educated and qualified just as thoroughly as possible to become practitioners in the delicate diseases which afflict women, that their secret parts should not be exposed to the notice of men. There should be a larger number of lady physicians educated not only to act as trained nurses, but also as physicians. It is a most horrible practice, this revealing the secret parts of women to men, or men being treated by women.

Women physicians should utterly refuse to look upon the secret parts of men. Women should be thoroughly educated to work for women, and men to work for men. Let men know that they must go to those of their own sex, and not apply to lady physicians. It is an insult to women, and God looks upon these things of commonness with abhorrence.

While physicians are called upon to teach social purity, let them practice that delicacy which is a constant lesson in practical purity. Women may do a noble work as practicing physicians; but when men ask a lady physician to give them examinations and treatments which demand the exposure of private parts, let her refuse decidedly to do this work.

In the medical work there are dangers which the physician should understand and constantly guard against. Truly converted men are the ones who should be employed as physicians in our sanitariums. Some physicians are self-sufficient, and consider themselves able to guard their own ways; whereas, if they but knew themselves, they would feel their great need of help from above.

Some medical men are unfit to act as physicians to women because of the attitude they assume toward them. They take liberties until it becomes a common thing with them to transgress the laws of chastity. Our physicians {24} should have the highest regard for the directions given By God to His church when they were delivered from Egypt. This will keep them from becoming loose in manners and careless in regard to the laws of chastity. All who will live by the laws that God gave from Sinai may be safely trusted.

It is not in harmony with the instruction given at Sinai that gentlemen physicians should do the work of midwives. The Bible speaks of women at childbirth being attended by women, and thus it ought always to be. Women should be educated and trained to act skillfully as midwives and physicians to their sex. It is just as important that a line of study be given to educate woman to deal with women's diseases as it is that there should be gentlemen thoroughly trained to act as physicians and surgeons. And the wages of the women should be proportionate to her services. She should be as much appreciated in her work as the gentleman physician is appreciated in his work.

Let us educate ladies to become intelligent in the work of treating the diseases of their sex. They will sometimes need the counsel and assistance of experienced gentlemen physicians. When brought into trying places, let all be led by supreme wisdom. Let all bear in mind that they need and may have the wisdom of the Great Physician in their work.

We ought to have a school where women can be educated by women physicians to do the best possible work in treating the diseases of women.

Among us as a people, the medical profession should stand at its highest. Physicians should bear in mind that it is their work to fit souls as well as bodies for healthy life. Their service for God is to be thoroughly uncorrupted by an evil practice

Every practitioner needs to study carefully the word of God. Read the story of the sons of Aaron in the tenth chapter of Leviticus, verses one to eleven. Here was a case where the use of wine benumbed the senses. The Lord demands that the appetites and all the habits of life of the physician be kept under strict control. While dealing with the bodies of their patients, they are to constantly remember that the eye of God is upon all their work.

The most exalted part of the physicians work is to lead the men and women under his care to see that the cause of disease lies in violation of the laws of health, and to encourage them to hold higher and holier views of life. Instruction should be given that will prove an antidote for the diseases of the soul as well as for the sicknesses of the body. Only that sanitarium will be a healthful institution where right principles are established. The physician who, knowing the remedy for the diseases of soul and body, neglects the educational part of his work, will have to give an account for his neglect in the day of judgment.

Ellen G. White

LESSONS FOR SANITARIUM WORKERS

November 11, 1907 {25}

Preparation for Trial

THE BURDEN IS UPON ME TO write that which will be a help to God's people in these closing days. A great crisis is just before us. To meet its trials and temptations, and to perform its duties, will require persevering faith. But we may triumph gloriously; not one watching, praying, believing soul will be ensnared by the enemy.

Christ sought to impart special instruction to the first disciples to prepare them for the trial of faith they must endure in His rejection and crucifixion by the Jews. "The Son of man shall be betrayed into the hands of men," He said, "and they shall kill Him; and the third day He shall rise again." "If any man will come after Me, let him deny himself, and take up his cross, and follow Me. For whosoever shall save his life shall lose it; and whosoever shall lose his life for My sake shall find it. For what is a man profited if he gain the whole world, and lose his own soul? or what shall a man give in exchange for his soul? For the Son of man shall come in the glory of His Father, with His angels; and then shall He reward every man according to his works. Verily I say unto you, There be some standing here, which shall not taste of death, till they see the Son of man coming in His kingdom."

"And after six days, Jesus taketh Peter, James, and John his brother, and bringeth them up into an high mountain apart."

The Saviour and His disciples have spent the day in traveling and teaching, and the mountain climb adds to their weariness. They follow where Christ leads the way, yet they wonder why their Master should lead them up this toilsome ascent when they are weary, and when He too is in need of rest.

Presently Jesus tells them that they are now to go no farther. Stepping a little aside from them, the Man of sorrows pours out His supplications with strong crying and tears. He prays for strength to bear the best in behalf of humanity. And He pours out His heart longings for His disciples, that in the hour of the power of darkness their faith may not fail.

At first the disciples unite their prayers with His in sincere devotion; but after a time they are overcome with weariness, and, even while trying to retain their interest in the scene, they fall asleep. The Saviour has seen the gloom of His disciples, and has longed to lighten their grief with the assurance that their faith has not been in vain. The burden of His prayer is that they may be given a manifestation of His glory that He had with the Father before the world was, that His kingdom may be revealed to human eyes, and that His disciples may be strengthened to behold it. He pleads that they may witness a manifestation of His divinity that will comfort them in the hour of His supreme agony with the knowledge that He is of a surety the Son of God, and that His shameful death is a part of the plan of redemption.

The Saviour's prayer was heard. He "was transfigured before them, and His face did shine as the sun, and His raiment was white as the light. And behold there appeared unto them Moses and Elias, talking with Him."

"Then answered Peter and said unto Jesus, Lord, it is good for us to be here; if Thou wilt, let us make here three tabernacles, one for Thee, and one for Moses, and one for Elias. While he yet spake, behold a bright cloud over-shadowed them, and behold a voice out of the cloud which said, This is My beloved Son in whom I am well pleased; hear ye Him. And when the disciples {26} heard it, they fell on their face and were sore afraid."

Through being overcome with sleep, the disciples heard little of what passed between Christ and the heavenly Messengers. Failing to watch and pray, they had not received the light that God desired to give them,—a knowledge of the sufferings of Christ and the glory that should follow. They lost the blessings that might have been theirs by sharing His self-sacrifice. Slow of heart to believe were these disciples, little appreciative of the treasure with which heaven sought to enrich them.

When Christ's predictions came to pass, and the disciples were brought over the ground of test and trial, they failed to endure the proving. Peter denied His Lord before His enemies. Had the disciples remained watching, they would not have lost their faith as they beheld the Son of God dying upon the cross. Amid the gloom of that terrible, trying hour, some rays of hope would have lighted up the darkness, and sustained their faith.

This experience of the disciples is recorded that we may learn its lesson. It is just as essential that the people of God today bear in mind how and where they have been tested, and where their faith has failed, where they have imperiled His cause by unbelief and self-confidence. Renouncing all self-dependence, they are to trust in God to save them from dishonoring His name.

God sends trials to prove who will stand faithful under temptation. He brings us into trying positions to see if we will trust in a power out of and above ourselves. Everyone has undiscovered traits of character that must come to light through trial. God allows those who are self-sufficient to be sorely tempted, that they may understand their helplessness. He suffers the deep waters of affliction to go over our souls, in order that we may know Him and Jesus Christ whom He has sent, in order that we may have deep heart longings to be cleansed from defilement, and may come forth from the trial purer, holier, happier. Often we enter the furnace of affliction with our souls darkened with selfishness; but if patient under the crucial test, we shall come forth reflecting the divine character. When His purpose in the affliction is accomplished "He shall bring forth thy righteousness as the light, and thy judgment as the noonday."

"Watch ye, and pray, lest ye enter into temptation." Watch against the stealthy approach of the enemy, watch against old habits and natural inclinations, lest they assert themselves; force them back, and watch. Watch the thoughts, watch the plans, lest they become self-centered. Watch over the souls that Christ has purchased with His own blood. Watch for opportunities to do them good.

How to be Great

Later the disciples were taught another lesson. On the journey through Galilee, Christ again tried to prepare their minds for the scenes before Him. He told them that He was to go up to Jerusalem to be put to death, and to rise again. The disciples did not even now comprehend His words. Although the shadow of a great sorrow fell upon them, a spirit of rivalry found a place in their hearts. They disputed among themselves which should be accounted the greatest in the kingdom. This strife they thought to conceal from Jesus, and they did not as usual, press close to His side, but loitered behind, so that {27} He was in advance of them when they entered Capernaum.

Jesus read their thoughts, and He longed to counsel and instruct them. But for this He awaited a quiet hour, when their hearts would be open to receive His words.

When He reached Capernaum, and had entered a house, the disciples came to Him saying, "Who is the greatest in the kingdom of heaven? And Jesus called a little child unto Him, and set him in the midst of them and said, Verily I say unto you, Except ye be converted, and become as little children, ye shall not enter into the kingdom of heaven."

Very tenderly, yet with solemn emphasis, Jesus tried to correct the evil. He showed what is the principle that bears sway in the kingdom of heaven, and in what true greatness consists, as estimated by the standard of the courts above. Those who were actuated by pride or love of distinction, were thinking of themselves, and of the rewards they were to have, rather than how they were to render back to God the gifts they had received. They would have no place in the kingdom of heaven, for they were identified with the ranks of Satan.

Before honor is humility. To fill a high place before men, Heaven chooses the worker who, like John the Baptist, takes a lowly place before God. The most child-like disciple is the most efficient in labor for God. The heavenly intelligences can co-operate with him who is seeking, not to exalt self, but to save souls. He who feels most deeply his need of divine aid will plead for it; and the Holy Spirit will give to him glimpses of Jesus that will strengthen and uplift the soul. From communion with Christ he will go forth to work for those who are perishing in their sins. He is anointed for his mission; and he succeeds where many of the learned and intellectually wise would fail.

The Lord has lessons for us all to learn regarding the position we should occupy toward each other and toward Him. Let no Pharisaical pride come into our ranks, but let us move humbly and wisely, putting from our hearts and minds every injurious thought and feeling. The spirit of selfishness that would lead a man to set himself above his brethren is evidence that he does not see the necessity of being a humble learner in Christ's school. The precious word of God is to be faithfully studied if God's professing people are to find a place among the redeemed.

"And whosoever receiveth one such little child in my name," the Saviour continued, "receiveth Me." "And whoso shall offend one of these little ones, it were better for him that a millstone were hanged about his neck and he were drowned into the depths of the sea."

The "little ones" are not children in years, but those who are young in the Christian life. Those who have newly come to the faith are to be treated with love and tenderness. They are to be instructed by precept and example in the way of the truth. "Take heed that ye despise not one of these little ones, for I say unto you, That in heaven, their angels do always behold the face of My Father which is in heaven. For the Son of man is come to seek and to save that which is lost." {28}

O, how different are the standards by which God and man measure character. God sees many temptations resisted of which the world, and even near friends, never know—temptations in the home, in the heart. He sees the soul's humility in view of its own weakness, the sincere repentance over even a thought that is evil. He sees the whole-hearted devotion to His service. He has noted the hours of hard battle with self—battle that won the victory. All this God and angels know. A book of remembrance is written for them that fear the Lord and that think upon His name.

Not in our learning, not in our position, not in our numbers or our entrusted talents, not in the will of man, is to be found the secret of success. Feeling our inefficiency, we are to contemplate Christ, and through Him who is the strength of all strength, the thought of all thought, the willing and obedient will gain victory after victory.

And however short our service or humble our work, if in simple faith we follow Christ, we shall not be disappointed of the reward. That which even the greatest and wisest cannot earn, the weakest and most humble may receive. Heaven's golden gate opens not to the self-exalted. It is not lifted up to the proud in spirit. But the everlasting portals will open wide to the trembling touch of a little child. Blessed will be the recompense of grace to those who have wrought for God in simplicity and faith and love.

Care for the Erring

"How think ye," the Saviour said, "if a man have an hundred sheep, and one of them be gone astray, doth he not leave the ninety and nine in the wilderness, and goeth into the mountains and seeketh that which is gone astray? And if so be that He find it, Verily I say unto you, he rejoiceth more over that sheep than over the ninety and nine which went not astray. Even so it is not the will of your Father that one of these little ones should perish."

My brethren and sisters, read this whole chapter, and let its instruction tender your hearts, and help you to understand your duty toward those who need your help. In every place angels of God are watching to see what kind of spirit is exercised in behalf of souls.

If the lost sheep is not brought back to the fold, it wanders until it perishes. And many souls go down to ruin for want of a hand stretched out to save. These erring ones may appear hard and reckless; but if they had received the advantages that others have had, they might have revealed far more nobility of soul, and greater talent for usefulness. Angels pity these wandering ones. Angels weep, while human eyes are dry and hearts are closed to pity.

There are many who err, and who feel their shame and folly. They look upon their mistakes and errors until they are driven almost to desperation. These souls we are not to neglect. When one has to swim against the stream, there is all the force of the current driving him back. Let a helping hand then be held out to him as was the Elder Brother's hand to the sinking Peter. Speak to him hopeful words, words that will establish confidence and awaken love. {29}

Thy brother, sick in spirit, needs thee as thou thyself hast needed a brother's love. He needs the experience of one who has been as weak as he, one who can sympathize with him and help him. The knowledge of our own weakness should help us to help another in his need. Never should we pass by one suffering soul without seeking to impart to him the comfort wherewith we ourselves are comforted of God.

It is fellowship with Christ, personal contact with a living Saviour, that enables the mind and heart and soul to triumph over the lower nature. Tell the wanderer of an almighty hand that will hold him up, of an infinite humanity in Christ that pities him. It is not enough for him to believe in law and force, things that have no pity, and never hear the call for help. He needs to clasp a hand that is warm, to trust in a heart full of tenderness. Keep his mind stayed on the thought of a divine presence ever beside him, ever looking upon him with pitying love. Bid him think of a Father's heart that ever grieves over sin, of a father's hand stretched out still, of a Father's voice, saying, "Let him take hold of My strength, and make peace with Me; and he shall make peace with Me."

As you engage in this work you have companions unseen by human eyes. Angels of heaven were beside the Samaritan who cared for the wounded stranger. Angels from the heavenly courts stand by the side of all who do God's service in ministering to their fellow-men. And you have the co-operation of Christ Himself. He is the restorer, and as you work under His supervision, you will see great results.

Physicians, nurses, and helpers, in all your dealings with the sick, let your words and actions be controlled by the Spirit of God. Precious words of comfort from the word of God may be spoken to the sick ones who come to our sanitariums, and earnest prayers be offered in their behalf. Hopeful words and cheerful countenances and helpful acts will reveal to the patients the love of God.

All the religious exercises of the home life should be of a cheering and encouraging nature. The physician or nurse who is easily offended, or who cherishes a jealous or suspicious disposition, is not prepared to take responsibilities in our institutions for the sick. Such influences will counterwork the best efforts that can be made to bring in a cheering and uplifting atmosphere. Our sanitariums are to be regarded as sacred places; the spiritual interests of the patients are to be carefully watched, and any influences that should injure should be removed. The men and women who care for the sick should be truly converted; then they will speak words that will help and uplift.

My fellow workers, keep your spiritual perceptions clear. Cherish the simplicity of the word of God. By the love of Jesus that is in your own hearts, draw these patients to the feet of Christ. One soul saved is of more worth in the sight of God than all the sanitarium buildings in the world.

Cooperation Between Our Schools and Sanitariums

I have been shown that there are decided advantages to be gained by having our schools located near our sanitariums, that the students may receive the benefits of the instruction given to the nurses, and may witness the {30} results of faithful work done for those who need help and counsel. The benefits of hearty co-operation extend beyond physicians and teachers, students and sanitarium helpers. When a sanitarium is built near a school, those in charge of the educational institution have a grand opportunity of setting a right example before those who all through their life have been easy-going idlers, and who have come to the sanitarium for treatment. The patient will see the contrast between the idle self-indulgent lives that they have lived, and the lives of self-denial and service lived by Christ's followers. They will learn that the object of medical missionary work is to restore, to correct wrongs, to show human beings how to avoid the self-indulgence that brings disease and death.

There is a great work to be done by our sanitariums and schools. Time is short; what is done must be done quickly. Let those who are connected with these important instrumentalities be wholly converted. Let them not live for self, for worldly purposes, withholding themselves from full consecration to God's service. Let them give themselves, body, soul, mind, and spirit to God, to be used by Him in saving souls. They are not at liberty to do with themselves as they please; they belong to God; for He has bought them with the life blood of His only begotten Son. And as they learn to abide in Christ, there will remain in the heart no room for selfishness. In His service, they will find the fullest satisfaction. The Lord would have His work move forward solidly. Let light shine forth as God designed that it should from His institutions, and let God be glorified and honored. This is the purpose and plan of heaven in the establishment of these institutions. Let physicians and nurses and teachers and students walk humbly before God, trusting in Him as the One who can make their work a success.

With Singleness of Heart

Christ is calling all who claim to believe in Him to reveal by their own example of self-denial and temperance in all things, the virtues of His character. He asks them, by an example of obedience to the truth, to bind souls to Him. The Saviour's example of self-denial and self-sacrifice is to be kept before the patients in the most attractive light. "God so loved the world, that He gave His only begotten Son, that whosoever believeth in Him should not perish, but have everlasting life." The Saviour's sacrifice, His taking human nature, His rejection by the people whom He came to bless, His uncomplaining sufferings, and especially His daily life of self-denial, are to be kept constantly before their minds.

In the work of restoring the moral image of God in man, everything depends upon the conversion of every power of the being of God. The saving grace of Christ is able to accomplish this for every soul. Those who would be soul-winners must study Christ's methods of reaching souls. Satan and his agencies are seeking to keep men and women in rebellion against God and the truth. When the workers in our sanitariums realize this as they should, every possible influence for good will be brought to bear upon those who come for treatment and rest.

If our institutions are rightly conducted they will be the means of bringing us in touch with the workers in the Women's Christian Temperance Union. Many of these noble souls in this organization need to learn that obedience to the fourth commandment is an experience that they need in order {31} to perfect a Christian character. When they will yield their will to His will in this matter, God will make their efforts more effectual to the saving of soul, body, and spirit of Himself.

My fellow-workers, keep on the armor of Christ's righteousness. Pleasant words, faithful attendance, a desire to relieve suffering, will win a way for you to turn the mind to the never failing source of healing, the One who died to pay the ransom price for lost and ruined men. The enemy will press the battle to the gates, but keep the armor on. Remember that everyone converted to the faith adds to our efficiency to give the truth to the world. The grace of Christ is promised us as we seek to turn souls to obedience to the commandments of God. We should be willing to undertake whatever He calls upon us to do.

In the Power of the Spirit

The Spirit of God is to be our efficiency in the work laid upon us. We must now move forward courageously; for we have no time to lose. Those who strive will win the victory. In His mediatorial work Christ gives to His servants the presence of the Holy Spirit. This means power and efficiency that will enable the human agent to represent Christ in the work of soul saving.

God has instructed me that our workers need to experience the deep moving of the Spirit of God; many are in need of a fuller conversion. On the day of Pentecost, in response to the continued prayers of the disciples, the Holy Spirit descended from heaven with the sound as of a rushing mighty wind. For ages the heavenly influences had been held in restraint; but in response to the fervent prayers of these humble men, they descended with power to co-operate with human agencies. Then what confessions came forth from human lips, what humiliation of soul was manifested. And what songs of praise and thanksgiving mingled with the voice of penitence and confession. All heaven bent to listen to the lowly seekers after God.

Through the grace of Christ, and under His direction, we can accomplish a grand and far-reaching work. Through the power that the Holy Spirit will impart, we can bring souls who are now living in rebellion to God, to see their need of Christ, and, accepting the provision made for them, become laborers together with God in the work of saving others.

God will withhold nothing from the soul who gives himself to Christ for service, but will give him ability to accomplish a work the results of which will be as measureless as eternity. The wounded hands of Christ are His pledge that grace sufficient will be given to every soul to work out the will of God. All power in heaven and in earth will co-operate with Him. Acting as Christ's instrumentality in the earth, day by day man becomes a partaker of the divine nature, escaping the corruption that is in the world through lust. The church on earth, having united with it the power of the church in heaven, will come off more than conqueror through the blood of the Lamb and the word of its testimony.

Ellen G. White

EXTRACTS FROM LETTERS CONCERNING FLESH EATING

July 26, 1896
Stanmore, Sydney, N.S.W. {32}

Dr. J. H. Kellogg:

THE PERFECTION OF CHRISTIAN character is attainable. As we approach the close of this earth's history, we will find that the whole world is becoming a lazar house of disease. The transgression of the law of God is bringing the sure result.

I present the word of the Lord God of Israel. Because of transgression, the curse of God has come upon the earth itself, upon the cattle and upon all flesh. Human beings are suffering the result of their own course of action in departing from the commandments of God. The beasts also suffer from under the curse.

Meat eating should not come into the prescriptions for any invalids from any physician from among those who understand these things. Disease in cattle is making meat eating a dangerous matter. The Lord's curse is upon the earth, upon man, upon beasts, upon the fish of the sea; and as transgression becomes almost universal, the curse will be permitted to become as broad and as deep as the transgression. Disease is contracted by the use of meat. The diseased flesh of these dead carcasses is sold in the market places, and disease among men is the sure result.

The Lord would bring His people into a position where they will not touch or taste the flesh of dead animals. Then let not these things be prescribed by any physician who has a knowledge of the truth for this time. There is no safety in the eating of the flesh of dead animals, and in a short time the milk of cows will also be excluded from the diet of God's commandment keeping people. In a short time it will not be safe to eat anything that comes from the animal creation. Those who take God at His word, and obey His commands with their whole heart will be blessed. He will be their shield of protection. But the Lord will not be trifled with. Distrust, disobedience, and alienation from God's will and way will place the sinner in a position where the Lord cannot give him His divine favor.

Again I refer to the diet question: We cannot now do as we have ventured to do in the past in regard to meat-eating. It has always been a curse to the human family, but now it is made particularly so in the curse which God has pronounced upon the herds of the field, because of man's transgression and sins. The disease upon animals is becoming more and more common, and our only safety now is in leaving meat entirely alone. The most aggravated diseases are now prevalent, and the very last thing that physicians who are enlightened should do, is to advise patients to eat meat. It is in eating meat so largely in the country that men and women are becoming demoralized, their blood corrupted and disease planted in their system. Because of meat-eating, many die, and they do not understand the cause. If the truth were known, it would bear the testimony it was the flesh of animals that passed through death. The thought of feeding upon dead flesh is repulsive, but there is something in meat-eating: we partake of diseased, dead flesh, and this sows its seed of corruption in the human organism.

I write to you, my brother, that the giving of prescriptions for the {33} eating of flesh of animals may no more be practiced in our sanitariums. There is no excuse for this. There is no safety in the after influence and results upon the human mind. Let us make known in our institutions that there is no longer a meat table, even for the boarders, and then the education given upon the discarding of a meat diet, will not only be saying, but doing. If patronage is less, so let it be. The principles will be of far greater value when they are understood, when it is known that the life of no living thing shall be taken to sustain the life of a Christian.

In this country we see the necessity of our words and deeds harmonizing. I had a decided talk with the physicians at just the right time, and I think I know the question will be settled with them. I spoke Sabbath upon this subject, and the church was full of believers. Of course, there must be an abundance of fruit and well-cooked grains.

Ellen. G. White

ELDER A. T. JONES

July 3, 1906
Sanitarium, California
(J -242- 1906)

Dear Brother,

AGAIN AND AGAIN YOUR CASE has been presented before me. I am now instructed to say to you, You have had a large knowledge of truth, and less, far less, spiritual understanding. When you were called to the important work at Washington, you had need of far more of the humble grace that becometh a Christian. Since the Berrien Springs meeting, your attitude and the attitude of several others has grieved the Spirit of God. You have been weighed in the balance and found wanting.

Though you had full confidence in yourself, you were out of the path of duty when, in order to criticize and reprove the work of your brethren, you, with others, interrupted the meeting called especially for prayer and confession and for seeking for a spirit of unity. Had you understood the work that needed to be done at that time, a very different presentation would have been made at that meeting. In the place of victory there was defeat. The Lord has said, "weighed in the balance and found wanting."

Self-exaltation is your great danger. It causes you to swell to large proportions. You trust in your own wisdom, and that is often foolishness.

Do you remember the counsel which I gave you in my letter of April, 1894? This was in answer to your letter expressing deep regret over the part you had taken in an unwise movement, and you appealed to me for instruction, that you might ever avoid such mistakes. Here is a portion of what I wrote you then:

"Your letter is received, and I would be glad to satisfy your mind on every point, but that is not in my power. While I can speak to you in words of warning, you may ask many questions that it is not my duty or in my power {34} to answer. I can tell you, and all our teachers of faith and doctrine, Stick to the Word. 'Preach the Word; be instant in season, out of season: reprove, rebuke, exhort with all longsuffering and doctrine.' But never, never make a place for A. T. Jones. Guard this point jealously. Do not even once take any advantage to employ ridicule or to bring against any person or any position a railing accusation. It is plainly revealed in the Word—that this is not God's plan.

"Always teach present truth as it is in Jesus. If you have a true sense of the sacredness of the work, you will be much with God in prayer. It is God only who can bruise Satan under your feet shortly. Walk steadily. Make straight paths for your feet, lest the lame be turned out of the way. Many are so weak in faith and experience that they will look to A. T. Jones, and what you say and do, they will say and do; for they will not look beyond you to Jesus, who is the Author and Finisher of our faith.

"At every step that we advance, if our advance is one of safety, we must lean wholly upon a power out of and above ourselves. The Lord is infinite. He has all resources at His command, and if we trust in Him implicitly, and not in our own capabilities, we shall walk softly and reverently before Him, and have less and less confidence in human capabilities. Nothing of the natural, the human, must take the place of the Spirit of God. No man, however much he may desire it, can use the Holy Spirit. The Holy Spirit is to use us.

Self must be placed at the disposal of the Spirit of God. This must be recognized as the working agent, to mold the man, and to teach him all things.

"In these times of special interest the guardians of the flock of God should teach the people that the spiritual powers are in controversy; it is not the human beings that are creating such intensity of feeling as now exists in the religious world. A power from Satan's spiritual synagogue is infusing the religious elements of the world, arousing men to decided action to press the advantages Satan has gained by leading the religious world in determined warfare against those who make the word of God their guide and the sole foundation of doctrine. Satan's masterly efforts are now put forth to gather in every principle and every power that he can employ to controvert the binding claims of the law of Jehovah, especially the fourth commandment, that defines who is the Creator of the heavens and the earth____

"God will inspire His loyal and true children with His Spirit. The Holy spirit is the representative of God, and will be the mighty working agent in our world to bind the loyal and true into bundles for the Lord's garner. Satan is also with intense activity gathering together in bundles his tares from among the wheat.

"The teaching of every true ambassador for Christ is a most solemn, serious matter now. We are engaged in a warfare which will never close until the final decision is made for all eternity. Let every disciple of Christ be reminded that "we fight not against flesh and blood; but against principalities, against powers, against the rulers of the darkness of this world, against spiritual wickedness in high places." O, there are eternal interests involved in this conflict, there must be no surface work, no cheap experience, to meet this issue. 'The Lord knoweth how to deliver the godly out of temptations, and to reserve the unjust to the day of judgment to be punished:.... whereas angels, which are greater in power and might, bring not railing accusation against them before the Lord.' {35}

"The Lord would have every human intelligence in His service withhold all severe accusations and railings. We are instructed to walk with wisdom toward them that are without. Leave with God the work of condemning and judging. Christ invites us, 'Come unto Me, all ye that labor and are heavy laden, and I will give you rest. Take My yoke upon you, and learn of Me;

for I am meek and lowly in heart; and ye shall find rest unto your souls.' Everyone who heeds this invitation will yoke up with Christ. We are to manifest at all times and in all places the meekness and lowliness of Christ. Then the Lord will stand by His messengers, and will make them His mouthpieces, and he who is a mouthpiece for God will never put into the lips of human beings words which the Majesty of heaven would not utter when contending with the devil.

"Our only safety is in receiving divine inspiration from Heaven. This alone can qualify finite men to be co-laborers with Christ. 'Seeing then that all these things shall be dissolved, what manner of persons ought ye to be in all holy conversation and godliness, looking for and hastening unto the coming of the day of God, wherein the heavens being on fire shall be dissolved, and the elements shall melt with fervent heat? Nevertheless we, according to His promise, look for new heavens, and a new earth, wherein dwelleth righteousness. Wherefore, beloved, seeing that ye look for such things, be diligent, that ye may be found of Him in peace, without spot, and blameless.' O that as a people bearing a solemn message to the world, we might heed every word of instruction given us of God for this time.

"My brother, I do not cease to remember you in my prayers. You were never in greater peril than at the present time. You are giving the last message of warning to our world, and Satan will weave his nets to entangle your feet if you are not praying, and watching, and relying every moment upon God to keep you and strengthen you to resist temptation. Your soul is in peril. Should I specify the particular temptations, Satan would shift his operations and prepare some temptation you are not expecting. Therefore watch with much prayer, watch your own spirit, and God will hold you up.

"'Little children, it is the last time: and as ye have heard that antichrist shall come, even now are there many antichrists; whereby we know that it is the last time.' They went out from us, but they were not of us.' And these apostates the apostles named antichrists. They are doing the work of Satan. 'If they had been of us, they would no doubt have continued with us: but they went out, that they might be made manifest that they were not all of us. But ye have an unction from the holy One, and ye know all things. I have not written unto you because ye know not the truth, but because ye know it, and that no lie is of the truth.'

"My brother, whom the Lord has honored by giving a message of truth for the world, in God alone can you maintain your integrity. 'But ye, beloved, building up yourselves on the most holy faith, praying in the Holy Ghost, keep yourselves in the love of God, looking for the mercy of our Lord Jesus Christ unto eternal life. And of some have compassion, making a difference: and others save with fear, pulling them out of the fire, hating even the garment spotted of the flesh.' While this hatred for the sin that spots and stains the soul is expressed, we are, with one hand, to lay hold of the sinner with the firm grasp of faith, while with the other we grasp the hand of Christ. 'Now unto Him that is able to keep you from falling, and to present you faultless before the presence of His glory with exceeding joy, to the only wise God {36} our Saviour, be glory and majesty, dominion and power, both now and forever. Amen.'"

When at the General Conference in Washington, I had a conversation with you, but it seemed to have no influence upon you. You appeared to feel fully capable of managing yourself. After that conversation scene after scene passed before me in the night season, and I was then instructed that you neither had been nor could be a help to Dr. Kellogg; for you were blind in regard to his dangers and his real standing. You cannot be a help to him; for you entirely misjudge his case. You consider the light given me of God regarding his position as of less value than your own judgment. You have upon your soul the guilt of confirming him in his wrong course of action, and building him upon a false foundation. You need the repentance that needeth not to be repented of; for in Dr. Kellogg's case, you have done a work that has encouraged him to resist the light given me of God for him. You are coming to be worked by the same spirit that has been working with Dr. Kellogg.

This I warned you of when I placed in your hands the written testimony for Dr. Kellogg. You need to become converted, and become as humble as a little child, else you will lose your soul. If you had possessed clear discernment, you could have helped Dr. Kellogg, but you have not the clear light that cometh from the Light of the world.

Brother Jones, I have a message for you. In many respects you are a weak man. If I were to write out all that has been revealed to me of your weakness, and of the developments of your work that have not been in accordance with the course of a true Christian, the representation would not be pleasing. This may have to be done if you continue to justify yourself in a course of apostasy. Until your mind is cleared of the mist of perplexity, silence is eloquence on your part.

I am so sorry that you are spoiling your record. Since the Berrien Springs meeting, you have received many warnings, but you have not heeded these. The fact, that while you were considered sound in the faith, you have done things that you were warned not to do, shows that you are not a safe leader.

You have gone farther than most of our people have supposed in strengthening Dr. Kellogg to continue in transactions against which the Lord has warned him. You are following in a false track. You are placing yourself in a position from which it will be difficult for you to recover yourself.

When in 1901 you came to the Pacific Coast, I hoped that the weight of responsibilities as president of the California conference would lead you to distrust your ability, and to take counsel with your brethren regarding the work to be done. But there was a growth of self-confidence, a rashness of spirit, and an abruptness of speech, which increased the existing lack of confidence in your judgment.

This was especially marked at the camp-meeting in Oakland. At that meeting I had a message to bear that there should be an earnest effort made to draw nigh to God. A coldness and a lack of spirituality had come into our ranks, and we should have made a most determined effort to seek the Lord in prayer, and to stand on vantage ground. Had there been full and free {37} confession of sin, and a clearing of the King's highway, the Spirit of the Lord would have come in, and the Lord would have been glorified.

But the words you had to speak at that time brought in feelings that thwarted the purpose of my message. At other times, and in other places, you manifested a domineering spirit that drove away the Spirit of God.

At the meeting in Fresno in 1902, a scene was presented before me in the night season. I was in a meeting where many spoke words of dissatisfaction with the record you had made as president of the California Conference. I saw there must be in your ministry a change, and received instruction for you and for the laborers in the Conference. This I presented at an early morning meeting. Here is a part of what I said at that meeting:}

"It is the pleasure of God that Brother A. T. Jones should serve this Conference another year as president. It is His pleasure that A. T. Jones should put away all appearance of a magisterial, domineering, authoritative manner. He is not to think that by virtue of his position as president of the conference, he has arbitrary authority. True, he is to have authority, but it is to be just such an authority as Jesus had, an authority that is hid in the meekness and lowliness of Christ.

"In the past, the work of Brother Jones has been represented to me in figures. He was holding out to the people a vessel filled with most beautiful fruit, but while offering the fruit to them, his attitude and manner were such that no one wanted any. Thus it has too often been with the spiritual truths that he offers to the people. In his presentation of these truths, a spirit sometimes crops out that is not heaven-born. Words are sometimes spoken, reproofs given, without due consideration, with a drive, a vim, that causes the people to turn away from the beautiful truths he has for them.

"I have seen Brother Jones when the melting Spirit of God was upon him. His love for the truth was genuine, and not something that he merely claimed to possess. He had cultivated and cherished this love, and it is still to be cherished in his heart. But our brother has a very poor way of manifesting the compassion, the tenderness, the lovable spirit of Christ_____

"It is not surprising that a man who has passed through the experience that Elder Jones passed through in Battle Creek should sometimes err, He has had to arm himself, and keep on the armor constantly, fighting the various evils that were continually creeping in. He has kept himself braced for so long that he must now make an effort to unlearn many things. He must be reconverted. In his manner of presenting the principles of truth he must reform. God has great love for Brother Jones as well as for every other mortal who in some respects fails of reaching the standard placed before him.

"The Lord by His Holy Spirit is going to strengthen Brother Jones, enabling him to endure the inconveniences and taxation of travel from place to place. He desires our brother to heed the messages that He has taken pains to send to him. He desires him to weave into the fabric of his character the threads of patience and kindness, that in heaven it can be said of him, He is complete in Christ Jesus. God desires every minister of the gospel to strive to attain to this perfection_____ {38}

"Brethren, let us all refrain from criticism. He who criticizes his brethren takes his position on the enemy's ground. Satan is an accuser of the brethren. Day and night he is accusing those who profess to follow Christ. Too often we think we could do better than those who are doing their best to carry on the work in right lines.

"When you think your brother is pursuing a wrong course go to him in kindness, telling him his fault 'between thee and him alone.' Ask him if he is sure that he is right in doing as he does. Invite him to compare notes with you. Often when you treat him in this way, light and blessing come to both of you. Not infrequently the supposed fault is found to be a virtue.

"Let us learn to follow the Bible rule for dealing with the erring. Let us do our part to answer Christ's prayer for unity among His people. During the coming year, let us obey the new commandment that Christ gave to His disciples in every age, 'Love one another, as I have loved you.' For our soul's sake let us serve Him with more zeal and earnestness than we have ever served Him before.

"Brethren, shall we not cease criticizing one another? Shall we not blend? Shall we not be determined so to unite that we shall be one strong whole? Shall we not bind heart to heart? Shall we not seek to subdue our hasty spirit, and learn to be as meek and lowly as the little children of whom Christ said to His disciples, 'Except ye be converted, and become as little children, ye shall not enter into the kingdom of heaven?'

"God desires His servants to stand with the whole armor on, in His might overcoming the powers of darkness, to His honor and glory. Let us begin this work today. 'With the heart man believeth unto righteousness; and with the mouth confession is made unto salvation.' Let us bring into our daily life, into all our words and works, belief unto righteousness, and confession unto salvation, in order that we may glorify the God of Heaven."

To this you responded most feelingly.

You said:

"In the nature of things, I should have something to say. I shall be brief; I shall be very brief: for you have been told it all, and it is all so. I thank God for the one great promise, that I am to be converted. That is the good, cheering news,—that I am to be converted; and I know it. I am glad that you know it, and so many of you; for I can have your help in making that thing effective. And, brethren, that is what I do want. You know that is what I asked for a year ago, at the beginning of my work in this conference; and I ask it still. So I just simply commit myself to God and to His word, and to His work, as has been described, and I ask your co-operation, your fellowship, and we shall go on together; and so let us pray;-}

(Praying) "Heavenly Father, we bow before Thee. Lord, we have heard Thy word. We submit all to Thee. O Lord, Thou hast called me by name, and hast told my failings and my sore need. Lord, I confess it all to Thee.

"O God, I thank Thee for Thy gracious word, Thy blessed, Thy special promise, that I, Lord, shall be converted unto Thee. And so, Lord, I put myself into Thy hands this moment, to be converted, to be molded and fashioned according to Thine own mind and by Thy Holy Spirit. O Lord, I pray that Thy {39} divine wish may be met, and that I shall ever be a channel for the flowing of that holy oil which Thou hast mentioned, and which Thou dost long to pour upon bereaved and sore and morning hearts. And Lord, I pray Thee that Thou wilt now convert me through and through. Make me, Lord altogether like Jesus, only like Jesus, that I shall be kind and courteous, gentle and careful, toward all my brethren and all to whom Thou dost send me.

"O Lord, Thou knowest all about it. I need not tell Thee anything. But Lord, I will confess all thou hast spoken. Take me, O Lord; Thou hast bought me; I am Thine. So I give myself to Thee, Lord, this morning, body, soul, and spirit to be devoted to Thee, to be consecrated to Thee, to be purified by Thee, to be cleansed by Thee, to be molded and shaped by Thee, conformed to the image of Thy dear Son, that I may walk worthy of Thee, dear Lord, and glorify Thee on earth, and finish the work which Thou hast given me to do.

"Lord, I pray Thee that the hearts of my brethren may not be pained any more by anything that I may do or say, but that they may be bound to Thee, Lord, and helped on the way.

"And so, now, Lord, we have committed all to Thee. We thank Thee that Thou dost accept everyone; and so, Lord, use us. Make us one, we pray Thee, O Lord, to help to make us one. Whomsoever Thou shalt choose as the band of men that shall go with me, make our hearts ones, our minds one, that we shall be workers together to unify the great work which Thou hast committed to us, to make Thy work prosperous, and carry it nobly and strongly.

"And so, Lord, I pray for this. I know, Lord, that Thou hast heard the prayer; and so answer, we pray Thee, in the multitude of Thy mercies, Lord, answer, that California may rise once more to the place that belongs to this Conference in this great work, that Thou mayest be glorified.

"Lord, I thank Thee for Thy Word; for Thy Spirit; for Thy promise. In Jesus' name. Amen."

The Spirit of the Lord was present, and His grace was freely bestowed. My heart was full of praise. After this experience I thought that you would be imbued with the Spirit of God, that you would move prayerfully and understandingly. But since that time you have again passed over the same ground. You have taken matters into your own hand, disregarding the counsel of the Holy Spirit, as though you possessed superior knowledge. The result of your course is seen in a clouding of your spiritual perceptions.

Brother Jones, you are acting the part of Aaron, and the Spirit of God is grieved. Dr. Kellogg has not been helped by you or his associate physicians; for your course has confirmed him in his blindness. You have done him great harm, but no good, and you are accounted as false watchmen.

You were entrusted with letters to be read to Dr. Kellogg. These letters contained instruction and warnings that should have been heeded by yourself. You should have prayed with Dr. Kellogg, and made every effort possible to obtain a spiritual influence over him, that you might convince him of his wrong course of action. He has had many schemes and devisings, with which the Lord had nothing to do. He was taking a course in some things that would ruin his influence. {40}

The Lord does not design that Battle Creek shall become a modern Jerusalem. The carrying out of the plans to make Battle Creek a great center would prove to be detrimental to the work of carrying the message to all the world. These things should be viewed by you in all their bearings.

"Enter ye in at the strait gate: for wide is the gate, and broad is the way, that leadeth to destruction, and many there be which go in thereat; because strait is the gate, and narrow is the way, which leadeth unto life, and few there be that find it."

In regard to the messages of warning given me regarding people being called to Battle Creek, you have worked contrary to the counsel of the Spirit of God. You were standing where you liked to be, and you have reasoned away the objections to being in Battle Creek. Standing, as did Aaron, directly opposed to the Word of the Lord, you have made of no effect the testimonies of warning sent to keep young men and young women from going to Battle Creek. You have allowed your influence to be used to lead people to do just what the Lord has warned them not to do, and the Lord pronounces you an unfaithful steward in your influence in Battle Creek. Whatever excuses you may make, it is thus charged against you. You have worked decidedly counter to the Lord's plans, and God says, "I will judge him for this, unless he repents."

Elder Tenney has departed from the faith, and is no help to Dr. Kellogg. He upholds him in a wrong course. You and he, ministers of the gospel, have stood directly in the way of the work of the Lord. You have confused the understanding of our people in Battle Creek, and now you are taking a course to confuse the people, leading some to move counter to the Lord's directions.

Elder Waggoner has not been a help in Battle Creek. In the European field he has sown seeds that bear evil fruit, leading some to depart from the faith.

There are others who might be mentioned as transgressors, and whose influence is a stumbling block to the youth. The spiritual conditions in Battle Creek are such that the youth cannot safely be encouraged to go there. For the past twenty years [FOOTNOTE: (1886-1906)] the Lord has been giving warnings that altogether too many people are settling in Battle Creek, leaving their small home churches, which should be kept alive by their earnest efforts. Educational centers should have been established in places wisely selected, and connected with them should be teachers who are settled in the

faith. Testimonies have been borne counseling our people to leave Battle Creek. And the Lord sent His judgments upon the institutions there to show His displeasure at the neglect of these warnings.

Brother Jones, you should realize that all the talent that has been entrusted to you is to be consecrated to your Redeemer. But..... {41}

A Physician's Opportunities

Every physician should be a Christian. In Christ's stead he is to stand by the suffering, working as Christ worked, ministering to the needs of the sin-sick soul as well as to the needs of the diseased body. The physician should look to his Saviour saying, "I sanctify myself through the grace freely given me, that those to whom I minister may also be sanctified."

An atheist or an irreligious man should never take up the work of a physician. The godless physician watches with human sympathy the sufferings of the afflicted: but he cannot do that which he might do did he realize that the One who gave his own life for the sufferer, even the Son of God, is watching the case with intense interest. How inconsistent for a physician to stand by the side of the suffering if he cannot point them to a sin-pardoning Saviour. How terrible not to be able to tell them of the Mighty One who can heal not only every physical disease but every spiritual malady.

The physician should look higher than himself. In simple, soothing words he should speak to the sufferer of the great Physician. He who cannot do this loses case after case which he might save if he were a Christian. If he could speak to the sufferer words that would inspire faith in the sympathizing Saviour, who feels every throb of anguish, the crisis would be passed safely. The sufferer would be strengthened to look and live.

The physician who has no practical knowledge of the great needs of the soul will look upon his patient merely from a scientific standpoint. He will trust to his own skill. If the patient recovers, he takes the praise, entirely forgetting the One who said, "Live, for I have taken pity on you, and will spare you that you may become acquainted with me and believe on my name."

Would that physicians might understand the greatness of the service they could render to humanity if they were able to speak simply and tenderly of the love of Jesus and of his willingness to save souls,

even at the last hour of life. Many physicians fail to see what a noble influence they might exert by accepting Christ and laying hold of eternal interests. They continue to live a hopeless life, a life in which God is not recognized. They refuse to be illuminated by the Light of the world, and are in a far worse condition than the one who is suffering from physical disease.

Great opportunities are given to the guardians of the sick. Knowing the Lord Jesus, it is the privilege of the Christian physician to introduce Him to the sickroom as the One who can speak peace to the soul and give strength to the body. He can point the sufferer to the Lamb of God, who taketh away the sin of the world. The Lord will give such a physician great wisdom in his work.

The physician should be a man of earnest prayer, that he may impart to others the light and hope and faith which he receives. He should himself possess the hope which is sure and steadfast, the hope that Jesus is a very present help in every time of trouble. He should reverence the Word of God. This Word is exceedingly precious to the receiver; for it sanctifies the soul. The Christian physician studies the Word of God, and is prepared to soothe those who are tossed by doubt and fear. He knows the value of the Redeemer's love and presence. He can speak with assurance of the soul hovering between {42} life and death. Who knows but in these last moments faith and hope may spring up in the heart and give inspiring energy to the apparently dying one. Who knows but that the compassionate Saviour may speak the word, "You shall live to sound forth my praises."

The physician needs to have a very close connection with God. Never is he to lose his hold of God's helpful, strengthening power. The fact, that the physician acts so important a part in bringing relief from suffering, will naturally place him where he will be regarded with feelings of love and gratitude by those whom he has helped. Let him not take the praise and glory to himself. Let him hide self in the Saviour, pointing to Christ as the One who is to receive all the praise.

When the sick are restored to health, the glory is often given to the physician, when it was the divine touch and healing balm of the Saviour that gave relief and prolonged life. If the one who has been restored gives praise to the physician, it is the physician's duty and privilege to point him to the compassionate Saviour as the

One who has spoken to him the word of life and given him a new lease of life to be used for a high and holy purpose. The Lord is the worker: the physician is only the instrument. "Without me," Christ declares, "ye can do nothing." He says to the faithful physician, "I will stand by your side, and as you tell those for whom you work that Christ is all and in all, that He died for their sins, in order that they should not perish, but have everlasting life, I will impress their heart."

Jesus is interested in every one who is in need of his healing, vitalizing power. "Are not five sparrows sold for a farthing, and yet not one of them is forgotten before God. But even the very hairs of your head are all numbered. Fear not, therefore, ye are of more value than many sparrows."

What a blessing the Christian physician can bring to sin tortured souls! What peace comes to the sufferer as he accepts the Saviour! What melody is awakened in the heavenly courts when Satan loses his prey!

The physician who is acquainted with Christ, who realizes the preciousness of pure and undefiled religion, is indeed a representative of the great Physician. The physician who tells the sick and suffering of the love that Christ has for them is a true teacher of righteousness. He bears to the afflicted the very balm of Gilead.

What a sacred work is this, and how earnestly should those who are preparing as physicians labor to fit themselves for it. They should make it their first business to become personally acquainted with the great Physician, that when in the sick room they may recognize His presence and receive His counsel.

To us as a people God has given advanced truth, and we are to seek to gain access to souls, that we may give them this truth. As the physicians and nurses in our sanitariums hold out to the patients the hope of restoration to physical health, they are also to present the blessed hope of the gospel, the wonderful comfort to be found in the mighty Healer, who can cure the leprosy of the soul. Thus hearts will be reached, and He who gives health to the body will speak peace to the soul. The Life Giver will fill the heart with joy that will work miraculously. {43}

Those thus born again will go from our institutions prepared to speak to others of the power of Him who has done so much for them. Jesus says of them, "Ye are my witnesses." God grants them a renewal of life and health that they may impart to others the knowledge they have obtained. They go forth as new born souls, converted and enlightened, knowing that by being temperate in all things and depending on Him who gave His life for them, they may work for God.

Our Sanitarium is to be established in harmony with God's appointment. Those who act a part in connection with this institution are to be themselves buildings for the Lord. Writing by the Holy Spirit, the apostle said, "Ye are God's husbandry; ye are God's building." God requires symmetry of character. His workers are ever to remember that self is to be hid in God. They are not to look to the men of the world for their strength, supposing that to gain a crumb of praise from them is something worth relating, even though those who give this praise are trampling God's commandments under their feet. When the great men of the world speak a word in toleration of the author of Christianity, what they say is repeated as though worthy of being immortalized. But words are cheap. They cost nothing. The Lord is honored only by those who love and obey His commandments.

Physicians should not suppose that it is right for them to make appointments or to travel on the Sabbath. Not only by precept but also by example they should honor the true Sabbath, which is to be immortalized as the evidence that God created the world in six days and rested on the seventh. God blessed the seventh day and hallowed it, placing the command concerning it in the very bosom of the Decalogue. It is to be sacredly observed.

Common, every day treatment should not be given on the Sabbath. Let the patients know that physicians must have one day on which to rest. Often it is impossible for physicians to take time on the Sabbath for rest and devotion. They may be called upon to relieve suffering. Our Saviour has shown us by His example that it is right to relieve suffering on the Sabbath. But physicians and nurses should do no unnecessary work on this day. Ordinary treatment and operations which can wait should be deferred till the next day.

MY DEAR BRETHREN
July 13, 1900

I WISH YOU TO UNDERSTAND me correctly. The Lord has given special light that you must not pattern after Dr. Kellogg in doing the line of work that he is doing; for God has not given you that work to do. Neither has he given to Dr. Kellogg the work in which he has spent much time and money, to the robbery of fields that were destitute of means and destitute of helpers. He is bringing in an accumulating burden, by which he is creating not producing, but consuming. God has not called upon us to use the treasures of His house thus, to set His money flowing in streams which call forth such an outlay of time, money and workers. {44}

God has given direction as to how to work is to be done. In our camp meetings we meet all classes of people, high and low, rich and poor. None are excluded. It is the Lord's desire that the very best of medical missionary physicians shall hold themselves in readiness to co-operate with the ministers of the gospel. They are to be one with Christ, men through whom God can work. The Lord desires His work to advance in a reformatory line. During our camp meetings genuine medical missionary work is to be done.

No line is to be drawn between the genuine medical missionary work and the gospel ministry. These two must blend. They are not to stand apart as separate lines of work. They are to be joined in an inseparable union, even as the hand is joined to the body. Those in our institutions are to give evidence that they understand their part in the genuine gospel medical missionary work. A solemn dignity is to characterize genuine medical missionaries. They are to be men who understand and know God and the power of His grace.

Whatever may be our ingathering or increase, the conference is to be kept free from every thread of selfishness. So also should the medical missionary be stripped of all selfishness, and carried forward after the order of God. The different lines of work are to sustain one another, but not in the way Dr. Kellogg has planned; for this is not God's way. Dr. Kellogg has misappropriated the Lord's money, investing it in a way he had no moral right to.

The work of preparing a people to know God and Jesus Christ whom He has sent is to go forward. This is the highest and most important work that it is possible for mortals to do. God desires medical missionary work to be represented in a way altogether different from the way in which it has been represented in Chicago. The work in Chicago has been a great hindrance to the harmonious action of the work God designed, giving the first, second, and third angels messages to all parts of our world. The work in Australia is not to be a second edition of the work done in Chicago. My heart is sore and grieved because the money which God designed to flow in currents of gifts and offerings to Australia, England, and other missionary fields has been obstructed by human devising and human planning. This must not be repeated in this country or in any other country; for it is not God's way to leave fields nigh and afar off without help. Thus the work of the gospel ministry is retarded. The last message of mercy is to be given to the world, to prepare a people for the second coming of our Lord and Saviour Jesus Christ, in power and great glory.

The establishment of sanitariums where they should be—in every new field that is opened,—will require means. God's money is not to be diverted into uncertain channels, but is to be used to accomplish a work which if done in the true order of God will accomplish a hundred fold more in making new plants in different localities.

"Sunnyside," Cooranbong, N.S.W.
May 19, 1897

"When thou saidst, seek ye my face; my heart said unto thee, Thy face, Lord will I seek."
"He that cometh to God must believe that he is; and that he is a rewarder of them that diligently seek him."

A CHRISTIAN! WHAT DOES the term comprehend? Our Saviour says, "If ye love me, keep my commandments. And I will pray the Father, and he shall give {45} you another comforter, that he may abide with you forever. Even the Spirit of truth, whom the world cannot receive, because it seeth him not, neither knoweth him." "But the natural man receiveth not the things of the Spirit of God: for they are foolishness unto him: neither can he know them, because they are spiritually discerned." "But ye know him, for he dwelleth with you, and shall be in you."

Thus the contrast between the two classes is presented. The world are those who receive not the drawing and invitation of Christ. Truth is that which they do not desire. They cannot desire Christ because they follow their own way and their own will. They do not see anything in Christ that they should desire Him. "Who hath believed our report? And to whom is the arm of the Lord revealed? For he shall grow up before him as a tender plant, and as a root out of a dry ground: he hath no form nor comeliness; and when we shall see him, there is no beauty that we should desire him. He is despised and rejected of men; a man of sorrows, and acquainted with grief: and we hid as it were our faces from him; he was despised, and we esteemed him not. Surely he hath born our griefs, and carried our sorrows: yet we did esteem him stricken, smitten of God, and afflicted. But he was wounded for our transgressions, he was bruised for our iniquities: the chastisement of our peace was upon him; and with his stripes we are healed."

The natural growth cannot develop a symmetrical character. There must be a new birth. "As many as received him, to them gave he power to become the sons of God, even to them that believe on his name." "Which was born, not of blood, nor of the will of the flesh, but of God." "That which is born of the flesh is flesh; and that which is born of the Spirit is Spirit. Marvel not that I say unto thee, Ye must be born again." The believing soul is here represented in the words of Christ: "Ye know him, for he dwelleth with you, and shall be in you," and His promise to His followers is: "I will never leave you comfortless."

I would say to students in our schools, Know thyself. The obligation we owe to God, in presenting to Him clean, pure healthful bodies, are not comprehended. We have special duties resting upon us. We should become acquainted with our physical structure and the laws controlling natural life. While Greek and Latin, which is seldom of any advantage, is made a study by many, Physiology and Hygiene is barely touched upon. The study to which we should give thought is that which concerns the natural life, a knowledge of one's self.

There is not one in a thousand married or unmarried, who realize the importance of purity of habits, in preserving cleanliness of the body and purity of thought. Sickness and disease is the sure consequence of disobedience to nature's laws, and neglect of the laws of life and health. It is the house in which we live that we need to preserve, that it may do honor to God who has redeemed us. We need to know how to preserve the living machinery, that our soul, body, and spirit may be consecrated to His service. As rational beings we are deplorably ignorant of the body and its requirements. While the schools we have established have taken up the study of physiology, they have not taken hold of the matter with that decided energy which they should. They have not practiced intelligently that which they have received in knowledge. And they do not realize that unless it is practiced, the body will decay. {46}

Notwithstanding all the light shining forth from the Scriptures on this subject: notwithstanding the lessons given in the history of Daniel, Shadrach, Meshach and Abed-nego: notwithstanding the result of plain healthful diet, there is little regard for the lessons penned by men inspired of God. The dietetic habits of the people generally are neglected; there is an increase of tobacco using, liquor drinking, and subsisting on flesh meats. I see young boys here in this locality, bright-looking, intelligent youth, from ten to twelve years of age, following the example of their fathers. His habits and practices are educating his children to do as he does. When going to Cooranbong a few days since, two lads were sitting in a tram before me. They were about ten or eleven years of age. One was smoking a cigarette. He would use the vile, poisonous little roll of paper, then the other would take the same in his mouth and enjoy the luxury. Physical and moral ruin is seen everywhere. The question is asked, Have I not a right to do as I please with my own body?— No; you have no moral right, because you are violating the laws of life and health which God has given you. You are the Lord's property—His by creation and His by redemption. "Thou shalt love thy neighbor as thyself." The law of self-respect, for the property of the Lord is here brought to view. And this will lead to respect for the obligations which every human being is under to preserve the living machinery that is so fearfully and wonderfully made. This living machinery is to be understood. Every part of its wonderful mechanism is to be carefully studied. Self-preservation is to be practiced.

The human agent has been granted a second probation. "For God so loved the world, that he gave his only begotten Son, that whosoever believeth on Him, should not perish, but have everlasting life." As you look upon your body, you should remember, that you are every moment sustained by the Creator of all things, the preserver of life, the Giver of happiness and peace and grace in obeying His requirements. Any action in eating, drinking, or dressing that is unhealthful, injures the fine works of the human machinery, and interferes with God's order. There are obstructions created in bone, brain, and muscle, which are destroying this wonderful machinery that God has organized to be kept in order. Any misuse of the delicate workmanship results in suffering.

The transgression of the physical law is the transgression of God's law. Our Creator is Jesus Christ. He is the Author of our being. He has created the human structure. He is the Author of physical laws as He is the Author of the moral law. And the human being who is careless and reckless of the habits and practices that concern his physical life and health sins against God.

Many who profess to love Jesus Christ do not show proper reverence and respect for Him who gave His life to save them from eternal death. He is not reverenced or respected or recognized. This is shown by the injury done to their own bodies in violation to the laws of their being. Whoever in any way disregards the laws of their being, will suffer the sure consequence of their own course of action. And in their pain and suffering, they will under the suggestions of Satan, find fault with God for causing them to be afflicted. Should the Lord work a miracle to restore the wonderful fine machinery which human beings (have damaged) through their own carelessness and inattention, and their indulgence of appetite and passions, in doing the very things that the Lord has told them that they should not do? Should He do so, the Lord would be administering to sin, which is the transgression of His own law. {47} The moral sense of the human agent in our world is exceedingly low upon the subject of their own bodies and their own lives. But the Lord has placed before the human family the right way in His word. Will they keep the way of the Lord?

But with the world there is a sacrifice made that is amazing to the heavenly intelligences. Satan is master of their appetites and inclinations, and he leads them to gratify and indulge perverted, unnatural appetites. He leads them to suppose that this is the very sum and substance of their happiness. A created appetite is the only law that controls the tobacco devotee, and it will continue to be thus to the close of this earth's history. Men and women and children are corrupting their ways before the Lord. They are fast reaching the boundary line when the Lord will speak, and His words, going forth from His exalted throne, will not return unto Him void.

Read carefully Genesis 6:5-14. Matthew 24:37, 51; 2 Corinthians 10:4, 5. 2 Peter 1:1-6.

The Lord has inspired men to write the very things that are essential for this time in regard to the special attention we must give to the care of the body. We are the Lord's property. Christ has paid a sum for the ransom of man that in no way can be computed. He gave Himself a living offering unto God. He bore the sins of the transgressor that God might be just, and yet be the justifier of the repenting, believing sinner. In the wilderness of temptation He overcame every temptation on the point of appetite. He fasted forty days and forty nights, and in His weak condition Satan assailed Him. But he answered not with His own words; for Satan was ready to enter into controversy if He had done this. And yet His answer was His own words, traced by human pen under the inspiration of the Spirit of God. He met Satan with "It is written, man shall not live by bread alone, but by every word that proceedeth out of the mouth of God." The insinuating temptation was presented, "If thou be the Son of God, command that this stone, (in appearance exactly like bread) be made bread." But the "If' of unbelief was not accepted, and there was no ground left for controversy.

When the temptation was presented to Christ that the whole world should be given to Him if He should fall down and worship Satan, divinity flashed through humanity, and with a voice that Satan understood perfectly, He said, "get thee hence, Satan; for it is written, thou shalt worship the Lord thy God and Him only shalt thou serve." Thus Christ resisted every temptation.

Then the whole universe of heaven rejoiced. Christ had passed over the ground of test and trial that Adam had failed to endure. In His human nature He had redeemed Adam's disgraceful failure and fall. This meant everything to the human family. By overcoming in man's behalf, He was placing fallen man on the vantage ground with God. In His human nature, Jesus gave evidence that in every temptation wherewith Satan shall assail fallen man, there is help for him in God, if he will take hold of His strength, and through obedience make peace with Him.

Jesus stood forth in human nature a conqueror in behalf of the fallen race. He was an overcomer in behalf of every human being, and as a pledge that all who shall receive His name may resist the temptations of Satan, and overcome in their own behalf as Christ has overcome in theirs. There is not one of the feeblest of humanity but can be a conqueror by being a partaker of the divine nature. As the branch is united to the vine and becomes partaker of the {48} nourishment of the vine, so he who is one with Christ absorbs the elements of the life of Christ, and are branches of the living vine. Every member of the human family is honored by the achievements of His wonderful victory, making it possible for every soul to become a partaker of the divine nature if he will connect with Christ.

All heaven was watching the working of the enemy against Christ when tempted in behalf of man. And all heaven is watching the striving of every individual soul under every temptation by which man shall be beset. If he will resist the temptation, if he will not yield on any point Satan cannot have the victory. And in the books of heaven will stand registered against your name that on such a day Satan sought to overthrow and ensnare one of my redeemed ones, but the tempted one looked to me, the conqueror, and I gave him angels to press back the powerful foe.

Read Matthew 4:11; Hebrews 1:14; John 1:12.

In that day when all cases are decided, when sentences are passed upon those who are rejecters of His mercy and His great love provided for them by the sacrifice of the Son of the infinite God, who bore the sins of every son and daughter of Adam, each will be called to account for the talents in intellect, in earthly treasures to bestow upon the needy. And what will those answer that have turned away from light and from knowledge, and lived a careless, self-indulgent life? The amount of evidence a man has had presented before him, the number of talents which he has received, the returns made to the Master—those will determine his destiny for eternity.

Those who have had privileges and opportunities and light upon light will find themselves brought into comparison with those whose religious advantages have been limited, and who have made diligent, persevering effort to lay hold of eternal life. Over such the Lord rejoiceth with singing. The whole heathen world will rise up in judgment against those whom heaven has favored the most, but have placed themselves on Satan's side, and worked in his lines to bring their soul destroying narcotics to foreign lands, to pollute and destroy the heathen nations with their defiling and health-destroying drugs. For the sake of revenue, a professedly Christian nation have forced their traffic upon heathen nations at the point of the sword, and thus compel them to accept their merchandise, which would in using degrade the people below the level of the brute creation.

"Shall I not judge for these things," saith God.

Christ came to our world to restore the moral image of God in men; but the men who have had great light have given themselves over to Satan. They have worked out his plans in introducing tobacco, liquor and opium into foreign, heathen lands. And these things have been recognized by the intelligent heathen as a deadly evil that leads to all kinds of violence and crime, and stirs up the savage elements to delight in war. Thus ungovernable propensities are perpetuated, making it almost hopeless to send missionaries among them. And the heathen hate the white man for this kind of work.

Although the so-called Christian has heard of the message of warning, the message of mercy, he has misappropriated his talents and used them to advance the work of the first great apostate. His heart has become hardened to all the {49} mercies received of God. He has abused His goodness, and done despite to the Holy Spirit by his persistent refusal to follow Christ.

The Lord has made it part of His plan that man's reaping shall be according to his sowing. And this is the explanation of the misery and suffering in our world, which is charged back on God. The man who serves himself, and makes a God of his stomach, will reap that which is a sure result of the violation of nature's laws. Those who abuse any organ of the body to gratify lustful appetite and debased passions, in the married or unmarried life, will bear testimony of the same in his countenance. He has sown to fleshly lusts, and he will just as surely realize the consequence.

The licentiate and profligate is attended by an ever-wary fiend. He is like a haunted being. He is a slave to passion, the chains of which he is unwilling to break. And at last he is left of God without conviction, without mercy, without hope, to destroy himself. He is left to the natural process of corrupting practices which degrade him below the brute creation. His sinfulness has ruined his mechanism of the living machinery, and nature's laws transgressed become his tormentor.

Read Proverbs 4:11-18.

The Lord sees every human being: He denotes every phase of character. In the great day of judgment He will execute the sentence against the sinner. It will then be seen that the sinner's conduct has never stopped with himself. Every departure from righteousness has a vital relation to His divine laws. Had we eyes as the eyes of God we would be able to see in the tiny seed the flower or shrub or tree therein enclosed. God made it thus. He searches the heart. He will look into our motives as He looks into the seed and He will reveal what we are and what we should have been.

The last great day will be a triumph of law. The Lord is preparing for His last great work, and He will rise out of His place to punish the world for her iniquity. Then the earth will disclose her blood, and shall no more cover her slain. Who will prepare to hold up a light amid the moral darkness that exists in our world. The wretchedness that has been accumulating for ages and that is degrading humanity, is not sensed as it should be. "Thou shalt have no other gods before me" is the command of God. Idolatry exists in the church-goers today as verily as in the days of Noah. But when His commands are obeyed, the human family will be elevated, ennobled, and exalted.

(Signed) E. G. White

THE PHYSICIAN'S WORK A CURE OF SOULS

[Prior to July 1915]

EVERY MEDICAL PRACTITIONER may through faith in Christ have in his possession a cure of the highest value—a remedy for the sin-sick soul. The physician who is converted and sanctified through the truth is registered in heaven as a laborer together with God, a follower of Jesus Christ. Through the sanctification of the truth, God gives to physicians and nurses wisdom and skill in treating the sick, and this work is opening the fast closed door to many hearts. Men and women are led to understand the truth which is needed to save the soul as well as the body. {50}

This is an element that gives character to the work for this time. The Medical Missionary work is as the right arm to the third angel's message which must be proclaimed to a fallen world; and physicians, managers, and workers in any line, in acting faithfully their part, are doing the work of the message. From them the sound of the truth will go forth to every kindred, tongue and people. In this work the heavenly angels bear a part. They awaken spiritual joy and melody in the hearts of those who have been freed from suffering, and thanksgiving to God arises from the lips of many who have received the precious truth.

Every physician in our ranks should be a Christian. Only those physicians who are genuine Bible Christians can discharge aright the high duties of their profession.

The physician who understands the responsibilities and accountability of his position will feel the necessity of Christ's presence with him in his work for those for whom such a sacrifice has been made. He will subordinate everything to the higher interests which concern the life that may be saved unto life eternal. He will do all in his power to save both the body and the soul. He will try to do the work that Christ would do were He in his place. The physician who loves the souls for whom Christ died will seek earnestly to bring into the sickroom a leaf from the tree of life. He will try to break the bread of life to the sufferer. Notwithstanding the obstacles and difficulties to be met, this is the solemn, sacred work of the medical profession.

True missionary work is that which the Saviour's work is best represented, His methods most closely copied, His glory best promoted. Missionary work that falls short of this standard is recorded in heaven as defective. It is weighed in the balances of the sanctuary and found wanting.

Physicians should seek to direct the minds of their patients to Christ, the great Physician of soul and body. That which physicians can only attempt to do, Christ accomplishes. The human agent strives to prolong life. Christ is life itself. He who passed through death to destroy him that had the power of death is the source of all vitality. There is a balm in Gilead, and a physician there. Christ endured an agonizing death under the most humiliating circumstances that we might have life. He gave up His precious life that He might vanquish death. But He rose from the tomb, and the myriads of angels who came to behold Him take up the life He had laid down heard His words of triumphant joy as He stood above the rent sepulcher of Joseph proclaiming, "I am the resurrection and the Life."

The question, "If a man die, shall he live again"? Job 14:14 has been answered. By bearing the penalty of sin, by going down into the grave, Christ has brightened the tomb for all who die in faith. God in human form has brought life and immortality to light through the gospel. In dying He condemned the originator of sin and disloyalty to suffer the penalty of sin—eternal death.

The possessor and giver of eternal life, Christ was the only one who could conquer death. He is our Redeemer: and blessed is every physician who is in a true sense of the word a missionary, a Saviour of the souls for whom Christ gave His life. Such a physician learns day by day from the great Physician how to watch and work for the saving of the souls and bodies of men {51} and women. The Saviour is present in the sickroom, in the operating room: and His power for His name's glory accomplishes great things.

The Physician can do a noble work if he is connected with the great Physician. To the relatives of the sick, whose hearts are full of sympathy for the sufferer, he may find opportunity to speak the words of life. And he can soothe and uplift the mind of the sufferer, by leading him to look to the One who can save to the uttermost all who come to him for salvation.

When the Spirit of God works on the mind of the afflicted one, leading him to inquire for truth, let the physician work for the precious soul as Christ would work for it. Do not urge upon him any special doctrine, but point him to Christ as the sin-pardoning Saviour. Angels of God will impress the mind. Some will refuse to be illuminated by the light which God would let shine into the chambers of the mind and into the soul temple: but many will respond to the light, and from these minds deception and error in its various forms will be swept away.

Every opportunity of working as Christ worked should be carefully improved. The physician should talk of the words of healing wrought by Christ, of His tenderness and love. He should believe that Jesus is his companion, close by his side. "We are laborers together with God." 1 Corinthians 3:9. Never should the physician neglect to direct the minds of his patients to Christ. If he has the Saviour abiding in his own heart, his thoughts will ever be directed to the great Healer of soul and body. He will lead the minds of sufferers to Him who can restore, who when on earth restored the sick to health, and healed the soul as well as the body, saying, "Son, thy sins be forgiven thee." Mark 2:5.

Never should familiarity with suffering cause the physician to become careless or unsympathetic. In cases of dangerous illness, the inflicted one feels that he is at the mercy of the physician. He looks to that physician as his only hope, and that physician should ever point the trembling soul to One who is greater than himself, even the Son of God, who gave His life to save him from death, who pities the sufferer, and who by His divine power will give skill and wisdom to all who ask Him.

When the patient knows not how his case will turn is the time for the physician to impress the mind. He should not do this with a desire to distinguish himself, but that he may point the soul to Christ as a personal Saviour. If the life is spared, there is a soul for that physician to watch for. The patient feels that the physician is the very life of his life. And to what purpose should all this weight of confidence be employed? Always to win a soul to Christ and magnify the power of God.

When the crisis has passed, and success is apparent, be the patient a believer or an unbeliever, let a few moments be spent with him in prayer. Give expression to your thankfulness for the life that has been spared. The physician who follows such a course carries his patient to the One upon whom he is dependent for life. Words of gratitude may flow from the patient to the physician: for through God he has bound his life up with his own: but let the praise and thankfulness be given to God, as to One who is present, though invisible. {52}

On the sickbed Christ is often accepted and confessed, and this will be done oftener in the future than it has been in the past, for a quick work will the Lord do in the world. Words of wisdom are to be on the lips of the physician, and Christ will water the seed sown causing it to bring forth fruit unto eternal life.

Our Sanitariums are to be a blessing to high and low, rich and poor. Men and women are brought together in these institutions, and they become acquainted with one another. They learn to sympathize with their fellow-sufferers, and thus the partition wall between man and his fellowmen is broken down. Those who visit the sanitarium are to be taught the power of God in the restoration of the sick. This will make an impression on the mind that God is in the place.

It is God's purpose that those who visit our health institution shall become acquainted with the third angel's message. Though doctrinal subjects are not to be urged upon the sick, yet if these truths are lived out, the Spirit of God will bring conviction to hearts, and the faithful guardian of souls will understand when the opportunity has come to present the special truth for this time.

We lose the most precious opportunities by neglecting to speak a word in season. Too often a precious talent that ought to produce a thousand fold is left unused. If the golden privilege is not watched for, it will pass. Something was allowed to prevent the physician from doing his appointed work as a minister of righteousness.

There are none too many godly physicians to minister in their profession. There is much work to be done, and ministers and doctors are to work in perfect union. Luke, the writer of the Gospel that bears his name, is called the beloved physician, and those who do a work similar to that which he did are living out the gospel.

Our camp meetings should have the labors of medical men. These should be men of wisdom and sound judgment, men who respect the ministry of the word, and who are not victims of unbelief. These men are the guardians of the health of the people, and they are to be recognized and respected. They should give instruction to the people in regard to dangers of intemperance. This evil must be more boldly met in the future than it has been in the past. Ministers and doctors should set forth the evils of intemperance. Both should work in the gospel in perfect harmony with power to condemn sin and exalt righteousness.

Countless are the opportunities of the physician for warning the impenitent, cheering the disconsolate and hopeless and wisely prescribing for the health of mind and body. As he thus instructs the people in the principles of true temperance, and as a guardian of souls gives advice to those who are mentally and physically diseased, the physician is acting his part in the great work of making ready a people prepared for the Lord. This is what medical missionary work is to accomplish in its relation to the third angel's message.

At our camp meeting practical physicians can give instructions line upon line, precept upon precept, here a little and there a little. These ministers or doctors who do not open their lips to make personal appeals to the people {53} are remiss in their duty. They fail of doing the work which God has appointed them.

Ministers and physicians are to work harmoniously with earnestness to save souls that are becoming entangled in Satan's snare. They are to point men and women to Jesus, their righteousness, their strength, and the health of their countenance,—continually they are to watch for souls. There are those who are struggling with strong temptations, in danger of being overcome in the fight with Satanic agencies. Will you pass these by without offering them assistance? If you see a soul in need of help, engage in conversation with him, even though you do not know him. Pray with him, point him to Jesus.

This work belongs just as surely to the doctor as to the minister. By public and private effort the physician should seek to win souls to Christ.

In all our enterprises and in all our institutions God is to be acknowledged as the great Master Worker. The physicians are to stand as his representatives. The medical fraternity have made many reforms, and they should rise still higher. Those who hold the lives of human beings in their hands should be educated, refined, sanctified. Then will the Lord work through them in mighty power to glorify his name. He will reveal Himself as the Healer of the body and the soul.

Dangers and Duties of the Physicians and the Medical Missionary

[Prior to July 1915]

THE FOURTH CHAPTER OF THE Epistle to the Ephesians contains lessons given us by God. In this chapter one speaks under the inspiration of God, one to whom in holy vision God had given instruction. He describes the distribution of God's gifts to his workers, as saying:

"And he gave some, apostles; and some, prophets; and some, evangelists; and some, pastors and teachers; for the perfecting of the saints, for the work of the ministry, for the edifying of the body of Christ: till we all come in the unity of the faith, and of the knowledge of the Son of God, unto a perfect man, unto the measure of the stature of the fullness of Christ:" Ephesians 4:11-13. Here we are shown that God gives to every man his work, and in doing this work man is fulfilling his part of God's great plan.

This lesson should be carefully considered by our physicians and medical missionaries,- God establishes his instrumentalities among a people who recognize the laws of the divine government. The sick are to be healed through the combined effort of the human and divine. Every gift, every power, that Christ promised his disciples, he bestows upon those who will serve him faithfully. And he who gives mental capabilities, and who entrusts talents to the men and women who are his by creation and by redemption, expects that these talents and these capabilities shall be increased by use. Every talent must be employed in blessing others, and thus bringing honor to God. But physicians have been led to suppose that their capabilities were their own individual property: the powers given them for God's work they have used in branching out into lines of work to which God has not appointed them.

Satan works every moment to find an opportunity for stealing in. He tells the physician that his talents are too valuable to be bound up among Seventh-day Adventists, that if he were free, he could do a large work. The physician {54} is tempted to feel that he has methods which he can carry independent of the people for whom God has wrought that he might place them above every other people on the face of the earth. But let not the physician feel that his influence would increase if he should separate himself from this work: Should he attempt to carry out his plans, he would not meet with success.

Selfishness introduced in any degree into ministerial or medical work is an infraction of the law of God. When men glory in their capabilities, and cause the praise of men to flow to finite beings, they dishonor God, and he will remove that in which they glory. The physician connected with our Sanitariums and medical missionary work have by God's providence been bound to this people, whom he has commanded to be a light to the world. Their work is to give all that the Lord has given them — to give, not as one influence among many, but as the influence through God to make effective the truth for this time.

God has committed to us a special work, a work that no other people can do. He has promised us the aid of the Holy Spirit. The heavenly current is flowing earthward for the accomplishment of the very work appointed us: but this heavenly current is turned aside by our many diversions from the straightforward path marked out by Christ. Man's disregard of the Lord's instruction robs us of the strength he longs to impart.

Physicians are not to suppose that they can compass the world by their plans and efforts. God has not set them to embrace so much with their own labors merely. The man who invests his powers in many lines of work cannot take in hand the management of a Sanitarium and do it justice.

If the Lord's workers take up lines of work which crowd out that which should be done by them in communicating light to the world, God does not receive through their labors the glory that should accrue to His holy name. When God calls a man to do a certain work in His cause He does not also lay upon him burdens that other men can and should bear. The Lord does not want the minds of His responsible men strained to the utmost point of endurance by taking up many lines of work. All these lines may be essential: but God apportions to every man his duty according to his wisdom. If the worker does not take up his appointed work, that which the Lord sees is the very thing he is fitted to do, he is neglecting duties which, if properly executed, would result in the promulgation of the truth, and would prepare men for the great crisis before us.

God cannot give in greatest measure either physical or mental power to those who gather to themselves burdens which He has not appointed. When men take upon themselves such responsibilities, however good the work may be, their physical strength is overtaxed, their minds become confused, and they cannot attain the highest success.

Physicians in our institutions should not engage in numerous enterprises, and thus allow the work which should stand upon right principles and exert a worldwide influence, to flag. God has not set his co-laborers to embrace so many things, to make such large plans that they fail in their allotted place of accomplishing the great good He expects them to do in diffusing light to the world, in drawing men and women to where He is leading by His supreme wisdom. {55}

The enemy has determined to counterwork the designs of God to benefit humanity in revealing to them what constitutes true medical missionary work. So many interests have been brought in that the workers cannot do all things according to the pattern shown in the mount. I have been instructed that the work appointed to physicians is enough for them to do, and what the Lord required of them was to link up closely with the gospel missionaries and do their work with faithfulness. He has not asked our physicians to embrace so large and varied a work as some have undertaken. He has not made it the special work of our physicians to go into the worst dens of iniquity in our large cities. The Lord does not require impossibilities of men. The work which He gave to our physicians was to symbolize to the world the ministry of the gospel in medical missionary work. The Lord does not lay upon His people all the burden of laboring for a class so hardened by sin that many of them will neither be benefited themselves nor benefit others. If there are men who can take up the work of laboring for the most degraded, if God lays upon them a burden to labor for the masses in various ways, let these go forth and gather from the world the means required for doing this work. Let them not depend on the means which God intends shall sustain the work of the third angel's message.

Our sanitariums need the power of brain and heart of which they are being robbed by another line of work. Everything that Satan can do he will do to multiply the responsibilities of our physicians, for he knows that this means weakness instead of strength to the institutions with which they are connected.

Great consideration must be exercised in the work which we undertake. We are not to take large burdens in the care of infant children. This work is being done by others. We have a special work in caring for and educating the children more advanced in years. Let families who can do so, adopt the little ones, and they will receive a blessing in so doing. But there is a higher and more important work to engage the attention of our physicians in educating those who have grown up with deformed characters. The principles of health reform must be brought before parents. They must be converted, that they may work as missionaries in their own homes. This work our physicians have done and can still do if they will not sacrifice themselves by carrying such large responsibilities.

The head physician in any institution holds a difficult position and he should keep himself free from minor responsibilities: for these will give him no time to rest. He should have sufficient help: for he has trying work to perform. He must bow in prayer with the suffering ones, and lead his patients to the great Physician. If as a humble suppliant he seeks God for wisdom to deal with each case, his strength and influence will be greatly increased.

Of himself, what can man accomplish in the great work set forth by the infinite God? Christ says, "Without me ye can do nothing." John 15:5. He came to our world to show men how to do the work given them by God, and He says to us, "Come unto me, all ye that labor and are heavy laden, and I will give you rest. Take my yoke upon you, and learn of me; for I am meek and lowly in the heart: and ye shall find rest unto your souls. For my yoke is easy, and my burden is light." Matthew 11:28-30. Why is Christ's yoke easy and His burden light? Because He bore the weight of it upon the cross of Calvary.

Personal religion is essential for every physician if he would be successful {56} in his work for the sick. He needs a power greater than his own intuition and skill. God desires physicians to link up with Him, and know that every soul is precious in His sight. He who depends upon God, realizing that He alone who made man knows how to direct, will not fail in his appointed work, as a healer of bodily infirmities, or as physician of the souls for whom Christ gave His life.

One who bears the heavy responsibilities of the physician needs the prayers of the gospel minister, and he should be linked, soul, body and mind, with the truth of God. Then he can speak a word in season to the afflicted. He can watch for souls as one who must give an account. He can present Christ as the Way, the Truth, and the Life. The Scriptures come clearly to his mind, and he speaks as one who knows the value of the souls with whom he is dealing.

CONFORMING TO THE WORLD

[Prior to July 1915]

THE LORD JESUS HAS SAID, "If any man will come after me, let him deny himself, and take up his cross daily, and follow me." Luke 9:23. Christ's words made an impression on the minds of His hearers. Many of them, though not clearly comprehending His instruction, were moved by deep conviction to say decidedly, "Never man spake like this man." John 7:46. The disciples did not always understand the lessons which Christ wished to convey by parables, and when the multitude had gone away, they would ask Him to explain His words. He was ever ready to lead them to a perfect understanding of His word and His will; for from them, in clear, distinct lines, truth was to go forth to the world.

At times Christ reproached His disciples with the slowness of their comprehension. He placed in their possession truths of which they little suspected the value. He had been with them a long time, giving them lessons in clear lines, but their previous religious education, the erroneous interpretations which they had heard the Jewish teachers place on the Scriptures, kept their minds clouded. Christ promised them that He would send them His Spirit, who would recall His words to their minds as forgotten truths. "He shall teach you all things," Christ said, "and bring all things to your remembrance, whatsoever I have said unto you." John 14:26.

The way in which the Jewish teachers explained the Scriptures, their endless repetition of maxims and fiction, called forth from Christ the words, "This people draweth nigh unto me with their mouth, and honoreth me with their lips, but their heart is far from me." They performed in the temple courts their round of duties. They offered sacrifices typifying the great Sacrifice, saying by their ceremonies, "Come, my Saviour," yet Christ, the One whom all these ceremonies represented, was among them, and they would not recognize or receive Him. The Saviour declared, "In vain do they worship me, teaching for doctrines the commandments of men." Matthew 15:9.

Christ is saying to His servants today as He said to His disciples, "If any man will come after me, let him deny himself, and take up his cross daily, and follow me." But men are as slow now to learn the lesson as in Christ's day. God has given His people warning after warning, but the customs, habits, and practices of the world have had so great power on the minds of His professed people that His warnings have been disregarded. {57}

Those who act a part in God's great cause are not to follow the example of worldlings. The voice of God is to be heeded. He who depends upon men for strength and influence leans upon a broken reed.

Depending upon men has been the great weakness of the church. Men have dishonored God by failing to appreciate His sufficiency, by coveting the influence of men. Thus Israel became weak. The people wanted to be like the other nations of the world, and they asked for a king. They desired to be guided by human power which they could see, rather than by the divine, invisible power that till then had led and guided them, and had given them victory in battle. They made their own choice, and the result was seen in the destruction of Jerusalem and the dispersion of the nation.

We cannot put confidence in any man, however learned, however elevated he may be, unless he holds the beginning of his confidence in God firm unto the end. What must have been the power of the enemy upon Solomon, a man whom Inspiration has thrice called the beloved of God, and to whom was committed the great work of building the temple. In that very work Solomon made an alliance with idolatrous nations. And through his marriages he bound himself up with heathen women. Through their influence he in his later years forsook the temple of God to prepare groves for their idols.

So now, men set aside God as not sufficient for them. They resort to worldly men for recognition, and think that by means of the influence gained from the world they can do some great thing. But they mistake. By leaning on the arm of the world instead of the arm of God, they turn aside the work which God desires to accomplish through His chosen people.

When brought in contact with the higher classes of society, let not the physician feel that he must conceal the peculiar characteristics which sanctification through the truth gives him. The physicians who unite with the work of God are to cooperate with God as His appointed instrumentalities: they are to give all their power and efficiency to magnifying the work of God's commandment-keeping people. These who in their human wisdom try to conceal the peculiar characteristics that distinguish God's people from the world will lose their spiritual life, and will no longer be upheld by His power.

Never let the idea be entertained that it is essential to make an appearance of being wealthy. There will be a strong temptation to do this, with the thought that it will give influence. But I am instructed to say that it will have just the opposite effect.

All who seek to uplift themselves by conforming to the world set an example that is misleading. God recognizes as His those only who are to understand that their power lies in their meekness and lowliness of heart. God will honor those who make Him their dependence.

The style of a physician's dress, his equipage, his furniture, weigh not one jot with God. He cannot work by His Holy Spirit with those who try to compete with the world in dress and display. He who follows Christ must deny himself and take up his cross.

The Physician who loves and fears God will need to make no outward display in order to distinguish himself: for the Sun of Righteousness is shining in his {58} heart and is revealed in his life, and this distinguishes him. When men work in Christ's lines, they will be living epistles, known and read of all men. Through their example and influence men of wealth and talent will be turned from the cheapness of material things and lay hold on eternal realities. The greatest respect will ever be shown to the physician who reveals that he receives his directions from God. Nothing will work so powerfully for the advancement of God's instrumentality as for those connected with it to stand steadfast as His faithful servants.

It is God's plan that even worldly people who come to our sanitariums shall have a sense of security while there, because they are in a place where prayer is offered to God. They are to see that here is in the world a people who possess talent and knowledge, yet who are not vain and self-exalted.

The physician will find that it is for his present and eternal good to follow the Lord's way of working for suffering humanity. The mind that God has made He can mold without the power of man, but He honors men by asking them to co-operate with Him in this great work.

Many regard their own wisdom as sufficient, and they arrange things according to their own judgment, thinking to bring about wonderful results. But if they would depend on God and not on themselves, they would receive heavenly wisdom. Those who are so engrossed with their work that they cannot find time to press their way to the throne of grace and obtain counsel from God, will surely turn the work into wrong channels. Our strength lies in our union with God through His only begotten Son, and in our union with one another.

The surgeon most truly successful is he who loves God, who sees God in His created work, and worships Him as he traces His wise arrangement in the human organism. The most successful physician is he who fears God from his youth, as did Timothy, who feels that Christ is his constant companion, a friend with whom he can always commune. Such a physician would not change his position for the highest office the world can give. He is more anxious to honor God and secure His approval than to secure patronage and honor from the great men of the world.

Prayer

Every sanitarium established among Seventh-day Adventists should be made a Bethel. All who are connected with this branch of the work should be consecrated to God. Those who minister to the sick, who perform delicate, grave operations, should remember that one slip of the knife, one nervous tremor, and a soul may be launched into eternity. They should not be allowed to take so many responsibilities that they have no time for special seasons of prayer. By earnest prayer they should acknowledge their dependence upon God. Only through a sense of God's pure truth in the mind and heart, only through the calmness and strength, which He alone can impart, are they qualified to perform those critical operations which mean life or death to the afflicted ones.

The physician who is truly converted will not gather to himself responsibilities that interfere with his work for souls. Since without Christ we can do nothing, how can a physician or a medical missionary engage successfully in his important work without earnestly seeking the Lord in prayer? Prayer and a study of the Word brings life and health to the soul. {59}

The Lord will do wondrous things for the truth's sake, and that His name may be glorified. But He requires that the people who engage in His service shall keep their minds ever directed to Him. Every day they should have time for reading the word of God and for prayer. Every officer and every soldier under the command of the God of Israel needs time in which to consult with God and seek His blessing. If the worker allows himself to be drawn away from this, he will lose his spiritual power. Individually we are to walk and talk with God: then the sacred influence of the gospel of Christ will appear in all its preciousness.

A work of reformation is to be carried on in our institutions. Physicians, workers, nurses, are to realize that they are on probation, on trial for their present life, and for that life which measures with the life of God. We are to put to the stretch every faculty, every nerve and muscle, in order to bring saving truth to the attention of suffering humanity. This work must be carried on in connection with the work of saving the sick. Then the work will stand forth before the world in the strength which God designs it shall have. Through the influence of sanctified workers the truth will be magnified. It will go forth as a lamp that burneth.

Exo10rbitant Fees

Honesty, integrity, justice, mercy, love, compassion, and sympathy are embraced in medical missionary work. In all this work the religion of the Bible is to be practiced. The Lord does not want anyone to labor as His representative who follows the wrong customs and practice of worldly physicians in treating suffering humanity. Our physicians need to reform in the matter of making high charges for critical operations. And the reform should extend farther than this. Often an exorbitant fee is charged for even small services, because physicians are supposed to be governed in their charges by the practices of worldly physicians. There are those who follow worldly policy in order to accumulate means, as they say, for God's service. But God does not accept such offerings. He says, "I hate robbery for burnt offering." Isaiah 61:8. Those who deal unjustly with their fellow-men while professing to believe My word, I will judge for thus misrepresenting Me.

As those things were presented before me, my Teacher said, "The institutions that depend upon God and receive His co-operation must ever work according to the principles of the law of God." To charge a large sum for a few moments work is not just and right. Physicians who are under the discipline of the greatest Physician the world ever knew must let the principles of the gospel regulate every fee. Let mercy and the love of God be written on every dollar received.

When our sanitariums are conducted as they should be, a large medical missionary work will be done. Every worker will do his work in such a way and with such a spirit that he will shine as a light in the world.

God calls for the doing of practical, Christ-like work. The patients who come to our sanitariums are to see carried out the principles laid down in the fifty-eighth chapter of Isaiah. Those who have accepted the truth are to practice it because it is the truth. In the work of God in our institutions the truth is to be preserved in all its sacred influence. {60}

The medical practitioner should in all places keep his religious principles clear and untarnished. Truth should be paramount in his practice. He is to use his influence as a means of cleansing the soul by the healing beams of the Sun of Righteousness. When a time comes that physicians cannot do this, the Lord would have no more medical institutions established among Seventh-day Adventists.

The Tithe

The men connected with the institutions of God's appointment should be careful to acknowledge God in all their ways. They are to show that to Him they owe their intellect and all their capabilities. As did Abraham, they are to pay tithe of all they possess and all they receive. A faithful tithe is the Lord's portion. To withhold it, is to rob God. Everyone should freely, willingly, and gladly bring tithes and offerings into the storehouse of the Lord. In so doing he will receive a blessing. There is no safety in withholding from God His own portion.

The Lord says, "Will a man rob God? Yet ye have robbed me. But ye say, Wherein have we robbed thee? In tithes and offerings. Ye are cursed with a curse: for ye have robbed me, even this whole nation. Bring ye all the tithes into the storehouse, that there may be meat in mine house, and prove me now herewith, saith the Lord of hosts, if I will not open you the windows of heaven, and pour you out a blessing, that there shall not be room enough to receive it. And I will rebuke the devourer for your sakes, and he shall not destroy the fruits of your ground; neither shall your vine cast her fruit before the time in the field, saith the Lord of hosts. And all nations shall call you blessed: for ye shall be a delightsome land, saith the Lord of hosts." Malachi 3:8-12.

Observance of the Sabbath

Let no man, because he is a physician, feel at liberty to do those things which God has forbidden. He should not travel on the Sabbath unless this is a necessity in order to relieve suffering humanity. He should plan his work so as to obey God's requirements. The Lord says, "Verily, my Sabbaths ye shall keep: for it is a sign between me and you throughout your generations." Exodus 31:13. When there is real suffering to be alleviated, it is not a desecration of the Sabbath for physicians to travel upon it: but unimportant cases should be deferred. God sanctified and blessed the seventh day, and it is to be kept as His sacred memorial.

God created the world in six days, and rested upon the seventh. Therefore, He declares, "the children of Israel shall keep the Sabbath throughout their generations, for a perpetual covenant." Exodus 31:16. Those who keep God's commandments may claim the promises contained in Isaiah 58:11-14.

The instruction given in this chapter is full and decided. Those who refrain from labor on the Sabbath may claim divine comfort and consolation. Shall we not believe God? Shall we not call holy the day which He calls holy? Man should not be ashamed to acknowledge as sacred that which God calls sacred. He should not be ashamed to do that which God has commanded. Obedience will bring him a knowledge of what constitutes true sanctification. {61}

Let there be no robber of God in tithes and offerings, no desecration of God's holy time. Man is not to do his own pleasure on God's day. He has six days in which to work at secular business, and God claims the seventh as His own. "In it," He says, "thou shalt not do any work." Exodus 20:10. The servant of God will call sacred that which the Lord calls sacred. Thus he will show that he has chosen the Lord as his leader. The Sabbath was made for man in Eden when the morning stars sang together, and all the sons of God shouted for joy. God has placed it in our charge. Let us keep it pure and holy.

The Importance of Obedience

Subtle, dangerous temptations will come to the physicians who believe the truth for these last days. That which would be condemned in a worker of another class is supposed to be admissible in a physician. Thus a multitude of sins are covered up, sins which are registered in the books of heaven as a departure from Bible principles. These temptations the physician may resist if he understands his peril and stands fast by his Saviour. If true to the word of God, we are on the side of Christ, on the side of the loyal, holy angels: we stand under the shield of Omnipotence. Of whom, then, should we be afraid?

There are those who cannot appreciate the gospel of Christ sufficiently to practice it in every line of their work. These will criticize. Those who are superficial and selfish do not know God or Jesus Christ by an experimental knowledge, and they are always faithless. In their eyes small obstructions appear as mountains. There is always a lion in the way.

The Lord requires truth in the inward parts. He will give the Holy Spirit to all who ask Him in faith. He calls for men to act as gospel ministers, to act as physicians, whom no flattery can cause to swerve from the truth. Ministers and doctors are to be under the rule of God. He in whose heart the Spirit of God bears rule, will follow the example of Christ. The life, the character, will be so Christ-like that it will roll back the unjust reproach from the pure truth of Christ.

There must be no failure in God's work. Every thought, every plan, must be in harmony with God's expressed will. He is our Creator, our Redeemer, our Counselor; He is to be the first, and last and best in everything.

In obedience to the commandments of God the soul will receive the best of everything. Every blessing may be enjoyed with the favor of God when heart, mind, and life are consecrated to His service. If men would accept Christ, and see the binding claims of the law of God, they would not take a neutral position, but would stand out in full confidence, and say, The Lord is my helper. He is the only true God, and Jesus Christ whom He has sent is the supreme and everlasting Good. Thus they would secure for themselves the grand promises of God.

This is an individual work. Every worker in God's cause should strive to become more and more efficient. There must be no careless disregard of God's expressed will. The laborer together with God must live by every word that proceedeth out of the mouth of God. Let us individually draw nigh to the mount that we may understand what the Lord commands, and then obey. {62}

CORRECT SCHOOL DISCIPLINE

[Prior to July 1915]

WE HAD IN THE SCHOOL IN Melbourne unruly students, who were disposed to disregard the instructions given from the word of God, and by their course of action betrayed sacred trusts. The Lord looked down from heaven on them, and beheld their deceptive practices, and their false denial of their actions. They were labored for faithfully; but they were altogether too near the city, and temptations were constantly arising. They forgot to be true and loyal to God's holy law. They transgressed His commandments; they were infatuated, and revealed as students that they had not moral integrity to be true. There seemed to be a Satanic agency at work to discourage the teachers and demoralize the school. Some acting as teachers did not exert a correct influence. When every jot of influence should have been placed on the side of discipline and order, these teachers, though knowing all the trials that disorderly students were bringing on the principal and his co-workers, who were burdened and oppressed, and who were seeking the Lord most earnestly, showed sympathy for the ones who were serving the enemy most earnestly. The students—the wrong-doers, knew this. A few took courage to brave out their wrong course of action, until it was brought home so strongly to them that they acknowledged that they had disobeyed the rules of the school, and had then tried to hide behind falsehood.

The school faculty held private consultations to consider what was best to be done. There was a voice in these councils that tried to counter-work the plans introduced to keep discipline and order. By this sympathizing voice indiscreet words were dropped to the students in reference to the matters under consideration in the council. This was and will be oft repeated, a betrayal of sacred trust. These things were caught up by the students. They thought that such a teacher was all right; that she was a clever teacher. She would have sympathy for the wrongdoer. Thus the hands of these carrying a heavy load were not strengthened, but weakened. The efforts made to repress evil were looked upon as harsh and uncharitable. "Young folks must have their jolly times" was repeated, with other insipid speeches. A word dropped here and a word there left its baleful impression, and the wrongdoers knew that there were those in the school who did not think that their course of deception and falsehood was a great sin. But to continually take up the cause of the wrongdoer, making of no account his departure from righteousness and truth and steadfast integrity, is a grievous sin against God.

There were those in the school who were carried through the terms of study because they had no means themselves. These should have made every effort to obtain all the advantages possible and thus show their gratitude to God, for the kindness of the friends who had helped them.

When young men and young women are in deed and truth converted, a decided change will be seen by all who have any connection with them. Their frivolity will leave them; the continual desire for amusement and selfish pleasure, the longing for some kind of change, to be in parties and excursions will be no longer seen.

Hear the words of the great Teacher: "For the bread of God is he which cometh down from heaven, and giveth life unto the world." There is no need to be dull and indolent, to live only for common earthly excitement. Light is given to every believer, as well as comfort and sobriety. All may have joy, because of the satisfaction of having Christ as an abiding guest in the soul. {63}

When Christ said to the multitude, 'The bread of God is he which cometh down from heaven, and giveth life unto the world,' some in the multitude said, "Lord, give us more of this bread." The bread of heaven was in their midst, but they did not recognize Him as the bread of life. Jesus then stated plainly, "I am the Bread of Life; he that cometh to me shall never hunger, and he that believeth on me shall never thirst."

This sixth chapter of John contains the most precious and important lessons for all who are being educated in our schools. If they want that education that will endure through time and through eternity, let them bring the wonderful truths of this chapter into their practical lives. The whole chapter is very instructive, and is only faintly understood. We urge students to take in these words of Christ, that they may understand their privileges. The Lord Jesus teaches us what He is to us, and what advantage it will be to us individually to eat His word, realizing that He Himself is the great center of our life. "The words that I speak unto you," He said, "They are spirit, and they are life."

Having Christ in the heart, we have an eye single to the glory of God. We should strive to comprehend what it means to be in complete union with Christ, who is the propitiation for our sins, and for the sins of the whole world, our substitute and surety for the sins before the Lord God of heaven. Our life should be bound up in the life of Christ; we should draw constantly from Him, partaking of Him, the living bread that came down from heaven, drawing from a fountain ever fresh, ever giving forth its abundant treasures. When this is in truth the experience of the Christian, there is seen in his life freshness, a simplicity, humility, meekness, and lowliness of heart, that show all with whom he associates that he has been with Jesus, and learned of Him.

This experience gives every teacher the very qualifications that will make him a representative of Christ Jesus. The methods of Christ's teachings will, if followed, give a force and directness to his communication and to his prayers. His witness for Christ will not be a narrow, tame, lifeless testimony, but will be like plowing up the field, quickening the conscience, opening the heart and preparing it for the seeds of truth.

None who deal with the youth should be iron-hearted, but affectionate, tender, pitiful, courteous, winning, and compassionate; yet they should know that reproof must be given, and that even rebuke must be spoken to cut off some evildoing. Encourage the youth to glorify God by giving expression to their gratitude to the Lord for all His mercies. Let their thanks be spoken often in the heart and with the voice, and let self-denial and self-sacrifice be shown, if those who claim to be Christ's disciples will have eternal life. "I will raise him up at the last day," Christ says, "For my flesh is meat indeed, and my blood is drink indeed." "He that eateth my flesh and drinketh my blood, dwelleth in me and I in him."

"As the living Father hath sent me, and I live by the Father, so he that eateth me, even he shall live by me." How many have experienced this? How many realize the true meaning of these words? Will we individually seek to understand the word of God, and practice it? This word, believed, is to every truly converted soul, the free gift of grace. It cannot be bought with money. {64}

We should continually realize that we do not deserve grace because of our merit; for all that we have is God's gift. He says to us, "Freely ye have received, freely give."

The atmosphere of unbelief is heavy and oppressive. The giddy laugh, the jesting, and joking, sickens the soul that is feeding on Christ. Cheap, foolish talk is painful to Him. With a humble heart read carefully 1 Peter 1:13-18. Those who enjoy talking should see that their words are select and well chosen. Be careful how you speak. Be careful how you represent the religion you have accepted. You may feel it no sin to gossip and talk nonsense, but this grieves your Saviour, and saddens the heavenly angels.

What testimony does Peter bear? "Wherefore laying aside all malice, and all guile, and hypocrisies, and envies, and all evil speakings, as new born babes, desire the sincere milk of the word, that ye may grow thereby: if so be ye have tasted that the Lord is gracious." Here again the same principle is brought out distinctly. No one need make a mistake. If as new born babes you desire the sincere milk of the word, that you may grow thereby, you will have no appetite to partake of a dish of evil speaking, that all such food will be at once rejected, because those who have tasted that the Lord is gracious cannot partake of a dish of nonsense, and folly, and backbiting. They will say decidedly, "Take this dish away. I do not want to eat such food." It is not the bread from heaven. It is eating and drinking the very spirit of the devil; for it is his business to be an accuser of the brethren.

It is best for every soul to closely investigate what mental food is served up for them to eat. When those come to you who live to talk and who are all armed and equipped to say, "Report, and we will report it," stop and think if the conversation will give spiritual help, spiritual efficiency, that in spiritual communication you may eat the flesh and drink the blood of the Son of God, "to whom coming, as unto a living stone, disallowed indeed of men, but chosen of God, and precious." These words express much. We are not to be tatlers, or gossipers or tale bearers; we are not to bear false witness. We are forbidden by God to engage in trifling, foolish conversation, in jesting, in joking, or speaking any idle words. We must give an account of what we say to God. We will be brought into judgment for our hasty words, that do no good to the speaker or the hearer. Then let us all speak words that will tend to edification. Remember that you are of value with God. Allow no cheap, foolish talk, or wrong principles to compose your Christian experience.

"Chosen of God and precious." Consider, everyone who names the name of Christ, have you tasted that the Lord is gracious? Has this been an actual part of your experience, represented in John 6 as eating the flesh and drinking the blood of the Son of God? As new born babes are you learning to desire the sincere milk of the word that you may grow thereby? Have you at any time in your life been truly converted? Have you been born again? If you have not, then it is time for you to obtain the experience that Christ told one of the chief rulers that he must have. "Ye must be born again," He said, "Except a man be born again he cannot see the kingdom of God." That is, he cannot discern the requirements essential to having a part in that spiritual kingdom. "Marvel not that I say unto thee, ye must be born again." If you open your minds to the entrance of God's word, with a determination to practice that word, light will come; for the word gives understanding to the simple. {65}

This is the very education that every student needs. When this is obtained, if they are converted, the frivolous life they have heretofore lived will change. The universe and heaven will look upon characters that have been transformed. The frivolous, common level will be forsaken and their feet will be placed upon the first round of the ladder, which is Christ Jesus. They will mount step by step, one round after another, heavenward. Christ will be revealed in their spirit, their words, and in their actions.

"Ye also, as living stones, are built up a spiritual house, a holy priesthood, to offer up spiritual sacrifices acceptable to God by Jesus Christ." Will teachers and students study this representation, and see if they are in that class who, through the abundant grace given, are obtaining an experience which is in harmony with the real, genuine experience that every child of God must have if he enters the higher grade.

When Nicodemus came to Jesus, Christ laid before him the conditions of divine life, teaching him the very alphabet of conversion. Nicodemus asked, "How can these things be? Art thou a master in Israel?" Christ answered, 'And knowest not these things?' This question might be addressed to many who are holding positions of responsibility as teachers, but who have neglected the work essential for them to do, before they are qualified to be teachers. If Christ's words were received into the soul, there would be a much higher intelligence, and much deeper spiritual knowledge of what constitutes one a disciple and a sincere follower of Christ. When the test and trial comes to every soul, there will be apostasies, traitors, heady, highminded, and self-sufficient men, who will turn away from the truth, making shipwreck of the faith. Why?—because they did not dig deep and make their foundation sure. They were not riveted to the eternal book. When the words of the Lord, through His chosen messengers, are brought to them, they murmur, and think that the way is made too strait. Like those who were thought to be the disciples of Christ, but who were displeased with His words, and walked no more with Him, they will turn away from Christ. "No man can come to me, except the Father which hath sent me draw him: and I will raise him up at the last day." What is the drawing?—"It is written in the prophets, and they shall be all taught of God. Every man therefore that hath heard, and hath learned of the Father, cometh unto me." There are men that hear, and not learn the lessons as diligent students. They have a form of godliness, but are not believers. They know not the truth by practice. They receive not the engrafted word. "Wherefore lay apart all filthiness and superfluity of naughtiness, and receive with meekness the engrafted word, which is able to save your souls. But be ye doers of the word, and not hearers only, deceiving your own selves. For if any be a hearer of the word, and not a doer, he is like unto a man beholding his natural face in a glass: for he beholdeth himself, and goeth his way, and straightway forgetteth what manner of man he was." He did not perceive the impression made upon his mind when comparing his course of action with the great moral looking-glass. He did not see his defects of character. He did not reform, and forgetting all about the impression made, he went not God's way, but, "His way," continuing to be unreformed.

Here is the only correct way for each human being to do if he would have a safe all-round experience: "But whoso looketh into the perfect law of liberty, and continueth therein, he being not a forgetful hearer, but a doer of the work, (For there is a work to be done that is neglected at the peril of the soul) this man shall be blessed in his deed. If any man among you seem to {66} be religious, and bridleth not his tongue, but deceiveth his own heart, this man's religion is vain. Pure religion and undefiled before God and the Father is this, to visit the fatherless and widows in their affliction, and to keep himself unspotted from the world." Carry this out, as a test of pure and undefiled religion and the blessing of the Lord will surely follow.

"Wherefore it is contained in the Scripture, behold, I lay in Sion a chief corner stone, elect, precious: and he that believeth on him shall not be confounded." Mark the figure represented in verse five: "Ye also as lively stones, are built up a spiritual house, a holy priesthood, to offer up spiritual sacrifices, acceptable to God by Jesus Christ." Then these lively stones are exerting a tangible, practical influence in the Lord's spiritual house. There they are a holy priesthood performing pure, sacred service. They offer up spiritual sacrifices

acceptable to God.

The Lord will not accept a heartless service, a round of ceremonies that are really Christless. His children must be lively stones in God's building. If all would give themselves unreservedly to God, if they would cease to study and plan for their amusements, for excursions and pleasure loving associations, and would study the words, 'Ye are not your own, for ye are bought with a price; therefore glorify God in your body, and in your spirit, which are God's,' they would never hunger and thirst for excitement or change. If it is for our true interest to be spiritual, if the salvation of our soul depends on being riveted on the eternal book, had we not better be engaged in seeking for that which will hold the whole building to the chief corner stone, that we may not be confused and confounded in our faith?

"Unto you therefore which believe he is precious: but unto them which be disobedient, the stone which the builders disallowed, the same is made the head of the corner, and a stone of stumbling, and a rock of offense, even to them which stumble at the word, being disobedient: whereunto also they were appointed." All men and youth are appointed to do a separate work. But some stumble at the word of truth. It does not harmonize with their inclinations, and therefore they refuse to be doers of the word. They will not wear Christ's yoke of perfect obedience to the law of God. They look upon this yoke as a burden, and Satan tells them that if they will break away from it they will become as gods, no one shall rule or dictate to them; they will be able to do as they please, and have all the liberty they desire. True, they feel that they have been oppressed and cramped in every way in their religious life, but that religious life was farce. They were appointed to be co-laborers with Jesus Christ and yoking up with Christ was their only chance for perfect rest and freedom. Had they done this, they would never have been confounded.

"But ye are a chosen generation, a royal priesthood, a holy nation, a peculiar people; that ye should show forth (your own efficiency, and attract attention to yourself, and seek your own glory? No, No.) the praises of him who hath called you (to a distasteful, hard life of bondage?) out of darkness into his marvelous light."

Many who profess to believe in Christ do not wear His yoke. They think that they do, but if they were not deluded and de-

ceived by Satan, they would have thoughts corresponding with their faith, and with the great truths which they profess to believe. They would realize that the words of Christ mean something to them. "If any man will come after me, let him deny himself, and {67} take up his cross, and follow me." If you follow Jesus, you are His disciple: if you follow your own impulses, your own unsanctified heart, you plainly say, I want not thy way, O Lord, but my own way.

We are to take in the situation and decide what is our purpose. I have a deep interest in young men and young women who have enlisted in the army of the Lord. My love for Jesus Christ imbues me with a love for the souls of all for whom Christ died. The words, "Ye are laborers together with God," mean much. No one can make conditions with God. We are servants of the living God, and all who shall be educated in our schools, are to be trained to be workers. They labor to acquire correct principle. They are to connect with Christ by faith. Thus they can give great satisfaction to the heavenly universe. If each volunteer in the army of the Lord will do his best, God will do the rest. They are to call nothing their own. When striving for the victory they are to strive lawfully. The word is to be their teacher. Unholy ambition will not advance them, for God only can give true wisdom and understanding; but He will not work with Satan. If envy and unholy ambition are cherished, if they wrestle for the victory to obtain human glory, the mind will be filled with confusion. Do your best advance as fast as possible to reach a high standard in spiritual knowledge. Sink self in Jesus Christ, and aim ever to glorify His name. Bear in mind that talent, learning, position, wealth, and influence, are the gifts from God; therefore they should be consecrated to Him. Seek to obtain an education that will qualify you to be wise stewards of the manifold grace of Christ Jesus, servants under Christ to do His bidding.

Let all students seek to take as broad a view as possible of their obligations to God. They are not to look forward to a time after the school term closes, when they will do some large, noted work. But they are to study earnestly how they can commence practicing working their student life by yoking up with Christ. Let every impulse be on the Lord's side. Do not pull down or discourage those who are your teachers. Do not burden their souls by manifesting a spirit of levity and a careless disregard for rules.

Students, you can make this school first class in success by being laborers together with your teachers to help other students, and by zealously uplifting yourself from a cheap, common low standard. Let each see what improvement he can make in conforming his conduct to Bible rules. Those who will seek to be themselves elevated and ennobled are co-operating with Jesus Christ by becoming refined in speech and in temper, under the control of the Holy Spirit. They are yoked up with Jesus Christ. They will not flounce about, and become unruly, and self-caring, studying their own selfish pleasures and satisfaction. They bound all their efforts with Jesus Christ as the messengers of His mercy and to be ministering to others of His grace.

Their hearts throb in unison with Christ's heart. They are one with Christ in spirit, one with Christ in action. They seek to store the mind with the precious treasure of the word of God, that each may do the work appointed him by God, to gather in the bright rays of the Sun of Righteousness, that they may shine unto others.

If you will watch and pray, and make earnest efforts in the right direction, you will be thoroughly imbued with the spirit of Jesus Christ. "But put ye on the Lord Jesus Christ, and make not provision for the flesh, to fulfil the lusts thereof." Be determined that you will make this school a success; {68} and if you will heed the instruction given in the word of God, you may go forth with a development of intellectual and moral power that will cause even the angels to rejoice, and God will rejoice over you with singing. If you are under God's discipline, you will secure the harmony and the co-operation of the physical, mental and moral powers, and the fullest development of your God-given faculties. Let not the buoyancy and the lust of youth through manifold temptations make your opportunities and privileges a failure. Day by day put on Christ, and in the brief season of your test and your trial here below, maintain your dignity in the strength of God, as co-workers with the highest agencies during your scholastic life.

All should say, I will not fail. I will not through my influence betray myself or my companions into the hands of the enemy. I will heed the words of the Lord. "Let him take hold of my strength, that he may make peace with me; and he shall make peace with me." Ever remember that you have one by your side who says to you, "Be not afraid. I have overcome the world." Bear in mind that Christ came as the Prince of heaven, and engaged in the warfare against the principles of sin. All who will unite with Christ will be workers together with God in this warfare.

"For their sakes I sanctify myself," Christ said, "That they also might be sanctified through the truth." The Lord Jesus is the way, the truth and the life; and those who unite with Him, putting Him on, will work as co-laborers with Him, by conforming to the principles of truth. Thus to those in error and sin to show the force and power of truth. By beholding, they become imbued with truth, and unite with Christ to transform the living temple given to idols, that human beings may become cleansed, refined, sanctified temples for the indwelling of the Holy Spirit.

"I have declared unto them thy name," Christ said, "And will declare it; that the love wherewith thou hast loved me may be in them and I in them." The Lord has made abundant provision that His love may be given us as His free abundant grace, as our inheritance in this life, to enable us to diffuse the same by being yoked up with Christ. Jesus conveys the circulating vitality of a pure and sanctified Christlike love through every part of our nature. When this love is expressed in the character it reveals to all those with whom we associate that it is possible for God to be formed within, the hope of glory. It shows that God loves the obedient one as He loved Jesus Christ; and nothing less than this satisfies His desires in our behalf. As soon as the human agent comes united with Christ in heart, soul, and spirit, the Father loves that soul as a part of Christ, as a member of the body of Christ, He Himself being the glorious head.

Dear Brother and Sister

Feb. 17, 1884
Healdsburg, California

I HAVE BEEN THINKING MUCH of the Health Institute at St. Helena. My thoughts crowd into my mind, and I wish to express some of them to you. I am sure that_____ has a work to do for herself which she does not realize. All that she has thought and done, and all that her husband has thought and done, she has looked up as beyond criticism, as just right. I know that this is a deception of the enemy. If anything is said to question her course or his, it appears to both of you that you are treated unjustly. This deception of the enemy {69} will have to be broken before you will be right.

I have been calling to mind the light God has given me, and through me to you, on health reform. Have you prayerfully and carefully sought to understand the will of God in these matters? The excuse has been, that the outsiders would have a meat diet, but even if they had some meat, I know that with care and skill, dishes could be prepared to take the place of meat in a large degree. But if one performs the cooking whose main dependence is meat, she can encourage meat eating, and the depraved appetite will frame every excuse for this kind of diet. When I saw how matters were going,_____ that if_____ had not meat to cook, she knew not what to provide as a substitute, and that meat was the principle article of diet,_____ I felt that there must be a change at once. There may be consumptives who demand meat, but let them have it in their own rooms, and do not tempt the already perverted appetite of those who should not eat it.

I became satisfied that no reform could be while_____ was cooking at the Institute. All that we might try to do would be undone in one week, because the appetite of a few had control in this matter. Large expenses have resulted, for meat is the most expensive diet that can be had. I could not see how the Lord could bless either of you in the course you have pursued, for it was directly contrary to the light He has given for years.

Now as to my own experience; meat seldom appears on my table: for weeks at a time I would not taste it, and after my appetite had been trained, I grew stronger, and could do better work. When I came to the Retreat, I determined not to taste meat, but I could get scarcely anything else to eat, and therefore ate a little meat. It caused unnatural action of the heart. I knew it was not the right kind of food. I wanted to keep house by myself, but this was overruled. If I could have done as I wished, I should have remained at the institution several weeks longer. The use of meat while at the Retreat awakened my old appetite, and after I returned home, it clamored for indulgence. Then I resolved to change entirely, and not under any circumstances eat meat and thus encourage this appetite. Not a morsel of meat or butter has been on my table since I returned. We have milk, fruit, grains and vegetables. For a time I lost all desire for food. Like the children of Israel, I hankered after flesh meats. I firmly refused to have meat bought or cooked. I was weak and trembling, as everyone will be who subsists on meat when deprived of the stimulus. But now my appetite has returned. I enjoy bread and fruit, my head is generally clear, and my strength firmer. I have none of the goneness so common with meat eaters. I have had my lesson, and, I hope, learned it well.

We ought to have seen the evil of allowing certain ones to control the preparation of food for the Retreat. Hot biscuit and flesh meat are entirely out of harmony with health reform principles. If we would allow reason to take the place of impulse and love of selfish indulgence, we would not taste of the flesh of dead animals. That is more repulsive to the sense of smell than a shop where flesh meats are kept for sale. The smell of raw flesh is offensive to all whose senses have not been depraved by the culture of unnatural appetites. What more unpleasant sight to a reflective mind than the beasts slain to be devoured. Persons who live largely on a meat diet are in danger of putrefaction should they contract disease. If the light God has given in regard to Health reform is disregarded, He will not work a miracle to keep in health those who are pursuing a course to make themselves sick. {70}

Now had another stood just where you have stood, and had prepared the meals as you have done, and you two had been lookers on, I wonder what position you would have taken in regard to the matter. You would not have let things continue as they have been going, not one week. You would have had a reform, or discharged the cook. But I have learned that it is not an easy matter to change the ideas and plans of some persons. They are very set, and are not easily turned about. As I think of these things, I feel sad and sick at heart. I know that all that is said to change the order of things is taken as fault-finding.

I have thought it a hopeless undertaking to right matters at the Retreat. Then I have thought notwithstanding your ideas and feelings, and impressions, it must be done. Your influence, your appetite, has molded the Institute, but it can be so no longer. You must change your manner of living. You may think you cannot work without meat: I thought so once, but I know that in His original plan, God did not provide for the flesh of dead animals to compose the diet for man. It is a gross, perverted taste that will accept such food. To think of dead flesh rotting in the stomach is revolting. Then the fact that meat is largely diseased, should lead us to make strenuous efforts to discontinue its use entirely. My position now is to let meat altogether alone. It will be hard for some to do this, as hard as for the rum drinker to forsake his dram; but they will be better for the change.

To The General Conference Committee and the Medical Missionary Board

July 6, 1902
"Elmshaven" Sanitarium

Dear Brethren:

OVER AND OVER AGAIN instruction has been given me that all must be done that can be done to draw our people away from Battle Creek. I was shown that the Sanitarium there was deteriorating for the want of men of capability and consecration to carry it forward in pure, upward lines, in accordance with Bible principles. Very clearly it has been presented to me that it would be in God's order for the work of the Battle Creek Sanitarium to be divided, and plants made in many other places, in the cities that are in need of sanitariums. More true medical missionary work would then be done; and from many centers the light of truth would shine forth with saving power.

I am instructed to say that our people must not be drawn upon for means to erect an immense sanitarium in Battle Creek; the money that would be thus used in the erection of that one mammoth building should be used in making plants in many places. We must not draw all we can from our people for the establishment of a great sanitarium in one place, to the neglect of other places, which are unworked for the want of means. It is not the Lord's will for His people to erect a mammoth sanitarium in Battle Creek or in any other place. In many places in America, sanitariums are to be established. These sanitariums are not to be large establishments, but are to be of sufficient size to enable the work to be carried forward successfully.

Cautions have been given me in reference to the work before us. We are not to encourage students in large numbers to receive their education at Battle Creek. Battle Creek is not the only place to which we are to look for the {71} education of nurses and other medical missionary workers. In every sanitarium established, preparation must be made to train young men and young women to be medical missionaries. The Lord will open the way before them as they go forth to work for Him.

The evidence before us of the fulfillment of prophecy declares that the end of all things is at hand. There is much important work to be done out of and away from Battle Creek. There will be need of sanitariums in many of the cities of the south, as well as in other parts of America.

It is time for us to think soberly. Taking all things into consideration, we should read the providence of God in His movements. Was the Battle Creek Sanitarium consumed by fire in order that the plans might be enlarged, greater buildings erected, and more display made? I think if there were more praying, more earnest study of God's ways and purposes for the advancement of His work, we should see our brethren taking a course altogether different from the course that some are taking.

When we bring into a garden a stream of water to irrigate it, do we provide for the watering of one spot only, leaving the other parts dry and barren to cry, "Give us water"? This is a representation of the way in which work has been carried forward in Battle Creek, to the neglect of other places. Shall the desolate places remain desolate? No! Let the stream flow through every place, carrying with it fertility and gladness.

Never are we to rely upon worldly recognition and rank. Never are we, in the establishment of institutions, to try to compete with worldly institutions in size or splendor. We shall gain the victory, not by erecting massive buildings, in rivalry with our enemies, but by cherishing a Christlike spirit of meekness and lowliness. Better far the cross and disappointed hopes, than to live with princes and forfeit heaven.

The Saviour of mankind was born of humble parentage, in a sin-cursed, wicked world. He was brought up in obscurity at Nazareth, a small town of Galilee. He began His work in poverty, and without worldly rank. Thus God introduced the gospel in a way altogether different from the way in which many deem it wise to proclaim the same gospel in 1902. At the very beginning of the gospel dispensation He taught His church to rely not on worldly rank and splendor, but on the power of faith and obedience. The favor of God is above the riches of gold and silver. The power of His Spirit is of inestimable value.

Thus saith the Lord: "Buildings will give character to my work only when those who erect them follow my instruction in regard to the establishment of institutions. Had those who have managed and sustained the work in the past always been controlled by pure, unselfish principles, the selfish gathering of a large share of my means to one or two places, regardless of the requirements of other places equally needy, would never have been. Institutions would have been established in many places. Seeds of truth, sown in many more fields, would have sprung up and borne fruit to my glory.

"The plants in Battle Creek have been unduly increased, when centers of influence should have been made in many other cities. There should have been more of an equalizing of facilities. The institutions in one place are not to embrace the whole land, swallowing up the means required for other places. {72} The places that have never had the advantages that a few places have had are now to receive attention. My people are to do a sharp, quick work. Those who with purity of purpose fully consecrate themselves to me, body, mind, and spirit, shall work in my way and in my name. Everyone shall stand in his lot, looking to me, his Guide and Counselor.

"My name has been greatly dishonored. Let no one erect large, costly buildings, even in Battle Creek, for the managers of the work there have been reproved for doing this in the past. God does not make such plans, and He cannot endorse them. He has reproved and rebuked many for errors that they have made. Many wrongs have been corrected, but an earnest, thorough work is still to be done,

"I will instruct the ignorant, and anoint with heavenly eyesalve the eyes of many who are now in spiritual blindness. I will raise up agents who will carry out my will to prepare a people to stand before me in the time of the end. In many places that ought to have been provided before with sanitariums and schools, I will establish institutions, and these institutions will become educational centers for the training of workers."

The Lord will work upon human minds in unexpected quarters. Some who apparently are enemies of the truth will in God's providence invest their means to develop properties and erect buildings. In time, these properties will be offered for sale at a price far below their cost. Our people will recognize the hand of Providence in these offers, and will secure valuable properties for use in institutional work. They will plan and manage with humility, self-denial, and self-sacrifice. Thus men of means are unconsciously preparing auxiliaries that will enable the Lord's people to advance His work rapidly.

In various places properties are to be purchased to be used for sanitarium purposes. When opportunity offers, our people should purchase properties away from the cities, on which are buildings already erected and fruit orchards already in bearing. Land is a valuable possession. Connected with our sanitariums there should be lands, small portions of which can be used for the homes of the helpers and others who are receiving a training in medical missionary work.

In proclaiming the message, God's servants must wrestle with perplexities. Obstacles must be removed. Sometimes the work will go hard at the beginning, as it did when we were establishing institutions in Battle Creek, Michigan, and Oakland, California. In Cooranbong, Australia, we began in a very crude way, pitching our tents in the woods, felling trees, and clearing the land, preparatory to the erection of buildings. What conflicts we had! What victories we gained! Unconsecrated workers and false friends have at times been connected with our institutions in that country; but the Lord has set things in order. By the power of His Spirit a reformation has been brought about. All can see the stately steppings of the Lord God of Israel.

Work is to be done in all parts of the vineyard. In the early days of the message a right beginning was made, but work has not developed as God desired it to develop. Too much has been centered in Battle Creek and Oakland, and in a few other places. Our brethren should never have built so largely in one place as they have in Battle Creek. In many fields very little has been done to establish memorials for God. This is wrong. Years ago very many of our {73} workers and people had the spirit of self-denial and self-sacrifice. Success attended their efforts. The Lord has signified that His work should be carried forward in the same spirit in which it was begun. The world is to be warned. Field after field is still unworked. Shall we as a people, by our actions, our business arrangements, our attitude toward a world unsaved, bear a testimony altogether different from the testimony borne by us twenty or thirty years ago? Shall we give evidence of spiritual disease and a lack of wise planning? Upon us has shone great light in regard to the last days of this earth's history. The sight of the souls perishing in sin should arouse us to give the light of present truth to those now in darkness. God's messengers must be clothed with power. They must have for the truth a reverence that they do not now possess. The Lord's solemn, sacred message of warning must be proclaimed not merely in our churches, but in the most difficult fields and in the most sinful cities,—in every place where the light of the third angel's message has not yet dawned. Everyone is to hear the last call to the marriage supper of the Lamb.

My brethren, let your building plans be reconsidered. Bring your building within your means. The Lord sees the work that must be done. He sees the fields that are unworked and destitute of facilities. From all in His service He requires equity, just judgment. In all parts of the world there is a work to be done that ought to have been done long ago. A large amount of means is not to be absorbed in one place. Every building erected is to be erected with reference to the other places that will need similar buildings. God calls upon men in positions of trust in His work not to block the way of advance by selfishly using in one place or in one line of work all the means that can be secured.

A Peculiar People

It has been stated that the Battle Creek Sanitarium is not denominational. But if ever an institution was established to be denominational, in every sense of the word, this sanitarium was. Why are sanitariums established if it is not that they may be the right hand of the gospel in calling the attention of men and women to the truth that we are living amid the perils of the last days? And yet, in one sense, it is true that the Battle Creek Sanitarium is undenominational, in that it receives as patients people of all classes and all denominations.

Do not the following words point out a denominational people:-}

"The Lord spake unto Moses, saying, Speak thou also unto the children of Israel, saying, Verily, my sabbaths ye shall keep: for it is a sign between me and you throughout your generations; that ye may know that I am the Lord that doth sanctify you. Ye shall keep the sabbath therefore; for it is holy unto you. Everyone that defileth it shall surely be put to death: for whosoever doeth any work therein, that soul shall be cut off from among his people. Six days may work be done; but in the seventh is the Sabbath of rest, holy to the Lord; whosoever doeth any work in the sabbath day, he shall surely be put to death. Wherefore the children of Israel shall keep the sabbath, to observe the Sabbath throughout their generations, for a perpetual covenant. It is a sign between me and the children of Israel for ever: for in six days the Lord made heaven and earth, and on the seventh day he rested, and was refreshed." {74}

"What doth the Lord thy God require of thee, but to fear the Lord thy God, to walk in all his ways, and to love him, and to serve the Lord thy God with all thy heart, and with all thy soul, to keep the commandments of the Lord, and his statutes, which I command thee this day for thy good?"

Now and ever we are to stand as a distinct and peculiar people, free from all worldly policy, unembarrassed by confederating with those who have not wisdom to discern the claims of God, so plainly set forth in His law. We are not to take pains to declare that the Battle Creek Sanitarium is not a Seventh-day Adventist institution; for this it certainly is. As a Seventh-day Adventist institution it was established, to represent the various features of gospel missionary work, thus to prepare the way for the coming of the Lord.

We have come to a time when God has been greatly dishonored. Those who have long known our belief, and what we teach, have been surprised by the statement that the Battle Creek Sanitarium is not denominational. No one has a right to make this statement. It does not bear the witness that God wishes His people to bear before men, and angels. In the name of the Lord we are to identify ourselves as Seventh-day Adventists. If anyone among us is ashamed of our colors, and wishes to stand under another banner, let him do so as a private individual, not as a representative of Seventh-day Adventist medical missionary work.

Let us take our position as Seventh-day Adventists. The name is a true expression of our faith. I am instructed to call upon God's people to bring their actions into harmony with their name, of which they have no need to be ashamed. The Seventh-day Adventist faith will bless whenever it is brought into the character-building.

Recent movements made in connection with the Sanitarium enterprise at Battle Creek, make it necessary for us to take our position decidedly before the world as a people who have not changed their faith. We are to show that we are seeking to work in harmony with heaven in preparing the way of the Lord. We are to bear witness to all nations, kindreds, and tongues that we are a people who love and fear God, a people who keep holy the seventh-day Sabbath,—the sign between God and His obedient children that He sanctifies them. And we are to show plainly that we have full faith that the Lord is soon to come in the clouds of heaven.

We have been greatly humiliated as a people by the course that some of our brethren in responsible positions have taken in departing from the old landmarks. There are those who in order to carry out their plans have by their works denied their faith. This shows how little dependence can be placed on human wisdom and human judgment. Now, as never before, we need to see the danger of being led unguardedly away from loyalty to God's commands. We need to realize that God has given us a decided message of warning for the world, even as He gave Noah a message of warning for the antediluvians. Let our people beware of belittling the importance of the Sabbath, in order to link up with unbelievers. Let them beware of departing from the principles of our faith, making it appear that it is not wrong to conform to the world. Let them be afraid of heeding any man's counsel, whatever his position may be, who works counter to that which God has wrought in order to keep His people separate from the world. {75}

The Lord is testing and trying His people, to see who will be loyal to the principles of His truth. Our work is to proclaim to the world the first, second, and third angel's messages. In the discharge of our duties, we are neither to despise nor fear our enemies. To bind ourselves up by contracts with those not of our faith is not in the order of God. We are to treat with kindness and courtesy those who refuse to be loyal to God, but we are never, never to unite with them in counsel regarding the vital interests of His work; for this is not the way of the Lord. Putting our trust in God, we are to move steadily forward, doing his work with unselfishness, in humble dependence upon Him, committing ourselves and all that concerns our present and future to His wise providence, holding the beginning of our confidence firm unto the end, remembering that it is not because of our worthiness that we receive the blessings of heaven, but because of the worthiness of Christ, and our acceptance, through faith in Him, of God's abounding grace.

I pray that my brethren may realize that the third angel's message means much to us, and that the observance of the true Sabbath is to be the sign that distinguishes those who serve God from those who serve Him not. Let those who have become sleepy and indifferent awake. We are called to be holy, and we should carefully avoid giving the impression that it is of little consequence whether or not we retain the peculiar features of our faith. Upon us rests the solemn obligation of taking a more decided stand for truth and righteousness than we have taken in the past. The line of demarcation between those who keep the commandments of God and those who do not, is to be revealed with unmistakable clearness. We are conscientiously to honor God, diligently using every means of keeping in covenant relation with Him, that we may receive His blessings,—the blessings so essential for the people who are to be so severely tried. To give the impression that our faith, our religion, is not a dominating power in our lives, is greatly to dishonor God. Thus we turn from His commandments, which are our life, denying that He is our God and we His people.

Diary

August 20, 1900

SOME THINGS HAVE BEEN presented to me which are of great consequence to our people in Australia. The Lord has given me a message for Dr. Caro and Brother Sharp and for our ministers in this country. I was instructed that temptations would come to them which they did not suspect as temptations, and the import of which they did not discern. The message was given me that Dr. Kellogg would be displeased if the Medical Missionary work in this country were connected with the work of the Union Conference. But there is to be no separation in the different lines of missionary work done by Seventh-day Adventists. The different parts of the work are to combine to make a great whole. He who is the Strength of Israel has His army on earth. His soldiers are to stand united with the army of heaven in the work of giving truth to our world, in places nigh and regions afar off. His servants are to work in perfect harmony, those in a place which has been blessed with advantages supplying those in more destitute regions with facilities for the work.

Christ has given the divine principle by which His work is to be carried forward. Strength is to be continually added to it by the talent of means, the talent of speech, the talent of genius. These gifts are to be used to {76} advance the work as a whole.

In the fourth chapter of Ephesians God has given instruction regarding the management of His work as a whole. The variety of gifts are to blend. I was instructed to warn Dr. Kellogg that he was making a great mistake in treating God's ministers as he has done. They are doing the very work God has appointed them. When the medical missionary workers are educated to carry on their work independently of the ministry which God has ordained, they step off the Bible platform to devise human plans and methods, which cannot stand.

God's people have a great work to do. Seeds must be planted which will produce the right kind of harvest. The world must see in the church of God true order, true discipline, true organization. Paul wrote, "Brethren, I count not myself to have apprehended; but this one thing I do, forgetting those things which are behind, I press toward the mark for the prize of the high calling of God in Christ Jesus. Let us therefore, as many as be perfect, be thus minded; and if in anything ye be otherwise minded, God shall reveal even this unto you. Nevertheless, whereto we have already attained, let us walk by the same rule, let us mind the same thing. Brethren, be followers together of me, and mark them which walk so as ye have us for ensample. (For many walk, of whom I have told you often, and now tell you even weeping, that they are enemies of the cross of Christ.)"

There is to be no schism in the body of believers. No confederacy is to be formed that will bind about the work or place all the means in the hands of one man. I was shown that the plan of placing all the power in the hands of one man is not of God but of man.

When there is presented before any church or any company of believers in any country the proposition to bind those who handle the health foods to a contract to conform to certain restrictions which man has made, the answer is always to be, No. God's work is not to be bound.

If God has given Dr. Kellogg wisdom from his immense fountain of supplies,

if He has given him means and scientific knowledge to meet the emergencies of the present time, does this impartation give him a patent right to this gift, bestowed on him to show that God has not forgotten His people? This gift belongs not to Dr. Kellogg, but to the great power beyond. Dr. Kellogg has forgotten that he is a man who has to be trained and educated like other men. God has greatly honored him, and will continue to honor him as long as he will wear Christ's yoke and learn in Christ's school His meekness and lowliness. But Dr. Kellogg did not create himself. He is not the only one who can drink from the fountain of knowledge. The Lord has other man whom He will instruct. Dr. Kellogg was not given his knowledge from God the he might carry it as a product of his own creating.

If through the wisdom donated by God for the benefit of His people, Dr. Kellogg has discovered something in regard to health foods, why should he feel that these productions are his own? It is a part of God's work, and is very far from being perfect, yet everyone connected with the Lord is at liberty to devise and plan and experiment from the wisdom which the Lord in His bounty has given him. God will give knowledge regarding the way in which to prepare food in the best and most wholesome manner, and the Lord forbid that any of his people should make one stroke with the pen in signing a contract saying they {77} will do this or that in regard to the sale of these foods.

Great improvements will be made in the line of health foods. Some foods will be found not to be prepared in the best and most wholesome manner. The Lord calls for men and women who will not stop where they are, but will work until under heaven's guidance these productions are more perfect than they now are. Let skillful minds take up the matter of improvement. The Lord will give wisdom. But remember that when you begin to think that your wisdom is of your own creation, and that you have a right to bind about as you will the productions of this wisdom, you are off Christ's ground. You are making crooked paths for your feet, and many that are lame will be turned out of the way.

God calls for men who will receive to impart. The Lord's work is not to be done in a corner. Impartial, unselfish witnesses are to give to others that which the Lord has given them, bearing a spontaneous testimony. One success in reform is to lead on

to another and still another success. This result will be seen if Christ's workers are learning in the school of Christ. They will then realize that they are not to draw into their business transactions one thread of selfishness. God says, "Ye are the light of the world." We are to exhibit in our borders all the improvements that our God-given tact and knowledge have enabled us to make. Everything which has a practical bearing on the improvement of the work is not to become the property of one man; for it comes from the heavenly Father, who gave manna from heaven to the whole camp of Israel. That which men achieve by means of the wisdom God has given them is not to be used merely to advance one line of the work, but is to be used to promote the cause of God as a whole.

Sunnyside, Cooranbong.

I could not sleep tonight after half past eleven. After inviting sleep till half past one, I dressed, and commenced writing. Things which I could not interpret were presented before me. There has been a meeting, and the presentation of business matters in the meeting pained me to the heart. A company has assembled to make suggestions regarding the school at College View. The words and deportment and decisions of Dr. Kellogg and his associates grieved me beyond expression. "What does this mean?" I asked. Why are these men so manifestly walking away from Bible principles?

Last night a similar presentation was made to me. The business transactions were of such a character that I again turned away with a burden of soul so heavy that I exclaimed, "The Lord pity you if this is your idea of how a Christian should act toward his fellow Christians." A Christian is one who follows Christ through evil as well as good report. Christian discipleship in regard to business matters means more than many realize. Our Lord said, "I must be about my Father's business." If we follow in His footsteps, we must as His human agents, copy His divine example. We must be faithful financiers for the Father. True Christians will follow in Christ's footsteps. If in the business connected with the cause and in our dealing with our brethren, if we do not bring the principles of the teaching of Christ, if we fail to obey the instruction He has given us, in the Old Testament as well as in the New, we are not true followers of His.

We have a most important work to do,—the work of obeying Christ and bearing witness of Him. He said to His disciples, "And ye also shall bear {78} witness because ye have been with me from the beginning." The disciples were to be honored by bearing witness concerning Christ's mission. They had been with Him constantly and had gained a most valuable knowledge to impart to others. We cannot be with Christ in person, as were His first disciples, but He has sent His Holy Spirit to guide us into all truth, and through this power we too can bear witness for the Saviour.

The union of the branch to the vine is no more essential to the life and fruitfulness of the branch than a union with Christ is essential to the life and fruitfulness of the believer. Receiving Him by faith and trusting in Him, true believers become partakers of the divine nature. They not only bear testimony for Him with their lips; they witness for Him by their works. "If ye abide in me, and my words abide in you," He says, "ye shall ask what ye will, and it shall be done unto you. If ye keep my commandments, ye shall abide in my love; even as I have kept my Father's commandments and abide in his love. These things have I spoken unto you, that my joy might remain in you, and that your joy might be full. This is my commandment, that ye love one another, as I have loved you."

"Ye are my friends, if ye do whatsoever I command you." No one is to work evil to his brother's interest with the excuse that it is to help in a certain line of the work of God. In doing that certain work, he places his brethren in a position where they are hindered from doing the work the Lord would have them do in behalf of truth and righteousness. The Lord will not accept such an offering. It is gained by robbery, and He says, "I hate robbery for burnt offering."

No man will be condemned for not accepting light he has never received, or for violating a law he never heard. But when light comes to him from the word of God, and he neglects to live by it, but in his business transactions in connection with the work and cause of God, and in his dealing with his brethren, uses oppression, because he supposes he has power to oppress, he does himself great harm. He will not receive from his injustice and oppression the advantage he expects to receive.

"I hate robbery for burnt offering." A plea that it is to do good will not justify a man for working on wrong principles. God will bring those who deprive their fellow-workers of their rightful advantage to a strict account. There are those who think they can do this work if they choose. Men often do themselves that which they condemn in others, without asking themselves, "Am I advancing the Lord's work in right lines? Am I doing that which I would condemn if done by others? What would Christ do under such circumstances? Will the Lord be pleased if I bind about the work my brethren are doing in order to advance my own interests? Would this not be weaving into the web threads of selfishness which would spoil the pattern?"

Men make the cause of God an excuse for doing unjust actions when in reality they wish to advance their own interests. God condemns such actions; for they are a misrepresentation of Christ's character, a working out of Satan's principles. Those who do this work are taking advantage of God's patience and long-suffering to strengthen self-confidence and arbitrary exactions; they are encouraging others in sin rather than leading them to avoid it. By their actions they give the most decided evidence that they cannot be trusted as the Lord's stewards to do His business. He will not sanction the use of common {79} instead of sacred fire in His work, any more than He would not excuse Nadab and Abihu in their departure from His requirements. The Lord has not changed. Those in positions of trust who do anything that savors of oppression will find no favor from God in the action. They are using common fire, not the sacred fire of His kindling. To fill aright important positions of trust requires a baptism of the Holy Spirit. Only as they receive this baptism can men work the works of Christ and reveal pure, holy principles. The words and works reveal the spirit and principles which control the heart.

God will not endorse one act of selfishness, one unrighteous deed. Men may claim high honor for their labor in God's service, but the way in which they accomplish their work testifies to their value. If they obey the law of Jehovah and cooperate with Him, witness is borne of them before the heavenly universe that they are true workers with God. God's ordinances and works are given to man to promote holiness of heart and purity of life. If this result is not seen, the object sought for by a righteous God is not accomplished. However zealous men may be in certain lines of work, which receive praise from men, God reads beneath the surface, and if the work is not of such a character as He can approve, the workers are not accepted by Him.

Sharp, critical self-examination is needed. Worldly principles are not to be woven into the web and made a part of the fabric.

So close is the union between Christ and the Father that as men treat Christ so they treat the Father. The greater the light and evidence God has given men regarding His character and will, the greater will be their guilt and condemnation if they do not love and obey Him.

"If there be therefore any consolation in Christ, if any comfort of love, if any fellowship of the Spirit, if any bowels and mercies, fulfil ye my joy, that ye be like-minded, having the same love, being of one accord, of one mind. Let nothing be done through strife or vainglory; but in lowliness of mind let each esteem other better than themselves. Look not every man on his own things, but every man also on the things of others. Let this mind be in you, which was also in Christ Jesus."

The gospel inculcates universal humility and benevolence. It produces the virtues of Christ's character in all who savingly accept it. Christ made the sacrifice of Himself to furnish man with grace and power. All who receive His spirit become sons of God, one with Christ in God. Those who attain to eternal life must overcome by the blood of the Lamb and the word of their testimony. In order to be saved, men must work out their own salvation with fear and trembling, revealing a faith which works by love and purifies the soul. Love for God and man has been enjoined upon every human being. God works by His Holy Spirit in those who believe in Christ as their personal Saviour. He helps them to work out their own salvation giving them grace for the grace which they impart to others.

The ministers of God, by the holy example they set, are constituted messengers of righteousness, and they should receive love and respect from those who cooperate with them. Let him who cherishes a spirit which leads him to accuse his fellow-workers who are proclaiming the message the Lord has given them, beware, for he is treading on holy ground, and might better take his shoes from off his feet. {80}

God chooses His agents, and gives each an individual trial. He allows His workers to be tempted: thus He proves them to see whether they are building on the right foundation, whether they are doing what Christ would do under similar circumstances. Those whose lips are sanctified will utter no witticisms or sarcasms to hurt the Lord's purchased possession. Men and women are the Lord's heritage, and no man on the face of the earth has the shadow of a right to oppress those whom God has redeemed. Christ shed His blood to make it possible for them to be partakers of the divine nature. Human beings are very dear to God's heart of love, and when He makes up His jewels He will gather to Himself those who love and believe in Him. In that great day when every case is settled forever, He will spare them as a man spareth his own son that serveth him. His chosen ones, who appreciate the value of redemption, will live through all eternity with Him whom they have served faithfully on this earth.

DIARY,

[Prior to July 1915]
Summer Hill, Sydney

THIS HAS BEEN A TRYING day for me. Things have been presented to me since coming to Sydney, and I cannot feel at rest until I shall give expression to the representations.

Propositions may be made by Dr. Kellogg and some in Africa regarding money matters, that are not to be accepted. These propositions will arrange for bonds and a party negotiation, the profits to be under the control of certain individuals who are not and have not been for some time under the control of the great Head. The word was spoken, Beware. Consider well before you use your pen to subscribe to any conditions which will place matters under the control of minds which are not guided by the Lord. Beware. You will have trials that you do not foresee. Arrangements may be proposed by the brethren in America and Africa that the Lord declares to be a snare. Leave yourselves wholly under the jurisdiction of the great Head. The Lord's cause is too sacred to be trifled with. In no case are His people to subscribe to conditions which will lead to endless perplexity, jealousy, evil-surmisings, suspicions and temptations. God declares, "The gold and the silver is mine, from the first penny, to the last, and for the abuse or misappropriation of my money I will call men to account."

God's ministers, God's missionaries, are to unite with Him. If they put their trust in Him, and commit the keeping of their souls to Him as unto a faithful Creator, He will keep that which is committed to Him against that day. He will honor those who honor Him.

The Lord has a great work to be done. Changes are continually taking place. In our association with those of different nationality, education, and experience we shall find that it is, a life and death struggle to bear forward the gospel in all its purity. We are not to enter into confederacy with human agencies which will prove a snare.

Race is nothing in the sight of God. Christian experience and sanctification through the truth is everything in His estimation.

Venture nothing in business transactions unless the God of heaven signifies that such a venture will not prove a thorn in the religious life. {81}

I tell you that there is a life and death struggle before us, a contest with human agencies who are not abiding in Christ, who have not proved in any sense God's stewards. Men of strong temperament and almost unsubduable character will make propositions which God has shown me it will not be best to accept. Enter not into a confederacy with them, unless the propositions are conscientiously clear according to God's word.

The only safety for the strong temperaments in Africa is to begin an entirely new chapter in their experience. Hearts must be softened. They must accept Christ's yoke, else they will never enter the kingdom of heaven. A strong spirit bears sway in Africa, which needs to be surrendered to the Spirit of God. There are those there with strong passions, which are easily excited. They lose control of themselves, and become unreasonable. God's people must wait on Him. The welfare of the cause of God needs careful consideration. It must not, with its possibilities and probabilities, be bought or sold. We have one Master, even Christ.

The presentation before me is not encouraging. Divine foresight is needed to see the result of business transactions between parties that it is next to impossible to unify. The missionary work is a great and grand work, and those whom God has made stewards in trust must not feel at liberty to unite in any confederacy which God, who sees the end from the beginning, cannot justify and endorse as glorifying His holy name. God must be consulted as to how His work shall be advanced without having woven into it one thread of selfishness. God will work. He will furnish means for the carrying forward of His work without entanglement. His work is not to be bound about because men choose to act out perverse human nature instead of submitting to be molded and fashioned after the divine similitude.

In Africa as well as in America and Australia men have been quarried out of the world, not to be left as rough stones, but to be taken into the workshop of God, and placed under the axe and hammer and made ready for the heavenly polishing. The roughness has not yet been put away. Many are not yet subdued by the Spirit of God. Because of this, the work in America and Africa and other parts of the Lord's vineyard has not advanced as it should. We are doing what we can, according to the light given, for Australia. A direct necessity, is being met by the work of women who have given themselves to the Lord, and are reaching out to help a needy, sin-stricken world, who want the truth, but do not know that they want it. Personal evangelistic work is to be done. People are reached by house-to-house labor. The women who have taken up this work do everything but preach the gospel from the pulpit. They carry the gospel to the homes of the people in the highways and byways. They read and explain the word to families and individuals, praying with them, caring for the sick, relieving their temporal necessities, presenting before them the purifying, transforming influence of the truth. They show them that the way to find peace and happiness and joy is to follow Jesus.

The Lord has permitted Brother John Wessels to go to Africa and Elder Daniells to accompany him. But I have been shown that there is in the hearts of the people of Africa something that will not be easily overcome, something that shows that some are not converted. They are not under the discipline of God. They do not accept God's way of doing them good, but choose rather their own way. They have yet to learn in the school of Christ His meekness and lowliness. They have yet to learn with Paul that to suffer for the sake of Christ {82} is for their present and eternal good. Paul looked upon present suffering as not worthy to be compared with the glory which was to follow. He desired heavenly treasure rather than earthly advantages. He did not see anything in the world worth living for but the joy of doing the will of God from the heart, trusting all the consequences to God.

God desires to see the souls of His people in Africa mastered by heaven-born purposes. But what a work needs to be done there! The people have not learned of the great Teacher. Human nature, when unsubdued, unsanctified and depraved, is a very curious and wonderful thing. It assumes a great many forms because it is not worked by the Holy Spirit. But when the Lord Jesus is an abiding presence in the soul, none need to question the value of the human being, man or woman.

Paul wrote to Timothy, his son in the gospel, "For God hath not given us the spirit of fear; but of power, and of love, and of a sound mind. Be not thou therefore ashamed of the testimony of our Lord, nor of me his prisoner: but be thou partaker of the afflictions of the gospel according to the power of God; who hath saved us, and called us with a holy calling, not according to our works, but according to his own purpose and grace, which was given us in Christ Jesus before the world began".

Peter declares, "Wherefore laying aside all malice, and all guile, and hypocrisies, and envies, and all evil speakings, as newborn babes, desire the sincere milk of the word, that ye may grow thereby: if so be ye have tasted that the Lord is gracious. To whom coming, as unto a living stone, disallowed indeed of men, but chosen of God, and precious, ye also, as lively stones, are built up a spiritual house, a holy priesthood, to offer up spiritual sacrifices, acceptable to God by Jesus Christ. Wherefore also it is contained in the Scripture, Behold, I lay in Sion a chief corner stone, elect, precious: and he that believeth on him shall not be confounded. Unto you therefore which believe he is precious: but unto them which be disobedient, the stone which the builders disallowed, the same is made the head of the corner, and a stone of stumbling, and a rock of offense, even to them which stumble at the word, being disobedient: whereunto also they were appointed. But ye are a chosen generation, a royal priesthood, a holy nation, a peculiar people; that ye should show forth the praises of him who hath called you out of darkness into his marvelous light."

This entire chapter should be studied. It contains instruction which will sweep back the mist and fog of skepticism, the evil thing which Satan throws across the pathway to eclipse the light which comes from the Father of light.

THE KRESS COLLECTION

DEAR CHILDREN, EDSON AND EMMA WHITE

July 17, 1900
Sunnyside, Cooranbong

I HAVE BEEN SO FULLY occupied that I have not been able to write as I otherwise would have done. We have many things to settle in reference to the future of the work in this country before we can leave it with assurance. We have acted according to the wisdom which God has given His agencies here. {83}

Last Friday Brother Sharp and Brother Merrit Kellogg walked into W.C. White's house. I had just come in to speak to May. They brought with them a plan of the Sanitarium for examination. W.C. was not present, but we expected him every moment. The plan was laid upon the table and we examined it. Two plans had been prepared, one more expensive than the other. One was a three story building capable of accommodating one hundred patients. It was a nice design.

Then I inquired in regard to the material to be used in the building. The design was to use brick, which would be very expensive. I told them that from the light I had received for the last thirty years brick and stone buildings were not the most healthful, as they were generally cold and damp. They reasoned that the appearance which a brick building would present would be much more attractive, and that we wanted the building attractive. I said, "So do I; but we have not the money to build with brick. We need a roomy building, and if brick is too costly, we must build of wood. In all our buildings in this country economy must be our study. This is a necessity, because of the greatness of the work which must be done in many lines in this part of God's moral vineyard. Every calculation in erecting these buildings should be with reference to other plants which must be made in other localities."

Some thought that patients would not feel safe from fire in a wooden structure. At this point W.C.W. joined us. He reminded us that we were not in a city, where buildings were crowded together, and that if fire broke out it would originate from within not from without; therefore brick would not be a safeguard. This matter will need to be presented to patients in the correct light that for health a wooden building is much more preferable than one of brick, because in it we avoid all dampness.

We who lead out in our buildings must do as we design others should follow, Even if he had the money in sight we would not selfishly use more than is needed in building, because in all our designs we must conduct our work with reference to other portions of the Lord's vineyard. We are all members of the one family, children of one Father, and the use which we make of the Lord's revenue to carry forward and advance His work must be with reference to the general interests of the cause of God in other localities. There must be a cultivation of the Lord's vineyard as a whole.

If we build expensively and incur a burden of debt, that would be an example which we do not wish to encourage in other localities, because it would be wrong for them to do this. Then we must build in such a way that we shall not violate the great principle laid down in the word of God that we should love our neighbor as ourselves. We are not to be guilty of absorbing all the means in the treasury in our special portion of the field and thus make it impossible for the work to be built up in other places, and for new territory to be added to the Lord's kingdom. The Lord would have other parts of His vineyard furnished with facilities so that they shall be able to give character to the work. The Lord forbid us to use any selfish schemes in His service, schemes that shall rob our neighbor of facilities which would enable them to act their part in representing the advanced light and clear, decided truth that is to be presented in many places.

After we had freely exchanged ideas, I said, "We must ever consider that our works must ever represent our faith. We believe that the Lord is soon to {84} come, and should not our faith be represented by our works? Shall we put a great outlay of money into a building which will soon be consumed in the great conflagration? Our money means souls. We must use the Lord's money in various ways to bring a knowledge of the truth to souls, who, because of sin, are under the condemnation of God. Then let us bind about the edges and not in any way be improvident, lest the Lord's treasury become empty and the builders shall not have means to do their appointed work. The strength and joy of our benefiting humanity is not in an expensive building after the world's calculation. No; we must remember how many are starving for necessary food and clothing. If we will walk in the wisdom of this world, we shall divorce our souls from God. We will do our duty and leave the result with

God who can give the success."

This reasoning was sensible and met the minds of all that were in counsel. It was decided that we should have a thoroughly constructed, wooden building with every facility brought into the structure for the health of the patients. Then our works will correspond with our faith. Dr. Kellogg suggested a change in some portions of the plan that would be necessary if the structure were made of wood. We decided that an appearance of grandeur should not influence us in erecting the building, but that any extra means which we might have should be spent in providing proper health-restoring facilities.

The building should be so constructed as to secure the God-given sunshine, which is essential for cheerfulness and healthfulness. The Lord Jesus has shown us great love, and we are to impart to others the sunshine of His love. It will be the brightness and the joy of the presence of Jesus that will bring the healing balm into the Sanitarium.

The most marked and effectual evidence of the truth is revealed in the harmony which should exist among the Lord's builders, among His husbandry. We must all draw together. Our strength is in our unity. We are weak when we do not love one another, and when we love our own selves more than we love Jesus. Christ declares that the demonstration of this unity is the evidence to the world that God has sent His Son into the world. When all who love God and keep His commandments work unselfishly, each working to build up not merely that which is under his immediate supervision, regardless of his fellow-laborers who are tugging and toiling with very few facilities with which to do the work; when they, in harmonious love, in unity of heart and action, interestedly favor others as they themselves have been favored, they will reveal to our world the great principle of the love of Christ.

I am instructed to say that we are on test and trial to reveal whether, if under favorable circumstances, we would share with our neighbor brethren the supplies and rich gifts bestowed by God upon us, that they may be able to work having advantages equal to those of our own. We are to demonstrate here in this world how we would conduct ourselves in the heavenly courts; for the same characters we reveal here, the way with which we deal with our brethren here is the way we would deal with those who are to compose the fami-

ly in heaven. Now is our testing, proving time. Just as we treat one another we will treat Him who gave His life to save a perishing world from eternal ruin.

We know not when our Master will come to settle the account of His servants; therefore we are to be constantly prepared to meet Him in peace. The probation of anyone of us may cease in a moment. Death by accident may suddenly and unexpectedly close our earthly period. How stands the life record of {85} each one of us today? To every man God has given his work, the very work which the Master would have each to do.

The Sanitarium building is to be a memorial to the Lord, to honor and glorify His name. It is to be regarded as a temple where spiritual truth is acted.

DEAR BROTHER MURPHET

March 29, 1900
"Sunnyside," Cooranbong,

I RECEIVED YOUR LETTER. I thank you for your statement that you will help us. You ask how much the Sanitarium building will cost. I cannot tell you this; for I do not know. Dr. Caro tells me that the house they are occupying in Summer Hill is now sold, and that they will have to move out to vacate it in a few months. We are so glad that you can help us in establishing our new Sanitarium. We do not feel like specifying how much you should give. The Lord can make your heart willing to help us in our emergency.

The Sanitarium in Sydney is now full. But the higher class of patients, those who can afford to pay well, will only remain long enough to take their treatment. They do not like the building or the rooms, and they will not stay any longer than they can help.

My brother, we do not wish to make duties for you, but could I have seen you, I would gladly have presented our situation before you. I have been instructed that we should seek to reach all classes of people with the message of truth, the last message of warning to be given to the world. Twenty-five years ago the Lord revealed to me that the best way in which to reach the higher classes is through our sanitariums. These institutions are to be located away from the cities, and are to be surrounded with land enough to enable fruit and produce to be grown.

In the Sanitarium which we are about to erect in New South Wales, provision

must be made for all classes. The accommodation and treatment must be such that patients of the higher class will be attracted to the institution. Rooms must be fitted for the use of those who are willing to pay a liberal price. Rational methods of treatment must be followed. The patients must not be given alcohol, tea, coffee, or drugs; for these always leave traces of evil behind.

By their stay at the Sanitarium, the patients are to become acquainted with Seventh-day Adventists and the reasons of their faith. Physicians and nurses are to manifest a deep interest in the physical sufferings of those to whom they minister. As efforts are made to remove suffering and disease, the hearts of the patients will be softened. Every physician should be a Christian. In Christ's stead he is to stay by the suffering one, ministering to the needs of the sin-sick soul as well as to the needs of the diseased body.

To us as a people God has given advanced light, and we are to seek to gain access to souls, that we may give them this truth. As the physicians and nurses in our sanitariums hold out to the patients the hope of restoration to physical health, they are also to present the blessed hope of the gospel, the {86} wonderful comfort to be found in the Mighty Healer, who can cure the leprosy of the soul. Thus hearts will be reached, and He who gives health to the body will speak peace to the soul. The Life-giver will fill the heart with a joy that will work miraculously.

Those thus born again will go from our institution prepared to speak to others of Him who has done so much for them. Jesus says of them, "Ye are my witnesses." God grant them a renewal of life and health that they may go forth to impart to others the knowledge they have obtained, to tell their friends that they may keep well by eating temperately and drinking temperately, discarding tea, coffee, drugs of all kinds, and alcohol in all its forms. They go from the sanitarium as newborn souls, converted and enlightened, knowing that by being temperate in all things, and depending on Him who gave His life for them, they may work for God.

An atheist or irreligious man should never take up the work of a physician. How inconsistent for a physician to stand by the side of the sick and suffering if he cannot point them to a sin-pardoning Saviour. How terrible not to be able to tell them of the Mighty One who can heal not only every physical disease but every spiritual malady. Would that physicians might realize the greatness of the service they could render to humanity if they were able to speak simply and tenderly of the love of Jesus and of His willingness to save souls, even at the last hour of life. Many physicians fail to see what a noble influence they might exert by accepting Christ and laying hold of eternal interests. They continue to live a hopeless life, a life in which God is not recognized. They refuse to be illuminated by the light of the world, and are in a far worse condition than the one who is suffering from physical disease.

What a blessing the Christian physician can bring to the sin-tortured soul! What peace comes to the sufferer as he accepts the Saviour! What melody is awakened in the heavenly courts when Satan loses his prey!

Physicians are given the work of standing in Christ's stead to the sick and suffering, and they should not be loaded down with burdens of a secular character. They should be free from financial care.

A physician needs to have a very close connection with God. Never is he to lose his hold of God's helpful, strengthening power. He is to drink deeply of the water of life, and then lead others to the living stream. The fact that the physician acts so important a part in bringing relief from suffering will naturally place him where he will be regarded with feelings of love and gratitude by those whom he has helped. Let him not take the praise and glory to himself. Let him hide self in the Saviour, pointing to Christ as the One who is to receive all praise and thanksgiving. The Lord is the worker: the physician is only the instrument. "Without me," Christ declares, "ye can do nothing." He says to the faithful physician, I will stand by your side, and as you tell those for whom you work that Christ is all and in all, that He died for your sins, in order that they should not perish, but have everlasting life, it will impress their hearts.

It is that such work as this may be done that we wish to establish a sanitarium. We ask you to give us a liberal donation. A great work can be accomplished for the Lord by a well conducted sanitarium. We have demonstrated this in America. To our sanitarium in America have come lawyers, doctors, senators, {87} and judges, to be guarded day and night against the cruel appetite for alcohol, tobacco, and morphine. Eternity alone can reveal the good that has

been accomplished for them. They have gone forth to proclaim the glory of God and to do honor to His name.

We had hoped to have our sanitarium in running order ere this, but we have not received enough money to enable us to arise and build. We desire to erect a plain yet tasteful building, with roomy, well-lighted rooms. I feel so thankful that you can help us. I praise God that He has entrusted His means to some who believe the truth, who will use their talents in the Master's cause. You will receive your reward in heaven.

I have always used my money as fast as it comes in to forward the work. The word of the Lord still comes to me, Advance; add new territory to my kingdom; enter fields that have never heard the truth. Lift the standard higher and still higher. Now is the time to prepare a highway for the King.

I have just received word that a third baptismal service has been held in Maitland, and that many people are interested in the Bible readings given.

I will now close this letter, thanking you again for your willingness to help us.

Yours respectfully

DR. J. H. KELLOGG
December. 12, 1900
"Sunnyside," Cooranbong

My Dear Brother:

YOU SPEAK AS THOUGH YOU had no friends. But God is your friend, and Sister White is your friend. You have thought that I had lost confidence in you; but, my dear brother, as I have before written to you, I know that the Lord has placed you in a very responsible position, standing as you do,—a man to whom the Lord has given understanding and knowledge, that you may do justice and judgment, and reveal the true missionary spirit in the institution which is to represent truth in contrast with error.

My brother, the Lord has not left you to go on a warfare at your own charges. He has given you wisdom, and favor with God and man. He has been your helper. He has chosen you as His agent to exalt the truth in the Battle Creek Sanitarium, as it is not represented in other medical institutions. The Battle Creek Sanitarium was to be known as an institution where the Lord was daily acknowledged as the monarch of the universe. "He doeth according to his will in the army of heaven, and among the inhabitants of the earth: and none can stay his hand, or say unto him, What doest thou?"

The Lord designs that the proclamation of the third angel's message shall be the highest, greatest work carried on in our world at this time. He honored you by placing you in a very responsible position. You were not to separate your influence from the ministry of the gospel. In every line of your work you were to understand and practice the truth. You were to make God first, and ever obey His word. In this would be your strength. {88}

You were to be a faithful physician of the souls as well as of the bodies of those under your charge. Had you fulfilled this responsibility with all the keen talent God gave you in trust, you would not have worked alone. One who never makes a mistake was presiding. Only the Holy Spirit's power can keep your spirit sweet and fragrant, soft and subdued, ever trusting in God, ever speaking the right words at the right time.

You were not faultless. Often you lost control of yourself. Then your words were not what they should have been. At times you were arbitrary and exacting. But you were striving for the mastery over self, and angels of God cooperated with you, because through you, God was to work to exalt His truth, and cause it to receive honored recognition in the world. God gave you wisdom, not that your name should be magnified, but that those coming to the Sanitarium in Battle Creek might carry away with them favorable impressions of Seventh-day Adventists. The honor given you did not come to you because you were righteous above all men, but because God desired to use you as His instrument.

In His providence the Lord has drawn many to the Sanitarium that they may become acquainted with the truth, and be converted, and then carry away with them the evidence of the miraculous power of God on body and soul. This has stirred the ire of Satan. It does not please him that it should be shown that God is working to magnify the truth.

It was God's purpose that in the Sanitarium missionaries, teachers, and physicians should become acquainted with the third angel's message, which embraces so much. Angels of God were to be your strength in the work that was to be done in order that the Battle Creek Sanitarium might be known as an institution under the special supervision of God. The missionary feeling and sympathy that prevailed in this institution was a result of the work of invisible heavenly agencies there. God said, "I thought it good to show signs and wonders. In my might, I wrought to glorify my name." Many have gone away from the Sanitarium with new hearts. The change has been decided. These, returning to their homes, have been as lights in the world. Their voices have been heard saying, "Come, all ye that fear God, and I will make known to you what he hath done for my soul. I have seen his greatness, I have tasted his goodness."

The Lord has appointed the physicians in the Sanitarium to stand as faithful sentinels. Through them, God desires to do the work that must be done. Through them, impressions are to be made in regard to the work of relieving suffering humanity.

But you needed the counsel of others than your colleagues. Fresh, new ideas were needed in your councils; for not all your ideas bore the divine credentials. You have been swaying the minds of those connected with the medical missionary work, until you and others were becoming like men lost in the fog of uncertainty.

The dangers of your plan of operation in connection with the conference held in South Lancaster were presented before me. I saw that you could not plan and devise as you had been doing, or carry out your ideas, without injury to yourself and to the cause of God. I was instructed by the Lord that your temptation would be to make your medical missionary work stand independent of the Conference. But this plan was not right. You were tempted by the enemy, and I hastened to write to you. I sent a copy of the letter to Elder Irwin; {89} for it was necessary that someone besides yourself should know your danger, that efforts might be made to save you from the course of action you had premeditated.

I would help you if I could; but I do not know how to help you. I write to you as a mother would to her son. I would go to see you if I could feel it my duty to leave the work here; but I dare not do this. You have built up hopes and nurtured plans without due consideration of how the tower is to be finished and supported. As one who knows, as one who has been permitted to have an insight into the future and results of the work you have taken upon you, I call upon you to stop and consider. God knows your frame. He knows that you are dust, even the small dust of the balance. You will certainly need the counsel, not of those who have permitted you to go in the work which you deem so important, but the counsel

of men who at the present time are able to see more clearly than you do, the results that will follow various undertakings.

I wish to state, Dr. Kellogg, that if you will receive the messages of warning given you, it will save you from great trial and mortification, and will be to the saving of your soul. Cast not behind you as of no consequence the warnings which as yet you do not understand. I tell you plainly that you are carrying forward that which you call missionary work according to misconceived judgment and opinions. The Sanitarium will suffer because you have given yourself up to do a work for which God will call you to account, saying, "Who hath required this at your hands?" I have been instructed that you have been doing a variety of work which the Lord has never appointed you to do. Means have been drawn from the Sanitarium to erect buildings for the care of people who can never be relied on to fill places as reliable men in the ministry or on councils. They have not a knowledge of the work to be done in these last days in character-building, and they cannot be relied on as men of forethought. They have ruined their mental powers and nearly destroyed their spiritual discernment by the indulgence of appetite and passion, and this makes them weak. They are fickle and changeable.

The Lord has shown me that if the enemy can by any means divert the work into wrong channels, and thus hinder its advancement, he will do so. The place assigned you by the Lord was under Him in the divine Theocracy. You were to learn of Jesus, the great Teacher. You were to be and do after His character and example.

I have been forced to inquire why several of our canvassers in this field, who were canvassing for the Home Hand Book, have left the field having only paid their expenses. Some did not even do this. They stated that when the time came for them to deliver their books, they could not obtain copies to deliver. They were themselves greatly disappointed, and the people who were expecting the book were also disappointed. What shall we do about this? I have talked to the men in the Echo Office about it, and they say that they cannot obtain copies of The Home Hand Book.

At every camp meeting, we make special efforts to get before the people the light upon health reform, as contained in your publications. But while you have been consuming you have not been producing. Never was there a time when a

greater interest was shown in regard to questions relating to health. What is it that hinders your books from being supplied to our offices, to be furnished to the canvassers? Shall this delay continue? Shall the people still be disappointed? {90}

I have been instructed to say that you have drawn your time and strength and money away from enterprises which if they had been advanced, would have done tenfold more good than the enterprises that you have carried forward. Invention after invention has taken your time and means. Your money has been used in a way which has done more harm than good. The setting of men to work in various ways in what is called medical missionary work has consumed much time and money, but has produced next to nothing. The Lord entrusted capital to you, to be used in advancing His kingdom in our world, and if you misuse this capital, you must settle with Him.

Investments have been made without sitting down and counting the cost, without finding out whether there was enough money to carry forward the work started. A short-sightedness has been shown. Men have failed to see that the Lord's vineyard embraces the world. There is such a thing as investing in that which it is hard to say is not a good work, because explanation cannot always be made to the one whose brain has been constantly at work to create and invent, but who has not the income to sustain the enterprises started.

The income of the Sanitariums that have been established must not be drawn upon to sustain the work called medical missionary work. The means that has been used to sustain this large and ever-increasing work should, by the Lord's order, have been used in making plants in other countries, where the light of health reform has not shone. Sanitariums, less costly than the large ones erected in America, should have been built. Thus plants would have been made which would have produced fruit, and when strong, would have established plants in other localities.

The Lord is not partial. But He has been misrepresented. The work that should have been done in the different parts of His vineyard has been hindered because men have failed to see how the work could be advanced in these parts of the vineyard. In some parts the work has been overdone. In this way, money has been absorbed that should have been used to enable workers in other parts of the vineyard to move forward without hindrance in the work of elevating the standard of truth. Some portions of the vineyard are not to be robbed in order that the means may be absorbed in one spot.

Man judges in accordance with his finite judgment. God looks at the character of the fruit borne, and then judges the tree. In the name of the Lord, I call upon all to think of the work we are required to do, and how this work is to be sustained. The world is the Lord's vineyard, and it is to be worked. Suppose in every place where there is a large center, the work which has been done in America should be made the pattern. Where would be our memorials of truth, which are to make a proper impression on the world?

There are those who are in danger of bringing into the work the objectionable sentiments received in former education. They need to practice the principles laid down in the Word, else the work will be marred and spoiled by their preconceived ideas. When we work with all the sanctified ability God has given us, when we put aside our will for the will of God, when self is crucified day by day, then actual results are seen. We move forward in faith, knowing that our Lord has promised to undertake the work entrusted to Him, and that He will accomplish it; for He never makes a failure.

The Lord's servants are merely stewards. The Lord will work through them {91} when they surrender themselves to Him to be worked by the Holy Spirit. When by faith men place themselves in the Lord's hands, saying, "Here am I; send me," He undertakes this work. But men must get out of the Lord's way. They must not hinder His purposes by their devising. For years the Lord has had a controversy with His people because they have followed their own judgment, and have not relied on divine wisdom. If the workers get in God's way, hindering the advancement of the work, thinking that their brain power is sufficient for the planning and carrying forward of the work, the Lord will correct their error. By His divine spirit He enlightens and trains every worker. He shapes His own providences to carry forward His work according to His mind and judgment.

If men would only humble themselves before God, if they would not exalt their judgment as the all-controlling influence, if they would make room for the Lord to plan and work, the Lord would use the qualifications He has given them in a way which would glorify His name. He will pu-

rify His workers from all selfishness, trimming down their superfluous plans, cutting off the branches that would entwine around this and that undesirable object, pruning the vine so that it will produce fruit. God is the Husbandman. He will make everything in the lives of those who are laborers together with Jesus Christ subservient to His great purpose of growth and fruit-bearing. It is His plan, by conforming His servants day by day to the image of Christ, by making them partakers of the divine nature, to cause them to bear fruit abundantly. He desires His people, through actual experience in the truth of the gospel, to become true, solid, trustworthy, experimental missionaries. He would have them show results far higher, holier, and more definite than have been revealed in the last fifteen years.

The potter takes the clay in his hands, and molds and fashions it according to his own will. He kneads it and works it. He tears it apart and then presses it together. He wets it and then dries it. He lets it lie for a while without touching it. When it is perfectly pliable, he continues the work of making from it a vessel. He forms it into shape, and on the wheel, trims and polishes it. He dries it in the sun and bakes it in the oven. Thus it becomes a vessel unto honor, fit for his use. So the great Master desires to mold and fashion us. And as the clay is in the hands of the potter, so we are to be in His hands. We are not to try to do the work of the potter. Our part is to yield ourselves to the molding of the Masterworker.

It is not a great number of institutions, large buildings, and wonderful display that God requires, but the harmonious action of a peculiar people, a people chosen by God and precious, united with one another, their life hid with Christ in God. The Lord will never place one man as a controlling power over another man. Every man is to stand in his lot and in his place, exerting a right influence in thought, word, and judgment. When all God's workers do this, and not till then, will the work be a complete, symmetrical whole. Individually, we need a solid faith, which is in perfect harmony with the first declaration of the first, second, and third angels' messages. The work that the gospel embraces as missionary work is a straightforward, substantial work, which will shine brighter and brighter unto the perfect day. God does not want the faith of His peculiar people to take on the features or appearance of the work now called medical missionary work. The means and talents of His people are not

to be buried in the slums of New York or Chicago. God's work is to be carried on in right lines. Self-denial, self-sacrifice, and the true {92} missionary spirit are to be shown. We are to work as Christ worked, in simplicity and meekness, in lowliness and sanctified moral elevation. Thus we can do a work distinct from all other missionary work in our world.

My brother, you have not as much firmness and assurance as you have had. You have the most critical cases to handle, and at times a dread comes upon you. To perform these difficult duties, you know that rapid work must be done, that no false moves must be made. Again and again you have had to pass swiftly from task to task. Who has been by your side during these critical operations? Who has kept you calm and self-possessed in the crisis, giving you quick, sharp discernment, clear eyesight, steady nerves, and skillful precision? The Lord Jesus has sent His angel to your side, to tell you what to do. A hand has been laid upon your hand. Jesus, and not you, has guided the movements of your hand. At times you have realized this, and a wonderful calmness has come over you. You dared not hurry, and yet you worked rapidly, knowing that there was not a second to waste. The Lord has greatly blessed you. Others who knew not of the presiding Presence working with you, gave you all the glory. Eminent physicians have witnessed your operations and praised your skill. This has been pleasant to you. You have not always been able to endure the seeing of the Invisible by faith. You have been under divine guidance. You have been greatly honored by God, that His name, and not yours, should be magnified. But you have had a great desire to distinguish yourself; you have not placed your entire dependence upon God. You have not been willing to heed the counsel of the Lord's servants. With your own brain, you have planned many things. The Lord would have you respect the gospel ministry. At the very time you needed discerning eyes, that you might see, not only one side of the work, but all sides, you chose for counselors, men under the reproof of God, as did Elder Olsen. If they would second your propositions, you would link up with them, to start enterprises that the Lord placed no burden on you to start.

The Lord gave you your work, not to be done in a rush, but in a calm, considerate manner. The Lord never compels hurried, complicated movements. But you have gathered to yourself responsibilities that the Lord, the merciful Father, did not place upon you. Duties He has never ordained chase each other wildly. Never are His servants to leave one given duty marred or incomplete in order to seize hold of another. He who labors in the calmness of the fear of God does not work in a haphazard manner, for fear something will hinder an anticipated plan.

Praying and seeking the Lord, the surrender of yourself to the guidance of God, would have prevented the creating of many things which have been born, not of the will of God, but of the will of man. You were given your appointed work. But you have neglected things of great importance to take up, with impulsive spirit, unadvised of the Lord or by your brethren, things of minor importance. Your brethren could have given you counsel, but you despised any word that interfered with your schemes, which have placed you in an intricate position. Had you done your appointed work, God would have made you more and more a laborer together with Him.

The Lord wants your mind to blend with other minds. His servants have sometimes attempted to differ with you. This was the very thing God required them to do. But you treated their advice in such a way that they remained silent when they should have spoken. God desires those He has placed in positions of trust as stewards not to use your brains, but the talents He has {93} given them personally. They are to do justice and judgment in all wisdom.

You do not allow men to think and act on their individual responsibility. You and Brother Haskell and Brother Butler saw the difficulties in Elder James White and the necessity of uniting together to remove responsibilities from him. If he needed this, you have come to the place where you need it tenfold more. And yet no one associated with you dares to tell you this truth.

If you are determined to carry on the same kind of warfare that you have been carrying on, straining nerve, brain, and muscle to come out ahead, and prove that the message the Lord sent was not true, you will find that your plans will be counter-worked by Him who for years has been giving you warnings.

The Lord has not laid upon you the Burdens you have been carrying. The result of your carrying these burdens is felt all through the vineyard of the Lord. God has not called His people to ignore present truth for these last days, and take up a work that so absorbs workers and means that the Lord is not represented as He would otherwise be. Never would a rival sanitarium have been, through Satan's devising, planted close to the Lord's institution, if you had kept at your work for the class of people whom the Lord desires to become through the Sanitarium acquainted with present truth, with the message God has given to those who follow Him, to be communicated to the world. The sanitarium in Battle Creek was to bring the chosen people of God before men of high standing, to represent the ways, works, and power of God. It was to be His witness in behalf of truth, elevated, sanctifying truth. The Lord made you, my brother, His honored instrument. He has never required from you one task that would crowd out your work in connection with the institution that was to stand for the truth, to do a certain work for God, flashing light upon the pathway of thousands.

The Lord would have kept the sanitarium pure and true, to represent the truth for these last days. But the very ones who could have helped you to do this work, you have despised, and turned from as unworthy of your notice. God sees that His work is being lowered into the slums, as Satan wants it to be; that the elevated sanctification of the truth will become so mingled with tares that its peculiar, holy character will sink out of sight. The Lord saw how this would be, and He has been sending you warnings. Yet you are tempted to go right on in your own way and pick flaws in the message, just as others have done before you.

You have a great and sacred work to do. If you hold faithfully to the work God has assigned you, through the skill given you, you will be enabled to work swiftly, though never appearing to be in haste. When your eyes are opened, you will see the deep poverty of the mission fields. You will see that the workers there are hampered at every step, while the Lord's money is being used to sustain other inventions and institutions, so that the message which should be given to the world, the first, second, and third angels' messages, are lost sight of.

God impresses different men to be laborers together with Him. One man is not authorized to gather too many responsibilities upon himself. The Lord would have the physician, upon whom so much depends, so closely connected with Him, that his spirit will not be stirred by little things. The Lord desires Dr. Kellogg to be one of the most efficient workers in the medical profession, {94} slurring nothing, marring nothing, knowing that he has a Counselor close by his side, to sustain, to strengthen, to impart a quietness and calm to the soul. Feverishness of spirit and uncertainty will make the hand unskillful. The touch of Christ upon the physician's hand brings vitality, restfulness, confidence, and power.

God desires His institutions and His chosen and adopted children to do Him honor by representing the attributes of Christian character. Many of those who are supposed to be rescued from the pit into which they have fallen cannot be relied upon as counselors, as those who can be trusted to engage in the sacred work done in these last days. The enemy is determined to mix error with truth. To do this, he uses the opportunity given him by the debased class for whom so much money is expended, whose appetites have been perverted through indulgence, whose souls have been abused, whose characters are misshapen and deformed, whose habits and desires are groveling, who think habitually of evil. Such ones can be transformed in character; but few ever are. Many make a superficial change in their habits and practices, and then suppose that they are Christians. They are received into church fellowship; but they are a great trouble and a great care. Through them, Satan tries to sow in the church the seeds of jealousy, dishonesty, criticism, and accusing. Thus he tries to corrupt the other members of the church. The same disposition that mastered the man from childhood, led him to break away from all restraint, and brought him into the place where he was found. He is reported to be rescued. But time shows that the work done for him did not make him a submissive child of God. Resentful feelings rise at every supposed slight. He cherishes bitterness, wrath, malice. By his words and spirit, he shows that he has not been born again. His tendencies are downward, tending to sensuality. He is untrustworthy, unthankful, and unholy. Thus it is with all the debased who have not been soundly converted. Every one of these marred characters, untransformed, becomes an efficient worker for Satan, creating dissension and strife.

The Lord has marked out His way of working. As a people we are not to imitate and fall in with the Salvation Army methods. This is not the work the Lord has given us to do. Neither is it our work to condemn them and speak harsh words against them. There are precious, self-sacrificing souls in the Salvation Army. We are to treat them kindly. There are in the Army honest souls, sincerely serving the Lord, who will see greater light, and advance to the acceptance of all truth. Those in the Salvation Army are trying to save the neglected, down-trodden ones. Discourage them not. Let them do that class of work by their own methods and in their own way. The Lord has plainly stated what Seventh-day Adventists are to do. Camp meetings are to be appointed and a series of tent meetings held. All who can should work in connection with the camp meeting. There should be no hesitancy in preaching the truth applicable for this time. A decided testimony is to be borne. The discourses should be so simple that children can understand them. {95}

To the General Conference Committee and the Medical Missionary Board

August 11, 1902
"Elmshaven," Sanitarium, Calif.

Dear Brethren:

A WONDERFUL WORK COULD have been done for the vast company gathered in Battle Creek at the General Conference of 1901, if the leaders of our work had taken themselves in hand. Had thorough work been done at this conference; had there been, as God designed there should be, a breaking up of the fallow ground of the heart by the men who had been bearing responsibilities; had they, in humility of soul, led out in the work of confession and consecration, giving evidence that they received the counsels and warnings sent by the Lord to correct their mistakes, there would have been of the greatest revivals that there has been since the day of Pentecost.

But the work that all heaven was waiting to do as soon as men prepared the way, was not done; for the leaders in the work closed and bolted the door against the Spirit's entrance. There was a stopping short of entire surrender to God. Hearts that might have been purified from error were strengthened in wrong doing. The doors were barred against the heavenly current that would have swept away all evil. Men left their sins unconfessed. They built themselves up in their wrong doing,

and said to the Spirit of God, "Go thy way for this time; when I have a more convenient season, I will call for thee."

The Lord calls for the close self-examination to be made now that was not made at the last General Conference, when He was waiting to be gracious. The present is our sowing time for eternity. We must reap the fruit of the evil seed we sow, unless we repent the sowing, and ask forgiveness for the mistakes we have made. Those who, given opportunity to repent and reform, pass over the ground without humbling the heart before God, without putting away that which He reproves, will become hardened against the counsel of the Lord Jesus.

"The Lord, whom ye seek, shall suddenly come to his temple. . . Who may abide the day of his coming? and who shall stand when he appeareth? for he is like a refiner's fire, and like fullers' soap: and he shall sit as a refiner and purifier of silver." Soon every man will be judged according to his deeds. Wake up, my brethren, before Christ comes to your name in the record books of heaven, and passes judgment upon every unchristlike word and deed.

"Sunnyside," Cooranbong, N.S.W.

July 18, 1897

W E HAVE FELT DEEPLY OVER the condition of the young men who seem to have little sense of propriety in their association with one another. To be useful, companionable, and cheerful, is your privilege. But this hilarity and wicked nonsense is degrading to young men who have been given the talent of reason. Day after day you listen to the most solemn appeals from the word of God, and you reveal that you care nothing for truth or righteousness. But God lives and reigns, and from this time I bear a message to you from Him: Your course of action is an offense to Him. Even if there were a greater number associated together, this is no excuse for your low, cheap, common conversation and {96} heedless frivolity. The atmosphere surrounding your soul is malarious. You grieve away from the school the Holy Spirit.

The whole school, Principal and teachers, are regarded as guilty before God of your misdemeanors, which are apparent. You show that you have no respect for the word of God, no respect for your teachers or for the Principal of the school. This school was not established at great ex-

pense, and the rates of tuition placed at a very low figure, to accommodate a class of students who ought to know how to behave like gentlemen, if not for the credit of the school, for their own sakes, but who dishonor themselves and their Maker. This matter has been presented to me, and I cannot keep silent. If the teachers have not given decided commands, it is time that they did, that the respectability and credit of the school may be maintained. The Lord makes principal and teachers responsible for their students. But who is sufficient to assume the office of guide to a company of youth who are here, it is understood, to be instructed, and to behave like gentlemen and Christians, but who do not do this; they cannot; for they do not know what the name of Christian comprehends. They do not know what it means to love God, and to wear the yoke that restrains them from evil practices.

You each have capabilities. These have been entrusted to you by God. You are to wisely improve the talents lent you to serve and glorify Him. God knows you all by name; and your every transaction, your every word, is written in His books. This record you must meet in the day of judgment. A burden of responsibility rests upon you to help with all your God-given ability in making this school such as will meet the approval of God. But we have not established the school to be a place where students are permitted to give loose reign to their own ways and objectionable traits of character. If you do not and will not consent to be under control and behave yourselves as gentlemen, you have the privilege of returning to your homes. After we find that the school is of no benefit to you, we will arrange for you to leave by writing to your parents and friends, and those who have arranged for you to come, telling them the reason why you are sent home.

We want students to come to this school who will not disappoint their parents and friends, so that at the close of the term the humiliating fact will not have to be made known that a few who were heady, high-minded, lovers of pleasure more than lovers of God, took the lead, and the leaven of their spirit so influenced others that many were leavened. We established this school that this disorderly, insubordinate element should be placed under discipline and under obedience to the word of God, that the students might know how to value and respect themselves and realize that they did not come to school to do as they pleased, but to place themselves under the yoke of restraint and obedience.

No disorder should have been allowed without a decided rebuke and command to cease. It would not be allowed even in the common schools. The principal and teachers of the school have not authority and government sufficient to set things in order. Someone should take the management who will require obedience. It has been one desire that these young men should respect themselves, that they should seek to make the most of the opportunity given them to receive an all-round education, that they might be thoroughly equipped for the life-work before them. {97}

The truth of God is to give shape to each distinct branch of education; but shall the truth of God be of no account because its influence is not recognized by a few who lead, and who are rioters and tempters? Satan works his will through them, so that the truth is made a common thing. But should this be? There are those who prize these privileges of hearing the truth from the word of God, but are counteracted by the influence of those who have not cared and who do not care to be on the Lord's side. We desire that every youth shall realize the importance of the truth. We cannot countenance any frivolity. Those who give way to this are being educated under Satan's dictation, and this we cannot allow in the school.

Opportunity is here given for all to make valuable acquisition to their stock of knowledge by improving their talents. Now is the time for you to make your decision. What are you here for? Did you think that when you came, you would be allowed to act independently of all restraint? What are you here for? Are you here to improve, to become more retentive, that your mental, moral, and physical powers may become more susceptible of improvement? Every movement made by the teachers leaves its impression on the youth. The countenances upon which the students look, the voices they hear, the words they speak, the company they keep, the books they peruse, leave their impress on the mind, either preparing it to be useful in this world, with a prospect of being exalted to the higher school, or marring its chance of eternal life.

If one who is heedless and unappreciative of truth is associated with those who profess to be followers of Jesus Christ, he is to behave himself as a gentleman, remembering that it is inappropriate and unfair for him to jest and joke and make remarks that are calculated to divert the mind from pure and holy meditation. Thus one sinner can do much harm, even though he claims, and is thought, to be a saint. Profession is nothing. Faith without works is dead, being alone.

In the name of Jesus Christ of Nazareth, I ask, Who in this school is on the Lord's side? Who will stand as faithful soldiers of Jesus Christ, refusing to allow Jesus to be denied and lightly regarded in their company? Because you are in the company of some who do not cultivate the superior qualities of character that constitute Christian gentlemen, but jest and joke, do not follow their example. Some use strange words, that are unbecoming for any who attend the school. Who will maintain their Christian principles? Who will frown down this lawless, riotous, godless spirit, which has been tolerated, but which has greatly displeased God, and which has effaced the impression made upon human hearts by the Spirit of God?

Daily there is opened before you the divinely-inspired word of God. The truth of God is precious. Let no irreverent, careless, heedless spirit be imbibed. Just as soon as we understand from the Spirit of God that harm is being done to the minds of those who wish to preserve sobriety and to receive good in the place of evil, an effort should be made to counteract the wrong. Our duty is plain. That class who will not take heed how they hear and how they speak, who allow the enemy to lead them whichever way he chooses, that he may use them as his agents, should be allowed to leave the school, and associate with the society they choose. They are not inclined to be pure, uncorrupted, refined, and elevated. They will not get good themselves if their minds are set not to be benefited by the light; and to keep among the students one who is not getting good himself, but who is an agent for evil, would be very unwise. {98}

We would feel sad should anyone choose to pursue such a course, but it is the duty of the principal and teachers to demand perfect order and perfect discipline. Teachers are to blend in harmony in this matter. Those teachers who do not see the necessity of maintaining the rules that it is deemed essential to make, have simply made a mistake in thinking they were prepared to teach, and accepting the situation. One imprudent word or action from a teacher would counter-work the object or purpose of the school, and would also be injurious to their own present and eternal good; and the sooner such teachers resign the position of teacher and become learners, the better it will be for the future of the school. No experiments should be made in this matter, for it is too dangerous a business. He who attempts to teach should be connected with Christ, wearing His yoke of restraint himself, that he may be an example to the students.

The Lord has signified that the atmosphere surrounding the souls of the students must change. The truths of the word of God demand the most serious attention. This truth is not to be lightly regarded or trifled with. Our duties and privileges are not to be measured by the lightness or frivolity of anyone. The Bible is to be followed as God's word, inspired by heaven. Its revealed facts, which are of the most awful importance to teachers and students, are not to be lightly regarded. Its requirements are not to be tramped upon; for they impose the most weighty obligations. In the rich promises, the consolation of God is presented to those who wear the yoke of restraint and obedience; but those who refuse to wear this yoke will find their course of action bring its own punishment.

Trivial characters must be changed. They must be converted, and receive the new heart that God has promised. In this work they must go to the word of God for guidance. "All Scripture is given by inspiration of God, and is profitable for doctrine, for reproof, for correction, for instruction in righteousness: that the man of God may be perfect, thoroughly furnished unto all good works." Teachers, as well as students, need to learn each day from the word of God, which is the man of our counsel. It never makes a mistake. Its teaching will perfect in each individual a character that God can approve. It is the voice of God speaking to the soul.

The youth may all be workers together with God in the school if they will cherish every amiable trait of character. The darkened understanding may be enlightened by the bright beams of the Sun of Righteousness. All who will heed the instruction given in the word of God may perfect a character after the similitude of the character of Christ.

If some continue, as they have been doing, to speak idle, foolish, and — I am sorry to say — profane words, they will block the way to their advancement. "Obey them that have the rule over you, and submit yourselves for they watch for your souls, as they that must give account, that they may do it with joy, and not with grief: for that is unprofitable for you." Teachers have a responsibility that they do not sense as they should. As they see the spirit that is working in the children of disobedience, they have perplexity and heartache. They do not want to appear harsh and severe; but unless they watch for souls as they that must give account, unless they are faithful and true to their trust, they will prove themselves to be unfaithful stewards. Students, you can make it hard for them. By your conduct you can cause them sadness of heart as they carry the terrible load of responsibility, while you go on, {99} heedless and careless; or you can help your teachers to help you to advance in a knowledge of Christian obligations. Thus you can make this school one of the best that has ever been held. It rests with you to decide whether you will be thought unworthy and unfit to remain in the school, or whether you will be an ornament to it. One thing cannot be allowed. The rooms that have been dedicated to God must not be defiled by your improper conversation and lawless course of action. Let all heed the words spoken to the Hebrews: "Wherefore lift up the hands which hang down, and the feeble knees; and make straight paths for your feet, lest that which is lame be turned out of the way; but let it rather be healed. Follow peace with all men, and holiness, without which no man shall see the Lord: looking diligently lest any man fail of the grace of God: lest any root of bitterness springing up trouble you, and thereby many be defiled."

The charge given to Timothy, is given to each of you: "For therefore we both labor and suffer reproach, because we trust in the living God, who is the Saviour of all men, specially of those that believe. These things command and teach. Let no man despise thy youth; but be thou an example of the believers, in word, in conversation, in charity, in spirit, in faith, in purity." "Young men likewise exhort to be sober-minded. In all things showing thyself a pattern of good works: in doctrine showing uncorruptness, gravity, sincerity, sound speech, that cannot be condemned; that he that is of the contrary part may be ashamed, having no evil thing to say of you. Exhort servants to be obedient unto their own masters, and to please them well in all things; not answering again; not purloining, but showing all good fidelity; that

they may adorn the doctrine of God our Saviour in all things. For the grace of God that bringeth salvation hath appeared to all men, teaching us that, denying ungodliness and worldly lusts, we should live soberly, righteously, and godly, in this present world; looking for that blessed hope, and the glorious appearing of the great God and our Saviour Jesus Christ; who gave himself for us, that he might redeem us from all iniquity, and purify unto himself a peculiar people, zealous of good works.

THE MEDICAL MISSIONARY WORK AND GOSPEL MINISTRY

[Prior to July 1915]

AS THE MEDICAL MISSIONARY work becomes more extended, there will be a temptation to make it independent of our conferences. But it has been presented to me that this plan is not right. The different lines of our work are but parts of one great whole. They have one center.

In Colossians we read, "The body is of Christ. Let no man beguile you of your reward in a voluntary humility and worshipping of angels, intruding into those things which he hath not seen, vainly puffed up by his fleshly mind, and not holding the Head, from which all the body by joints and bands having nourishment ministered, and knit together, increaseth with the increase of God." Colossians 2:17-19. Our work in all its lines is to demonstrate the influence of the cross. The work of God in the plan of salvation is not to be done in any disjointed way. It is not to operate at random. The plan that provided the influence of the cross provided also the methods of its diffusion. This method is simple in its principles and comprehensive in its plain distinct lines. Part is connected with part in perfect order and relation. {100}

God has brought His people together in church capacity in order that they may reveal to the world the wisdom of Him who formed this organization. God knew what plans to outline for the efficiency and success of His people. Adherence to these plans will enable them to testify of the divine authorship of God's great plan for the restoration of the world.

Those who take part in God's work are to be led and guided by God. Every human ambition is to be submerged in Jesus Christ, who is head over all the institutions that God has established. He knows how

to set in operation His own agencies. He knows that the cross must occupy the central place, because it is the means of man's atonement, and because of the influence it exerts on every part of the divine government. The Lord Jesus, who has been through all the history of our world, understands the methods that should be invested with power over human minds. He knows the importance of every agency, and understands how the varied agencies should be related to one another.

"None of us liveth to himself." Romans 14:7. This is a law of God in heaven and on earth. God is the great center. From Him all life proceeds. To Him all service, homage and allegiance belong. For all created beings there is the same great principle of life—dependence upon and co-operation with God. The relationship existing in the pure family of God in heaven was to exist in the family of God on earth. Under God, Adam was to stand at the head of the earthly family, to maintain the principles of the heavenly family. This would have brought peace and happiness. But the law that none liveth to himself Satan was determined to oppose, He desired to live for self. He sought to make himself a center of influence. It was this that brought rebellion in heaven, and it was man's acceptance of this principle that brought sin on earth. When Adam sinned, man broke away from the heaven-ordained center. A demon became the central power in the world. Where God's throne should have been, Satan had placed his throne. The world laid its homage, as a willing offering, at the feet of the enemy.

Who could bring in the principles ordained by God in His rule and government to counterwork the plans of Satan, to bring the world back to its loyalty? God said, I will send My Son. "God so loved the world that he gave his only begotten son that whosoever believeth in him should not perish but have everlasting life." John 3:16. This is the remedy for sin. Christ says, Where Satan has set his throng there shall stand My cross. Satan shall be cast out, and I will be lifted up to draw all men unto Me. I will become the center of the redeemed world. The Lord shall be exalted. Those who are now controlled by human ambition, human passions, shall become workers for Me. Evil influences have conspired to counterwork all good. They have confederated to make men think it righteous to oppose the law of Jehovah. But My army shall meet in conflict with the Satanic force. My Spirit shall combine with every heavenly agency to oppose them. I will engage every sanctified human agency in the universe. None of My agencies are to be absent. I work for all who love Me. I have employment for every soul who will work under my direction. The activity of Satan's army, the danger that surrounds the human soul, call for the energies of every worker. But no compulsion shall be exercised. Man's depravity is to be met by the love, the patience, the long-suffering of God. My work shall be to save those who are under Satan's rule.

Through Christ, God works to bring man back to his first relation to his Creator, and to correct the disorganizing influences brought in by Satan. {101} Christ alone stood unpolluted in a world of selfishness, where men would destroy a friend or brother in order to accomplish a scheme put into their minds by Satan. Christ came to our world, clothing His divinity with humanity, that humanity might touch humanity, and divinity grasp divinity. Amid the din of selfishness He could say to men, Return to your center, God. He Himself made it possible for man to do this by carrying out in this world the principles of heaven. In humanity He lived the law of God. To men in every nation, every country, every clime, He will impart heaven's choicest gifts if they will accept God as their Creator and Christ as their Redeemer.

Christ alone can do this. His gospel, in the hearts and hands of His followers, is the power which is to accomplish His great work. "O the depth of the riches both of the wisdom and knowledge of God!" Romans 11:33. Christ made it possible for the work of redemption to be accomplished by Himself becoming subject to Satan's misrepresentations. Thus was Satan to show himself to be the cause of disloyalty in God's universe. Thus was to be forever settled the great controversy between Christ and Satan.

Satan strengthens the destructive tendencies of man's nature. He brings in envy, jealousy, selfishness, covetousness, emulation, and strife for the highest place. Evil agencies act their part through the devising of Satan. Thus the enemy's plans, with their destructive tendencies, have been brought into the church. Christ comes with His own redeeming influence proposing through the agency of His Spirit to impart His Spirit to impart His efficiency to men, and to

employ them as His instrumentalities, laborers together with Him in seeking to draw the world back to its loyalty.

Men are bound in fellowship, independence, to one another. By the golden links of the chain of love they are to be found fast to the throne of God. This can be done only by Christ's imparting to finite man the attributes which man would have ever possessed had he remained loyal and true to God.

Those who, through an intelligent understanding of the Scriptures, view the cross aright, those who truly believe in Jesus, have a sure foundation for their faith. They have that faith which works by love and purifies the soul from all its hereditary and cultivated imperfections.

God has united believers in church capacity in order that one may strengthen another in good and righteous endeavor. The church on earth would indeed be a symbol of the church in heaven if the members were of one mind and one faith. It is those who are not worked by the Holy Spirit that mar God's plan. Another spirit takes possession of them and they help to strengthen the forces of darkness. Those who are sanctified by the precious blood of Christ will not become the means of counter-working the great plan which God Himself has devised. They will not bring human depravity into things small or great. They will not do anything to perpetuate division in the church.

It is true there are tares among the wheat; in the body of Sabbathkeepers evils are seen; but because of this shall we disparage the church? Shall not the managers of every institution, the leaders of every church take up the work of purification in such a way that the transformation in the church shall make it a bright light in a dark place? {102}

What may not even one believer be in the exercise of pure, heavenly principles if he refuses to be contaminated, if he will stand as firm as a rock to a "Thus saith the Lord?" Angels of God will come to his help, preparing the way before him.

Paul wrote to the Romans, "I beseech you, therefore, brethren, by the mercies of God, that ye present your bodies a living sacrifice, holy, acceptable unto God, which is your reasonable service. And be not conformed to this world, but be ye transformed by the renewing of your mind, that ye may prove what is that good and acceptable and perfect will of God." Romans 12:1, 2. This entire chapter is a lesson which I entreat all

who claim to be members of the body of Christ to study.

Again, Paul writes, "If the first fruits be holy, the lump is also holy; and if the fruit be holy so are the branches. And if some of the branches be broken off, and thou, being a wild olive tree, were grafted in among them, and with them partaketh of the root and fatness of the olive tree, boast not against the branches, but if thou boast, thou bearest not the root, but the root thee. Thou wilt say then, The branches were broken off that I might be grafted in. Well, because of unbelief they were broken off, and thou standest by faith. Be not high minded, but fear; for if God spared not the natural branches, take heed lest he also spare not thee. Behold therefore the goodness and severity of God, on them which fell, severity, but toward thee, goodness, if thou continue in His goodness; otherwise thou also shall be cut off." Romans 11:16-22. Very plainly these words show that there is to be no disparaging of the agencies which God has placed in the church.

Sanctified ministry calls for self-denial. The cross must be uplifted, and its place in the gospel work shown. Human influence is to draw its efficacy from the One who is able to save and to keep saved all who recognize their dependence upon him. By the union of church members with Christ and with one another, the transforming power of the gospel is to be diffused throughout the world.

In the work of the gospel the Lord uses different instrumentalities, and nothing is to be allowed to separate these instrumentalities. Never should a Sanitarium be established as an enterprise independent of the church. Our physicians are to unite with the work of the ministry of the gospel. Through their labors, souls are to be saved, that the name of God may be magnified.

Medical missionary work is in no case to be divorced from the gospel ministry. The Lord has specified that the two shall be as closely connected as the arm is connected with the body. Without this union, neither part of the work is complete. The medical missionary work is the gospel in illustration.

But God did not design that the medical missionary work should eclipse the work of the third angels message. The arm is not to become the body. The third angel's message is the Gospel message for these last days, and in no case is it to be overshadowed by other interests and made to appear as an unessential consideration. When in our institutions anything is placed above the third angel's message, the gospel is not there, the great leading power. {103}

The cross is the center of all religious institutions. These institutions are to be under the control of the spirit of God; in no institution is any one man to be the sole head. The divine mind has men for every place.

Through the power of the holy spirit, every work of God's appointment is to be elevated and ennobled, and made to witness for the Lord. Man must place himself under the control of the eternal mind, whose dictates he is to obey in every particular.

Let us seek to understand our privilege of walking and working with God. The gospel, though it contains God's expressed will, is of no value to men, high or low, rich or poor, unless they place themselves in subjection to God. He who bears to his fellowmen the remedy for sin, must first be worked himself with the spirit of God. He must not ply the oars unless he is under divine direction. He cannot work effectually, he cannot carry out the will of God in harmony with the divine mind, unless he finds out, not from human sources, but from infinite wisdom, that God is pleased with his plans.

God's benevolent design embraces every branch of his work. The law of reciprocal dependence and influence is to be recognized and obeyed. None of us liveth to himself." The enemy has used the chain of dependence to draw men together. They have united to destroy God's image in man. To counter work the gospel by perverting its principles. They are represented in God's word as being bound up in bundles to be burned. Satan is uniting his forces for perdition. The unity of God's chosen people has been terribly shaken. God presents a remedy. This remedy is not one influence among many influences, and on the same level with them: it is an influence above all influences upon the face of the earth, corrective, uplifting and ennobling. Those who work in the Gospel should be elevated and sanctified; they are dealing with God's great principles. Yoked up with Christ, they are laborers together with God. Thus the Lord will bind His followers together, that they may be a power for good, each acting his part, yet all cherishing the sacred principles of dependence on the Great Head.

THE KRESS COLLECTION

[Counsel for Young Ministers]

January 22, 1900

LET OUR MINISTERS consecrate themselves to God. We need so much, O so much! humble men, who feel it a pleasure to do their very best. A glorious gospel work opens before the converted, faithful minister. He is to help his fellow men to a better understanding of the Word. The influence exerted by the minister with whom God works is weighty and momentous. The Lord is highly pleased with the minister who works humbly and willingly. Those who are wholly consecrated to God will ever seek wisdom from on high to enable them to bear their heavy responsibilities. They will be patient, forbearing, courteous, knowing that they are Christ's representatives. They will show a deep earnestness and fervor in prayer and in their appeals to individuals and congregations.

There are in the ministry young men who have been receiving wages from the conference, yet whose labors bring nothing in, who are only consumers. I have been instructed that this need not be. It would not be if our young ministers were worked by the spirit of God.

Some of our ministers might better stop and consider. Let them ask themselves how much they have received from the conference, and how much their {104} labors have been blessed in the conversion of souls. If you are not producers as well as consumers, what is the value of your work? How can the cause of God sustain as workers those who are not sanctified by the truth? Begin at the beginning of this year to consecrate yourselves to God. Wait not. Make an entire surrender.

Should not our ministers study this question? Many of our young ministers, if truly converted, would do much good by entering the canvassing field. They would there obtain an experience in faith. Their knowledge of the Scriptures would greatly increase, because as they imparted to others the light given them, they would receive more to impart. Let them enter the canvassing fields, and see what they can do in the way of producing. By meeting people and presenting to them our publications, they will gain an experience which they would not gain by simply preaching. As they go from house to house, they can converse with those whom they meet, carrying with them the

---

fragrance of Christ's life.

The faithful, youthful Timothy was taught by experienced men of God's appointment how to read the Word and how to explain it to others. Paul, his father in the gospel, addressed him in the words, "Thou therefore, my son, be strong in the grace that is in Christ Jesus. And the things that thou hast heard of me among many witnesses, the same commit thou to faithful men, who shall be able to teach others also. Thou therefore endure hardness, as a good soldier of Jesus Christ."

It is the canvasser's duty to cultivate the talents God has given him, to maintain his connection with God, to help always where he can. He has positive and constant need of the angelic ministration; for he has an important work to do, a work that he cannot do in his own strength. Thanks be unto God which always causeth us to triumph through our Lord Jesus Christ, and maketh manifest the savor of his knowledge by us in every place. For we are unto God as a sweet savor in Christ, in them that are saved and in them that perish. To the one we are a savor of death unto death; and to the other the savor of life unto life. And who is sufficient for these things?"

In his work the canvasser will be brought in contact with those who are in feeble health, who need the light on health reform, and with those who are dissatisfied with their religious experience, who are longing for something which they have not. To these he is to open the word of truth, rightly interpreting its meaning. "For we are not as many who corrupt the word of God, but as of sincerity, but as of God, in the sight of God speak we in Christ."

Ever remember that there are those who teach for doctrine the commandments of men. They make void the law of God by their traditions, like the Pharisees whom Christ exposed, saying, "Ye do err, not knowing the Scriptures, nor the power of God." The precious gems of truth are buried beneath a mass of error. By the sophistry of religious teachers the meaning of the plain, clear word of God is hidden. The people are left in perplexity.

By his work, the converted, consecrated canvasser is sowing the seeds of truth. This work must be done without delay; for we have but a short time in which to work. Everything that can be done to reach the people must be done. Speak to them in a way that will win their confidence. Pray for the sick. Ask {105} the Lord to restore and heal suffering humanity. He has declared, "These signs shall follow them that believe."

Men and women are wandering in the mist and fog of error. They want to know what is truth. Tell them; not in high-flown language, but with the simplicity of children of God. Satan is on your track. He is an artful opponent, and the malignant spirit which you meet in your work, is inspired by him. Those whom he controls echo his words. If the vail should be rent away from our eyes, those thus worked would see Satan plying all his arts to win them from the truth. There are those who do not believe in the personality of Satan. These do not oppose his work in their hearts. They are ignorant of his devices.

Instead of becoming like the world, we are to become more and more distinct from the world. Satan has combined and will continue to combine with the churches in making a masterly effort against the truth of God. Everything that is done by God's people to make inroads upon the world will call forth determined opposition from the powers of darkness. The enemy's last great conflict will be a most determined one. It will be the last battle between the powers of darkness and the powers of light. Every true child of God will fight bravely on the side of Christ. Those who in this great crisis allow themselves to be more on the side of the world than of God, will eventually place themselves wholly on the side of the world. Those who become confused in their understanding of the word, who fail to see the meaning of antichrist, will surely place themselves on the side of antichrist. There is no time now for us to assimilate with the world. Daniel is standing in his lot and in his place. The prophecies of Daniel and of John are to be understood. They interpret each other. They give to the world truths which everyone should understand. These prophecies are to be witness in the world. By their fulfillment in these last days, they will explain themselves.

The Lord is about to punish the world for its iniquity. He is about to punish religious bodies for their rejection of the light and truth which has been given them. The great message, combining the first, second, and third angel's messages, is to be given to the world. This is to be the burden of our work. Those who truly believe in Christ will openly conform to the law of Jehovah. The Sabbath is the sign between God and His people, and we are to make visible our conformity to the law of God by observing the Sabbath. It is to be the mark of distinction between God's chosen people and the world. It means much to be true to God. This embraces health reform. It means that our diet must be simple, that we must be temperate in all things. The many varieties of food so often seen on tables is not necessary, but highly injurious. Mind and body are to be preserved in the best condition of health. Only those who have been trained in the knowledge and fear of God should be chosen to take responsibilities. Those who have been long in the truth, yet who cannot distinguish between the pure principles of righteousness and the principles of evil, whose understanding in regard to justice, mercy, and the love of God is beclouded, should be relieved of responsibility.

God has important lessons for his people to learn. Had these lessons been learned before, his cause would not be where it is today. One thing must be done. The truth is not to be withheld from ministers or men in positions of responsibility for fear of incurring their displeasure. There are to be {106} connected with our institutions men who with meekness and in wisdom will declare the whole counsel of God. God's wrath is kindled against those who in carnal security and price have shown contempt for his management. They are endangering the prosperity of the cause.

Every false way is a deception, and if sustained, will in the end bring destruction. Thus the Lord permits those who maintain false plans to be destroyed. At the very time when praise and adulation is heard, sudden destruction comes. There are those who, notwithstanding they know of the reproof received by others, because of unfaithfulness, turn away from admonition. These are doubly guilty. They knew the Lord's will and did it not. Their punishment will be proportionate to their guilt. They would not take heed to the word of the Lord.

ELDERS JONES, WILCOX, AND IRWIN

April 18, 1900
"Sunnyside," Cooranbong

Dear Brethren:

IT IS NOT ALWAYS BEST TO MEET the Sunday question in Parliament or among a large crowd of people, where are talented men and women who are moved by a power from beneath, inspired with Satan's venomous spirit. When the Seventh-day Adventists at the heart of the work show uncorrupted principles, when the word of God, straight as an arrow, goes to the mark to kill the unjust and unholy principles which are so displeasing to the Lord, the God can bless his people. But God's favor will not be restored until decided work is done to cleanse our institutions from the evils existing in them. When this work is done, it will be shown by the softening, subduing influence of the Spirit of God, which will teach men how to use pen and voice with the eloquence Christ had when He was upon this earth. But stay your pen and voice in judging and condemning others until that work is accomplished which God would have done in our very midst, lest the leprosy of Gehazi come upon the cause because of those who while handling sacred things are mingling the sacred and the common.

God is dishonored, and the whole work is marred and retarded; for God will not serve with man's selfishness and unholy principles. Let Jesus come in and cleanse the temple from all fraud and injustice. Then we shall know how to work for such bodies as the Women's Christian Temperance Union.

Please read the nineteenth chapter of first Kings. "Jezebel sent a message unto Elijah, saying, So let the gods do by me and more also if I make not thy life like the life of one of them tomorrow about this time. And when he saw that, he arose, and went for his life, and came to Beersheba, which belongeth unto Judah."

However bold and successful and courageous the people of God may have been in doing a special work, unless they constantly look to God and continue to have confidence in the work he has given them, they will lose their courage. After God has given them a wonderful revelation of his power, bracing them up to do {107} his work, circumstances will arise to test their faith, and they will fail unless they trust implicitly in the Lord.

Thus it was with Elijah. He had by the help of God defeated the prophets of Baal. But he was disappointed as to the result of the manifestation of God. Under the threats of the wicked queen, he lost his courage and his faith. He lost sight of Him in whose keeping he was, and without being sent, he fled for his life. He was terribly depressed; for he had hoped much from the miracle wrought before all the people.

Had Elijah, knowing he had done the divine will, maintained his confidence in God, had he made God his refuge and strength, standing steadfast and immovable for the truth, the impression made upon the king and the people would have wrought a reformation. Elijah had been braced for trial under the inspiration of God, but when Jezebel's threatening message was brought to him, and shouted in his ear, awakening him from a deep sleep, he lost his hold on God. He had been exalted above measure, and the reaction was tremendous.

This was the time when he should have had courage in the Lord, showing a living, active faith. He should not have fled from his post of duty. God had given him a wonderful manifestation of his power to assure him that he would not forsake him, that his power was wholly sufficient to sustain him; for he was the Lord of the powers of heaven and earth.

But Elijah forgot God and fled. He went to Beersheba, and going a day's journey into the wilderness, sat down under a juniper tree. "And he requested for himself that he might die; and said, It is enough; now, O Lord, take away my life; for I am not better than my fathers. And as he lay and slept under a juniper tree, behold, an angel from Heaven touched him, and said unto him, Arise and eat. And he looked and behold there was a cake baken on the coals, and a cruise of water beside his head. And the angel of the Lord came again the second time, and touched him, and said, Arise and eat; because the journey is too great for thee."

My heart melts within me as I read the words of Holy Writ, and see the interest that the heavenly family has in the faithful servants of the Most High.

"And he arose, and did eat and drink, and went in the strength of that meat forty days and forty nights unto Horeb, the mount of God."

"And he came thither unto a cave, and lodged there; and behold, the word of the Lord came to him, and he said unto him, What doest thou here, Elijah? And he said, I have been very jealous for the Lord God of hosts; for the children of Israel have forsaken thy covenant, thrown down thine altars, and I, even I only, am left; and they seek my life to take it away."

"And he said, Go forth and stand upon the mount before the Lord. And, behold, the Lord passed by, and a great and strong wind rent the mountains, and brake in pieces the rock before the Lord; but the Lord was not in the wind; and after the wind an earthquake; but the Lord was not in the earthquake; and after the earthquake a fire; but the Lord was not in the fire; and after the fire a still, small voice. And it was so when Elijah heard it, that he wrapped his face in his mantle, and went out, and stood at the entering in of the cave."

His petulance was silenced. The Lord desired him to understand that boisterous, noisy elements are not always producers of the best results. The still small voice could subdue and soften, and accomplish great things. {108}

"And behold there came a voice unto him, and said, What doest thou here, Elijah? And he said, I have been very jealous for the Lord God of hosts; because the children of Israel have forsaken thy covenant, thrown down thine altars, and slain thy prophets with the sword; and I, even I only am left; and they seek my life, to take it away." The Lord convinced Elijah that the wrong doers would not always go unpunished. He told him to go to the land of Horeb and appoint three persons who were to fulfil the Lord's purpose in punishing idolatrous Israel. All working in different ways, these three were to avenge the controversy God had with Israel.

Then he who knows the hearts of all men corrected the impression held by Elijah that he was the only one left who was true to the worship of God. "I have left me," God said, "seven thousand in Israel, all the knees which have not bowed unto Baal, and every mouth which hath not kissed him."

The Lord desired to teach his servant that it is not the thing which makes the greatest show, the most powerful representation, that is the most successful in doing his work. It is not always the most powerful presentation, by pen or voice that accomplished the most good.

Faithful Stewardship

June 26, 1900

Unity Among Believers

I SPEAK TO THOSE WHO are acting as stewards in the cause of God. In your work for the advancement of the cause, act in such a way that the truth will be properly represented, in all its lines. The ministry is not to be given an inferior position. Those who disparage the gospel ministry give sure evidence that they have lost their spiritual discernment. They need a better understanding of the claims of God. The Lord's servants are to be given ample room to do their appointed work. As teachers of men, women, and children, they are to see and understand the work for this time.

We are all workers for the Master. The instruction given in the eighteenth chapter of Matthew shows how this work is to be done. Self is to be kept under the control of the great Teacher. Study your Bibles. I have been charged to tell you all to study your Bibles with an intense interest. Practice its teachings. When this is done, less human wisdom will be seen and more of the wisdom of God. A large amount of time and strength will be saved.

The world by wisdom knows not God. The men and women of the world do not realize that they are daily deciding their own destiny, and that it becomes them as believers in His word, to walk very softly before God. Immortality,—a life that measures with the life of God,—is not obtained through human beings, but through Christ, "who will render to every man according to his deeds; to them who by patient continuance in well doing seek for glory, and honor, eternal life."

Christians will discern Christ in their fellowmen. They will not pull apart. Strife for the supremacy is after the working of Satan. Satan was the {109} most beautiful angel in the heavenly courts, the most highly gifted, the most richly endowed. But he fell through jealousy and selfish ambition. Why, I ask, are men not afraid of themselves? Why are they so anxious to do something wonderful, something that will lead people to say, This is the work of a great man? This is all vanity. Of ourselves we are weak and helpless. If the Lord has entrusted us with capabilities, let us remember that our gifts come from God. They are lent to us by him, that by this he may test and try us. Let those who desire to win God's approval walk humbly before him. Remember that you are only one among the Lord's agents. There are others whom he recognizes and whose work he endorses.

Our institutions will be safely conducted only when those who are carrying the responsibilities in them fear their own weakness. Let them not feel highly exalted because they receive praise from men who do not see the truth in the living oracles of God. Those who know the truth should show these commandment-breakers that they regard the law of God as a savor of life unto life. All who know the truth are to honor the truth. God says, Them that honor me I will honor.

We are to respect God's faithful servants, who preach his word, and who seek to win souls to the truth. Let us not link up with unbelievers, giving them honor because we suppose that they have great wisdom . Let us not cherish their words of praise in our hearts, while at the same time we show disrespect for the Lord's chosen instruments, regarding their counsel as unworthy of our notice. Association with those who believe not the truth will prove in time of temptation a savor of death unto death.

Those who claim to believe the truth should obey the word of God just as it reads, practicing its instruction. Remember that those who love not their brethren deny the faith. Many because their brethren do not follow their leading, manifest toward them a spirit of hatred. Is their leading right? Is it wrong? God has never bidden us follow the leading of any man, and he has said, "He that saith he is in the light, and hateth his brother, is in darkness even until now. He that loveth his brother abideth in the light, and there is none occasion of a tumbling in him. But he that hateth his brother is in darkness, and walketh in darkness, and knoweth not whither he goeth, because that darkness hath blinded his eyes." Can we not see from this what it means to be at variance?

Christ declares, "I am the light of the world; he that followeth me shall not walk in darkness, but shall have the light of life." This light is all contained in the great commandment of love. "A new commandment I give unto you," Christ said, "that ye love one another; as I have loved you that ye also love one another." By this shall all men know that ye are my disciples, if ye have love one to another."

The union between Christ and his people is to be living, true, and unfailing, resembling the union that exists between the Father and the Son. This union is the fruit of the indwelling of the Holy Spirit. All true children of God will reveal to the world their union with Christ, and their brethren. Those in whose hearts Christ abides will bear the fruit of brotherly love. They will realize that as members of Christ's family they are pledged to cultivate, cherish, and perpetuate Christian love and fellowship, in spirit, words, and action. {110}

To be children of God, members of the royal family, means more than many suppose. Those who are accounted by God as his children will reveal Christlike love for one another. They will live and work for one object,—the proper representation of Christ to the world. By their love and unity they will show to the world that they bear the divine credentials. By the nobility of love and self-denial, they will show those around them that they are true followers of the Saviour. "By this shall all men know that ye are my disciples, if ye have love one to another."

In the Old Testament are recorded the laws which the Lord gave for the guidance of his people. He would have his people today study these laws. "The Lord spake unto Moses, saying, Speak unto all the congregation of the children of Israel, and say unto them, Ye shall be holy; for I the Lord your God am holy. . . . When ye reap the harvest of your land, ye shall not wholly reap the corners of your field, neither shalt thou gather the gleanings of thy harvest. And thou shalt not glean thy vintage, neither shalt thou gather every grape of thy vineyard; thou shalt leave them for the poor and the stranger; I am the Lord. Ye shall not steal, neither deal falsely, neither lie one to another. . . . Thou shalt not defraud thy neighbor, neither rob him; the wages of him that is hired shall not abide with thee all night until the morning. Thou shalt not curse the deaf, nor put a stumbling block before the blind, but shalt fear the Lord thy God; I am the Lord. Ye shall do no unrighteousness in judgment; thou shalt not respect the person of the poor, nor honor the person of the mighty; but in righteousness shalt thou judge thy neighbor. Thou shalt not go up and down as a tale bearer among thy people; neither shalt thou stand against the blood of thy neighbor; I am the Lord. Thou shalt not hate thy brother in thine heart; thou shalt in any wise rebuke thy neighbor, and not suffer sin upon him. Thou shalt not avenge nor bear any grudge against the children of thy people, but thou shalt love thy neighbor as thyself; I am the Lord."

Christ is deeply grieved when his professed followers, his disciples, neglect to cultivate Christian love, when they act in a way that causes pain to the hearts of their brethren in the faith. They injure their religious experience, laying stumbling blocks in their own way and in the way of others. They dishonor the truth they claim to believe. By their passionate words and overbearing actions in dealing with their brethren, they show that they are controlled by the spirit of the enemy of all righteousness. They use common fire in the place of the sacred.

The most powerful evidence that a man can give that he has been born again and is a new man in Christ Jesus, is the manifestation of love for his brethren, the doing for them of Christlike deeds. This is the most powerful witness that can be borne in favor of Christianity, and will win souls to the truth.

In his prayer for His disciples Christ said, "Neither pray I for thee alone, but for them also which shall believe on me through their word; that they all may be one, as thou, Father, art in me, and I in thee, that they also may be one in us; and that the world may believe that thou hast sent me."

Christ brings all true believers into complete oneness with himself, even the oneness which exists between himself and his Father. The true children of God are bound up with one another and with their Saviour. They are one with Christ in God. {111}

"And the glory which thou gavest me, I have given them; that they may be one, even as we are one: I in them and thou in me, that they may be made perfect in one; and that the world may know that thou hast sent me, and hast loved them as thou hast loved me. Father, I will that they also, whom thou hast given me, be with me where I am; that they may behold my glory, which thou hast given me, for thou lovest me before the foundation of the world. O righteous Father, the world hath not known thee, but I have known thee, and these have known that thou hast sent me. And I have declared unto them thy name, and will declare it; that the love wherewith thou hast loved me may be in them, and I in them."

These are indeed wonderful words. They need to be thought of, studied, and brought into the practical life. They are to be lived out in the daily experiences. Only thus can the result for which Christ prayed be produced.

The Spirit of Christ never leads those of the same faith to separate into distinct, independent parties. When such a separation takes place, an impression exactly opposite from that for which Christ prayed is given to the world.

Why do those who profess to believe in Christ, who profess to keep the commandments, make such feeble efforts to answer the Saviour's prayer: Why do they seek to have their own way, instead of choosing the way and will of the Spirit of God? Those who do this will one day see the harm they have done to the cause of God by pulling apart. Instead of co-operating with God, instead of laboring together with Christ, many who occupy positions of trust are working in opposition to Christ. The Lord has presented this to me in a most decided manner to present to His people.

If God's followers would seek in their religious life to answer Christ's prayer, revealing by the transformation in their lives the power of the truth, what a wonderful testimony would be borne to the world. How powerfully the character and work of Christ would be made known and the glory of God be revealed.

It is our God given duty to love one another as Christ has loved us. The performance of this duty brings with it the blessedness of peace and quietude in the Lord and the ennobling and uplifting of the whole being. Those who love as Christ loved are born of God, and are "kept by the power of God through faith unto salvation ready to be revealed in the last time."

"Wherefore laying aside all malice, and all guile, and hypocrisy, and envies, and all evil-speakings, as new born babes desire the sincere milk of the word, that ye may grow thereby: if so be that ye have tasted that the Lord is gracious. To whom coming as unto a living stone, disallowed indeed of men, but chosen of God, and precious, ye also, as lively stones are built up a spiritual house, an holy priesthood, to offer up spiritual sacrifices acceptable to God by Jesus Christ. . . .Ye are a chosen generation, a royal priesthood, an holy nation, a peculiar people; that ye should show forth the praises of him who hath called you out of darkness into his marvelous light."

I am instructed to say to our people, "Be ye doers of the word, and not hearers only, deceiving your own selves." (James 1:22) There are many who are unprepared to meet Christ. "For if any be a hearer of the word, and not a doer, he is like unto a man beholding his natural face in a glass: For he beholdeth himself, and goeth his way, and straightway forgetteth what manner of man he was. But whoso looketh into the perfect law of liberty, and continueth therein, he being not a forgetful hearer, but a doer of the work, this man shall be blessed in his deed. (James 1:23-25) {112}

A sacred relationship exists between Christ our Saviour and the believer. He says, "I will betroth thee unto me forever; yea, I will betroth thee unto me in righteousness, and in judgment, and in loving kindness, and in mercies. I will even betroth thee unto me in faithfulness; and thou shalt know the Lord." "Thou shalt know."

Is not this the desire of the soul? There are many who ridicule the idea of there being any certainty in religious experience. Some cannot bear to hear sanctification and the higher attainments spoken about. But the Word says, "Thou shalt know" the Lord, and this means holiness and sanctification.

How may we know God? By doing his word. We have the assurance of this. Read the first chapter of Second Peter. The entire chapter is an assurance of the true believer. "Grace and peace be multiplied unto you through the knowledge of God and of Jesus our Lord. (to verse 7.)

We must work upon the plan of addition, adding to our character the graces here mentioned.

"If, these things be in you and abound, they make you that ye shall neither be barren nor unfruitful. This is our life insurance policy.

"That by these ye might be partakers of the divine nature, having escaped the corruption that is in the world through lust." The lust here mentioned does not only mean a perverse, base passion. It includes an unholy desire for riches, for praise, for the possession of power. To fear God and obey his word is the only way to gain true exaltation. But forgetting this, man presumptuously craves more and still more worldly power and honor. He devises and plans in every way to accomplish certain results, losing sight of justice and equity and love for God and his brethren. With a perversity that is blind to results, he sacrifices his peace of mind, his assurance of knowing God and Christ.

"When Ephraim spake trembling, he exalted himself in Israel; but when he offended in Baal, he died. And now they sin more and more, and have made them molten images of their silver, and idols according to their own understanding, all of it the work of the craftsmen: they say of them, Let the men that sacrifice kiss the calves. Therefore they shall be as the morning cloud, and as the early dew that passeth away, as the chaff that is driven with the whirlwind out of the floor, and as the smoke out of the chimney. Yet I am the LORD thy God from the land of Egypt, and thou shalt know no god but me: for there is no saviour beside me." (Hosea 13:1-4.)

"O Israel, return unto the LORD thy God; for thou hast fallen by thine iniquity. Take with you words, and turn to the LORD: say unto him, Take away all iniquity, and receive us graciously: so will we

render the calves of our lips." "I will heal their backsliding, I will love them freely: for mine anger is turned away from him. I will be as the dew unto Israel: he shall grow as the lily, and cast forth his roots as Lebanon. His branches shall spread, and his beauty shall be as the olive tree, and his smell as Lebanon." "Who is wise, and he shall understand these things? prudent, and he shall know them? for the ways of the LORD are right, and the just shall walk in them: but the transgressors shall fall therein." (Hosea 14:1-2, 4, 5, 9.)

The Lord is infinitely merciful and gracious. He is waiting for us to repent and turn to him with humble confession, saying, "We will take thy way, O Lord: we will no longer walk in the way of our own counsels. Have mercy on us and save us, and those who have erred in following a path not cast up for the ransomed of the Lord.

The time has come for the renunciation of all self-confidence. The time has come to follow the Lord's way. He has given instruction for all who will be guided by him, who have faith in his word and courage to go forward. God calls upon those who have walked in paths of their own choosing to return to him. "Seek ye the LORD while he may be found, call ye upon him while he is near: Let the wicked forsake his way, and the unrighteous man his thoughts: and let him return unto the LORD, and he will have mercy upon him; and to our God, for he will abundantly pardon. For my thoughts are not your thoughts, neither are your ways my ways, saith the LORD. For as the heavens are higher than the earth, so are my ways higher than your ways, and my thoughts than your thoughts." Isaiah 55:6-9. {113}

"BE YE THEREFORE PERFECT"

[Prior to July 1915]

THE LORD ESTIMATES AS OF supreme value the holiness of his people, and He permits reverses to come upon individuals, upon families, and upon churches, that his people may see their danger and humble their hearts before him in repentance. He will treat his backslidden ones with tenderness. He will speak pardon to them, and clothe them with the garments of Christ's righteousness. He will honor them with his presence.

In this, the great day of atonement, it is our duty to confess our sins and acknowledge God's mercy and love in pardoning our transgressions. Let us thank the Lord for the warnings he has given to save us from our perverse ways. Let us witness to his goodness by revealing a change in our lives. If those to whom the Lord has sent reproof, warning them that they are not walking in his way, will repent and with humility and contrition of heart make confession, the Lord will surely receive them again into favor. If they will honor God by obeying his commandments, they will be exalted by him. He will teach them what constitutes true honor and strength and victory. Those who despise the word of the Lord, who, although they have the oracles of God to reprove wrong and encourage righteousness, continue to walk in their own way, indulging their desire for self-exaltation and leading those who have confidence in them into wrong paths will, unless utterly forsaken by God, become weary of themselves.

God chastens his people, with the hope of saving their souls. The defections among God's people are keenly felt by Him who died to ransom them from Satan's power. The church is burdened and saddened. A cloud hangs over her. Let every soul seek God, inquiring, "Lord, is it I who have brought this discouragement upon thy people? Is it because of my perversity that Zion is burdened? Have I given occasion for our enemies to triumph—If so, Lord, have mercy upon thy sinful child, and save me for thy mercies' sake.

Let there be a close examination of self. Do not seek to hide yourself under your citizen's dress, saying that you are doing as others do, and therefore you cannot be far out of the way. Yes, you may do as many apostates who live today have done. Some are even now travelling over this ground. But is the picture a pleasant one? If with the experience of others before us we walk contrary to the way of the Lord and are punished, whom have we to blame but ourselves?

O that a deep realization of the importance of these things may come to the people of God! O that all departure from the narrow path of obedience and holiness may be seen as it is! O that men and women may seek the Lord as they have never done before!

A season of great trial is before us. It becomes us now to use all our capabilities and gifts in advancing the work of God. The powers the Lord has given us are to be used to build up, not to discourage and tear down.

Those who are ignorantly deceived are not to remain in these conditions. The Lord says to his messengers, Go to them, and declare unto them what I have said, whether they will hear, or whether they will forbear. "Thou shalt speak my words unto them," God said to the prophet, "whether they will hear or whether they will forbear; for they are a most rebellious house. But thou, O son of man, hear what I say unto thee: be not thou rebellious like that rebellious house." {114}

There are those claiming to be children of God whose course of action the Lord does not justify. Faithful work is to be done in giving reproof, as well as in giving encouragement. The cross is not to be shunned. No unchristlike course of action to your brethren is to be justified. The time is right upon us when persecution will come to those who proclaim the truth. Those who teach the truth, opening the word of God to others, must surrender self entirely to God. To them the truth will bring its own reward, filling the soul with joy.

Will the people of God now humble their hearts before him, confessing and forsaking their sins, that they may receive the forgiveness and favor of God, and come into complete harmony with him? It is not because of a lack of evidence that sinners perish, but because of their unwillingness to appropriate the means whereby God designs they shall learn his will. The ignorance of many is voluntary and inexcusable.

The outlook is not flattering, but notwithstanding this, let us not give up our efforts to save those who have had an experience but are ready to perish, for whose ransom the Prince of heaven offered up his precious life. When one means fails, try another way. Our efforts must not be dead and lifeless. As long as life is spared, let us work for God. In all ages of the church God's appointed messengers have exposed themselves to reproach and persecution for the truth's sake. But wherever God's people may be forced to go, even though, like the beloved disciple, they are banished to desert islands, Christ will know where they are, and will strengthen and bless them with peace and joy.

Soon there is to be trouble all over the world. It becomes everyone to seek to know God. We have no time to delay. With earnestness and fervor the message must be given: "Ho, every one that thirsteth, come, ye to the waters, and he that hath no money; come ye, buy wine and milk without money and without price." "Thus saith the Lord, Keep ye judgment, and do justice. Isaiah 56:1-5.

God's love for his church is infinite. His care over his heritage is unceasing. He suffers no affliction to come upon the church but such as is essential for her purification, her present and eternal good. He will purify his church even as he purified the temple at the beginning and close of his ministry on earth. All that he brings upon the church is test and trial comes that his people may gain deeper piety and more strength to carry the triumphs of the cross to all parts of the world. He has a work for all to do. There must be constant enlargement and progress. The work must extend from city to city, from country to country, and from nation to nation, moving continually onward and upward, established, strengthened, and settled.

"By their fruits ye shall know them." The inward adorning of a meek and quiet spirit is priceless. In the life of the true Christian, the outward adorning is always in harmony with the inward peace and holiness. Thus in the righteousness of the members shall the church be established. God's people are to show a faith, orderly, steadfast, and immovable. The Bible is their standard. Rich currents of grace from heaven will produce light in them which they are to impart to others. In all its power the truth is to be proclaimed. Those who faithfully do this work, keeping the commandments of God in deed and in truth will be acknowledged as laborers together with God. {115}

"The work of righteousness shall be peace, and the effect of righteousness quietness and assurance forever." From the beginning to the end of the history of the church, Christ will be to his people all that these words express, if they will heed the invitation, "Come unto me all ye that labor. Matthew 11:28-30. Christ is to his people life and strength, efficiency and power, wisdom and holiness. When we realize this as we should the prayer will go from unfeigned lips, "The LORD is exalted; for he dwelleth on high: he hath filled Zion with judgment and righteousness. And wisdom and knowledge shall be the stability of thy times, and strength of salvation: the fear of the LORD is his treasure." "The sinners in Zion are afraid; fearfulness hath surprised the hypocrites. Who among us shall dwell with the devouring fire? who among us shall dwell with everlasting burnings? He that walketh righteously, and speaketh uprightly; he that despiseth the gain of oppressions, that shaketh his hands from holding of bribes, that stoppeth his ears from hearing of blood, and shutteth his eyes from seeing evil; He shall dwell on high: his place of defense shall be the munitions of rocks: bread shall be given him; his waters shall be sure. Thine eyes shall see the king in his beauty: they shall behold the land that is very far off. Isaiah 33:5, 6, 14-17.

THE REGIONS BEYOND

(D.E.R. Aug. 24, 1900.)

OUR WORLD IS A FIELD OF missionary toil. We are to present before the people the love of God, not only as the motive of effort, but as the model of all our plans. We must work in the way Christ worked. His example is to be our pattern.

The Lord has given men and women capabilities and tact and skill to be used to His name's glory. When sincere, earnest efforts are put forth to win souls to God, we shall see of the salvation of God. Those who claim to be Christians should make an unreserved surrender of all they have to the Lord. Their time, their substance, and their influence as a savor of life unto life are required of them by Him who willingly gave himself to save to the uttermost all who come to him. Those who claim to be children of God should throw the whole weight of their influence on the side of Christ, for his sake practicing his self-denial and self-sacrifice. There is need of close communion with God and entire conformity to his will. This is the secret of gaining the power that will convict and convert sinners. The church has failed because she has not come up to the help of the Lord, to the help of the Lord against the mighty influence of the Satanic force. Church members have not as they should pressed back the powers of darkness. This is the reason for the deficiency in the church today. The quickening power of God is needed. Men and women who love God supremely and their neighbor as themselves are needed, men and women who crave the power of God, that they may bear witness to the love of Jesus.

Church members are to be God's instruments in seeking to save those ready to perish. Be they many or few, they are to confer together, laying before one another their designs and plans, and obtaining the benefit of one another's perception and foresight as to the best plan for securing success in the work. There are to be found no separate parties, who shall supply themselves with all the facilities for ensuring success, at the same time leaving those who should have equal encouragement and means with which to carry on the work, with nothing with which to do the work which means the adding of new territory to the Lord's kingdom.

The many fields in the Lord's vineyard which have not been touched call upon the places in which institutions are already established to understand the situation. Let men curtail their ambition to branch out in a field which God's appointment has already been worked. Let there not be on the part of churches, families, or individuals any withholding of the means needed to furnish God's servants with facilities for doing the work in regions beyond. Let not those in the fields where the work is established think of the great things they can do, and continue to expand self to large proportions, while other portions of the Lord's vineyard are destitute of the advantages by which the work might be {116} properly done. This is a religion of selfishness, and is offensive to God. It is a selfish ambition which leads men to call for more facilities in a field already possessing ample facilities, while missionary fields are in need of the advantages which these worked fields have in abundance.

The Lord's work in new territories is to be carried forward to a successful accomplishment. In this work God's plan is to be followed, not the inclinations of those who would gather into the section over which they have supervision, every possible advantage, to give, as they say, character to the work, while the utter destitution of other parts of the Lord's vineyard is forgotten. Every work is tested of God. Every selfish thread drawn into it he will cut out.

After nine years of struggling, we begin to see some signs of success in this country. But the advancement has been made under the most trying circumstances. In order to advance the work we have been obliged to borrow thousands of dollars. I tell you in the name of the Lord that this need not have been. If our institutions, our sanitariums and publishing houses had bound about their desire for more facilities, and had shown an unselfish interest in the work so constantly set before them, the cause in foreign fields would have certainly made much more advancement, and marked success would have attended the business of which they were stewards. The selfish desire which some have shown to use all the means to enrich one portion of the Lord's vineyard reveals unfaithful stewardship; and I am charged to make this appeal to God's people.

The great Head of the church has given talents to the company of believers. He has given his word to mold the character and his Spirit to bring all things to their remembrance. He desires his people to bring into their work the true abiding principles of missionary effort. Many of the Lord's servants are numbered with those of whom John wrote, "Blessed are the dead which die in the Lord from henceforth: Yea, saith the Spirit, that they may rest from their labors, and their works do follow them." Those who are left to plant the standard in new places are to have a keen, sanctified interest in every plan which is related, directly or indirectly, to the great work of warning the world. Those who have stood in positions of trust, faithful men who have been led and guided by God, are to thank him for his molding, fashioning power. They are to carry his work onward and upward to perfect accomplishment. They are to move with careful, prayerful consideration, lest they mar the influence of the work by changing the order which the Lord has said should be followed. As they advance step by step they are to mind the same things, to advance in the same lines, that the truth may ever be honored or lose its sacred, holy influence in the sight of the world.

As those who took up the work at the beginning of the message have advanced by self-denial and self-sacrifice, God has given them his blessing. They have had much to learn, they have made mistakes, they have needed continual guidance and counsel; but they have had reason for constant gratitude, because the work has gone forward in spite of poverty and a lack of facilities. They strained every nerve to make the work a success, to establish those buildings which were necessary for the proper development of the work; and under all circumstances the Lord guided them.

Those who come into the work later and find things ready to their hand should at least attempt to pay the debt they owe the Lord and the workers who went before them, by carrying the truth into new territories, until it has gone to every nation, kindred, tongue, and people. In every country men and women are to be {117} raised up to carry forward the very work begun by those who have been laid away to rest. The memory of these pioneer workers is to be guarded, and from their treasure of experience the workers are to learn to pass from one line of work to another, following the methods declared by the Holy Spirit to be in the order of God, asserting the principles enjoined in the word, carrying the aggressive warfare into new fields.

Home and foreign missions are to share equally of God's trust money. In planning for the work, the difficulties to be met in foreign fields are to be considered. Let not those who have every advantage be niggardly in appropriating means for the advancement of the work in mission fields. For Christ's sake willing support is to be given to the work of the gospel, which is to be carried to all parts of the world. And by the work of the press the work is to be established and confirmed.

Christ should never again be dishonored and his cause put to shame by a lack of the true missionary spirit. A great mistake has been made. In their selfishness men have grasped means and advantages for their own field, though knowing the need of help in new fields. They have not supplied that which was necessary for the progress of the work. They have not helped their brethren fight the battle which once had to be fought in the fields they now occupy.

The work all over the world is to receive consideration. New fields are to be entered. Let those at the heart of the work remember that much means and much hard labor is required to accomplish the work in new fields. Let them be faithful stewards of the Lord's goods. Let them not feel that they are rich and increased with goods and have need of nothing, but let them practice true Bible religion, which enjoins self-sacrifice at every step. They are to closely examine the needs of the work, reviewing the needs of all the fields; for they are God's agents to do this. They are set for the extension of the truth in all parts of the world. They are not excusable if they remain in blindness and ignorance regarding the needs of the work. They are to know the advantage and defects of each field, and then with a true spirit of unselfish interest they are to work for the accomplishment of the work as a whole.

In this work all the churches which have been established are to have a part, according to their several ability. If diffi-

culties come up in missionary fields, let interested investigation be made without delay, lest the path of duty be hid or made obscure. As these questions come up before those who are wise in God's wisdom, examination will be united with the exercise of prudence. By using the knowledge God has given them men will gain a clear, sharp experience. By exercising their God-given ability in helping to plant the standard of truth in new territory, they will receive great blessing. After they have unselfishly tried to gain a right understanding of the situation, they are to approach the mercy seat, asking for clear intuition and an unselfish purpose, that they may see the necessities of far off fields. As they ask the Lord to help them to advance the work in regions beyond, they will receive grace from on high. Never will they seek the Lord in vain.

America was long the field of missionary conflict. God has prospered the work in that country. If those there had cherished the spirit of self-sacrificing missionary effort, fewer unnecessary buildings would have been erected, and the kingdom of Christ would have been extended to many regions. There would {118} have been shown a missionary zeal which has not yet been developed by those whose duty it is to carry the needs of the work on their souls. Much more would have been done to plant the standard in other places beside America.

But selfishness so abhorrent to God came in. The work was neglected, when there was plenty of means to send missionaries abroad to preach the gospel, raise up churches, and erect meeting houses. If men had worked actively on the Lord's plan, laboring earnestly and unselfishly to impart what God had given them, churches would have been established in many places. The standard would have been planted in new fields. Witness would have been borne to the truth in many more cities. God's memorial of creation, the seventh day Sabbath would have been honored.

The great head of the church permitted a parable to be enacted in your midst at the last General Conference. You were led to expect from one claiming to be converted, a large donation, pledged to different branches of the work. Apparently the one who was pledged to make this donation was as sincere as any man in the Conference, but he disappeared, and all came to nothing.

Just in this way has God been disap-

pointed in his people, whom He has enriched abundantly with all good things, but who have failed to fulfil his expectations.

A straightforward plan is to be followed in dealing with believers in home and foreign fields. An unselfish equality is to be maintained among the working forces. Money is to be provided to support missionaries. An agent should be appointed to investigate the situation in foreign countries and to report. Those in places where the work has been established should bind about their supposed wants, that the work in foreign fields may go forward. In the institutions which have been established there will be a desire to grasp more and still more advantages. To make a larger plant, let them work economically, till they themselves succeed in doing this. But the Lord declares that this should not be. The means in his treasury is to be used in building up the work in the places where there are no conveniences. The workers in foreign fields should not be left to beg. The condition of every new mission field should be examined, that there may be equality in the distribution of means which come into our conference and benevolent institutions.

Such high wages should not be paid to the men in our publishing institutions. The payment of such high wages has been a mistake. The extra money paid to a few should have been paid to missionaries in new fields, who were at a loss to know where the means to advance the work is coming from. The extra amount drawn from the treasury for men who did not need it should have been appropriated for the benefit of fields which had no resources, to support laborers to open and plant and sow the fields with truth.

The workers God sends into his field will if they have the true missionary spirit be more anxious to do their work than to get the wages. But because of this, they should not be neglected. The work of those in missionary fields calls for more self-denial than the work of those employed in our institutions, who are not obliged to travel from place to place. Many calls are made upon those who begin work in a new field, and these workers are to be supported in accordance with their work. There should be more equality between the wages of those in our institutions and those who in missionary fields where there is no resources to draw from, are wrestling with difficulty, doing the hardest and most laborious work. {119}

God is not pleased with the way in which these things have been managed. He has a controversy with those who have shown no practical interest in the work of foreign missions, even though they knew what was required to make a beginning in a new field. The discernment of some at the heart of the work has been clouded. Their hands have been opened to grasp all the means they could possibly get, while in other parts of the Lord's vineyard the workers have been obliged to do with poor food and poor clothing, while at the same time some were told, You must sustain yourselves.

God calls sternly for an adjustment of these matters; for his name is reproached. He marks every move made by his missionary workers in improving his vineyard. He sees the unfair way in which these workers have been treated. There is need of a recognition of the rights of the missionaries sent by God to carry the gospel message to all parts of the world. These men and women take their lives into their hands, and for Christ's sake endure trials and hardships. Let men realize that God is a God of justice. His actual presence follows his missionaries from place to place as they try to do his will, devoting all their time and energy to his service.

Let those who have every convenience at hand for the work they are doing ask themselves, How is it with those who are breaking new fields? Can I not help those who are working in new fields, where the standard of truth has not been lifted? God requires those in our institutions to have their conception sharpened, their minds enlarged. He will be pleased to have foreign missionary work become a burden that will weigh so heavily upon their minds that they will know the difference between the work of those in places where the work has been established and the work of those who engage in aggressive warfare. Let the true spirit of self-denial be learned out of the Word and brought into the practical life.

A work has been started in some cities which has absorbed much means, but which will bring small returns; for it has been done for a class who are not producers but consumers. The money invested in this work should have largely been used in other channels, supplying the regions beyond with facilities for the work of the Lord. In the lines of work which God has not appointed much liberality has been shown, while his work in foreign fields has been left to languish. In a short time, if this management is continued, how will the cause of God in the third angel's message stand before the world?

Into foreign fields the Lord has sent experienced workers who are capable for leading out in enterprises for the advancement of the work. But enough consideration has not been given by those at the heart of the work to foreign mission fields. Unless a decided change is made, we shall stand before the world humiliated, crippled, and disordered, because Christ's principles have not been carried into the work.

Among the people of God there is to be cooperation but not confederacy. The work is not to be bound about by bonds, limitations, or restrictions. Christian unity is not Free Masonry. The love of Christ is the golden chain which is to bind us to one another and to God.

Our offerings are not to be entrusted to any one person. We are to make no one man our steward. The third angels' message is to go to all parts of the {120} world, and we are not to help in the creation of any interests which will absorb God's money in a work which has in it much which belongs not to the work for this time.

There is a power in the truth. When allowed to operate under favorable conditions, the gospel will gather a harvest of souls. Every truly converted man, firmly established in the truth, is a light bearer to the world; for Christ shines through him. He shines in a world enshrouded in moral darkness. A few truly converted souls are of infinitely more value than a large number who are unconverted, dead in trespasses and sins.

A work is to be done in the Lord's vineyard which will testify to the genuineness and value of the truth, and will glorify God. We are to labor for those who when converted will be a help in the work, producers not consumers. But the work done for the lowest class of outcasts is a very uncertain matter. Those who spend their time and strength in work for those who will never do anything but hang upon them for help, disqualify themselves for the position God would have them fill in His army. Workers are greatly needed to labor for those who rightly handled will come to a knowledge of the truth, and will then do valuable service in the cause. But those who after being prayed with say, I am saved, have no real understanding of what it means to receive Christ. No man can say, I am saved, until he has endured test and trial, until he has shown that he can overcome temptation. Those who fail to do the work which God has said should be done soon lose the right perception of spiritual things, and become blinded as to the character of the truth. They are unfitted to do the work which would make them complete in Christ.

The churches must arouse. The members must awake out of sleep and begin to inquire, How is the money which we put into the treasury being used? The Lord desires that a close search be made. Are all satisfied with the history of the work for the past fifteen years? Where is the evidence of the co-working with God? Where has been heard throughout the churches the prayer for the help of the Holy Spirit? Dissatisfied and disheartened, we turn away from the scene.

Our churches and institutions must return to where they were before the backsliding commenced, when they began trusting in man and making flesh their arm. Have we not seen enough of human wisdom? Shall we not now seek God in earnestness and simplicity, and serve him with heart and mind and strength?

The children of Israel beheld the awful semblance of God's presence in the mount; but before Moses had been forty days away from them, they substituted a golden calf for Jehovah. Things similar to this have been done among us as a people. Let us now return to God in penitence and contrition. Let us trust in Him, not in man.

DEAR BROTHER DANIELLS

June 18, 1900
"Sunnyside" Cooranbong

I WISH TO WRITE YOU A few lines, which I may not be able to get copied. I have within the last half hour learned that a mail leaves for Africa tomorrow morning. It is now fifteen minutes past three in the afternoon. I wrote yesterday and this morning some nineteen pages of letter paper, and no less than ten {121} pages in my diary. A few pages have been copied, a letter to Dr. Kellogg.

A letter has been received from John Wessels, but it contained nothing regarding the condition of things in Capetown, so we are left in complete darkness and ignorance, as you have not written us one line. Have you written and has the letter miscarried? What does this silence mean?

When attending the meeting at Parramatta, I was in the night season passing through some exciting scenes in Africa. There were laid out some formulated arrangements and plans which were presented for acceptance; but Elder Daniells did not feel prepared to accept these plans, because they had in them some things which meant more than all could see. And while some would have accepted them, Elder Daniells said, "I cannot subscribe my name to them." This refusal greatly disappointed the framers of the articles of agreement. But no one who has had an experience in the rise and progress of the cause of God would without special advice from the Source of all wisdom concede to the terms of agreement or bind themselves to the conditions laid down, which the Lord could not favor.

Our brethren in Africa will have to drink deeper of the clear, flowing springs of Lebanon before they can see all things clearly. From the light given me I know that we must enter into contracts very cautiously. We must have special light from God before we do this. Every problem which has any reference to the cause and work of God should be studied with earnest prayer. It is the privilege of every man who claims to be a Christian, who is walking in the path of duty, to have confidence in God's presence. The Lord is able to make that which is dark plain.

We are today in great peril of following in false paths. If negotiations are made with the Wessels family, God must give direction as to how they shall be framed. Let all remember that this is a time when Satan is working to lead the Lord's people in various countries to tie themselves up as his people in America have done. There there is little freedom and little means because the conference, which in the fear of the Lord should have stood steadfast to principle, departed from the right way. Alliances with men need prayerful adjustment. We are God's stewards and are dealing with his money, with his talents. That which in our human judgment would appear to promise much at the beginning may through the unwise movements of someone in the alliance create much disappointment and endless perplexity.

I consider that the Wessels family have a right to be cautious. For in the workers that were sent from America, they have had to deal with some who were not straightforward. I would say to them, Sanctify yourselves by a new consecration to God. Regard the Lord as ready and willing to help you. A wrong was done to the Wessels family in the use made of their means by those who came from America. Their money was used extravagantly, and ways were devised to draw upon them. It would have been better if this money had never been placed in the hands of those who received it.

The Wessels family have made large donations of money to Dr. Kellogg, as though he was the one who was to be steward of their means. The means that the Wessels family gave so abundantly in America should not have been handled by one man as he pleased, but by faithful stewards, who would have appropriated the money for the opening of the work in Africa. A great work might have been done {122} in that field. Books should have been translated for use in fields needing strong missionary effort. Had the work been done that should have been done, the religious experience of the Dutch people would have been materially changed.

This is where the young men of the Wessels family made a mistake. Mission fields in Africa were in their destitution crying to God for help and relief. They were starving for the light that should have shone in the dark places in regions beyond. This cruel, treacherous war would not have come at this time had the missionary work been done that the people of Africa were in suffering need of. The things which ought to have been done, but which have not been done testify to a neglect of duty.

Let it never be forgotten that true Christianity comes through the engraving of Bible principles upon the heart and character. This must be an individual work, visibly expressed. Then true missionary work will be done. The Lord's means will be carefully invested.

A class of workers should have been sent to Africa who would have tried by every means in their power to educate the people they came over to help. But some of those sent to Africa as missionaries needed the converting power of God upon their hearts. Before they could teach others the truth, they needed to yoke up with Christ to learn of Him, His meekness and lowliness. In every department of God's economy he works through instruments that will be worked. Preaching the word is one great means, and furnishing the people with reading matter is another. The Lord has appointed that the preaching of the gospel and the press shall act in harmony.

Tuesday, June 19. I have just looked at my watch; it is two o'clock. I dress, seek the Lord, and try to write a few words to go in the mail to Africa this morning. May the Lord help me in tracing each line.

From the light God has given me, I know that he has not inaugurated such a work for our people to do as Dr. Kellogg had started in Chicago. In every city there should be missionaries, evangelists, appointed to work for the lower classes, who through abuse are ruining themselves. But all the resources are not to be used in this work, or the work of bringing the truth to other cities and missionary fields afar off from America will not be accomplished. God's money has been used lavishly in some places, so that there is not means to invest in sustaining the gospel ministry in all parts of the world by voice and by the press. Both must be linked together, and God's standard must be raised in new territory. New fields must be worked, the warning must be given. A representation of the work to be done is given in the fifty-eighth chapter of Isaiah.

The cause of God is nearly bankrupt through man's devising, by their lack of wisdom in bringing in consumers and not producers. Thus God names it. The question to be treated is a large one. God calls for decided changes to be made. Self-denial and self-sacrifice will be called for in all who undertake the work now.

Our brethren in America, before carrying out their plans for such an extensive and wonderful work in certain lines, might far better have considered the words of Christ, "Which of you intending to build a tower, sitteth not down first and counteth the cost, whether he have sufficient to finish it?" Had they done {123} this, acting under the direction of God, men's ideas would not have been carried thus far in building the tower. Thousands of dollars that have been invested in Chicago for the lowest and most unpromising specimens of humanity, would have gone to open new fields, annexing new territory, planting standard in new places.

In many new fields there should be camp-meetings of two, three, or four weeks in a place, if the circumstances demand it. And all through these meetings there is to be much personal effort, not only in the exposition of the word in the meetings, but by individuals. Follow up every advantage in the very height of the surprise of the people to find out that there are important, wonderful things in the word that they have not known were there at all, because the shepherds of the flock have not searched the Scriptures as diligent students of the Word. There is to be diligent work done. The testing truth for this time is to be made known, and the explanation given. All classes, the higher as well as the most lowly, come to these meetings, and we are to work for all. After the warning message has been given, let those who are specially interested be called to the tent by themselves, and there labor for their conversion. This kind of labor is missionary work of the highest order.

The temperance question is to have special attention. Work in this line may be called medical missionary work, but that work in its relation to the work of the third angel's message is ever to be recognized as the hand to the body. In America it has been made the head and not the hand. The gospel ministry is not to be treated as it has been treated,—as something hardly worthy to be recognized. It is God's appointed means, the very means which has made us what we are, and its work is to be carried forward in the same lines and in the same way, because it is God's. Nothing is to be devised to stand as a memorial of man's greatness or woman's greatness.

See Isaiah 49. I cannot write out this whole chapter. Read it carefully and solemnly. What words are these, "And he said, Thou art my servant, O Israel, in whom I shall be glorified." How many after they have done their best under most trying circumstances, suffering for the want of facilities and from dearth of means, are ready to say, in the words of Scripture, "I have labored in vain, I have spent my strength for naught, and in vain; yet surely my judgment is with the Lord, and my work with my God."

All the warnings must be given. The truth, Bible truth, is to be proclaimed in our large camp-meetings, and the churches can hear the truth. They have the opportunity. All may not desire to hear. Many oppose anything that calls for self-denial. They are not willing to accept the Sabbath. In Exodus 31:12-18, is clearly marked out in definite lines what God expects from his people, and the decided consequence of rejecting is death. Notwithstanding this many will refuse obedience because the truth involves self-denial and self-sacrifice.

Many of the ministers will not hear and be convinced. They will not enter the sanctuary of truth to receive the knowledge of truth from the word, but will take away the key of knowledge from the people by perversion of the Scriptures, wresting the word of God from its true meaning. Thus every step gained in reaching the people to save them from being lost in error and disobedience requires a hard, constant battle. But shall it stop? No; lift up the standard. Plan memorials of God's truth in every place possible, and conversions will be made. {124} Some who do not take their stand at once will help advance the work with their means and with their sympathy.

"And now saith the Lord that formed thee from the womb to be his servant, to bring Jacob again to him, though Israel be not gathered, (who is Israel? the church members of today.) yet will I be glorious in the eyes of the Lord, and my God shall be my strength." The message must go from east to west, and from west to east again. A great shaking up must come. The professed believers in the truth for this time are asleep. They need to awake, and shine anew because the light of truth has not only flashed upon them, but rightly done its work. God will have representatives in every place in all parts of the world.

The message of the angel following the third is now to be given to all parts of the world. It is to be the harvest message, and the whole earth will be lighted with the glory of God. The Lord has this one more call of mercy to the world, but the perversity of men diverts the work from its true bearing, and the light has to struggle amid the darkness of men who feel themselves competent to do a work which God has not appointed them to do.

Read verses 13-16. What is the matter with those who claim to believe the truth of the third angel's message? Why has it lost its power with the very ones whom God has honored for the sake of making it known to all people. Self has interposed; Satan has so wrought upon human agencies, and self has grown to such large proportions that it will not recognize a Thus saith the Lord, through his appointed channels.

God has spoken he has said that his work is one, that his workers are to keep in solid union. Even though men may sell themselves for a song, God continues to carry forward his work in his own appointed way in the light shining forth in the redemption of his people. Those who hold fast the beginning of their confidence firm unto the end will sing the song, "We overcame by the blood of the Lamb, and by the word of our testimony." The work of truth will go forward in the hearts of the true seekers because God sees in them his own name and the word of truth magnified.

For the glory of his own name God will continue to bear with the perversity of men that they may repent, lest his and their enemies shall triumph in their positive destruction. He bears long with their waywardness and folly. He disciplines them, that they should seek him, and if they will humble their hearts before him, he will not bring them to shame, but through their suffering and their turning unto the Lord, he will make them the eternal monuments of his mercy. His almighty power alone can avail in behalf of any human agency through his abiding grace. Wholehearted obedience God requires of his people as their only means of happiness and prosperity. Only through humbling themselves and exalting God by their devotion to him can they find true prosperity. Yet this is the most difficult lesson for them to learn. Christ and his body, the church, are to become one as is represented in John 1:17—Christ and his people united to God the great Head. The ministry, which has been belittled, will be the power and energy of Christ in word and doctrine. These are they whom man despiseth, whom the nation abhorreth, because they bear the sign of the original Sabbath. Exodus 31:12-18. God's commandment keeping people are made to be a servant to rulers, they are required by man-made laws to disregard the law of God. {125}

"Listen, O isles, unto me; and hearken, ye people, from far; The LORD hath called me from the womb; from the bowels of my mother hath he made mention of my name. And he hath made my mouth like a sharp sword; in the shadow of his hand hath he hid me, and made me a polished shaft; in his quiver hath he hid me; And said unto me, Thou art my servant, O Israel, in whom I will be glorified. Then I said, I have labored in vain, I have spent my strength for nought, and in vain: yet surely my judgment is with the LORD, and my work with my God. And now, saith the LORD that formed me from the womb to be his servant, to bring Jacob again to him, Though Israel be not gathered, yet shall I be glorious in the eyes of the LORD, and my God shall be my strength. And he said, It is a light thing that thou shouldest be my servant to raise up the tribes of Jacob, and to restore the preserved of Israel: I will also give thee for a light to the Gentiles, that thou mayest be my salvation unto the end of the earth. Thus saith the LORD, the Redeemer of Israel, and his Holy One, to him whom man despiseth, to him whom the nation abhorreth, to a servant of rulers, Kings shall see and arise, princes also shall worship, because of the LORD that is faithful, and the Holy One of Israel, and he shall choose thee. Thus saith the LORD, In an acceptable time have I heard thee, and in a day of salvation have I helped thee: and I will preserve thee, and give thee for a covenant of the people, to establish the earth, to cause to inherit the desolate heritages; That thou mayest say to the prisoners, Go forth; to them that are in darkness, Shew yourselves. They shall feed in the ways, and their pastures shall be in all high places. They shall not hunger nor thirst; neither shall the heat nor sun smite them: for he that hath mercy on them shall lead them, even by the springs of water shall he guide them. And I will make all my mountains a way, and my highways shall be exalted. Behold, these shall come from far: and, lo, these from the north and from the west; and these from the land of Sinim. Sing, O heavens; and be joyful, O earth; and break forth into singing, O mountains: for the LORD hath comforted his people, and will have mercy upon his afflicted. But Zion said, The LORD hath forsaken me, and my Lord hath forgotten me. Can a woman forget her sucking child, that she should not have compassion on the son of her womb? yea, they may forget, yet will I not forget thee. Behold, I have graven thee upon the palms of my hands; thy walls are continually before me. Thy children shall make haste; thy destroyers and they that made thee waste shall go forth of thee. Lift up thine eyes round about, and behold: all these gather themselves together, and come to thee. As I live, saith the LORD, thou shalt surely clothe thee with them all, as with an ornament, and bind them on thee, as a bride doeth. For thy waste and thy desolate places, and the land of thy destruction, shall even now be too narrow by reason of the inhabitants, and they that swallowed thee up shall be far away." Isaiah 49:1-19.

The hidden ones have been scattered because of man's enmity against the law of Jehovah. They have been oppressed by all the powers of the earth. They have been scattered in the dens and caves of the earth through violence of their adversaries, because they are true and obedient to the laws of Jehovah. But deliverance comes to the people of God. To their enemies God will show himself as a God of just retribution.

"And when he had opened the fifth seal, I saw under the altar the souls of them that were slain for the word of God, and for the testimony which they held: And they cried with a loud voice, saying, How long, O Lord, holy and true, dost thou not judge and avenge our blood on them that dwell on the earth? And white robes were given unto every one of them; and it was said unto them, that they should rest yet for a little season, until their fellow servants also and their brethren, that should be killed as they were, should be fulfilled. And I beheld when he had opened the sixth seal, and, lo, there was a great earthquake; and the sun became black as sackcloth of hair, and the moon became as blood; And the stars of heaven fell unto the earth, even as a fig tree casteth her untimely figs, when she is shaken of a mighty wind. And the heaven departed as a scroll when it is rolled together; and every mountain and island were moved out of their places. And the kings of the earth, and the great men, and the rich men, and the chief captains, and the mighty men, and every bondman, and every free man, hid themselves in the dens and in the rocks of the mountains; And said to the mountains and rocks, Fall on us, and hide us from the face of him that sitteth on the throne, and from the wrath of the Lamb: For the great day of his wrath is come; and who shall be able to stand?" Revelation 6:9-17. From the dens and caves of the earth, that have been the secret hiding places of God's people, they are called forth as his witnesses, true and faithful.

The people who have braved out their rebellion will fill the description given in Revelation 6:15-17. In these very caves and dens they find the very statement of truth in the letters and in the publications as witnesses against them. The shepherd who leads the sheep in false paths will hear the charge made against them, "It was you who made light of the truth. It was you who told us that God's law was abrogated, that it was a yoke of bondage. It was you who voiced the false doctrines when I was convicted that these Seventh-day Adventists had the truth. The blood of our souls is upon your priestly garments. The persecution brought upon those who kept God's commandments did not destroy them or their influence. I could not read my Bible with its condemnatory words, and I laid it aside. Now will you pay the ransom for my soul. You said you would stand between my soul and God, but you are now full of anguish yourself. What shall we do who listened to your garbling of the Scriptures and your turning into a lie the truth that if obeyed would have saved us?

When Christ comes to take vengeance on those who have educated and trained the people to trample on God's Sabbath, to tear down his memorial, and tread down with their feet the feed of his pastures, lamentations will be in vain. Those who trusted in the false shepherds had the word of God to search for themselves, and they find that God will judge every man who has had the truth and turned from light because it involved self-denial and the cross. Rocks and mountains cannot screen them from the indignation of him that sitteth on the throne and from the wrath of the Lamb.

DEAR BROTHER AND SISTER HASKELL

July 4, 1900
"Sunnyside" Cooranbong,

I SIT HERE IN MY BED, this cold July morning trying to write to you. I have woolen mits on my hands, leaving my fingers free to write. I place my lamp on one side at my left hand, rather than behind me, and then the light shines on my paper in just the right way. Sitting on the bed is the easiest position for me, and I call this my throne. It is a little past two o'clock. I continue to be an early riser, and I write every day. There has been considerable rainy weather here this winter, and this has kept me indoors.

Although I carry a heavy burden for the work in Australia and America, yet I also have a thankful heart for the mercy and gracious loving kindness of my God. {126} Notwithstanding the fact that there is war and bloodshed, and nations are preparing for battle, thanksgiving should arise from our hearts because the Sun of Righteousness never sets. The mightiest earthly potentates may be engaged in battle for the supremacy, but the children of God, whose life is hid with Christ, in God have nothing to fear. Their refuge is safe and sure.

Christ has declared, "All power is given unto me in heaven and in earth. Go ye therefore and teach all nations, baptizing them in the name of the Father, and of the Son, and of the Holy Ghost, teaching them to observe all things whatsoever I have commanded you; and lo, I am with you alway, even unto the end of the world."

This is the work for God's watchmen at the present time.

My brother, there is danger of those in our ranks making a mistake in regard to receiving the Holy Ghost. Many suppose an emotion or a rapture of feeling to be an evidence of the presence of the Holy Spirit. There is danger that right sentiments will not be understood, and that Christ's words, "Teaching them to observe all things whatsoever I have commanded you," will lose their significance. There is danger that original devisings and superstitious imaginings will take the place of the Scriptures. Be not anxious to bring in something not revealed in the Word. Keep close to Christ. Remember his words, "Teaching them to observe all things whatsoever I have commanded you; and lo, I am with you alway, even unto the end of the world." He is with us as we teach the words he spoke in the Old Testament as well as in the New. He who gave commandment in the New Testament is the One also who gave the instruction contained in the Old Testament. The Old and the New Testaments are both sacred; for they both contain the words of Christ. All communication from heaven to earth since Adam's fall has come through Christ. He who believes the instruction contained in the New Testament and in the Old, doing those things which Christ has commanded therein, has the Saviour always with him.

In his record of the giving of the commission Mark says, "He said unto them, Go ye into all the world, and preach the gospel to every creature. He that believeth and is baptized shall be saved; but he that believeth not shall be damned. And these signs shall follow them that believe: In my name shall they cast out devils; they shall speak with new tongues; they shall take up serpents; and if they drink any deadly thing, it shall not hurt them: they shall lay hands on the sick, and they shall recover." These words are to be literally fulfilled. This is the work the Lord Jesus Christ will do through his appointed agencies. "So then, after the Lord had spoken unto them, he was received up into heaven, and sat on the right hand of God. And they went forth and preached everywhere, the Lord working with them, and confirming the word with signs following."

Let us remember that the word Christ has commanded us to preach to all nations, kindreds, tongues, and peoples is confirmed by the Holy Spirit. This is God's plan of work. Christ is the mighty power which confirms the word, bringing men and women, through conversion to the truth, to an understanding faith, making them willing to do whatsoever he has commanded them. The human agent, the seen instrument, is to preach the word, and the Lord Jesus, the unseen agency, by his Holy Spirit is to make the word efficacious and powerful.

The law of the Lord is to be presented in its true bearing. Paul bears testimony regarding this law. "What shall we say then?" he asks. "Is the law sin? God forbid. Nay, I had not known sin but by the law," which is the {127} detector of sin. "For I had not known lust except the law had said, Thou shalt not covet. But sin, taking occasion by the commandment, wrought in me all manner of concupiscence. For without the law sin was dead. For I was alive without the law once; but when the commandment came, sin revived, and I died. And the commandment, which was ordained to life, I found to be unto death. For sin, taking occasion by the commandment, deceived me, and by it slew me." Because of this does Paul say, Have nothing to do with the law? Oh no, this is not his conclusion. Sin is the transgression of the law, and by the law is the knowledge of sin. Paul saw sin in all its hideous deformity. The law pointed him to Christ, the healer of sin which is repented of and confessed. "Wherefore," Paul declared, "the law is holy, and the commandment holy, and just, and good." Why then do men in their transgression curse the law of God? Because it condemns sin.

DEAR BROTHER AND SISTER HASKELL

August 22, 1900

TODAY SARA, MAGGIE, AND I drove up from Cooranbong with our faithful horses, Jasper and Jessie. We came to attend a general meeting for the Newcastle, Maitland, and Cooranbong churches. Quite a number are coming from Cooranbong and Maitland.

I am staying at the Baths with Brother and Sister Louis Currow. Our medical work in Newcastle gives every promise of success. Some weeks ago we rented the building in Hamilton known as the Turkish Baths. This building is provided with facilities for giving Turkish baths and hot and cold water baths. It is surrounded by open grounds, and is only a few minutes walk from our church in Hamilton.

As soon as we saw the advantages of this place, we decided that the best thing we could do was to secure it. We feel very thankful to the Lord for this opening in Newcastle. Work at the Baths was begun about two weeks ago, and thus far success has attended it. Several prominent men are taking treatment and yesterday three Catholic priests came in for a bath. Brother Currow, who is in charge of the bath work, is an excellent nurse. His wife who used to be Miss Lizzie Hubbard, and he are both doing well.

In the building there are four rooms upstairs, and four downstairs. Two are unfurnished. When we have sufficient means they will be furnished ready for patients.

If properly conducted, this institution will be the means of doing much good, both in relieving physical suffering and in making known the truth. Idolatry prevails in our cities. Everything that Satan can do he is doing to keep his dark shadow between sinners and God. He desires to keep the minds of men fixed upon the things of earth. By means of medical work a class of people may be reached who would otherwise never hear present truth. Souls ready to perish may be saved.

Friday, Apr. 27. We thank the Lord for pleasant weather. Quite a number have come from Cooranbong to attend the meeting. Most of these will be accommodated at the Baths.

April 28, Sabbath. The Lord gave me strength to speak to the people this afternoon. I felt indeed that physical and spiritual strength was given me. I {128} spoke from John 16:1-6. Christ's words are plain and definite: "These things have I spoken unto you that ye should not be offended." Before this, some of the disciples had been offended because Christ had said, "I am the bread of life: he that cometh to me shall never hunger; and he that believeth on me shall never thirst." "I am the living bread which came down from heaven; if any man eat of this bread he shall live forever; and the bread that I will give is my flesh, which I will give for the life of the world."

"The Jews therefore strove among themselves, saying, How can this man give up his flesh to eat? Then Jesus said unto them, Verily, verily, I say unto you, Except ye eat the flesh of the Son of man, and drink his blood, ye have no life in you. . . . He that eateth my flesh and drinketh my blood dwelleth in me and I in him. As the living Father hath sent me, and I live by the Father, so he that eateth me, even he shall live by me."

"Many therefore of his disciples, when they heard this, said, This is an hard saying; who can hear it? When Jesus knew in himself that His disciples murmured at it, he said unto them, Doth this offend you? What and if ye shall see the Son of man ascend up where he was before? It is the Spirit that quickeneth; the flesh profiteth nothing; the words that I speak unto you, they are spirit and they are life."

In Christ God was manifest in the flesh, justified in the Spirit, seen of angels, preached unto the Gentiles, believed on in the world, received up into glory." This we are to believe. These words are not merely to be read as a lesson. They are to be received in the heart, understood, believed, and lived. They will bring us spiritual life. Christ's teachings are to be brought into the daily experience. We have redemption through his blood, even the forgiveness of our sins. Spiritual life comes to us as we receive and practice his words.

The disciples of Christ are to bring the perfections of his character into their character. He has given us his word as spiritual food. As we eat this word, we shall grow up into him, manifesting unselfishness, integrity, kindness, and love. In all we do, Christlikeness is to be revealed. Thus we may show that we are eating the bread of heaven and drawing the living water from the wells of salvation.

As our physical life is sustained by natural food, so our spiritual life is to be sustained by spiritual food,—the words of Christ. The gospel, believed and lived, means eternal life. It gives spiritual health and vigor. It enables us to bear in the daily life the fruits of the Spirit.

Sunday, April 29. The meetings close tonight. They have been well attended, and we feel very much encouraged. We believe that it was in the order of God for them to be held at this time.

The work at Maitland is still going forward. Some very precious souls have taken their stand for the truth. Others are convinced, and we hope that they will soon demonstrate their faith. We are praying earnestly that the Lord will give them courage to do this. Mr. Scott, one of those who are convinced, works for his brother, who is an infidel. Although fully convinced of the truth, he is slow to take his stand before the world as a Seventh-day Adventist. His wife and two daughters have been baptized. Mr. Scobi is the only one of a large family of {129} brothers who used tobac-

co. On one occasion his father and brothers offered him L50 if he would give up tobacco, but he did not accept the offer. When he heard at the meetings in the tent the truth in regard to the evil effects of tobacco upon the system, he stopped using it.

A young man and his wife have lately taken their stand with us. He was employed in a bakery, but lost his position when he began keeping the Sabbath. He has been entrusted with the sale of the Health Foods. We hope that he will be able to do good work in this line. He and his wife are both young and strong, and they will be able, we hope, to manage the health food business in Maitland successfully.

Another young man and his wife, Baker by name, have commenced keeping the Sabbath. He is employed as a salesman in a boot and shoe shop. He says that if he loses his position, he will go into the business for himself.

Twenty persons have been baptized in Maitland and soon several more will be baptized. Those who have taken their stand for the truth seem to be fully and thoroughly converted. We pray for more Sabbath-keepers in Maitland.

The tent has been taken down, and Brother Colcord is holding meetings in a small hall connected with the house in which the mission family live. Brother and Sister James from Ballaret have charge of the mission home. They both labor as they can to instruct the people. Sisters Wilson and Robertson have been and are doing a good work in Maitland. The Lord sustains them, and they have many friends. In the past they have had to walk three and four miles to give their readings, but now they have a horse and buggy.

Brother and Sister Hickox are working in East Maitland. Brother and Sister Colcord are working in West Maitland. Sister Colcord, having a family, does not work much among the people. But it is altogether better to have married people in the work. Workers who are married can work to much greater advantage in the families they visit than can those who are unmarried.

Brother and Sister James are going to take into the mission home an old lady who embraced the truth at the camp meeting. She was, I believe, the first one to keep the Sabbath. She is an invalid, and will be one as long as she lives, but she is always cheerful and will not accept charity. She supports herself by her own handiwork. She will be a blessing in the mission house.

A church must be built in Maitland as soon as the money for it can be raised. When all those who are now convinced decide for the truth, an effort will be made to raise some money for the church. The ministers in Maitland are still very bitter, and keep up the most determined opposition. But if our workers will only walk humbly before God, he will make them vessels unto honor. All who have embraced the truth in Maitland have had to take their stand in the face of decided enmity. Canright's falsehoods have been circulated, and have been met by his own statements.

Our laborers in Maitland are doing good work. All are working in concert, watching for souls as they that must give an account.

Union is strength, and in the work of God unity must be preserved. Strength is not to be wasted in desultory, meaningless efforts but is to be consecrated to a high and holy purpose. {130}

There is much work to be done in and around Newcastle and Maitland, and we feel that the next camp meeting in New South Wales should be held between Maitland and Newcastle, or in East Maitland. I see no way to carry forward the work except by camp meetings. It is of little use to attempt to hold tent meetings without first awakening a general interest. It may be well, where the opposition has been very bitter, to hold two camp meetings in one place. Let the ministers exhaust their opposition, and then let the truths which they have misstated and misinterpreted be presented again in the Spirit and power of God.

The field around Maitland Newcastle is so large that we could use twenty workers, all working in concert under one supreme leader. The Lord will work with every sincere, devoted soldier of the cross. But no man can be a good soldier who thinks he must work independently of his fellow worker, who regards his own judgment as the best. God's workers must blend together, one supplying what the other lacks.

God has given to his church a diversity of gifts. Paul writes, "He gave some, apostles; and some, prophets; and some, evangelists; and some, pastors; and some, teachers; for the perfecting of the saints, for the work of the ministry, for the edifying of the body of Christ, till we all come in the unity of the faith, and of the knowledge of the son of God, unto a perfect man, unto the measure of the fullness of the stature of Christ. . . . I therefore the prisoner of the Lord, beseech you that ye walk worthy of the vocation wherewith ye are called, with all lowliness and meekness, with long-suffering, forebearing one another in love, endeavouring to keep the unity of the Spirit in the bonds of peace. . . . That we henceforth be no more children, tossed to and fro, and carried about with every wind of doctrine, and cunning craftiness, whereby they lie in wait to deceive; but speaking the truth in love, may grow up into him in all things, which is the head, even Christ: from whom the whole body fitly framed together, and compacted by that which every joint supplieth according to the effectual working in the measure of every part, making increase of the body unto the edifying of itself in love."

This instruction is given for our help. Those who will obey will find that the Lord knows what is best for them. The people of God are to work as a perfect whole.

We have not money to pay more workers, but the Lord can work by few as well as by many. He can do a great work through two or three who labor, "not with eye service, as men pleasers, but as the servants of Christ, doing the will of God from the heart, with good will doing service as to the Lord and not to man."

"Finally my brethren be strong in the Lord and in the power of his might." Do not trust in your own strength. "Put on the whole armor of God, that ye may be able to stand against the wiles of the devil." Do we make the preparation it is our privilege to make to stand against the wiles of the enemy? Do we realize the sacred character of God's work and the necessity of watching for souls as they that must give account? We must be vigilant, "knowing the time that now it is high time to awake out of sleep; for now is our salvation nearer than when we believed." "The night is far spent; the day is at hand: let us therefore cast off the works of darkness, and let us put on the armor of light."

Are we learning to forego our own wishes? Or is self still consulted so much that in labor with our brethren we regard our judgment as best of all? God {131} forbid that we should allow self-supremacy to withhold from us the blessings God gives to the meek and lowly. Those who truly glorify God will hide self in Christ, rejoicing if God can be glorified by the labors of those connected with them. No one can succeed in the work of God who has too high an appreciation of himself. As time goes on, his feeling of supremacy grows, and soon he comes to think that he would rather not unite with his brethren in labor but would prefer to work alone.

Such a man is not prepared to do efficient service as a soldier of the cross. He has developed such sensitiveness that he does not wish to be criticized, feeling that it is for his best good to be let alone. He takes offense if his brethren do not work in harmony with his ideas and plans. What can God do with such material?

Let us put far from us every feeling of self-exaltation. Let us prepare to be good soldiers of the cross by learning the lesson Christ gave when he said, "Take my yoke upon you, and learn of me, for I am meek and lowly in heart, and ye shall find rest unto your souls."

He who has crushed down all desire for self-recognition will most surely be recognized by the unselfishness of his actions. In order to help and encourage others, he is willing to put aside his own wishes, becoming all things to all men that he may by some means save some. Such a man is a noble leader in Christ's army.

Look at the Saviour's patient endurance in suffering and trial. Yoke up with him in unselfish service. We are engaged in a severe and trying warfare. "We wrestle not against flesh and blood, but against principalities, against powers, against the rulers of the darkness of this world, against spiritual wickedness in high places." "Wherefore take unto yourself the whole armor of God, that ye may be able to withstand in the evil day, and having done all, to stand."

"Judgment is turned away backward, and justice standeth afar off: for truth is fallen in the street and equity cannot enter. Yea, the Lord saw it, and it displeased him that there was no judgment. . . . According to their deeds, accordingly he will repay, fury to his adversaries, recompence to his enemies; to the islands he will repay recompence. So shall they fear the name of the Lord from the west, and his glory from the rising of the sun. When the enemy shall come in like a flood, the Spirit of the Lord shall lift up a standard against him."

Let us walk carefully and prayerfully before the Lord, not serving self, but serving the Prince of heaven. Read and obey the instruction contained in the second chapter of Philippians. As you do this, you will certainly see the salvation of God.

"Let nothing be done through strife of vain glory; but in lowliness of mind let each esteem other better than himself. . . . Let this mind be in you which was also in Christ Jesus: who being in the form of God, thought it not robbery to be equal with God: but made himself of no reputation, and took upon him the form of a servant, and was made in the likeness of men. . . . Work out your own salvation with fear and trembling: for it is God that worketh in you both to will and to do of his good pleasure. Do all things without murmurings and disputings: that ye may be blameless and harmless, the sons of God, without rebuke, in the midst of a crooked and perverse nation, among whom ye shine as lights in the world." {132}

THE HEALTH FOOD QUESTION

June 16, 1902

I MUST NOW GIVE TO MY brethren the instruction that the Lord has given me in regard to the health food question. By many the health foods are looked upon as of man's devising, but they are of God's originating, as a blessing to His people. The health food work is the property of God, and is not to be made a financial speculation for personal gain. The light that God has given and will continue to give on the food question is to be to His people today what the manna was to the children of Israel. The manna fell from heaven, and the people were told to gather it, and prepare it to be eaten. So in the different countries of the world, light will be given to the Lord's people, and health foods suited to these countries will be prepared.

The members of every church are to cultivate the tact and ingenuity that God will give them. The Lord has skill and understanding for all who will use their ability in striving to learn how to combine the productions of the earth so as to make simple, easily-prepared, healthful foods, which will take the place of flesh meats, so that the people will have no excuse for eating flesh meat.

Those who are giving a knowledge of how to prepare such foods must use their knowledge unselfishly. They are to help their poor brethren. They are to be the producers as well as consumers.

It is God's purpose that health foods shall be manufactured in many places. Those who accept the truth are to learn how to prepare these simple foods. It is not the Lord's plan that the poor shall suffer for the necessaries of life. The Lord calls upon His people in the different countries to ask Him for wisdom, and then to use aright the wisdom He gives. We are not to settle down in hopelessness and discouragement. We are to do our best to enlighten others.

I am instructed to say that we must not look to any human being for power or experience, depending on them for strength and guidance. Christ says, "Look unto Me. I am the Light of the world. He that followeth Me shall not walk in darkness, but shall have the light of life." I speak to those who claim to be children of God. Is it not time that we know the source of our strength and the source of our power? Shall we not, from this time forward, make a record more pleasing to the Lord? Scenes are presented to me that I can find no language to describe. Trials will come that will humble all hearts that are lifted up. Let no one feel that he is safe in following his own way, or in making man his trust. The Lord calls for men of experience, men who will carry responsibilities in His name and in His strength, men who will receive His grace with a realization of their accountability to impart it to others.

It has been most distinctly presented to me that as a people we must walk and work as men and women accountable to God. We must depend upon Him, not on human beings, for, if we depend on human beings, we shall be brought into bondage. The Word of the Living God is to be our guide. Each one is to realize his dependence upon Him whose he is by creation and by redemption. Read and study the statements made in the sixth chapter of John. Pray for an understanding of these truths. I am alarmed as I see the spiritual weakness of those who have had such great light. Had they walked in this light, they would have been strong in the Lord. But they have not, and those who come into the truth through their efforts look to human beings for wisdom, instead of looking to Jesus Christ, {133} "the true Light, which lighteth every man that cometh into the world." When those who claim to believe in Christ receive Him by faith, He will be to them their sanctification, their righteousness, and their exceeding great reward.

The Lord's agencies, the men of His appointment, are individually to receive wisdom from Him. They greatly dishonor Him when they trust in human devising as assurance. They are to see Him distinctly as their sufficiency, their strength.

Are you representing Christ? Have you broken away from the spirit and influence of worldly policy plans and from human devising? Are you eating daily of the bread of life?

Pray that those who have been entrusted with the management of the work of God shall not allow worldly plans to gain the pre-eminence. Let the prayer come from unfeigned lips, "Make me to understand the ways of Thy precepts; so shall I talk of Thy wondrous works." "Thy Word have I hid in mine heart that I might not sin against Thee." "Thy Word is true from the beginning: and every one of Thy righteous judgments endureth forever."

THE MANUFACTURE OF HEALTH FOODS

March 10, 1900
Cooranbong

DURING THE PAST NIGHT MANY things have been opened before me. The production and sale of health foods will require careful consideration. This is a definite subject, and one that needs to be prayerfully and thoughtfully considered.

The Lord does not give to one man only the talent of preparing health foods. There are many minds in many places to whom the Lord will surely give knowledge of how to make foods that are healthful and palatable, if He sees that they will use this knowledge righteously. Animals are becoming more and more diseased, and it will not be long till the use of animal food will be given up by many besides our people. Foods that are healthful and life-sustaining are to be prepared so that men and women will not need to eat meat. The Lord will teach many in all parts of the world to combine fruits, grains, and vegetables into foods that will sustain life and will not bring disease.

Those who have not seen the recipes of how to make the health foods now on the market will make experiments with the food productions of the earth, and will be given light regarding the use of these productions. The Lord will show them what to do. He who gives skill and understanding to His people in one part of the world will give skill and understanding to His people in other parts of the world. It is His design that the food treasures of each different country shall be prepared in such a way that they can be used in the countries for which they are suited.

As God gave manna from heaven to sustain the children of Israel, so He will give His people in different places skill and wisdom to use the productions of these countries in making foods that will take the place of meat. These foods {134} must be made in the different countries; for to transport foods from one country to another makes them so expensive that the poor cannot afford to buy them. It will never pay to depend upon America for the supply of health foods for foreign countries. Men will find great difficulty in handling the imported goods without financial loss.

No selfishness is to be shown in this line of work. Everyone is to work for the benefit of his fellow men. Unless men allow the Lord to guide their minds, untold difficulties will arise as God gives to different ones the knowledge of how to make health foods. When the Lord gives skill and understanding, let that one remember that this wisdom was not given to him for his benefit only, but that with it he might help others.

No man is to think that he is the possessor of all knowledge regarding the preparation of health foods, or that he has the sole right to use the Lord's treasures of earth and tree in making health foods. The Lord will give skill and understanding to many minds. No man is to feel free to use according to his own pleasure the knowledge God has given him on this subject.

It is our wisdom to prepare simple, inexpensive health foods. Many of our people are poor. Healthful foods are to be provided that can be supplied at prices that the poor can afford to pay. It is the Lord's design that the poorest people in every place shall be supplied with inexpensive, healthful foods. In many places industries for the manufacture of these foods are to be established. That which is a blessing to the work in one place, helping its advancement, will be a blessing in another place where money is very much harder to obtain.

God is working in behalf of His people. He does not desire them to be without resources. He is bringing them back to the diet originally given to man. Their diet is to consist of the foods made from the materials He has provided. He will teach them how to make healthful foods. The materials principally used in these foods will be fruits and grains and nuts, but various roots will also be used.

The profits on these foods are to come principally from the world, and not from the Lord's people. God's people have to sustain His work and cause by tithes and offerings. They have to enter new fields and establish churches. On them rest the burdens of many missionary enterprises.

No yokes are to be put upon their necks, and to them no oppression is to be manifested. To His people the Lord is a present help in every time of need.

Some of the specially prepared foods now being made can be improved, and our plans regarding their use will have to be modified. Some have used the nut preparations too freely. Great care should be exercised by those who prepare the recipes for our health journals.

Many have written to me, "I cannot use the nut foods; what shall I use in the place of meat?" One night I seemed to be standing before a company of people, telling them that nuts are used too freely in their preparation of nut foods, and that if they were used more sparingly the results would be more satisfactory; for the system cannot take care of them as combined in some recipes given. {135}

The Lord desires those living in countries where fresh fruits can be obtained during a large part of the year to awake to the blessing they have in this fruit. The more that we learn to depend upon the fresh fruit just as it is plucked from the tree, the greater the blessing will it prove to be.

Some, after adopting a vegetarian diet, return to the use of flesh meat. In this they are foolish indeed; for the animal creation is becoming more and more diseased. But in many cases the reason for this is that they do not know enough about true health reform to substitute proper food in the place of meat.

Cooking schools, conducted by wise instructors, are to be held in America and in other lands. Everything that we can do should be done to show the people the value of the reform diet.

THE MANUFACTURE OF HEALTH FOODS II

February 16, 1901
St. Helena, California

LAST NIGHT I SEEMED TO BE speaking to our people, telling them that as Seventh-day Adventists we must cultivate love, patience, and true courtesy. Jesus will strengthen the leaders of His people if they will learn of Him. God's people must strive to teach the very highest standard of excellence.

I have a most earnest desire that in every place the work shall be carried forward in accordance with His commands. I see trouble as high as mountains ahead for our people in the way in which some things are now being done, and especially in regard to the health food business. As we advance we shall have to meet very difficult problems of human invention, which will bring much perplexity.

With great skill and with painstaking effort, Dr. Kellogg and his associates have prepared a special line of health foods. Their chief motive has been to benefit humanity, and the blessing of God has rested upon their efforts. If they walk in the counsel of God, they will continue to advance; for God will give skill and understanding to those who seek Him unselfishly. In some respects improvements can be made in the health foods sent out from our factories. The Lord will teach His servants how to make food preparations that are more simple and less expensive. There are many whom God will teach in this line if they will walk in His counsel and in harmony with their brethren.

To Our Brethren in All Lands

The Lord has instructed me to say that He has not confined to a few persons all the light on the best preparations of health foods. He will give to many minds in different places tact and skill that will enable them to prepare health foods suitable for the countries in which they live.

God is the author of all wisdom, all intelligence, all talent. He will magnify His name by giving to many minds wisdom in the preparation of healthful foods. And when He does this, the making of these new foods is not to be looked {136} upon as an infringement of the rights of those who are already manufacturing health foods, although in some respects the foods made by the different ones may be similar. God will take ordinary men and women and will give them skill and understanding in the use of the fruits of the earth. He deals impartially with His workers. Not one is forgotten by Him. He will impress business men who are Sabbathkeepers to establish industries that will provide employment for His people. And He will teach His servants to prepare less expensive health foods, which can be purchased by the poor.

In all our plans we should remember that the health food work is the property of God, and that it is not to be made a financial speculation for personal gain. This business is God's gift to His people, and the profits are to be used for the good of suffering humanity everywhere.

An Evil Work

Some of our brethren have done a work that has wrought great injury to the cause. The knowledge of how to manufacture health foods, which God gave to His people as a means for helping to sustain the cause, these men have disclosed to worldly businessmen, who will use this knowledge as a means of personal gain, giving none of the glory to God. Those who have thus disclosed the secrets in their possession in regard to the preparation of health foods, have abused a God-given trust. As they see the result of this betrayal of trust, some will sorely regret that they did not keep their own counsel, and wait for the Lord to lead His servants and to work out His plans in His own way.

The health food business should not be borrowed or stolen from those who by its management are endeavoring to build up and advance the cause. Dr. Kellogg, with the help of others, has, at a large outlay of means, studied out the processes for the preparation of certain foods, and has provided expensive facilities for their manufacture. This work has taken a great deal of precious time; for many experiments have had to be made. Is it not right that those who have thus labored and invested their means, should be allowed to reap the fruit of their labor? Should not Dr. Kellogg, as the Lord's steward, be allowed to control a reasonable income from the special products that he, by the blessing of God, has been enabled to produce?

I understand that Dr. Kellogg has entered into agreement with our medical institutions in various places that they may handle the foods in their localities for the benefit of sanitarium work. I understand that the profits on some lines of foods are used for the support of such benevolent institutions as the Orphans' Home and the Old People's Home at Battle Creek.

Under these circumstances, how unreasonable it is for some of our brethren to follow the course that they are following. They take up the preparation of these special foods, and sell them for personal profit, while at the same time they give the impression that they are working in harmony with those who in the first place prepared these foods for sale. No one has a right to engage in the manufacture of the health foods in any such way.

I have a warning for those who have a knowledge of the methods of manufacturing health foods. They are not to use their knowledge for selfish purposes, or in a way that will misrepresent the cause. Neither are they to make the {137} knowledge of how to prepare these foods a public matter. Let the churches take hold of this, and show these brethren that such a course is a betrayal of their trust, and that it will bring reproach upon the cause.

Let not those who have been and are employed in the work of making the health foods first prepared by Dr. Kellogg, or by any other pioneer in this work, open up all that they know; for thus they defraud the cause of that which should be used for its advancement. I beseech you, my brethren, to make straight paths for your feet, lest the lame be turned out of the way. Do not place information in the hands of unbelievers,—persons who from lack of conscientious regard for health reform, may place impure articles on the market, under the name of health foods.

Stand on the side of righteousness in all your transactions; then you will not appear to disadvantage before God or man. Do not enter into any dishonest practices. Those who take up the preparation and sale of health foods for personal profit are taking a liberty to which they have no right. Thus great confusion is brought into the work. Some manufacture foods professing to be health foods which contain ingredients which health reform condemns. Then again, the foods are often of such an inferior quality that much harm is done to the cause by their sale, those who buy them supposing that all health foods are similar.

No one has any right to take advantage of the business arrangements that have been made in regard to health foods. Those who handle these foods should first come to an understanding with Dr. Kellogg or others who are working in harmony with him, and learn the best methods of handling the health foods. He who enters selfishly into this work, at the same time giving his customers the impression that the profits on the goods he sells are used for personal interest, is under the displeasure of God. By and by their business will fail, and they will get things into such a tangle that their brethren will have to buy them out to save disgrace being brought on the cause.

The Lord is greatly displeased when His service is dishonored by the selfishness of those engaged in it. He wills that every part of His work shall be in harmony with every other part, joint connecting with joint.

The Lord wants His people to stand far above selfish interests. He wants them to conquer the temptations they meet. He calls for the communion of saints. He desires His workers to stand under His supervision. He will plane and polish the material for His temple, preparing each piece to fit closely to the other, so that the building will be perfect and complete, wanting nothing.

Heaven is to begin on this earth. When the Lord's people are filled with meekness and tenderness, they will realize that His banner over them is love, and His fruit will be sweet to their taste. They will make a heaven below in which to prepare for heaven above. {138}

MEDICAL MISSIONARY WORK IN THE CITIES OF CALIFORNIA

December 12, 1900
San Francisco, California

THERE IS WORK TO BE DONE in California that has been strangely neglected. Let this work be no longer delayed. As doors open for the presentation of truth, let us be ready to enter. Some work has been done in the large city of San Francisco, but as we study the field, we see plainly that only a beginning has been made. As soon as possible, well-organized efforts should be put forth in different sections of this city, and also in Oakland. The wickedness of San Francisco is not realized. Our work in this city must broaden and deepen. God sees in it many souls to be saved.

In San Francisco a hygienic restaurant has been opened; also a food store and treatment rooms. These are doing a good work, but their influence should be greatly extended. Other restaurants similar to the one on Market Street should be opened in San Francisco and in Oakland. Concerning the effort that is now being made in these lines of work, we can say, Amen and amen. And as soon as possible other lines of work that will be a blessing to the people will be established. Medical missionary evangelistic work should be carried on in a most prudent and thorough manner. The solemn, sacred work of saving souls is to advance in a way that is modest and yet ever elevated.

Where are the working forces? There are precious souls to be won to Christ. Thoroughly converted men and women of discernment and keen foresight should act as directors of this work. To do this special work, good judgment must be exercised in employing persons who love God and who walk before Him in all humility,—persons who will be effective agencies in God's hand for the accomplishment of the object He has in view,—the uplifting and saving of human beings.

Medical missionary evangelists will be able to do excellent pioneer work. The work of the minister will blend fully with that of the medical missionary evangelist. Christian physicians are not to regard their missionary work as inferior to that of the ministry. A consecrated physician bears a double responsibility; for in him are combined the qualifications of the physician with those of the gospel minister. His is a grand, a sacred, and a very necessary work.

The physician and the minister should realize that they are engaged in the same work. They should work in complete harmony. They are to counsel together. By their unity they will bear witness that God has sent His only begotten Son into the world to save all who will believe in Him as their personal Saviour.

Physicians whose professional abilities are above those of the ordinary doctor, should engage in the service of God in the large cities. They should seek to reach the higher classes. Something is being done in this line in San Francisco. But much more should be done. Let there be no misconception of the nature and the importance of this work. San Francisco is a large and an important portion of the Lord's vineyard.

Medical missionaries who labor in evangelistic lines are doing a work of as high an order as are their ministerial fellow workers. The efforts put forth by these workers are not to be limited to the poorer classes. The higher classes {139} have been strangely neglected. In the higher walks of life will be found many who will respond to the truth because it is consistent, because it bears the stamp of the high character of the gospel. Not a few of the men of ability thus won to the cause will enter energetically into the Lord's work.

We are to do a special work for those who are in high positions of trust. The Lord calls upon those to whom He has entrusted His precious gifts to use in His service their talents of intellect and means. Some will be impressed by the Holy Spirit to invest the Lord's means in a way that will advance His work. They will fulfil His purpose by helping to create centers of influence in the large cities. Our workers should present before these men a plain statement of our needs, letting them know what they need in order to help the poor and needy and to establish this work on a firm basis.

Shall we not do all in our power to advance the work in San Francisco and Oakland, and in all the other cities of California? Thousands upon thousands who live in the cities close by us, need help in various ways. Let the ministers of the gospel remember that the Lord Jesus Christ said to His disciples, "Ye are the light of the world. A city that is set on an hill cannot be hid." "Ye are the salt of the earth; but if the salt have lost his savor, wherewith shall it be salted?"

In our cities interested workers will be led to offer themselves for various lines of missionary effort. Hygienic restaurants will be established. But with what carefulness should this work be done! Those working in these restaurants should be constantly studying, always experimenting, that they may make progress in the preparation of healthful foods. Every hygienic restaurant should be a school for the workers connected with it. In the cities this line of work may be done on a much larger scale than in the smaller places. But in every place where there is a church, instruction should be given in regard to the preparation of healthful, inexpensive foods. Thus the poor will be encouraged to adopt the principles of health reform. They will become industrious.

I saw also that there were several young men and young women, and also those of more mature age,—men and women of capability,—who were being taught of God how to prepare wholesome, palatable foods in an acceptable manner. I was instructed to encourage the establishment of cooking schools in all places where medical missionary work is done. Every inducement to lead the people to reform must be held out before them. Let as much light as possible shine upon them. Teach them to make every improvement that they can in the preparation of food, that they may teach others.

The Lord Jesus will work miracles for His people. In the sixteenth of Mark we read: "So then after the Lord had spoken unto them, He was received up into heaven, and sat on the right hand of God. And they went forth and preached everywhere, the Lord working with them, and confirming the word with signs following." Here we are assured that the Lord was qualifying His chosen servants to take up medical missionary work after His ascension.

From the record of the Lord's miracles in providing wine at the wedding feast and in feeding the multitude, we may learn a lesson of the highest importance. The food business is one of the Lord's own instrumentalities, to supply a necessity. The heavenly Provider of all foods will not leave His people in ignorance in regard to the preparation of the best foods for all times and occasions. {140}

Our workers should exercise their ingenuity in the preparation of healthful foods. None are to pry into Dr. Kellogg's secrets. Yet I have been shown that the Lord is teaching many minds in many places to make healthful foods. There are many products which, if properly prepared and combined, can be made into foods that will be a blessing to those who cannot afford to purchase the more expensive health foods. He who in the building of the tabernacle gave skill and understanding in all manner of cunning work, will now give skill and understanding in the combining of natural food products, thus showing His people how to secure a wholesome, healthful diet. The work of combining fruits, grains, and roots into wholesome foods, is the Lord's work.

No one is to strive to become a great manufacturer of health foods, or to establish a monopoly in this business. Let no one seek to control the food business. But let everyone do his God-appointed work in combining natural products to make healthful foods.

REPORT OF COUNCIL ABOUT MEDICAL MISSIONARY WORK

Chapter I. The Health Food Work
April 13, 1902
"Elmshaven," St. Helena, California

Present: Mrs. E. G. White, W. C. White, N. C. McClure, M. E. Cady, Brethren Loper, Boeker, Fulton, Bowen, Haynes, Morian, and others.

W. C. WHITE: I esteem it a great privilege that we may meet together for counsel in regard to the work of the Food Company. I know that mother is weary, and yet I trust that the Lord will bless us with instruction that has been given to her. Here are Brethren Fulton and Haynes, from San Francisco, Brethren Cady, McClure, and Lashier, from Healdsburg; Brother Loper from the Sanitarium; and Brethren Boeker, Bowen, and others from the Food Company. In a very short time we shall enter meetings in which we ought to present to our people plans and ideals in regard to the work. It is certainly our privilege to ask and receive counsel and enlightenment from God.

[Prayer by Brethren McClure and W. C. White]

W. C. WHITE: If I understand the matter correctly, we have come to believe that the Lord would be pleased to have us make the health food business a great missionary agency, a means of reaching the people with the truths and reforms of this generation. To do this, we must reach out and establish the business in as many localities as we can. As a matter of first importance is to bring right principles of dealing into our homework, so that our employees shall be trained aright and be enabled to develop Christian character, so that when they go out they may correctly represent a Christian enterprise.

In the development of plans the managers of the Food Company have been studying how to place the foods in the hands of our people at prices which they can afford to pay,—how to free the foods consumed by our people from those high prices which are necessary when we give a liberal salary to the man who {141} travels to sell the goods, and a commission to the grocery-man who retails them. To accomplish this, it has been proposed that we organize a business connected with the college, operating under the name of the Healdsburg College Food Company, or some similar name, and that instead of dealing with agents or grocery-men, we sell to our people direct at a net rate. We have discussed more or less the question of how the Food Company should connect with the college—whether we should ask the college to conduct this business upon plans which we could approve, or whether the Food Company should conduct the business on plans which the college could approve; or whether the two should unite hand in hand in a partnership.

Here are the propositions prepared for consideration:

First:

That we organize a department of the food business for the direct supply of the manufactured health foods, also fruits, legumes, health appliances, literature, etc., to all members of the California Medical Missionary and Benevolent Association, stockholders of Healdsburg College and Pacific Press, and the members of the Adventist Church generally.

Second:

That for this work we organize under the name of the "Healdsburg College Food

Company," said company to be an equal partnership of the St. Helena Food Company and the Healdsburg college.

Third:

(A) That we encourage the St. Helena Sanitarium Food Company to incorporate under the supervision of the Pacific Medical Missionary Association.

(B) That we encourage the Food Company to undertake the establishment of vegetarian restaurants in connection with its food stores and in other places as may seem advisable.

(C) That we encourage the Food Company to establish food stores in the principal cities on the coast.

Fourth:

That we establish in San Francisco a purchasing and supply agency for the assistance and convenience of our various missionary enterprises, food stores, restaurants, etc.

In the afternoon meeting these plans were discussed and approved.

W. C. WHITE: Another question, mother, that we have been considering is, what is our duty in the matter of establishing restaurants? We have heard you say in private and in public, and have read in what you have written, something with reference to the advantages to the cause, of establishing vegetarian restaurants. Recently there have seemed to be some good openings. The difficulty that we have been considering is the expense. To establish a restaurant according to the plan on which they are usually conducted, means an investment of from seven hundred to a thousand dollars. {142}

When Dr. Kellogg was here last, he was much interested in our food stores, and the doctor suggested that we consider the advisability of establishing restaurants in an inexpensive way in connection with these stores. We have thought that such beginnings could be made with an outlay of two or three hundred dollars in a place. What would you think of that plan?

MRS. E. G. WHITE: That would be a very small outlay, would it not? Could you limit the expenditure to that amount? I should think that you would have to expend a little more than that.

W. C. WHITE: If the restaurants succeed at all, they would grow and require more. That is the case with our children,—as they grow larger, and we see them develop, we are ready to spend more on them.

There is a question in our minds as to whether it would be right to make the Food

Company more independent, more self-reliant, than it has been in the past, and then encourage it to take up the restaurant business, and introduce restaurants in connection with its stores?

Heretofore our restaurants have been separate enterprises,—often established by individuals,—one person here, one person there, or two persons in some place, or by an agent of an association sent out to do this kind of work. Each restaurant had to work out most of the problems for itself.

In the establishment of food stores, one man has gone out and opened stores, and all have been managed on a uniform plan. We have been thinking of letting the same company undertake the establishment of small restaurants. It could have a number of them. If they grew too large to be operated to advantage in connection with the food stores, then another place could be found. We have thought that as you said we should begin small and let things grow, perhaps it would be in harmony with right principles to follow this plan in the establishment of restaurants.

Hygienic Restaurants

MRS. E. G. WHITE: I have much to say in regard to hygienic restaurants, sanitariums, and the health foods. I am perplexed to know where to begin.

The light given me is, that instead of presenting the subject of health reform abruptly to a congregation of unbelievers, our laborers should first reach the hearts by presenting Christ and Him crucified. Many unbelievers know no more of health reform than do babies. True, the laborers must dwell on reforms; but let them first endeavor to touch and tender the hearts of the people and lead them to be converted. After conversion, men and women will be ready to receive instruction in regard to further reforms, and will permit their teachers to lead them along step by step into the full light of the present truth.

While in New York last winter, I received light in regard to hygienic restaurants. Night after night the course that our brethren should pursue in that city, passed before me. They have a vegetarian restaurant in Brooklyn. They should go forward in the establishment of other hygienic restaurants. Instead of resting satisfied with having only the one that has been opened, they are to open other restaurants in various sections of the city. The people living in one part of Greater New York do not usually know what is going on in the other {143} parts of that great city; and

therefore it is necessary to establish many restaurants. As men and women eat at these places, they will become conscious of an improvement in health. Their confidence once gained, they are more ready to accept God's special message of truth.

Whenever in our large cities there is a strong educational missionary work being carried forward, there should be some sort of hygienic restaurant established, which shall demonstrate to the people right methods in the selection and preparation of food.

When in Los Angeles, I was shown that not only in various sections of that city, but in San Diego and in smaller tourist resorts of Southern California, health restaurants and treatment rooms should be established. Our efforts should include the great seaside resorts.

H. H. HAYNES: Here is a question that has been asked me by a great many of our people within the last year. They say, "We could open a health boarding house; but would it be right to do this and serve guests on the Sabbath, and have them around on that day as we should in an ordinary boarding-house

MRS. E. G. WHITE: I have had no special light in regard to its being the duty of our people to conduct boarding-houses something after the order of hotels. Years ago the brethren began to work in that line in Battle Creek, but the Lord forbade them to continue.

It began in the Sanitarium before Dr. Kellogg came into the institution. Persons who came there to board and room brought in chess playing and many other amusements. This was not right, and the Lord rebuked the management. Our Sanitariums are not to cater to the perverted tastes of worldly people. The same evils have existed in the Sanitarium on the hillside. A few years ago the managers made it more of a hotel than an institution for healing the sick. In the rooms of the guests could be seen the wine bottles that they had brought with them. The boarders indulged appetite for many harmful things. God was not at all pleased with the course pursued by the management in allowing such indulgence; for His purpose in the establishment of the institution was not being carried out. He sent light in regard to it, and the result was that some in leading positions withdrew. They said, "If we refuse to serve meat, we cannot hold the patrons." But whether patronage increases or decreases, right principles must be upheld in the Lord's institutions. In all our work we are to show the advantage of a health reform diet. Between us and the world there is to be a distinct line of demarcation.

We are not building sanitariums for hotels. Receive into sanitariums only those persons who desire to conform to right principles. Let them use the foods that we place before them. If we should allow them to have intoxicating liquors in their rooms, or should serve them with meat, how can we give them the help they should receive in coming to our sanitariums? We must let them know that we have principle enough to keep such articles out of the institution. The same is true in the hygienic restaurants. We must be as true to principle as the needle to the pole. We have no time to dally. Do we not have a desire to see our fellow-being freed from disease and infirmity and in the enjoyment of health and strength? {144}

Hygienic Restaurants in Connection with Treatment Rooms

To return to the question concerning boarding-houses: I have not seen, and cannot now see, any light in opening a boarding-house for the purpose of taking in every tourist that desires merely food and lodging. I have had light, however, that in many cities it is advisable for a restaurant to be connected with treatment rooms. The two can work in harmony, and uphold right principles. In connection with our treatment rooms and restaurants in the cities, it is sometimes advisable to have rooms where we can provide lodgings for the sick. But we are not to erect in the cities immense buildings in which to care for the sick, because of God does not want them to remain in the cities.

Instruction on the Health Food Question

In the early days of health reform among our people, some of our sisters were on the alert for opportunities to show the people how to prepare hygienic foods. On the occasion of large gatherings, some in Battle Creek, thirty years ago, went to the fair-ground—the very place where Dr. Kellogg's house now stands—and, setting up their stoves, they baked and cooked in the presence of the people, and served the food free of charge. This cost time and money, but the result was well worth the effort. Many sampled the foods, pronounced them good, and asked how they were prepared. Gladly they were taught how to prepare the various dishes.

Wherever the truth goes, the people should be given instruction in the preparation of healthful foods. God desires that in every place the people shall be taught to use the products that can be readily obtained. Skillful teachers should show the people how to prepare the products that they can raise or secure in their section of the country. Thus the poor, as well as those in better circumstances, can learn to live healthfully.

All the way along from the beginning, we have found it necessary to educate, educate, educate. God desires us to continue the work of educating the people. We are not to neglect this work because of the effect we may fear it will have on the sales of the goods prepared in the health food factories. That is not the most important matter. Our work is to show the people how they can obtain and prepare wholesome food, how they can co-operate with God in restoring His moral image in themselves. In the effort to help them, difficulties will arise. Some have written to me about the recipes for using the nut preparations, saying that the foods as prepared do not agree with them, and that they have written to the Sanitarium and to others, but have not learned the cause of the difficulty. In replying to such inquiries, I have suggested that they use only one-fifth part of the nut preparations called for in the recipes. This is the instruction given me. It would be a blessing if our cookbooks were pruned of some of the recipes appearing in them.

In the use of foods we should exercise good judgment, and sound sense. When we find that something does not agree with us, we need not write letters of inquiry to learn the cause of the disturbance. We are to use our reason. Change the diet; use less of some of the foods; try other preparations. Soon we shall know the effect that certain combinations have on us. We are not machines; we are intelligent human beings; and we are to exercise our common sense. We can experiment with different combinations of foods. {145}

There are persons who would be more benefited by abstinence from food for a day or two every week than by any amount of medicine or treatment or medical advice. To fast one day a week would be of incalculable benefit to them. It is foolish for one to keep on eating day after day, and yet wonder why he is in distress. Let such an one relieve himself from distress by changing his diet or by eating less. If he wills to do so, he can soon obtain relief.

God never intended that the manufacture of health foods should be committed to any one man or set of men. Knowledge in regard to the preparation of health foods is God's property, and has not been entrusted to a few men only, to be kept to themselves. God communicates to men in order that man may communicate to his fellow men. In saying this, I do not refer to the special preparations that it has taken Dr. Kellogg and others long study and much expense to perfect. I refer especially to the simple preparations that all can make for themselves, instruction in regard to which should be given to those who desire to live healthfully, and especially to the poor.

There is one thing that our brethren have done, which has wrought great injury to the work. God has given us knowledge in the manufacture of foods, as a means of helping to sustain the cause; yet there are some who have been so indiscreet as to disclose to worldly men secrets in regard to the preparation of health foods. Thus they have abused their God-given trust. They ought to have kept their own counsel, and allowed the Lord to lead.

It is the Lord's design that in every place men and women shall have the privilege of developing their talents by preparing healthful foods from the natural products of their section of the country. No man is to forbid them. If they look to God, exercising their skill and ingenuity under the guidance of His Spirit, they will learn how to prepare natural products into healthful foods. Thus they will be able to teach the poor how to prepare foods that will take the place of flesh meat. Those thus helped can in turn instruct others. Such a work will yet be done. If it had been done before, there would today be many more people in the truth than there are, and we should have had many more who could give instruction, than we have. Let us learn what our duty is, and then do it. We are not to be dependent and helpless, trusting in human beings.

In reform movements, too often our leaders do not take the people with them. My husband was very particular in regard to this point. He tried to move no faster than he could lead the people. He regarded it as beneficial to the cause of truth to counsel with his brethren and sisters, as we have met for counsel today. After laying his plans before the council, he would say, "If you all agree to these plans, we will place them before our people. They support the work in the field, and we must bring these things to their attention, that we may all move understandingly, working to one point."

In connection with the food question, the Southern field was opened before me in a special manner. In some sections of the South the people will find it necessary to obtain some of the health foods from places outside of that field. But many of the products raised in the South may be utilized in making wholesome foods. In some parts of that field there is a good supply of fruit.

I cannot enter into the minute in regard to the health food business. The details must be worked out by others, and these must be men and women of consecration and common sense. Many ask, "What would you do in such and such a case?" {146} My brethren and sisters, find out what to do when you come to the perplexity. You cannot learn everything at once. You must learn as you advance. Constantly advance. There should be a gradual development. Learn from one another. Pray for divine enlightenment. God has skill and understanding for His people. He who gave manna to the Israelites for forty years, who kept their shoes and clothing from waxing old and worn, still has a care for His children. If we place ourselves in right relation to Him, and daily commune with Him, we shall be taught of Him, and shall receive His blessing.

"Herein is My Father glorified, that ye bear much fruit; so shall ye be My disciples. . . . If ye keep My commandments, ye shall abide in My love, even as I have kept My Father's commandments, and abide in His love." These things have I spoken unto you, that My joy might remain in you, and that your joy might be full." Into every department of God's work there is to be brought hope, courage and joy,—the joy of Christ. Then spiritual things will be spiritually discerned. The joy of the Lord is as far above every other joy as holiness is above unholiness. It gives strength to the physical, mental, and spiritual powers.

_____

MY BROTHER

July 10, 1900

I WRITE TO YOU AT THIS TIME to set before you our great necessity. The Lord has entrusted to you the talent of means to use and improve to his name's glory. There is a great work to be done. The last message of mercy is being given to the world. Everything in the political world is being stirred with agitation. There are wars and rumors of wars. The nations are angry, and the time of the dead has come that they should be judged.

A most solemn and important work is to be done in our world by God's people. This work is represented by the third angel flying in the midst of heaven. The third angel's message is preceded by the messages of the first and second angels. The first angel's message proclaims the hour of God's judgment. The second declares the fall of Babylon.

John writes, "I saw another angel fly in the midst of heaven, having the everlasting gospel to preach unto them that dwell on the earth, and to every nation, and kindred, and tongue, and people, saying with a loud voice, Fear God, and give glory to him: for the hour of his judgment is come; and worship him that made heaven, and earth, and the sea, and the fountains of waters.

"And there followed another angel, saying, Babylon is fallen, is fallen, that great city, because she made all nations drink of the wine of the wrath of her fornications."

"And the third angel followed them, saying with a loud voice, If any man worship the beast, and his image, and receive his mark in his forehead, or in his hand, the same shall drink of the wine of the wrath of God, which is poured out without mixture into the cup of his indignation; and he shall be tormented with fire and brimstone in the presence of the holy angels, and in the presence of the Lamb." {147}

These messages must go to all the inhabitants of the world. The Lord is soon to come, and he calls upon all to whom he has entrusted his capital of means to invest it in his work as it demands help. His money is not to be shut up in banks and buildings and lands when there is such a great work to be accomplished. The Lord will not send His judgments for disobedience and transgression upon the world until he has sent his watchmen to give the message of warning.

The Lord has been pleased to give his people the third angel's message as a testing message to bear to the world. John beholds a people distinct and separate from the world, who refuse to worship the beast or his image, who bear God's sign, keeping holy his Sabbath, the seventh day, to be kept holy as a memorial of the living God, the Creator of heaven and earth. Of them the apostle writes, "Here are they that keep the commandments of God and the faith of Jesus."

"After these things I saw another angel come down from heaven, having great power, and the earth was lightened with his glory. And he cried mightily with a strong voice, saying, Babylon is fallen, is fallen, and is become the habitation of devils, and the hold of every foul spirit, and the cage of every unclean and hateful bird. For all nations have drunk of the wine of the wrath of her fornication, and the kings of the earth have committed fornication with her, and the merchants of the earth are waxed rich through the abundance of her delicacies. And I heard another voice from heaven, saying, Come out of her, my people, that ye be not partakers of her sins, and that ye receive not of her plagues. For her sins have reached unto heaven, and God hath remembered her iniquities."

What is sin? "The transgression of the law." God denounces Babylon, "because she made all nations drink of the wine of the wrath of her fornications." This means that she has disregarded the only commandment which points out the true God, and has torn down the Sabbath, God's memorial of creation.

God made the world in six days and rested on the seventh, sanctifying this day, and setting it apart from all others as holy to himself, to be observed by his people throughout their generations.

But the man of sin, exalting himself above God, sitting in the temple of God, and showing himself to be God, thought to change times and laws. This power, thinking to prove that it was not only equal to God, but above God, changed the rest day, placing the first day of the week where the seventh should be. And the Protestant world has taken this child of the Papacy to be regarded as sacred. This is called in the word of God her fornication.

God has a controversy with the churches today. They are fulfilling the prophecy of John. "All nations have drunk of the wine of the wrath of her fornication." They have divorced themselves from God by refusing to receive his sign. They have not the spirit of God's true commandment keeping people. And the people of the world in giving their sanction to a false sabbath, and in trampling under their feet the Sabbath of the Lord, have drunk of the wine of the wrath of her fornication.

God set the seventh day apart as the day of his rest. But the man of sin has set up a false sabbath, which the kings and merchants of the earth have accepted and exalted above the Sabbath of the

Bible. In doing this they have chosen a religion like that of Cain, who slew his brother Abel. Cain and Abel {148} both offered sacrifice to God. Abel's offering was accepted because he complied with God's requirements. Cain's was rejected because he followed his own human inventions. Because of this he became so angry that he would not listen to Abel's entreaties or to God's warnings and reproofs, but slew his brother.

By accepting a spurious rest day the churches have dishonored God. The people of the world accept the falsehood, and are angry because God's commandment keeping people do not respect and reverence Sunday. The Lord sanctified and blessed the seventh day. God says, "Her sins have reached unto heaven, and God hath remembered her iniquities. Reward her even as she rewarded you, and double unto her double according to her works; in the cup which she hath filled, fill to her double. How much she hath glorified herself, and lived deliciously, so much torment and sorrow give her; for she saith in her heart, I sit a queen, and am no widow, and shall see no sorrow. Therefore shall her plagues come in one day, death, and mourning, and famine; and she shall be utterly burned with fire; for strong is the Lord who judgeth her."

God declares, "If any man worship the beast and his image, and receive his mark in his forehead, or in his hand, the same shall drink of the wine of the wrath of God." God will punish those who attempt to compel their fellow men to keep the first day of the week. They tempt them to deny their allegiance to God. They accept the fruit of the forbidden tree, and try to force others to eat it. They will try to compel their fellowmen to work on the seventh day of the week and rest on the first. God says of them, "They shall drink of the wine of the wrath of God, which is poured out without mixture into the cup of his indignation."

"Verily my sabbaths ye shall keep," the Lord says, "for it is a sign between me and you throughout your generations, that ye may know that I am the Lord that doth sanctify you." Some will seek to place obstacles in the way of Sabbath observance, saying, You do not know what day is the Sabbath. But they seem to understand when Sunday comes, and have manifested great zeal in making laws for compelling its observance, as though they could control the conscience of man.

God has given men the Sabbath as a sign between him and them, as a test of their loyalty. Those who, after the light regarding God's law comes to them, continue to disobey, and exalt human laws above the law of God in the great crisis before us, will receive the mark of the beast.

The prosperity of God's people is dependent on their obedience. The Lord declares, "It shall come to pass, if ye shall hearken diligently unto my commandments, which I command you this day, to love the Lord your God, and to serve him with all your heart and with all your soul, that I will give you the rain of your land in his due season, the first rain and the latter rain, that thou mayest gather in thy corn, and thy wine, and thine oil. And I will send grass in thy fields for thy cattle, that thou mayest eat and be full. Take heed to yourselves that your heart be not deceived, and ye turn aside, and serve other gods, and he shut up the heaven, that there be no rain, and that the land yield not her fruit, and lest ye perish quickly from off the good land which the Lord giveth you."

God's curse for disobedience is upon man and beast and the fruit of the earth. Why do not those who claim to obey God, study his word, and learn there {149} why the earth does not produce as it once did. Why are the cattle all so full of disease?

"Behold I set before you this day a blessing and a curse: a blessing if ye obey the commandments of the Lord your God, which I command you this day; and a curse if ye will not obey the Lord your God, but turn aside out of the way which I command you this day, to go after gods, which ye have not known.

"Thou art an holy people unto the Lord thy God: the Lord thy God hath chosen thee to be a special people unto himself, above all people that are upon the face of the earth. The Lord did not set his love upon you, nor choose you, because ye were more in number than any people; but because the Lord loved you, and because he would keep the oath which he had sworn unto your fathers, hath the Lord brought you out with a mighty hand, and redeemed you out of the house of bondmen, the hand of Pharaoh King of Egypt. Know therefore that the Lord thy God, he is God, the faithful God, which keepeth covenant and mercy with them that love him, and keep his commandments to a thousand generations; and repayeth them that hate him to their face, to destroy them; he will not be slack to him that hateth him, he will repay

him to his face. Thou shalt therefore keep the commandments, and the statutes, and the judgments, which I command thee this day, to do them."

These words should be as distinctly stamped upon every soul as though written with a pen of iron. Obedience brings its reward; disobedience its retribution.

"Thou shalt remember all the way which the Lord thy God led thee these forty years in the wilderness, to humble thee, and to prove thee, to know what was in thine heart, whether thou wouldest keep his commandments or no. And he humbled thee, and suffered thee to hunger, and fed thee with manna, which thou knewest not, neither did thy fathers know, that he might make thee know that man doth not live by bread alone, but by every word that proceedeth out of the mouth, (not of man, but) of God. Thy raiment waxed not old upon thee, neither did thy foot swell, these forty years. Thou shalt also consider in thine heart, that, as a man chasteneth his son, so the Lord thy God chasteneth thee. Therefore thou shalt keep the commandments of the Lord thy God, to walk in his ways, and to fear him."

God has given his people positive instruction and has laid upon them positive restrictions, that by obtaining a perfect experience in his service they may be qualified to stand before the heavenly universe and before the fallen world as overcomers. They are to overcome by the blood of the Lamb and by the word of their testimony. Those who fall short of making the preparation essential will be numbered with the unthankful and the unholy.

The Lord brings his people by ways which they know not, that he may test and try them. This world is our place of proving. Here we decide what our eternal destiny will be. God never exalts his people. He humbles them, that his will may be wrought in them. Thus God dealt with the children of Israel as he led them through the wilderness. He told them what their fate would have been had he not laid his restraining hand upon that which would have hurt them. He speaks to them. Hear what he says. It is a revelation of the ministration of angels. "Who led thee through that great and terrible wilderness, wherein were fiery serpents, and scorpions, and drought, where there was no water; who brought {150} thee forth water out of the rock of flint; who fed thee in the wilderness with manna, which thy fathers knew not, that he might humble thee, and that he might prove thee, to do thee good at thy latter end: and thou say in thine heart, My power and the might of mine hand hath gotten me this wealth. But thou shalt remember the Lord thy God; for it is he that giveth thee power to get wealth, that he may establish his covenant which he sware unto the fathers, as it is this day. And it shall be, if thou do at all forget the Lord thy God, to walk after other gods, to serve them, and worship them, I testify against you this day that ye shall surely perish. As the nations which the Lord destroyeth before your face, so shall ye perish; because ye would not be obedient unto the voice of the Lord your God."

"At that time the Lord said unto me, Hew thee two tables of stone like unto the first, and come up into me into the mount, and make thee an ark of wood. And I will write on the tables the words that were in the first tables which thou brakest, and thou shalt put them in the ark. And I made an ark of shittim wood, and hewed two tables of stone like unto the first, and went up into the mount, having the two tables in mine hand. And he wrote on the tables according to the first writing, the ten commandments, which the Lord spake unto you out of the mount, out of the midst of the fire, in the day of the assembly; and the Lord gave them unto me. And I turned myself, and came down from the mount, and put the tables in the ark which I had made; and there they be, as the Lord commanded me." Yes: there they were to be hidden and preserved, to justify the obedient and condemn the disobedient. Those who choose to disobey will surely receive sentence according to their works.

I present these things before you that ye may know and understand. Our present course of action is deciding our destiny for eternity. This is indeed a solemn thought. Those who know the truth are to practice the truth, realizing that the fear of the Lord is of more value than gold or silver. The world is the Lord's vineyard. He says, Go work today in my vineyard." As I have cared for you and blessed you, so you are to care for my honor and my name's glory.

In his dealing with ancient Israel God has given us an illustration of the result that will follow an unrighteous, disobedient course. He will punish all who make his glory to be reproached, even as he punished the children of Israel. Those who exalt themselves will be humbled, even as Jerusalem, by her own course of action, was humiliated and brought low. Her people

chose Barabbas, and God left them to their choice. They would not submit to God's way, and he permitted them to have their own way, and to carry out the purposes of their unsanctified hearts.

Christ warned the Jews of their danger, and entreated them to return to God, but they were too proud to accept his overtures of mercy. They persisted in a course of rebellion, and as a result the protection of God's heavenly intelligences was withdrawn from them.

When Christ predicted the destruction of Jerusalem, he predicted also the destruction of the world; for he saw that till the end of this earth's history men would continue to refuse God's mercy.

By love of money, desire for the supremacy, dishonesty, we not only rob God of the fruit of his vineyard, but we practice selfishness toward our brethren {151} and toward those who are weighing and measuring the influence exerted by the one who claims to love God and obey the truth. God has placed men and women in positions of trust that they may represent him. He has given them talents that they may work in his service. But in their selfishness men misuse these talents. The talent of means is the most dangerous and the most deceptive when put to a wrong use. God's word declares that the love of money is the root of all evil.

He who is unjust in small matters will be unjust in matters concerning his eternal interest. Those who will rob their fellow men will rob God. The Lord gives men talents that they may benefit and bless their fellow men. He has made men his stewards in trust, that they may relieve the temporal and spiritual necessities of those for whom Christ had died. Those who faithfully do this work labor in Christ's stead.

God blesses the work of men's hands. They are to act their part as faithful stewards by returning to the Lord his portion. They are to devote their means to his service, that his vineyard may not remain a barren waste. They are to study what course the Lord would pursue were he in their place. They are to take all difficult matters to the Lord in prayer. They are not to use all the means at their command in supplying with an overabundance of facilities the portion of the vineyard in which they are placed. They are to unselfishly impart that which they have to the Lord's workers in hard places. They are to study methods and ways whereby their fellow workers shall have opportu-

nity to improve their portion of the Lord's vineyard. All God's workers are to reveal an unselfish interest in the building up of the work in all parts of the vineyard. The Lord's principles are to be carried out with clear, sharp discernment.

The true workers will count the cost of every method and plan. He will say, I am receiving a larger portion of the Lord's goods than many others of the Lord's workers. I will not lay plans to gather more responsibility to myself than I can carry. The goods entrusted to me are the Lords, and they could be used to greater advantage in more destitute portions of his vineyard than in this place. I will impart to my fellow workers that which the Lord has given me. I will also impart of the foresight and judgment to help the work in places where the necessity is great.

Willingly and cheerfully the true Christian will bind about his own inclinations to invest his means, God's own relief fund, in a larger work than he could possibly manage. If he sees that his fellow laborers in other portions of the field are pained and perplexed by a lack of proper facilities, he will willingly impart to them a portion of what the Lord has entrusted to him. As he shows by his unselfishness that he loves his neighbor as himself, the Lord says of him in the councils of heaven, "He is faithful steward. I can trust him to handle my goods. He keeps my fear before him. His works of righteousness will be a continual stream flowing to the desert portions of my vineyard. He will not claim what he has as his own, to use as the human agent pleases. He will heed my counsel, and do with my goods as I shall choose."

Unwise generalship is an offense to God, because it involves many others in difficulties. The Lord proves and tests every man, to see whether he will deal wisely with the Master's goods. If he grasps in his arms all he can possibly obtain, to manage according to his own wisdom, if he uplifts himself as very wise, and neglects to take hold in the places where God's work is in the greatest need of help, he fails to do God's will. The heavenly universe watches his course with sadness; for he robs the Lord of the glory due to him, in establishing churches in new territories, and deprives his fellow workers of the means the Lord God designed should be given to them. {152}

He who is unfair in the least will be unfair also in much. Those who grasp all the advantages they can for the work in their portion of the field, selfishly refusing to help their fellow workers, are unwise stewards. They help that portion of the vineyard in which they are interested, allowing other portions to get along as they can. They say, I will take care of the things under my supervision. But the Lord is greatly displeased by this course of action. He has given them his means for wise consideration of all doing his service and wise distribution. His workmen pray to him for facilities with which to work, while those to whom he has given his means, the very means to answer these prayers, neglect his work, allowing his workers to lose their time and wear out their strength in working against disadvantages which need not be. These selfish stewards have not the mind of Christ. They do not say, All we are brethren. We will share our blessings, that our fellow-workers, whom God has sent into the new field, may have a chance to invest the Lord's abundant provision in other portions of the vineyard. We will help our fellow workers out of their difficulty, that the Lord's work may be a praise in all parts of the earth.

There are those who are improvident in their handling of the Lord's property, who do many things which are really in need of undoing, who swerve the work out of the humble, self-sacrificing lines in which it should be kept. By this wrong use of money, workers together with God are brought to a standstill. In some places means have been expended profusely, while in others the workers could only stand and wait, in deep distress because they had not the means the Lord designed them to have for the work. The Lord is displeased and his name is dishonored because men work in accordance with their finite impulses. They claim as their own that which the Lord has entrusted to them to be used with equity and judgment, that the holy Sabbath may be known in all parts of the world.

These things mean much to those who have had a knowledge of the leadings of God from the beginning of their responsibility. "If therefore ye have not been faithful in the unrighteous mammon, if you have not had wisdom to do in my way the work appointed you, who will commit to you the true riches? You would act an independent part in heaven as you have acted on the earth. If you cannot be faithful in that which is another man's, who will give you that which is your own?

Money and goods, houses and lands, are the Lord's, entrusted to human agents to be used for the advancement of the work of God. Those who spend this money in luxury and show are not following Christ's footsteps. Outside show and parade is the fruit of self-exaltation. This influence hinders the work the Lord desires to go forward in triumph.

Some of the supposed advantages for which the Lord's money is spent are concocted by Satan, to confuse God's people and lead them in false paths. As he succeeds in inducing the workers to leave the right track, he comes closer and closer, framing lies for their acceptance. He insinuates the thought that the gospel ministry is standing in the way of the great and grand work that might be done. Dissension, strife and disunion are the result. The work may be good in itself, but men have become exalted in regard to their own wisdom. Thus great trial is brought upon God's workers. Wearing, vexatious issues are brought about that should never come up.

The elevated character of the work of God is to be maintained. The Lord desires his chosen elect people to stand superior in this Theocracy, shining amid {153} the moral darkness of a hollow insincere formalism. The children of God are not to pull one another to pieces. The work must be carried forward in Christ's lines. He has left us an example of humility and unselfishness. He is our Pattern, and he says, "He that will come after me, let him deny himself, and take up his cross, and follow me." Let all remember the words, "Ye are laborers together with God, ye are God's husbandry; ye are God's building." You are not wise enough to work by yourself. He has made you his steward in trust, to prove and try you, even as he did ancient Israel. He will not have his army composed of undisciplined, unsanctified erratic soldiers, who would misrepresent his order and purity.

Serving mammon.

How few realize what this really means! It is Satan's work to lead men into false paths. He will if possible bring in false issues, which lead to a denial of the truth for this time. Those who in thought, word, or deed belittle or disparage the gospel ministry because it does not sustain them in erratic movements are on perilous ground. They need to study the lesson God teaches in the parable of the two sons. Unbelievers do not pretend to obey God. More dangerous are those who regard their disobedience as obedience. God will have order in his work. There are unfaithful men in the ministry, but this does not make the ministry any less the Lord's means for doing a great work. Those who accuse and disparage the ministry because the work done does not appear to be the work that should be done, are not wise men.

Those who think they are pleasing God by obeying some other law than his, and by performing works other than those the gospel has enjoined, are mocking God. They are insulting the Holy One of Israel. Warning after warning has been given. Appeal after appeal is made in the last message of mercy given to the world. Loath to give up, hoping, sorrowfully hoping, Christ knocks for the last time at the door of the heart. Men and women are given a final test. The worst of sinners are to hear the message of mercy. God will prove who will receive his seal or mark.

When Christ saw in the Jewish people a nation divorced from God, he saw also a professed Christian church united to the world and the Papacy. And as he stood upon Mount Olivet, weeping over Jerusalem till the sun sank behind the western hills, so he is watching over and pleading with sinners in these last moments of time. Soon he will say to the angels who are holding the four winds, "Let the plagues loose; let darkness, destruction, and death come upon the transgressors of my law." Will he be obliged to say to those who have had great light and great knowledge, as he said to the Jews, "O that thou hadst known, even thou in this thy day, the things which belong unto thy peace. But now they are hid from thine eyes."?

TO EVERY MAN HIS WORK
[Prior to July 1915]

WE ARE LABORERS TOGETHER with God. We must have spiritual workers, not only laborers who labor in the pulpit for the churches but those who will do personal work among the people. Too much time is devoted to the churches in preaching. This is not attended with the best results. The work of the Lord's ambassadors is to organize a company of workers to hunt for souls who need help, but hours are spent in preaching that had better be devoted to personal house to house labor. In the Spirit of Christ, with the heart all aglow with his love, seek to win the hearts of those in the family. Give faithful admonitions and {154} instructions from the Word of God. There are appropriate and applicable Scriptures that need to be presented, and to be presented in love for souls for whom Christ has died. "All Scripture is given by inspiration of God, and is profitable for doctrine, for reproof, for correction, for instruction in righteousness; that the man of God may be perfect, thoroughly furnished unto all good works." But many souls have had no personal labor. Words of kindly instruction in the application of Scriptures have not been spoken to them.

When a church is visited by wise and experienced workmen, let these men find out if there is not something for them to do for that church that will be a blessing to families. Converse with them in regard to their spiritual advancement. Show them that they are under obligations to work as those who have received the grace of God. The missionary spirit must be kept awake, and in order for this spirit to live, the members of the church must be laborers together with God. It is time that unselfish consecrated workmen should enter into families who have already accepted the truth, and yet have not worked for its advancement. It is time that our preaching brethren should minister not only to the congregation, but in families. Come close to your brethren; seek for them; come close to the hearts, as one touched with the feelings of their infirmities. Thus may we achieve victories that our small faith has not grasped. The members of these families should be given some labor to perform for the good of souls. Mutual love and confidence will give them moral force to be laborers together with God.

Pastors of churches are remiss in ministering, in educating faithfully the members of the church. If they are not acquainted with their duty in this respect, they need a teacher to instruct them. "Let a man so account of us, as of the ministers of Christ, and stewards of the mystery of God. Moreover it is required in stewards, that a man be found faithful." "Who then is a faithful and wise servant, whom his Lord hath made ruler over his household, to give them meat in due season? Blessed is that servant, whom his Lord when he cometh will find so doing. Verily, I say unto you, that he shall make him ruler over all his goods. But, and if that servant shall say in his heart, My lord delayeth his coming; And shall begin to smite his fellowservants, and to eat and drink with the drunken; The Lord of that servant shall come in a day when he looketh not for him, and in an hour that he is not aware of, and

shall cut him asunder, and appoint him his portion with the hypocrites: there shall be weeping and gnashing of teeth."

A steward identifies himself with his master. His master's interests become his. He has accepted the responsibilities of a steward and he must act in the master's stead doing as the master would do if he were presiding over his own goods. The position is one of dignity in that his master trusts him. If a steward in any wise acts selfishly, and turns the advantages gained in trading with his lord's goods to his own advantage, he has perverted the trust reposed in him. The master can no longer look upon him as a servant to be trusted, one on whom he can depend.

Every Christian is a steward of God, and entrusted with his goods. Ministers and laymen have a work committed to them as individuals. All who are connected by faith with our Lord Jesus Christ have a ministry to perform. Those who do not take their position on the Lord's side, ought to without delay; for they will have to give an account of themselves to God. Christ paid the ransom for {155} them as verily as for every professed Christian. If they despise the gift, the question will be asked, Who bewitched you, that you should not obey the truth, before whose eyes Jesus Christ has been evidently set forth, crucified among you?"

Whether you are believers or unbelievers, you are the Lord's property, bought with a price. You may ignore your relationship with God as His children. Whose children then are you? Children of the devil, and his deeds you are content to do. But all the influence you might have exercised by using your talents in behalf of truth, and by co-operating with God, all the improvements your talents would have made if put into actual service through the provisions made for you to cooperate with God, will be charged to your account. You stubbornly held yourself on Satan's side giving your influence to the great apostate; and all the good you might have done through the atoning sacrifice, but did not do, will be charged against you when you are weighed in the balances and found wanting. You had a work to do. A special stewardship was entrusted to you, but you would not accept the trust. Christ crucified was presented to you. The spirit of God pled with you. By being lifted up on the cross Christ sought to draw you to himself. But your stubborn will would not yield to his invitations. His appeals were resisted.

You are stewards notwithstanding; but unfaithful, dishonorable stewards, burying your talents in the world, serving Satan in the place of serving the Lord. Impenitent sinner, what excuse will you give to God for your wasted opportunities.

Ministers of Jesus Christ, are you faithful in setting before families by personal effort their accountability to seek and to save that which is lost? Do you enter into this work, educating young men by taking them with you, and teaching them how to work? "It is required of stewards, that a man be found faithful." He may not be an eloquent speaker, but he can present the truth in the clearest simplicity. He can work intelligently, doing his best according to his ability; and if he is faithful, God will give him wisdom, and increase his talents.

To some are entrusted larger responsibilities than to others. But if you have only one talent, you can increase it by use, to two. Then by working humbly, trustingly, you may add to the two, two more. Thus the work in your charge may be continually growing. But there are a large number of idle stewards. Those are to be found among those who bear credentials as ministers. But they do not minister, carrying the burden of souls. Dishonest, idle shepherds, they do not have travail for the souls that are perishing all around them.

Let every church member carefully consider his responsibilities, and look himself in the face. Become acquainted with yourself. Urge home upon your own hearts that you are not to seek to make yourself a specialty, for effect, for praise, but a specialty in seeking first the kingdom of God and his righteousness, inquire seriously, "Am I faithful?" Be first a most faithful steward over yourself. Search your own heart, and often compare it with the great mirror of the word of God, until tried and searched by God, you will be approved of him, not having your own righteousness, but the righteousness of Jesus Christ. Strengthened by his might in the inner man you will be accepted as a vessel unto honor.

You may say, I have not large means and can do but little with the little I have. All the Lord asks of you is to be a faithful steward, to render to God {156} a tenth of all your increase without stopping to measure the matter to see how you are coming out. You have but little means, render back to him the portion belonging to him; for it is not yours. It is a serious matter to rob God. Thus you deprive yourself of the blessing he has promised to bestow if you exercise faithful stewardship. If you have been untrue to God, if you show that you will not do according to the agreement he has made with you, will he bless you with facilities of obtaining more means? You keep yourself under condemnation as unfaithful stewards by working contrary to a "Thus saith the Lord." You deprive the treasury of God of your proportion of his agreement with you, because you choose to walk in the light of the sparks of your own kindling. In your finite wisdom, you think you are making better terms with yourself than God has made with you. How then, if you are unfaithful steward with the least, can the Lord entrust to you larger responsibilities?

God wants all his stewards to be exact in following divine arrangements. They are not to offset the Lord's plans with some deed of charity, some gift, or some offering, done or given when and how, the human agents, shall see fit. God has made his plan known, and all who co-operate with him will carry out his plan, instead of daring to attempt to improve on it, by their own arrangements. Those who honor a "Thus saith the Lord," who accept exactly what the Lord has devised, will be according to God's plan. God will honor them, and work in their behalf: For we have his pledged word that he will open the windows of heaven and pour us out a blessing, such as there will not be room enough to receive.

It is a very poor policy for men to seek to improve on God's plan, and invent a makeshift, averaging up their good impulses in this and that instance, and offsetting them against all that is required of God. God calls upon you to give every jot of influence to his own arrangement and ordinances. We are to strike true and faithful figures in tithing and then say to the Lord, I have done as thou hast commanded me. If you will honor me by trusting me with thy goods to trade upon, I will be thy faithful steward, doing all in my power to bring meat to thy house, and I will seek to instruct others how to work in the same lines.

Bear in mind, "Moreover, it is required of a steward that he be found faithful." Men who have large responsibilities are to be sure that they are not robbing God in any jots or tittles, when so much is involved, as is plainly stated in Malachi. Here we are told that a blessing is given for a faithful disposition of the tithes, and a curse for covetous retention of the money which should flow into the treasury. Then ought we not to be sure to work on the safe side, so dealing with God in handling the property lent us on trust, that no shadow of reproach will fall on us?

"Will a man rob God? Yet ye have robbed me. But ye say, Wherein have we robbed thee. In Tithes and offerings. Ye are cursed with a curse, for ye have robbed me, even this whole nation. Bring ye all the tithes into the storehouse, that there may be meat in mine house and prove me now herewith, saith the Lord of hosts, if I will not open you the windows of heaven, and pour you out a blessing that there shall not be room enough to receive it: And I will rebuke the devourer for your sake, and he shall not destroy the fruits of your ground; neither shall your vine cast her fruit before the time in the field, saith the Lord of hosts. And all nations shall call you blessed: for ye shall be a delightsome land, saith the Lord of hosts." I need not ask, Will not God bless {157} those who are faithful? We have his pledged word. But the blessing of God is withdrawn from dishonest, covetous church members in this life. God says it, and what God says is true. Who of you claiming to be the children of God will venture to meet your delinquencies when the books shall be opened, and every man judged according to the deeds done in the body. The first point we need to settle is that we are not to look upon the property we are handling as our own with which we may do as we please. It is the Lord's, to be administered in accordance with his prescribed plans. Be faithful in giving to the Lord the specified amount he has directed you to give. Then present the great mystery of godliness, lifting up Christ, and saying, Behold the Lamb of God, who taketh away the sins of the world.

Every church member who has been truly converted is to be given some work. "The case that I knew not, I searched out," Job declared. Consideration is to be given as to what service for God means. It means that we are to do the same kind of ministry that Christ did when he was in our world. In this work, whether we are rich or poor, we are called upon to wear Christ's yoke, and learn of him to be meek and lowly in heart. Some more may especially be given the work of setting forth Christ from the pulpit, opening the oracles of God to the churches. Yet they should not exclude themselves from visiting families, talking with them, praying with them, exhorting them, encouraging those who need encouraging, and presenting a "Thus saith the Lord" to meet every case of deficiency. Altogether too little of this work is done. Personal labor is greatly needed. Many, many souls might be saved if those who claim to be followers of Christ would work as Christ worked living not to please self, but to glorify God, acting as missionaries, showing genuine love for the Master by making every possible use of their entrusted talents. From the very nature of work in Christ's lines, those who do it will lose sight of self. We are called upon to love souls as Christ loved them, to feel a travail of soul that sinners shall be converted. Present the matchless love of Christ. Hide self out of sight. Oh, what care should be taken by all who claim to be Christians that they do not call their passions and self-importance religion. By showing vanity, by longing for distinction, many hide the person of Christ, and expose themselves to view. There is such self-importance in their own ideas and way, and they cherish such a pleasing sense of their smartness, that the Lord cannot bestow his Holy Spirit upon them. If he did, they would misinterpret it, and exalt themselves still higher because of it. Their self pleasing ideas are a great hindrance to the advancement of the work. Whatever part they act self is the main picture presented. Their own zeal and devotion is thought to be the great power of truth. Unaware to themselves, all such are unfaithful stewards. They swerve the work in wrong lines. Self-importance leads them where they will be left to make false moves.

We are not to exalt the work of any man, magnifying him and praising his judgment. The first rising of self is the beginning of your fall, your separation from Christ. We cannot in any degree exalt self without being humbled. As Christians, we are to make the light of Christ's truth shine. Self is to be kept out of sight. Christ is the truth and the Light. He is the mirror from which we reflect truly every work done to his name's glory. The world needs light. "Let your light so shine before men that they may see your good works, and glorify your Father which is in heaven."

What makes it so hard for a rich man to enter into the kingdom of heaven? Why are riches, instead of becoming a precious treasure to be used to advance {158} the work and cause of God, made a curse, separating the soul from God? Why allow them to lead to the idolatry of self? God wants you, rich men, to use your goods as a sacred trust not your own. He has made you stewards over these goods. You are to calculate wisely, employing your powers to use to the very best advantage the means entrusted.

But oh, how many of God's gifts have been misused, because those to whom they are given did not have the fervor of the love of Christ in the soul. There is a great need of each one doing his best. There are those who would have used wisely the talents given to them, if they had been left to struggle and depend on their capabilities. But they become the possessors of means, and they lost the incentives to cultivate their talents, and make all possible of themselves by communicating what they had. An abundance of money has spoiled them for faithfully fulfilling their stewardship.

All who claim to be Christians should deal wisely with the Lord's goods. God is making an inventory of the money lent you and the spiritual advantage given you. Will you as stewards make careful inventory? Will you examine whether you are using economically all that God has placed in your charge, or whether you are wasting the Lord's goods by selfish outlay in order to make a display? Would that all that is spent needlessly, were laid up as treasure in heaven.

God gives more than money to his stewards. Your talent of imparting is a gift. What are you communicating of the gifts of God, in your words, in your tender sympathy? Are you allowing your money to go into the ranks of the enemy to ruin the ones you seek to please? Then again, the knowledge of truth is a talent. There are many souls in darkness that might be enlightened by true, faithful words from you. There are hearts that are hungering for sympathy, perishing away from God. Your sympathy may help them.

The Lord has need of your words, dictated by his Holy Spirit. He has need of the investment of your means. He needs your work for the salvation of souls. You can permit your means to be taken out of your hands to please your children. You may allow the enemy to rob you of the means that God has called for, to be used in lifting up the standard of truth in places where the people have not yet heard the message. Your means may be sunk in worldly investments, and turned into worldly channels. They may be used to do no one any

good. But the Lord the owner of all, will call you to render your account to him.

The first work for all Christians to do is to search the Scriptures with most earnest prayer, that they may have that faith that works by love, and purifies the soul from every thread of selfishness. If the truth is received into the heart, it works like good leaven, until every power is brought into subjection to the will of God. Then you can no more help shining than the sun can help shining. You have striven to separate from every kind of rubbish, and to let the peace of Christ rule in your heart. But if you do not have the bright beams of the Sun of Righteousness, you will reveal this by your outward insincerity. You will show this by revealing a heart that is pleased with vanity and outward adornment, by using the means that come into your hands, to gratify the unsanctified soul with idols of some order. How small is the treasure laid up in heaven by such. How little do they communicate to others in sacred ministry.

All natural gifts are to be sanctified as precious endowments. They are to be consecrated to God, that they may minister for the Master. All social advantages {159} are talents. They are not to be devoted to self-pleasing, amusements, or self-gratification. Money and estate are the Lord's, to be used wholly to honor him; for he has pledged his word that if we use his entrusted goods as faithful stewards, we shall be rich in blessings, of which we shall have a supply to bless others. But if we regard the advantages given us as our own, to be used according to our pleasure, to make a display, to create a sensation, the Lord Jesus our Redeemer, is put to shame by the characters of his professed followers.

Has God given you intellect? Is it for you to manage according to your inclinations? Can you glorify God by being educated to represent characters in plays, and to amuse audiences with fables? Has not the Lord given you intellect to be used to his name's glory in proclaiming the gospel of Christ. If you desire a public career, there is a work that you may do. Help the class you represent in plays. Come to the reality. Give your sympathy where it is needed by actually lifting up the bowed down. Satan's ruling passion is to pervert the intellect and cause men to long for shows and theatrical performances. The experience and character of all who engage in this work will be in accordance with the food given to the mind.

The Lord has given evidences of his

love for the world. There was no falsity, no acting, in what he did. He gave a lifting gift, capable of suffering humiliation, neglect, shame, reproach. While human beings are instituting schemes and methods to destroy him. The Son of the infinite God came to our world to give an example of the great work to be done to redeem and save men. But today the proud and disobedient are striving to acquire a great name and great honor from their fellowmen by using their God-given endowments to amuse. This they do instead of calling upon them to behold the Lamb of God, who taketh away the sins of the world.

God's great and wonderful work is to redeem and save, and thus repair the ruin that sin has made. Some see many things in the Bible that to them sanction a course of action that God will never approve. But when God converts human agents, they will flee to Christ, to be hid with Him in God. They will lift up their eyes to the perpetual.

CHRIST'S MISSION

[Prior to July 1915]

CHRIST IS THE GREATEST missionary the world has ever known. How did he come? What was his message? John, his forerunner, came with a message. His voice was lifted up in the wilderness of Judea, saying, "Repent ye, for the kingdom of heaven is at hand; for this is he which was spoken of by the prophet Esaias, saying, the voice of one crying in the wilderness, Prepare ye the way of the Lord." "Make straight in the desert a highway for our God. Every valley shall be exalted, and every mountain and hill shall be brought low: and the crooked shall be made straight, and the rough places plain. And the glory of the Lord shall be revealed, and all flesh shall see it together: for the mouth of the Lord hath spoken it. The voice said, Cry, and he said, what shall I cry? All flesh is as grass, and all the goodness thereof is as the flower of the field. The grass withereth, the flower fadeth: because the Spirit of the Lord bloweth upon it. Surely the people is grass. Grass withereth, flower fadeth, but the word of our God shall stand forever. O Zion, that bringeth good tidings, get thee up into the high mountain; O Jerusalem, that bringeth good tidings, {160} Behold your God; behold the Lord God will come with strong hands, and his arm shall rule for him: behold, his reward is with him, and his work before him. He shall feed his flock like a shepherd: he shall gather the lambs in his arms, and carry them to his bosom, "From that time Jesus began to preach, and to say, Repent: for the kingdom of heaven is at hand." This was the work and mission of Christ. The very same message that John bore, Christ bore. But while John preached in the wilderness, Christ's work was among the people, that he might reach the people where they were, he encircled the race with his long, human arm, while with his divine arm, he grasped the throne of the infinite, uniting finite man with the infinite God, and connecting earth with Heaven.

"And Jesus walking by the sea of Galilee, saw two brethren, Simeon called Peter, and Andrew and his brother, casting their net into the sea; for they were fishers. And he saith unto them, follow me, and I will make you fishers of men. These were first disciples Christ called. They were not chosen from among the Pharisees, but from among the lowly. With these humble men he could cooperate. He could educate and train them to do the highest work ever given to mortals.

"Behold my servant, whom I uphold, mine elect in whom my soul delighteth. I have put my Spirit upon him: he shall bring forth judgment to the Gentiles. He shall not cry, nor lift up, nor cause his voice to be heard in the streets. A bruised reed shall he not break and a smoking flax shall he not quench: he shall bring forth judgment unto truth. He shall not fail nor be discouraged till he hath set judgment in the earth: and the Isle shall wait for his law. Thus saith God the Lord, he that created the heavens, and stretcheth them out: He that spread forth the earth, and that which cometh out of it: He that giveth breath unto the people upon it, and Spirit to them that walk therein. I the Lord hath called thee in righteousness and will hold thy hand and will keep thee, and give thee for a covenant of the people, for a light of the Gentiles; to open the blind eyes, to bring out the prisoners from the prison, and them that sat in darkness from the prison house. I am the Lord: that is my name, and my glory will I not give to another, neither my praise to graven images. Behold, the former things have come to pass, and new things do I declare: before they spring forth I tell you of them. And I will bring the blind by a way that they knew not; I will lead them in paths that they have not known: I will make darkness light before them, and crooked things straight. These things will I do unto

them, and not forsake them. The Lord is well pleased for his righteousness sake: he will magnify the law and make it honorable. "And Jesus went about all Galilee, teaching in their synagogues, and preaching the gospel of the kingdom." Connected with this work was his ministry of healing. He went about "healing all manner of sickness and all manner of disease among the people, and his fame went throughout all Syria: and they brought unto him all sick people that were taken with divers diseases and torments and those which were possessed with devils, and those which were lunatic, and those which had the palsy, and he helped them. And there followed him a great multitude of people from Galilee, and from Decapolis, and from Jerusalem, and from Judea, and from beyond Jordan." "And seeing the multitude, he went up into a mountain and when he was set, his disciples came unto him." On this mountain the beatitudes were given to the people.

Here I wish to impress upon all interested in missionary work that first the truth is to be presented, and the warning given to the people, "The kingdom {161} of God is at hand." Nothing will so impress the people as the lifting up of the Saviour before them as Christ and him crucified. "As Moses lifted up the serpent in the wilderness, even so must the Son of man be lifted up." In the wilderness the word was given, sounded by the trumpet, caught up by appointed men, and the trumpet was given a certain sound. Everyone today who is bitten by the sting of the serpent is to look and live. This is the special work that is to be accomplished. Said John as he saw Jesus, "Behold the Lamb of God, which taketh away the sin of the world." All who look upon him will live. Then the question, "What shall I do to be saved?" is answered.

The message that God gives to his longing, starving people, is the same that Jesus gave to the palsied man, who was brought to him, and let down through the roof, as the only way in which he could reach the Great Physician, is given us. "Behold, they brought to him a man sick of the palsy, lying on a bed." There was a crowd about the house, and the sick man's friends sought means to bring him directly to Christ, that they might lay him before Him." "And when they could not find by what way they might bring him in, because of the multitude, they went upon the housetop, and let him down through the tiling with his couch into the midst before Jesus." Christ saw the man suffering with bodily disease. He also

saw him suffering with a sin-sick soul. In order to heal the bodily maladies, he must bring relief to the mind, and cleanse the soul from sin. The Saviour was not unmindful of the efforts that had been made to bring the man to him. His heart of love and pity was at once moved. "When he saw their faith, "It was enough." He said to the sick man, "Son, thy sins are forgiven thee." Many were watching with bated breath every movement in this strange transaction. Many felt that Christ's words were an invitation to them. Were they not soul-sick because of sin? Were they not anxious to get rid of this burden?

But the anger and the frowning countenance of the Pharisees could not be concealed. Apparently their looks expressed holy horror. They began to reason, saying, "Who is this which speaketh blasphemy? Who can forgive sin but God alone?" But who was it that had uttered the words, "Thy sins are forgiven thee?"—The Son of the Living God. Had the Pharisees not been blinded, they would have seen that God alone could forgive sin, and that he was Christ that was before them. Christ was in the Father and the Father in Christ, "I and my Father are one," he declared.

Christ took the very course he designed to take toward the afflicted one. He needed health of soul before he could appreciate health of body. "When Jesus perceived their thoughts, he answering said unto them, why reason ye in your hearts? Whether is it easier to say, Thy sins be forgiven thee; or to say, Rise up and walk. But that ye may know that the Son of God hath power upon earth to forgive sins, (he said unto the sick of the palsy,) I say unto you, Arise, take up thy couch, and go into thine house. And immediately he arose up before them, and took up that whereon he lay, and departed to his own house glorifying God." He was healed of the leprosy of sin, healed of the maladies that afflicted his body, healed every whit. "And they were all amazed, and they glorified God, and were filled with fear, saying, we have seen strange things today." What an evidence was this to the priests, rulers and Pharisees.

Christ said to the reasoning Pharisees, "That ye may know that the Son of God hath power upon earth to forgive sins." He had that power in heaven. {162}

"And after these things he went forth, and saw a publican named Levi sitting at the receipt of custom; and he said unto him, Follow me. And he left all, arose up, and followed him." Just such invitations will be given by Christ's ambassadors. General invitations are given; but not definite and personal invitations, as in this case. If more personal calls were given, more decided movements would be made to follow Christ.

"And Levi made him a great feast in his own house. He felt himself highly honored by Christ's call, and gave expression to his feelings, by making an effort in calling his friends; for he was to be no longer engaged in the business he had followed. Jesus and his disciples were invited, and "many publicans and sinners came and sat down with his disciples." Jesus never refused invitations of this kind, because here he could ask and answer questions that would diffuse light. He came to sow the seeds of truth in human hearts, knowing that the time would come when hearts would respond to the truth that fell from his lips.

"But the Scribes and Pharisees murmured against his disciples, saying, Why do ye eat and drink with sinners and publicans and sinners? And Jesus answered and said unto them, They that are whole (or claim to be whole) need not a physician; but they that are sick. I came not to call the righteous, but sinners to repentance."

This is a lesson for all our churches. The Lord went into the busy thoroughfares of travel that he might find souls, that he might speak words that would reach sinners. They needed a Saviour. They were sick, and needed a physician that could portray before them in parables their true condition. Thus Christ reached to the very depths of human woe and misery.

The Lord has not sent his people at great expense to different parts of the globe, among idolatrous and heathen nations, in order that they may use large amounts of money in building medical missionary hospitals. Their first work is to bear the message, Christ the crucified one is our risen Saviour. They are to awaken a decided interest in Christ's power to forgive sins. "This is life eternal that they might know thee, the only true God, and Jesus Christ whom he hath sent." Christ's work was a marked work. People flocked and crowded around him wherever he went. His first work was to teach the truth, then to mingle with his teaching, by demonstration of the Spirit, the work of healing.

"And when he had called unto him his twelve disciples, he gave them power against unclean spirits, to cast them out, and to heal all manner of sickness and all manner of disease." "And as ye go," he said, "preach, saying, the kingdom of heaven is at hand. Heal the sick, cleanse the lepers, raise the dead, cast out devils: freely ye have received, freely give. Provide neither gold, nor silver, nor brass in your purses." "And they departed, and went through the towns, preaching the gospel, and healing everywhere."

This is the work that is being done today. Missions should be established, not merely in one or two cities in America, but in various localities. These buildings should be as inexpensive as possible. It is not the expensive buildings that give character to our work; it is the spirit of the workers who show that they have the cooperation of the Holy Spirit that gives power to their influence. It is the spirit revealed in those who bear the message of truth, through whom God works, that give character to the work. {163}

Jesus gave to his disciples an example of the work they should do. In the New Testament is recorded the life of Christ and his way of working. "And from thence he arose, and went into the borders of Tyre and Sidon, and entered into a house, and would have no man know it, but he could not be hid; for a certain woman, whose daughter had an unclean Spirit, came and fell at his feet." This woman was a Greek. Her daughter was possessed by an evil Spirit. She followed Jesus and besought him to cast the devil out of her daughter. In answer Jesus said, let the children first be filled; for it is not meat to take the children's bread, and to cast it unto the dogs. This was the sentiment of the disciples. And she answered and said unto him, yes, Lord: yet the dogs under the table eat of the children's crumbs. And He said unto her, for this saying, go thy way. The devil is gone out of thy daughter. And when she was come to her house she found the devil gone out, and her daughter laid upon the bed.

"And again, departing from the coasts of Tyre and Sidon, he came unto the sea of Galilee, through the midst of the coasts of Decapolis. And they bring unto him one that was deaf, and had an impediment in his speech. And they beseeched him to put his hand upon him. And he took him aside from the multitude, and put his fingers into his ears, and he spit, and touched his tongue; and looked up to heaven, he sighed, and saith unto him, Ephphatha, that is, be opened. And straightway his ears were opened and the spring of his tongue loosed, and he spake plain." The deaf was made to hear, the blind to see.

"And he charged them that they should tell no man, but the more he charged them, so much the more the great deal they published it; and were beyond measure astonished, saying, he hath done all things well: he maketh both the deaf to hear and the dumb to speak.

This was Christ's work. Our churches have not filled their place in cooperating with God in this great work. Every position in life is permitted in the providence of God. Every sphere of action requires most thorough consecration to God. Those who are hid with Christ in God will become instruments in God's hands for the development of Christian virtues. All classes have a part to act. God's people are not to sit, Sabbath after Sabbath hearing the word, and then do nothing to communicate to others what they have heard. They are to be laborers together with God. The Lord has given every one a work to do. Not one will He excuse who cherishes the least inclination to fold his hands and make himself a center. Truth is to be proclaimed. It is to go forth as a lamp that burneth. Not a thread of selfishness is to be woven into the work. We must see light in God's light.

Dr. D. H. Kress

November 18, 1909
Sanitarium (Napa County) California
Dear Brother:

YESTERDAY I RECEIVED and read a letter from you, and I thank you for explaining your convictions and feelings so fully as you have done. I am glad that you and your wife can be united in your labors. With your varied gifts, you can unitedly do an excellent work. {164}

The work that you have been doing in connection with Brother and Sister Starr has had a good influence. I am assured that it is right for you and Sister Kress to unite with them in labor. You can be a great help to them and they to you.

The work you have been doing in the cities is meeting heaven's approval. This experience is to be a lesson to others besides Elder Starr and Dr. Kress. What you have done demonstrates that if our physicians and our ministers can work together in the presentation of truth to the people, more can be reached than could be influenced by the minister laboring alone. I trust that your example in this respect may be followed by other physicians.

Brother Starr has capabilities that fit him to labor in the large cities. I see no light in his being taken from that work.

I am sorry for your perplexities regarding leaving Washington. You say that your wife and others feel that you ought not to leave the Sanitarium, and that you do not feel clear to leave. I do not urge that you and your wife separate entirely from the Sanitarium. Your connection with the institution will increase your influence in the field. During your absence, other physicians must carry largely the responsibilities in the Sanitarium.

You need not feel that the Lord has separated you from the Sanitarium because you have made more direct efforts to reach the souls in our cities, who need to be converted. You have a burden for this work of presenting the message to the people. Present Christ as the Healer of the sin-sick soul. In your work in the field, you will gain a broader and more extended influence than if you were confined to an institution.

Whoever is medical superintendent of the institution, there should be associated with him wise counselors. No one man is to try to carry the responsibility of the Sanitarium at Takoma Park. One man's mind is not infallible. Capable men are to cooperate. It is safer in most matters to follow the united judgment of several men than of one man.

It is not the Lord's plan that you should wholly disconnect from the Sanitarium; but it is His plan that in connection with your wife, you should go into the cities and seek to reach the people with the message of present truth. This work will help to make known the work at the Sanitarium, and it will also establish confidence in the minds of the people in the institution. The acquaintances you make as you attend meetings and present the truth from the physician's standpoint, will help to give you an influence; and this line of work will be the means of bringing to our sanitariums a class of people who can be greatly benefited. Arrange your plans so that you can engage in this line of work with freedom, and so that your absence will not hurt the work of the institution.

Present before the people the need of resisting the temptation to indulge appetite. This is where many are failing. Explain how closely body and mind are related, and show the need of keeping both in the very best condition. The health talks which you give in the meetings will be one of the best ways of advertising our sanitariums. This is a work that I have been shown you should do. (This was to reach the higher class). {165}

I am instructed to say to our sanitarium workers that their light is to go forth as a lamp that burneth. There are ministerial duties devolving upon the head physicians of our sanitariums outside of the purely medical work. They must give heed to the urgent calls that come for soul-winning efforts. Every jot of influence that the Lord has given them is to be used for Him. Our medical superintendents should so live and labor as to be recognized as men who place their trust in God, men who fear the Lord, and depend upon His divine power.

The God-fearing surgeon, when required to operate in critical cases, will call upon God for wisdom and help. And the Lord will honor His servant at such times, guiding the instrument he handles in the fear of God. At such times it is of the greatest importance that the physician be calm and able to speak words of faith and trust in the One who is our Creator and our King. Many times this manifestation of calm trust in God will decide the case favorably, for the confidence of the physician in unseen agencies, his faith that his prayers in behalf of the afflicted one will be heard, will give confidence, and balance the mind of the one who is passing through the crisis. And the faith that will lay hold upon the Lord in the hour of peril will be respected.

The minds of the suffering ones must be led to grasp the hope of deliverance from special peril. Speak to them hopeful words, words of courage. There are those patronizing our sanitariums whom the Lord will heal if they will abstain from the use of liquor and drugs, and will use simple and safe remedies to counteract disease brought on through perverted appetite. If they will act their part to break the spell of the enemy by firmly resisting temptation and will surrender themselves to the One who gave His life for sinful souls, they will become sons and daughters of God.

All who indulge the appetite, waste the physical energies, and weaken the moral power, will sooner or later feel the retribution that follows the transgression of physical law.

Christ gave His life to purchase redemption for the sinner. The world's Redeemer knew that indulgence of appetite was bringing physical debility and deadening the perceptive faculties so that sacred and eternal things could not be discerned. He knew that self-indulgence was perverting the moral powers, and that man's great need was conversion—in heart and mind and soul, from the life of self-indulgence to one of self-denial and self-sacrifice. May the Lord help you as His servant to appeal to the ministers and to arouse the sleeping churches. Let your labors as a physician and a minister be in harmony. It is for this that our sanitariums are established, to preach the truth of true temperance.

In your letter you speak of the rescue work in the poorer parts of the city. I am glad that you feel a burden to help the very ones who need help. Christ desires His work to become the light of the world. He Himself came to make known to all classes the gospel of salvation. But it is not your special duty to make great efforts among the worst classes of society. There may be associated with you some who should work among the unfortunate and the degraded, but you are especially fitted to labor for the higher classes. Your influence with them would be lessened should you be associated largely with the rescue work for those who are generally regarded as outcasts. {166}

Christ entered upon the test on the point of appetite, and for nearly six weeks resisted temptation in behalf of man. That long fast in the wilderness was to be a lesson to fallen man for all time. Christ was not overcome by the struggling against temptation. Christ has made it possible for every member of the human family to resist temptation. All who would live godly lives may overcome as Christ overcame, by the blood of the Lamb, and the word of their testimony. That long fast of the Saviour strengthened Him to endure. He gave evidence to man that He would begin the work of overcoming just where ruin began—on the point of appetite.

As a people, we need to reform, and especially do ministers and teachers of the Word need to reform. I am instructed to say to our ministers and to the presidents of our conferences:—Your usefulness as laborers for God in the work of recovering perishing souls, depends much on your success in overcoming appetite. Overcome the desire to gratify appetite, and if you do this, your passions will be easily controlled. Then your mental and moral powers will be stronger. "And they overcame by the blood of the Lamb and the word of their testimony."

We need the influence of the right example of our physicians and our ministers. Let them exercise their powers for the control of appetite, that mental and moral powers may be strengthened. As far as possible, let them adopt such habits of life that the physical and mental powers shall be equally taxed. The exercise of the voice in speaking is a healthful exercise. Teach and live carefully. Hold firmly to the position that all, even our leading men, need to exercise good common sense in the care of their health, securing equal taxation of the body and the brain.

(Signed) Ellen G. White

COUNSELS FROM LEADERSHIP

[Prior to 1956]
By Dr. D. H. Kress

AFTER COMING TO the sanitarium at Takoma Park, I received communications from Sister White, directing me as to how to carry forward the work of the sanitarium, and in the field along educational lines. It may be of interest to learn how the Lord opened the way for me to leave Australia, a field to which I felt I was called.

Sister White, in addressing a letter to Elder O. A. Olsen, who was then President of the Union Conference of Australia, on February 2, 1907, said: "Our Sanitarium at Takoma Park is nearing completion. We should have a strong medical faculty at the Washington Institution, but where are they to be found? Elder Irwin has spoken to me several times about his convictions that Drs. H. H. and Lauretta Kress were needed in Washington to give a mold to the medical and spiritual work to be done there and to influence our medical work throughout the field. I gave my sentence that the time is not yet. The work in Australia must not be crippled.

"In my last interview with Elder Irwin I said, if Dr. Kress could be spared from Wahroonga without crippling the work in Australia it would be well to call him to Washington. The work there is very important. It has been delayed too long. Strong physicians will there do much to strengthen our work throughout the field. Therefore, if good, faithful workers can be secured to take their place in Wahroonga, and if their minds are drawn toward Washington to work, secure their transfer if possible. I believe that the Lord has been working to bring about changes that would open the way

for Dr. Kress to come to Washington. We need him there very much, and we need him just now at the opening of the work. {167} I have written to you as early as possible, and have written hurriedly. I wish that Dr. Kress could get there before the opening of the Sanitarium."

In a letter addressed to me by Elder Daniells, he said: "I may say that some months ago it became very apparent to the members of the board that we ought to secure a man of experience and loyalty to head our Washington Sanitarium. As we studied and prayed over the matter we were continually impressed that if you could be spared from Australia you would be the man to take the place. At last the board passed a resolution requesting me to place the matter fully before Sister White. I did so, with the result that she advised us to call you to this position." I had just received their letter when your communication came. As soon as these were received, Elder Evans, the vice-president of Washington Sanitarium board, called the members together, and it was unanimously voted that you should be chosen superintendent of the Washington Sanitarium, that we should send you a cable requesting you to come immediately."

After the work was well started here at Takoma Park, I received a communication from Sister White, urging me to give attention to the large cities of the East; especially New York, Boston, and Portland, Maine, were mentioned. She said: "I have been shown that Dr. Kress is too closely confined to his work at the Washington Sanitarium. He should be given an opportunity to have his influence more widely felt."

On the strength of this I aimed to arrange my work so that I could do some work in the field, especially in connection with the large gatherings of our people and in conducting special efforts in the cities. While at the camp meeting in New York City, Sister White called me into her room. She was lying upon a cot. She looked up into my face and said: "Doctor, this is the work that I have been shown that you should do." I said to her: "Sister White, do you think that I had better sever my connection from the Sanitarium in order to be able to do this work?" She replied: "No, that is not it. Your connection with the Sanitarium will give you an influence in the field, and your work in the field will bring patients to the Sanitarium. But ar-

range the work in such a way that you can leave it without it being harmed during your absence."

February 22, 1909, she said: "The Lord will bless Brother and Sister Kress if they will in the name of the Lord go forth in connection with the gospel ministry to labor in the cities. The cities in the East should now receive special attention." "It is the Lord's plan that physicians well versed in the Bible truths shall unite with ministers laboring in the cities and aid in giving as a whole the harmonious message of warning that should be given to the world. Some of the very best qualified men in our institutions should be chosen for this work. To some it may seem unwise to take men qualified for the position of head physician and put them to labor in the cities and choose men to take their places in the institution; but we need to take a broader view of the work, and to consider that the Lord is calling for a special line of work to be done in the cities,—a work which requires the efforts of men of clear perception and who in the power of the Holy Spirit can present before large congregations the principles of health reform. The presenting of Bible principles by intelligent physicians will have great weight with many people. The efficiency and power of one who can combine in his influence the work of a physician and of the gospel minister who can estimate? This work commends itself to the good judgment of the people. If Dr. Kress will labor as a medical evangelist under the Lord's direction and go forward in humility, a good work will be accomplished." {168}

In response I arranged my work so as to carry out this instruction, Elder G. B. Starr united with me in a medical missionary effort, in New York City. My wife and daughter, and Miss Cornor, from the Sanitarium, assisted in this effort in conducting a real school of health, giving special attention to diet. The daily papers gave liberal space, devoting in some instances almost a full page in writing "Kress gatherings." Later a letter came from Sister White in which she said: "The work you have been doing in the city is meeting Heaven's approval. This experience is to be a lesson to others besides Elder Starr and Dr. Kress. You have demonstrated that if our physicians and our ministers would work together in the presentation of truth to the people, more can be reached than could be influenced by the ministers laboring alone. I trust that your example in this respect may be followed by other physicians. I do not urge that you and your wife separate entirely from the Sanitarium. Your connection with the institution will increase your influence in the field. During your absence, other physicians must carry largely the responsibilities in the Sanitarium. In your work in the field you will gain a broader and more extended influence than if you were confined to an institution. It is not the Lord's plan that you should wholly disconnect from the Sanitarium, but it is His plan that in connection with your wife you should go into the cities and seek to reach the people with the message of present truth. This work will help to make known the work of the Sanitarium and will also establish confidence in the minds of the people in the institution. The acquaintances you make as you attend meetings and present the truth from a physician's standpoint will help to give you an influence, and this line of work will then be the means of bringing to your sanitarium a class of people who can be greatly benefited. Arrange your plans so that you can engage in this line of work with freedom and so that your absence will not hurt the work of the institution. The health talks which you give in the meetings will be one of the best ways of advertising our Sanitarium. This is the work that I have been shown you should do."

In a letter dated January 15th, 1910, she said: "My mind has been burdened in behalf of the large cities of the East, like New York City, where you labored last summer. There is the important city of Boston, near which is situated the Melrose Sanitarium. I know of no place where there is greater need of rebuilding of the first works than in Boston, and in Portland, Maine, where the first messages were given in power, but where now there is but a little handful of our people. . . . I have not a word to say to hinder you from following the guiding hand of God, but I beg of you to bear in mind the neglected cities. The Lord God of Israel is calling for these cities now to be worked. Results will be seen as an interest is created."

I must admit that I felt rather perplexed in knowing just how to arrange my work in the sanitarium so that I could engage in this city work with freedom.

Before graduating from the University of Michigan, during the last year I spent three months in the city of Chicago, where we opened up a medical mission and aimed to help the outcasts and neglected, known as the down-and-outs in the worst part of the city of Chicago. I enjoyed this work, and in my perplexity I thought possibly I should take up that work again. I wrote Sister White telling her of what I had been thinking, and in reply she said, (Nov. 18, 1909) "In your letter you speak of the rescue work in the poorer parts of the city. I am glad that you feel a burden to help the very ones that need help. Christ desires His work to become the light of the world. He Himself came to make {169} known to all classes the gospel of salvation. There may be associated with you some who should work among the unfortunate and the degraded, but you are especially fitted to labor for the higher classes. Your influence with them would be lessened should you be associated largely with the rescue work for those who are generally regarded as outcasts."

Again, on February 9, 1910, in a communication, she said: "The Lord will assuredly guide you if you will seek to do His will, even though it should interfere with some of your desires and plans. If you walk and work in the counsel of God doors will be opened before you of opportunities for uniting the work of the ministry and that of the physician." "If in the city of Boston and other cities of the East you and your wife will unite in medical evangelistic work, your usefulness will increase; there will open before you clearer views of duty."

I am fully convinced that the medical work today would advance more rapidly among our own people as well as on the outside by placing it in its proper setting in the message

Never has my confidence in the spirit of prophecy been more decided than it is at the present time. I have witnessed to some extent the possibilities of our health message, when combined with the third angel's message of which it is a vital part.

D. H. Kress, M. D.

————————

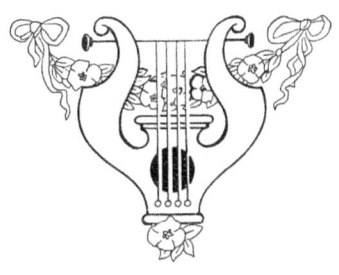